Measurement of Joint Motion
A Guide to Goniometry

Cynthia C. Norkin, EdD, PT
Former Associate Professor and Director
School of Physical Therapy
College of Health and Human Services
Ohio University
Athens, Ohio

D. Joyce White, DSc, PT
Associate Professor of Physical Therapy
College of Health Professions
University of Massachusetts Lowell
Lowell, Massachusetts

Measurement of Joint Motion
A Guide to Goniometry
THIRD EDITION

Photographs by Jocelyn Greene Molleur and Lucia Grochowska Littlefield

Illustrations by Timothy Wayne Malone

Additional illustrations provided by Jennifer Daniell and Meredith Taylor Stelling

F. A. Davis Company • Philadelphia

F.A. Davis Company
1915 Arch Street
Philadelphia, PA 10103
www.fadavis.com

Printed in the United States of America

Last digit indicates print number : 10 9 8 7 6 5 4 3 2 1

Acquisitions Editor: Margaret Biblis
Manager, Creative Development: Susan Rhyner
Developmental Editor: Anne Seitz
Cover Designer: Louis J. Forgione

As new scientific information becomes available through basic and clinical research, recommended treatments and drug therapies undergo changes. The author(s) and publisher have done everything possible to make this book accurate, up to date, and in accord with accepted standards at the time of publication. The author(s), editors, and publisher are not responsible for errors or omissions or for consequences from application of the book, and make no warranty, expressed or implied, in regard to the contents of the book. Any practice described in this book should be applied by the reader in accordance with professional standards of care used in regard to the unique circumstances that may apply in each situation. The reader is advised always to check product information (package inserts) for changes and new information regarding dose and contraindications before administering any drug. Caution is especially urged when using new or infrequently ordered drugs.

Library of Congress Cataloging-in-Publication Data

Norkin, Cynthia C.
Measurement of joint motion : a guide to goniometry / Cynthia C. Norkin,
D. Joyce White ; photographs by Jocelyn Greene and Lucia Grochowska
Littlefield ; illustrations by Timothy Wayne Malone ; additional
illustrations provided by Jennifer Daniell and Meredith Taylor Stelling.—
3rd ed.
        p. cm.
Includes bibliographical references and index.
  ISBN 0-8036-0972-8
1. Joints—Range of motion—Measurement. I. White, D. Joyce. II. Title.
  RD734.N67 2003
  612.7′5–dc21

2003046244

To Alexandra, Taylor, and Kimberly.
CCN

To Jonathan, Alexander, and Ethan.
DJW

Preface

The measurement of joint motion is an important component of a thorough physical examination of the extremities and spine, one which helps health professionals identify impairments and assess rehabilitative status. The need for a comprehensive text with sufficient written detail and photographs to allow for the standardization of goniometric measurement methods—both for the purposes of teaching and clinical practice led to the development of the first edition of the *Measurement of Joint Motion: A Guide to Goniometry* in 1985. Our approach included a discussion and illustration of testing position, stabilization, end-feel, and goniometer alignment for each measurable joint in the body. The resulting text was extremely well received by a variety of health professional educational programs and was used as a reference in many clinical settings.

In the years following initial publication, a considerable amount of research on the measurement of joint motion appeared in the literature. Consequently, in the second edition, which was published in 1995, we created a new chapter on the reliability and validity of joint measurement and added joint-specific research sections to existing chapters. We also expanded the text by adding structure, osteokinematics, arthrokinematics, capsular and noncapsular patterns of limitation, and functional ranges of motion for each joint.

The expanded third edition includes new research findings to help clarify normative range of motion values for various age and gender groups, as well as the range of motion needed to perform common functional tasks. We added current information on the effects of subject characteristics, such as body mass, occupational and recreational activities, and the effects of the testing process, such as the testing position and type of measuring instrument, on range of motion. New to the third edition is the inclusion of muscle length testing at joints where muscle length is often a factor affecting range of motion. This addition integrates the measurement procedures used in this book with the American Physical Therapy Association's *Guide to Physical Therapy Practice*. Inclinometer techniques for measuring range of

motion of the spine are also added to coincide with current practice in some clinical settings. We introduce illustrations to accompany anatomical descriptions so that the reader will have a visual reminder of the joint structures involved in range of motion. New illustrations of bony anatomical landmarks and photographs of surface anatomy will help the reader align the goniometer accurately. In addition, over 180 new photographs replace many of the older, dated photographs.

Similar to earlier editions, the book presents goniometry logically and clearly. Chapter 1 discusses basic concepts regarding the use of goniometry to assess range of motion and muscle length in patient evaluation. Arthrokinematic and osteokinematic movements, elements of active and passive range of motion, hypomobility, hypermobility, and factors affecting joint motion are included. The inclusion of end-feels and capsular and noncapsular patterns of joint limitation introduces readers to current concepts in orthopedic manual therapy and encourages them to consider joint structure while measuring joint motion.

Chapter 2 takes the reader through a step-by-step process to master the techniques of goniometric evaluation, including: positioning, stabilization, instruments used for measurement, goniometer alignment, and the recording of results. Exercises that help develop necessary psychomotor skills and demonstrate direct application of theoretical concepts facilitate learning.

Chapter 3 discusses the validity and reliability of measurement. The results of validity and reliability studies on the measurement of joint motion are summarized to help the reader focus on ways of improving and interpreting goniometric measurements. Mathematical methods of evaluating reliability are shown along with examples and exercises so that the readers can assess their reliability in taking measurements.

Chapters 4 to 13 present detailed information on goniometric testing procedures for the upper and lower extremities, spine, and temporomandibular joint. When appropriate, muscle length testing procedures are also included. The text presents the anatomical landmarks, testing position, stabilization, testing motion, normal end-feel, and goniometer alignment for each joint and motion, in a format that reinforces a consistent approach to evaluation. The extensive use of photographs and captions eliminates the need for repeated demonstrations by an instructor and provides the reader with a permanent reference for visualizing the procedures. Also included is information on joint structure, osteokinematic and arthrokinematic motion, and capsular patterns of restrictions. A review of current literature regarding normal range of motion values; the effects of age, gender, and other factors; functional range of motion; and reliability and validity is also presented for each body region to assist the reader to comply with evidence-based practice.

We hope this book makes the teaching and learning of goniometry easier and improves the standardization and thus the reliability of this assessment tool. We believe that the third edition provides a comprehensive coverage of the measurement of joint motion and muscle length. We hope that the additions will motivate health professionals to conduct research and to use research results in evaluation. We encourage our readers to provide us with feedback on our current efforts to bring you a high-quality, user-friendly text.

CCN

DJW

Acknowledgments

We are very grateful for the contributions of the many people who were involved in the development and production of this text. Photographer Jocelyn Molleur applied her skill and patience during many sessions at the physical therapy laboratory at the University of Massachusetts Lowell to produce the high-quality photographs that appear in this third edition. Her efforts combined with those of Lucia Grochowska Littlefield, who took the photographs for the first edition, are responsible for an important feature of the book. Timothy Malone, an artist from Ohio, used his talents, knowledge of anatomy, and good humor to create the excellent illustrations that appear in this edition. We also offer our thanks to Jessica Bouffard, Alexander White, and Claudia Van Bibber who graciously agreed to be subjects for some of the photographs.

We wish to express our appreciation to these dedicated professionals at F. A Davis: Margaret Biblis, Publisher, and Susan Rhyner, Manager of Creative Development, for their encouragement, ingenuity, and commitment to excellence. Thanks are also extended to Sam Rondinelli, Production Manager; Jack Brandt, Illustration Specialist; Louis Forgione, Design Manager; Ona Kosmos, Editorial Associate; Melissa Reed, Developmental Associate; Anne Seitz, Freelance Editor; and Jean-Francois Vilain, Former Publisher. We are grateful to the numerous students, faculty, and clinicians who over the years have used the book or formally reviewed portions of the manuscript and offered insightful comments and helpful suggestions.

Finally, we wish to thank our families: Cynthia's daughter, Alexandra, and Joyce's husband, Jonathan, and sons, Alexander and Ethan, for their encouragement, support, and tolerance of "time away" for this endeavor. We will always be appreciative.

Reviewers

Suzanne Robben Brown, MPH, PT
Associate Professor & Chair
Department of Physical Therapy
Arizona School of Health Sciences
Mesa, AZ

Larry Chinnock, PT, EdD
Instructor/Academic Coordinator
Department of Physical Therapy
Loma Linda University
School of Allied Health Professions
Loma Linda, CA

Robyn Colleen Davies, BHSCPT, MAPPSC, PT
Lecturer
Department of Physical Therapy
University of Toronto
Toronto, Canada

Jodi Gootkin, PT
Site Coordinator
Physical Therapy Assistant Program
Broward Community College
Ft. Myers, FL

Deidre Lever-Dunn, PhD, ATC
Assistant Professor
Department of Health Sciences
Program Director
Athletic Training Education
University of Alabama
Tuscaloosa, AL

John T. Myers, PT, MBA
Instructor/Program Director
Physical Therapy Assistant Program
Lorain County Community College
Elyria, OH

James R. Roush, PhD, PT, ATC
Associate Professor
Department of Physical Therapy
Arizona School of Health Science
Mesa, AZ

Sharon D. Yap, PTA, BPS
Academic Coordinator of Clinical Education
Physical Therapy Assistant Program
Indian River Community College
Fort Pierce, FL

Contents

PART I
Introduction to Goniometry 1

CHAPTER 1
Basic Concepts 3
  GONIOMETRY
  JOINT MOTION
    Arthrokinematics
    Osteokinematics
  RANGE OF MOTION
    Active Range of Motion
    Passive Range of Motion
    Hypomobility
    Hypermobility
    Factors Affecting Range of Motion
  MUSCLE LENGTH TESTING

CHAPTER 2
Procedures 17
  POSITIONING
  STABILIZATION
    EXERCISE 1: Determining the End of the Range of Motion and End-feel
  MEASUREMENT INSTRUMENTS
    Universal Goniometer
    Gravity-dependent Goniometers (Inclinometers)
    Electrogoniometers
    Visual Estimation
    EXERCISE 2: The Universal Goniometer
  ALIGNMENT
    EXERCISE 3: Goniometer Alignment for Elbow Flexion
  RECORDING
    Numerical Tables
    Pictorial Charts
    Sagittal-frontal-transverse-rotation Method
    American Medical Association Guide to Evaluation Method
  PROCEDURES
    Explanation Procedure
    Testing Procedure

  EXERCISE 4: Explanation of Goniometry
  EXERCISE 5: Testing Procedure for Goniometric Evaluation of Elbow Flexion

CHAPTER 3
Validity and Reliability 39
  VALIDITY
    Face Validity
    Content Validity
    Criterion-related Validity
    Construct Validity
  RELIABILITY
    Summary of Goniometric Reliability Studies
    Statistical Methods of Evaluating Measurement Reliability
    Exercises to Evaluate Reliability
    EXERCISE 6: Intratester Reliability
    EXERCISE 7: Intertester Reliability

PART II
Upper-Extremity Testing 55

CHAPTER 4
The Shoulder 57
  STRUCTURE AND FUNCTION
    Glenohumeral Joint
    Sternoclavicular Joint
    Acromioclavicular Joint
    Scalpulothoracic Joint
  RESEARCH FINDINGS
    Effects of Age, Gender, and Other Factors
    Functional Range of Motion
    Reliability and Validity
  RANGE OF MOTION TESTING PROCEDURES: THE SHOULDER
  LANDMARKS FOR GONIOMETER ALIGNMENT
    Flexion
    Extension

Abduction
Adduction
Medial (Internal) Rotation
Lateral (External) Rotation

CHAPTER 5

The Elbow and Forearm............................**91**

STRUCTURE AND FUNCTION
Humeroulnar and Humeroradial Joints
Superior and Inferior Radioulnar Joints
RESEARCH FINDINGS
Effects of Age, Gender, and Other Factors
Functional Range of Motion
Reliability and Validity
RANGE OF MOTION TESTING PROCEDURES: ELBOW AND
FOREARM
LANDMARKS FOR GONIOMETER ALIGNMENT
Flexion
Extension
Pronation
Supination
MUSCLE LENGTH TESTING PROCEDURES: ELBOW AND
FOREARM
Biceps Brachii
Triceps Brachii

CHAPTER 6

The Wrist **111**

STRUCTURE AND FUNCTION
Radiocarpal and Midcarpal Joints
RESEARCH FINDINGS
Effects of Age, Gender, and Other Factors
Functional Range of Motion
Reliability and Validity
RANGE OF MOTION TESTING PROCEDURES: WRIST
LANDMARKS FOR GONIOMETRIC ALIGNMENT: THE
WRIST
Flexion
Extension
Radial Deviation
Ulnar Deviation
MUSCLE LENGTH TESTING PROCEDURES: WRIST
Flexor Digitorum Profundus and Flexor Digitorum
Superficialis
Extensor Digitorum, Extensor Indicis, and Extensor
Digiti Minimi

CHAPTER 7

The Hand **137**

STRUCTURE AND FUNCTION
Fingers: Metacarpophalangeal Joints
Fingers: Proximal Interphalangeal and Distal
Interphalangeal Joints
Thumb: Carpometacarpal Joint
Thumb: Metacarpophalangeal Joint
Thumb: Interphalangeal Joint

RESEARCH FINDINGS
Effects of Age, Gender, and Other Factors
Functional Range of Motion
Reliability and Validity
RANGE OF MOTION TESTING PROCEDURES: FINGERS
LANDMARKS FOR GONIOMETER ALIGNMENT
Metacarpophalangeal Flexion
Metacarpophalangeal Extension
Metacarpophalangeal Abduction
Metacarpophalangeal Adduction
Proximal Interphalangeal Flexion
Proximal Interphalangeal Extension
Distal Interphalangeal Flexion
Distal Interphalangeal Extension
RANGE OF MOTION TESTING PROCEDURES: THUMB
LANDMARKS FOR GONIOMETER ALIGNMENT
Carpometacarpal Flexion
Carpometacarpal Extension
Carpometacarpal Abduction
Carpometacarpal Adduction
Carpometacarpal Opposition
Metacarpophalangeal Flexion
Metacarpophalangeal Extension
Interphalangeal Flexion
Interphalangeal Extension
MUSCLE LENGTH TESTING PROCEDURES: FINGERS
Lumbricals, Palmar and Dorsal Interossei

PART III

Lower-Extremity Testing **181**

CHAPTER 8

The Hip **183**

STRUCTURE AND FUNCTION
Iliofemoral Joint
RESEARCH FINDINGS
Effects of Age, Gender, and Other Factors
Functional Range of Motion
Reliability and Validity
RANGE OF MOTION TESTING PROCEDURES: HIP
LANDMARKS FOR GONIOMETER ALIGNMENT
Flexion
Extension
Abduction
Adduction
Medial (Internal) Rotation
Lateral (External) Rotation
MUSCLE LENGTH TESTING PROCEDURES
Hip Flexors (Thomas Test)
The Hamstrings: Semitendinous, Semimembranosus,
and Biceps Femoris (Straight Leg Test)
Tensor Fascia Latae (Ober Test)

CHAPTER 9

The Knee..**221**

STRUCTURE AND FUNCTION
Tibiofemoral and Patellofemoral Joints

RESEARCH FINDINGS
    Effects of Age, Gender, and Other Factors
    Functional Range of Motion
    Reliability and Validity
RANGE OF MOTION TESTING PROCEDURES: KNEE
LANDMARKS FOR GONIOMETER ALIGNMENT
    Flexion
    Extension
MUSCLE LENGTH TESTING PROCEDURES: KNEE
    Rectus Femoris: Ely Test
    Hamstring Muscles: Semitendinosus, Semimembranosus,
      and Biceps Femoris: Distal Hamstring Length Test

CHAPTER 10
The Ankle and Foot 241

STRUCTURE AND FUNCTION
    Proximal and Distal Tibiofibular Joints
    Talocrural Joint
    Subtalar Joint
    Transverse Tarsal (Midtarsal) Joint
    Tarsometatarsal Joints
    Metatarsophalangeal Joints
    Interphalangeal Joints
RESEARCH FINDINGS
    Effects of Age, Gender, and Other Factors
    Functional Range of Motion
    Reliability and Validity
RANGE OF MOTION TESTING PROCEDURES: ANKLE
    AND FOOT
LANDMARKS FOR GONIOMETER ALIGNMENT:
    TALOCRURAL JOINT
    Dorsiflexion: Talocrural Joint
    Plantarflexion: Talocrural Joint
LANDMARKS FOR GONIOMETER ALIGNMENT: TARSAL
    JOINTS
    Inversion: Tarsal Joints
    Eversion: Tarsal Joints
LANDMARKS FOR GONIOMETER ALIGNMENT: SUBTALAR
    JOINT (REARFOOT)
    Inversion: Subtalar Joint (Rearfoot)
    Eversion: Subtalar Joint (Rearfoot)
    Inversion: Transverse Tarsal Joint
    Eversion: Transverse Tarsal Joint
LANDMARKS FOR GONIOMETER ALIGNMENT:
    METATARSOPHALANGEAL JOINT
    Flexion: Metatarsophalangeal Joint
    Extension: Metatarsophalangeal Joint
    Abduction: Metatarsophalangeal Joint
    Adduction and Metatarsophalangeal Joint
    Flexion: Interphalangeal Joint of the First Toe and
      Proximal Interphalangeal Joints of the Four Lesser Toes
    Extension: Interphalangeal Joint of the First Toe and
      Proximal Interphalangeal Joints of the Four Lesser Toes
    Flexion: Distal Interphalangeal Joints of the Four Lesser
      Toes
    Extension: Distal Interphalangeal Joints of the Four
      Lesser Toes
MUSCLE LENGTH TESTING PROCEDURES:
    Gastrocnemius

PART IV
Testing of the Spine and
Temporomandibular Joint 293

CHAPTER 11
The Cervical Spine 295

STRUCTURE AND FUNCTION
    Atlanto-occipital and Atlantoaxial Joints
    Intervertebral and Zygapophyseal Joints
RESEARCH FINDINGS
    Effects of Age, Gender, and Other Factors
    Functional Range of Motion
    Reliability and Validity
RANGE OF MOTION TESTING PROCEDURES:
    CERVICAL SPINE
LANDMARKS FOR GONIOMETER ALIGNMENT
    Flexion
    Extension
    Lateral Flexion
    Rotation

CHAPTER 12
The Thoracic and Lumbar Spine 331

STRUCTURE AND FUNCTION
    Thoracic Spine
    Lumbar Spine
RESEARCH FINDINGS
    Effects of Age, Gender, and Other Factors
    Functional Range of Motion
    Reliability and Validity
RANGE OF MOTION TESTING PROCEDURES
ANATOMICAL LANDMARKS: FOR TAPE MEASURE
    ALIGNMENT
    Thoracic and Lumbar Flexion
    Lumbar Flexion
    Thoracic and Lumbar Extension
    Lumbar Extension
    Thoracic and Lumbar Lateral Flexion
    Thoracic and Lumbar Rotation

CHAPTER 13
The Temporomandibular Joint................365

STRUCTURE AND FUNCTION
    Temporomandibular Joint
RESEARCH FINDINGS
    Effects of Age, Gender, and Other Factors
    Reliability and Validity
RANGE OF MOTION TESTING PROCEDURES:
    TEMPOROMANDIBULAR JOINT
LANDMARKS FOR RULER ALIGNMENT MEASURING
    Depression of the Mandible (Mouth Opening)
    Protrusion of the Mandible
    Lateral Deviation of the Mandible

APPENDIX A
**Normative Range of Motion
Values** 375

APPENDIX B
**Joint Measurements by Body
Position**......................................381

APPENDIX C
Goniometer Price Lists...........................383

APPENDIX D
Numerical Recording Forms 387
Index..393

PART I

Introduction to Goniometry

Objectives

ON COMPLETION OF PART 1 THE READER WILL BE ABLE TO:

1. Define:

   goniometry
   planes and axes
   range of motion
   end-feel
   muscle length testing
   reliability
   validity

2. Identify the appropriate planes and axes for each of the following motions:

   flexion-extension, abduction-adduction, and rotation

3. Compare:

   active and passive ranges of motion
   arthrokinematic and osteokinematic motions
   soft, firm, and hard end-feels
   hypomobility and hypermobility
   capsular and noncapsular patterns of restricted motion
   one-, two-, and multijoint muscles
   reliability and validity
   intratester and intertester reliability

4. Explain the importance of:

   testing positions
   stabilization
   clinical estimates of range of motion
   recording starting and ending positions

5. Describe the parts of universal, fluid, and pendulum goniometers

6. List:

   the six-step explanation sequence
   the 12-step testing sequence
   the 10 items included in recording

7. Perform a goniometric evaluation of the elbow joint including:

   a clear explanation of the procedure
   positioning of a subject in the testing position
   adequate stabilization of the proximal joint component
   a correct determination of the end of the range of motion
   a correct identification of the end-feel
   palpation of the correct bony landmarks
   accurate alignment of the goniometer
   correct reading of the goniometer and recording of the measurement

8. Perform and interpret intratester and intertester reliability tests including standard deviation, coefficient of variation, correlation coefficients, and standard error of measurement.

CHAPTER 1

Basic Concepts

This book is designed to serve as a guide to learning the technique of human joint measurement called goniometry. Background information on principles and procedures necessary for an understanding of goniometry is found in Part 1. Practice exercises are included at appropriate intervals to help the examiner apply this information and develop the psychomotor skills necessary for competency in goniometry. Procedures for the goniometric examination of joints and muscle length testing of the upper extremity, lower extremity, and spine and temporomandibular joint are presented in Parts 2, 3, and 4, respectively.

Goniometry

The term **goniometry** is derived from two Greek words, *gonia*, meaning angle, and *metron*, meaning measure.

Therefore, goniometry refers to the measurement of angles, in particular the measurement of angles created at human joints by the bones of the body. The examiner obtains these measurements by placing the parts of the measuring instrument, called a goniometer, along the bones immediately proximal and distal to the joint being evaluated. Goniometry may be used to determine both a particular joint position and the total amount of motion available at a joint.

EXAMPLE: The elbow joint is evaluated by placing the parts of the measuring instrument on the humerus (proximal segment) and the forearm (distal segment) and measuring either a specific joint position or the total arc of motion (Fig. 1–1).

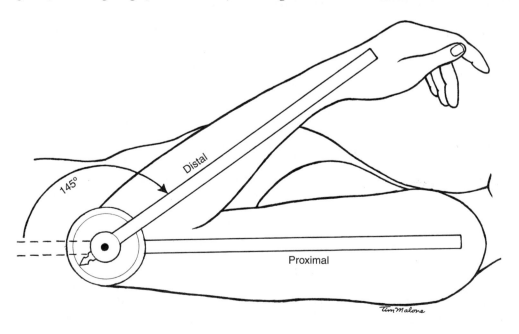

145°

Distal

Proximal

Tim Malone

FIGURE 1–1 The upper left extremity of a subject in the supine position is shown. The parts of the measuring instrument have been placed along the proximal (humerus) and distal (radius) components and centered over the axis of the elbow joint. When the distal component has been moved toward the proximal component (elbow flexion), a measurement of the arc of motion can be obtained.

Goniometry is an important part of a comprehensive examination of joints and surrounding soft tissue. A comprehensive examination typically begins by interviewing the subject and reviewing records to obtain an accurate description of current symptoms; functional abilities; occupational, social and recreational activities; and medical history. Observation of the body to assess bone and soft tissue contour, as well as skin and nail condition, usually follows the interview. Gentle palpation is used to determine skin temperature and the quality of soft tissue deformities and to locate pain symptoms in relation to anatomical structures. Anthropometric measurements such as leg length, circumference, and body volume may be indicated.

The performance of active joint motions by the subject during the examination allows the examiner to screen for abnormal movements and gain information about the subject's willingness to move. If abnormal active motions are found, the examiner performs passive joint motions in an attempt to determine reasons for joint limitation. Performing passive joint motions enables the examiner to assess the tissue that is limiting the motion, detect pain, and make an estimate of the amount of motion. Goniometry is used to measure and document the amount of active and passive joint motion as well as abnormal fixed joint positions. Resisted isometric muscle contractions, joint integrity and mobility tests, and special tests for specific body regions are used in conjunction with goniometry to help identify the injured anatomical structures. Tests to assess muscle performance and neurological function are often included. Diagnostic imaging procedures and laboratory tests may be required.

Goniometric data used in conjunction with other information can provide a basis for:

- Determining the presence or absence of impairment
- Establishing a diagnosis
- Developing a prognosis, treatment goals, and plan of care
- Evaluating progress or lack of progress toward rehabilitative goals
- Modifying treatment
- Motivating the subject
- Researching the effectiveness of therapeutic techniques or regimens; for example, exercises, medications, and surgical procedures
- Fabricating orthoses and adaptive equipment

Joint Motion

Arthrokinematics

Motion at a joint occurs as the result of movement of one joint surface in relation to another. **Arthrokinematics** is the term used to refer to the movement of joint surfaces. The movements of joint surfaces are described as slides (glides), spins, and rolls.[1] A slide (glide), which is a translatory motion, is the sliding of one joint surface over another, as when a braked wheel skids. A spin is a rotary (angular) motion, similar to the spinning of a toy top. All points on the moving joint surface rotate at a constant distance around a fixed axis of motion. A roll is a rotary motion similar to the rolling of the bottom of a rocking chair on the floor, or the rolling of a tire on the road. In the human body, glides, spins, and rolls usually occur in combination with each other and result in movement of the shafts of the bones.

Osteokinematics

Osteokinematics refers to the movement of the shafts of bones rather than the movement of joint surfaces. The movements of the shafts of bones are usually described in terms of the rotary motion produced, as if the movement occurs around a fixed axis of motion. Goniometry measures the angles created by the rotary motion of the shafts of the bones. However, some translatory motion usually accompanies rotary motion and creates a slightly changing axis of motion during movement. Nevertheless, most clinicians find the description of osteokinematic movement in terms of rotary motion sufficiently accurate and use goniometry to measure osteokinematic movements.

Planes and Axes

Osteokinematic motions are classically described as taking place in one of the three cardinal **planes** of the body (sagittal, frontal, transverse) around three corresponding **axes** (medial-lateral, anterior-posterior, vertical). The three planes lie at right angles to one another, whereas the three axes lie at right angles both to one another and to their corresponding planes.

The **sagittal plane** proceeds from the anterior to the posterior aspect of the body. The median sagittal plane divides the body into right and left halves. The motions of flexion and extension occur in the sagittal plane (Fig. 1–2). The axis around which the motions of flexion and extension occur may be envisioned as a line that is perpendicular to the sagittal plane and proceeds from one side of the body to the other. This axis is called a medial-lateral axis. All motions in the sagittal plane take place around a medial-lateral axis.

The **frontal plane** proceeds from one side of the body to the other and divides the body into front and back halves. The motions that occur in the frontal plane are abduction and adduction (Fig. 1–3). The axis around which the motions of abduction and adduction take place is an anterior-posterior axis. This axis lies at right angles to the frontal plane and proceeds from the anterior to the posterior aspect of the body. Therefore, the anterior-posterior axis lies in the sagittal plane.

The **transverse plane** is horizontal and divides the body into upper and lower portions. The motion of rota-

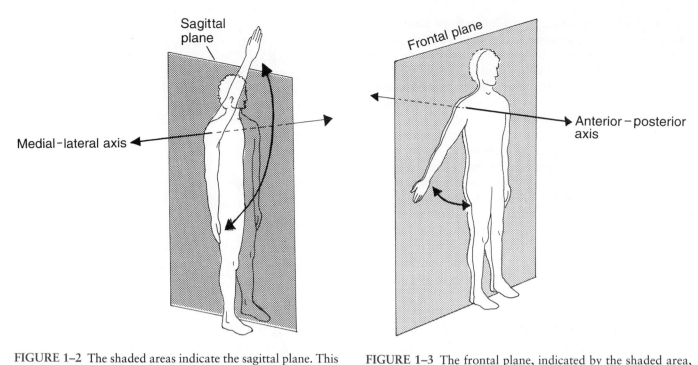

FIGURE 1–2 The shaded areas indicate the sagittal plane. This plane extends from the anterior aspect of the body to the posterior aspect. Motions in this plane, such as flexion and extension of the upper and lower extremities, take place around a medial-lateral axis

FIGURE 1–3 The frontal plane, indicated by the shaded area, extends from one side of the body to the other. Motions in this plane, such as abduction and adduction of the upper and lower extremities, take place around an anterior-posterior axis.

tion occurs in the transverse plane around a vertical axis (Fig. 1–4A and B). The vertical axis lies at right angles to the transverse plane and proceeds in a cranial to caudal direction.

The motions described previously are considered to occur in a single plane around a single axis. Combination

motions such as circumduction (flexion-abduction-extension-adduction) are possible at many joints, but because of the limitations imposed by the uniaxial design of the measuring instrument, only motions occurring in a single plane are measured in goniometry.

The type of motion that is available at a joint varies

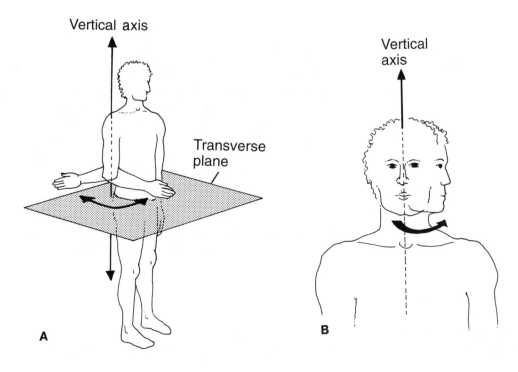

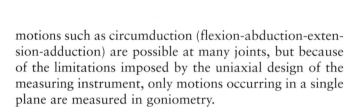

FIGURE 1–4 (A) The transverse plane is indicated by the shaded area. Movements in this plane take place around a vertical axis. These motions include rotation of the head (B), shoulder, (A), and hip, as well as pronation and supination of the forearm.

according to the structure of the joint. Some joints, such as the interphalangeal joints of the digits, permit a large amount of motion in only one plane around a single axis: flexion and extension in the sagittal plane around a medial-lateral axis. A joint that allows motion in only one plane is described as having 1 **degree of freedom of motion.** The interphalangeal joints of the digits have 1 degree of freedom of motion. Other joints, such as the glenohumeral joint, permit motion in three planes around three axes: flexion and extension in the sagittal plane around a medial-lateral axis, abduction and adduction in the frontal plane around an anterior-posterior axis, and medial and lateral rotation in the transverse plane around a vertical axis. The glenohumeral joint has three degrees of freedom of motion.

The planes and axes for each joint and joint motion to be measured are presented for the examiner in Chapters 4 through 13.

Range of Motion

Range of motion (ROM) is the arc of motion that occurs at a joint or a series of joints.[2] The starting position for measuring all ROM, except rotations in the transverse plane, is the anatomical position. Three notation systems have been used to define ROM: the 0- to 180-degree system, the 180- to 0-degree system, and the 360-degree system.

In the **0- to 180-degree notation system,** the upper and lower extremity joints are at 0 degrees for flexion-extension and abduction-adduction when the body is in anatomical position (Fig. 1–5A). A body position in which the extremity joints are halfway between medial (internal) and lateral (external) rotation is 0 degrees for the ROM in rotation (Fig. 1–5B). An ROM normally begins at 0 degrees and proceeds in an arc toward 180 degrees. This 0- to 180-degree system of notation, also called the *neutral zero method,* is widely used throughout the world. First described by Silver[3] in 1923, its use has been supported by many authorities, including Cave and Roberts,[4] Moore,[5,6] the American Academy of Orthopaedic Surgeons,[7,8] and the American Medical Association.[9]

> **EXAMPLE:** The ROM for shoulder flexion, which begins with the shoulder in the anatomical position (0 degrees) and ends with the arm overhead in full flexion (180 degrees), is expressed as 0 to 180 degrees.

In the preceding example, the portion of the extension ROM from full shoulder flexion back to the zero starting position does not need to be measured because this ROM represents the same arc of motion that was measured in flexion. However, the portion of the extension ROM that is available beyond the zero starting position must be

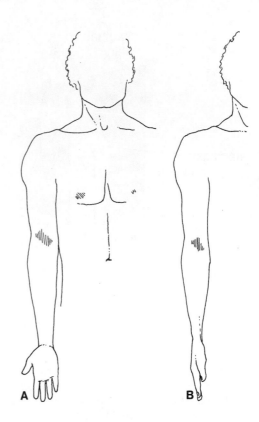

FIGURE 1–5 (A) In the anatomical position, the forearm is supinated so that the palms of the hands face anteriorly. (B) When the forearm is in a neutral position (with respect to rotation), the palm of the hand faces the side of the body.

measured (Fig. 1–6). Documentation of extension ROM usually incorporates only the extension that occurs beyond the zero starting position. The term **extension,** as it is used in this manual, refers to both the motion that is a return from full flexion to the zero starting position and the motion that normally occurs beyond the zero starting position. The term **hyperextension** is used to describe a greater than normal extension ROM.

Two other systems of notation have been described. The **180- to 0-degree notation system** defines anatomical position as 180 degrees.[10] An ROM begins at 180 degrees and proceeds in an arc toward 0 degrees. The **360-degree notation system** also defines anatomical position as 180 degrees.[11,12] The motions of flexion and abduction begin at 180 degrees and proceed in an arc toward 0 degrees. The motions of extension and adduction begin at 180 degrees and proceed in an arc toward 360 degrees. These two notation systems are more difficult to interpret than the 0- to 180-degree notation system and are infrequently used. Therefore, we have not included them in this text.

Active Range of Motion

Active range of motion is the arc of motion attained by a subject during unassisted voluntary joint motion. Having

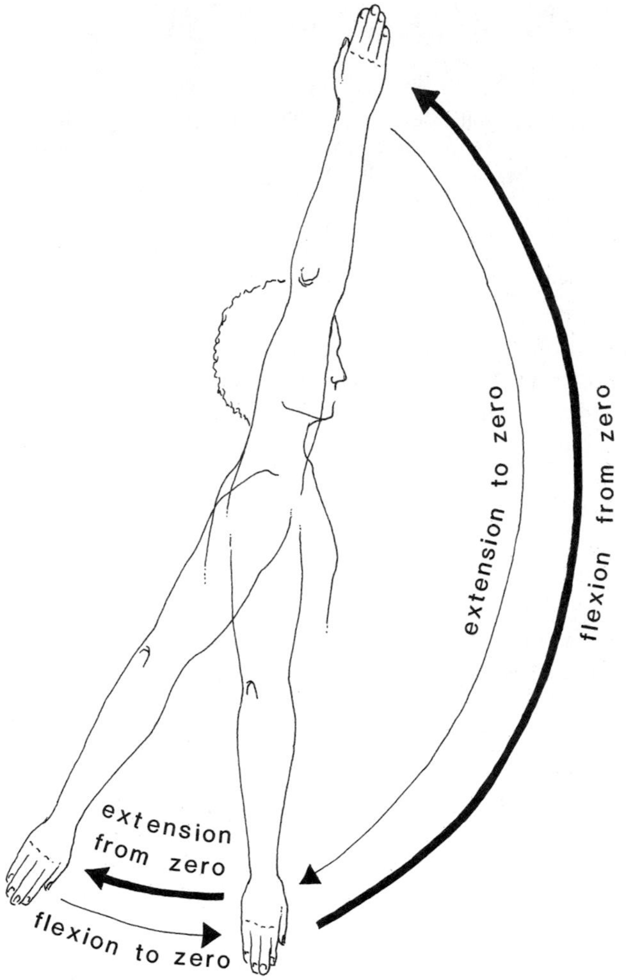

Passive Range of Motion

Passive range of motion is the arc of motion attained by an examiner without assistance from the subject. The subject remains relaxed and plays no active role in producing the motion. Normally passive ROM is slightly greater than active ROM [13,14] because each joint has a small amount of available motion that is not under voluntary control. The additional passive ROM that is available at the end of the normal active ROM is due to the stretch of tissues surrounding the joint and the reduced bulk of relaxed muscles. This additional passive ROM helps to protect joint structures because it allows the joint to absorb extrinsic forces.

Testing passive ROM provides the examiner with information about the integrity of the articular surfaces and the extensibility of the joint capsule, associated ligaments, muscles, fascia, and skin. To focus on these issues, passive ROM rather than active ROM should be tested in goniometry. Unlike active ROM, passive ROM does not depend on the subject's muscle strength and coordination. Comparisons between passive ROMs and active ROMs provide information about the amount of motion permitted by the joint structure (passive ROM) relative to the subject's ability to produce motion at a joint (active ROM). In cases of impairment such as muscle weakness, passive ROMs and active ROMs may vary considerably.

EXAMPLE: An examiner may find that a subject with a muscle paralysis has a full passive ROM but no active ROM at the same joint. In this instance, the joint surfaces and the extensibility of the joint capsule, ligaments, and muscles are sufficient to allow full passive ROM. The lack of muscle strength is prevents active motion at the joint.

The examiner should test passive ROM prior to performing a manual muscle test of muscle strength because the grading of manual muscle tests is based on completion of a joint ROM. An examiner must know the extent of the passive ROM before initiating a manual muscle test.

If pain occurs during passive ROM, it is often due to moving, stretching, or pinching of noncontractile (inert) structures. Pain occurring at the end of passive ROM may be due to stretching of contractile structures as well as noncontractile structures. Pain during passive ROM is not due to active shortening (contracting) of contractile tissues. By comparing which motions (active versus passive) cause pain and noting the location of the pain, the examiner can begin to determine which injured tissues are involved. Having the subject perform resisted isometric muscle contractions midway through the ROM, so that no tissues are being stretched, can help to isolate contractile structures. Having the examiner

FIGURE 1–6 Shoulder flexion and extension. Flexion begins with the shoulder in the anatomical position and the forearm in the neutral position. The ROM in flexion proceeds from the zero position through an arc of 180 degrees. The long, bold arrow shows the ROM in flexion, which is measured in goniometry. The short, bold arrow shows the ROM in extension, which is measured in goniometry.

a subject perform active ROM provides the examiner with information about the subject's willingness to move, coordination, muscle strength, and joint ROM. If pain occurs during active ROM, it may be due to contracting or stretching of "contractile" tissues, such as muscles, tendons, and their attachments to bone. Pain may also be due to stretching or pinching of noncontractile (inert) tissues, such as ligaments, joint capsules, bursa, fascia, and skin. Testing active ROM is a good screening technique to help focus a physical examination. If a subject can complete active ROM easily and painlessly, further testing of that motion is probably not needed. If, however, active ROM is limited, painful, or awkward, the physical examination should include additional testing to clarify the problem.

TABLE 1–1	Normal End-feels	
End-feel	**Structure**	**Example**
Soft	Soft tissue approximation	Knee flexion (contact between soft tissue of posterior leg and posterior thigh)
Firm	Muscular stretch	Hip flexion with the knee straight (passive elastic tension of hamstring muscles)
	Capsular stretch	Extension of metacarpophalangeal joints of fingers (tension in the anterior capsule)
	Ligamentous stretch	Forearm supination (tension in the palmar radioulnar ligament of the inferior radioulnar joint, interosseous membrane, oblique cord)
Hard	Bone contacting bone	Elbow extension (contact between the olecranon process of the ulna and the olecranon fossa of the humerus)

perform joint mobility and joint integrity tests on the subject can help determine which noncontractile structures are involved. Careful consideration of the end-feel and location of tissue tension and pain during passive ROM also adds information about structures that are limiting ROM.

End-feel

The amount of passive ROM is determined by the unique structure of the joint being tested. Some joints are structured so that the joint capsules limit the end of the ROM in a particular direction, whereas other joints are so structured that ligaments limit the end of a particular ROM. Other normal limitations to motion include passive tension in soft tissue such as muscles, fascia, and skin, soft tissue approximation, and contact of joint surfaces.

The type of structure that limits a ROM has a characteristic feel that may be detected by the examiner who is performing the passive ROM. This feeling, which is experienced by an examiner as a barrier to further motion at the end of a passive ROM, is called the **end-feel**. Developing the ability to determine the character of the end-feel requires practice and sensitivity. Determination of the end-feel must be carried out slowly and carefully to detect the end of the ROM and to distinguish among the various normal and abnormal end-feels. The ability to detect the end of the ROM is critical to the

safe and accurate performance of goniometry. The ability to distinguish among the various end-feels helps the examiner identify the type of limiting structure. Cyriax,[15] Kaltenborn,[16] and Paris[17] have described a variety of normal (physiological) and abnormal (pathological) end-feels.[18] Table 1–1, which describes normal end-feels, and Table 1–2, which describes abnormal end-feels, have been adapted from the works of these authors.

In Chapters 4 through 13 we describe what we believe are the normal end-feels and the structures that limit the ROM for each joint and motion. Because of the paucity of specific literature in this area, these descriptions are based on our experience in evaluating joint motion and on information obtained from established anatomy[19,20] and biomechanics texts[21–27] There is considerable controversy among experts concerning the structures that limit the ROM in some parts of the body. Also, normal individual variations in body structure may cause instances in which the end-feel differs from our description.

Examiners should practice trying to distinguish among the end-feels. In Chapter 2, Exercise 1 is included for this purpose. However, some additional topics regarding positioning and stabilization must be addressed before this exercise can be completed.

Hypomobility

The term **hypomobility** refers to a decrease in passive

TABLE 1–2	Abnormal End-feels	
End-feel		**Examples**
Soft	Occurs sooner or later in the ROM than is usual, or in a joint that normally has a firm or hard end-feel. Feels boggy.	Soft tissue edema Synovitis
Firm	Occurs sooner or later in the ROM than is usual, or in a joint that normally has a soft or hard end-feel.	Increased muscular tonus Capsular, muscular, ligamentous, and fascial shortening
Hard	Occurs sooner or later in the ROM than is usual or in a joint that normally has a soft or firm end-feel. A bony grating or bony block is felt.	Chondromalacia Osteoarthritis Loose bodies in joint Myositis ossificans Fracture
Empty	No real end-feel because pain prevents reaching end of ROM. No resistance is felt except for patient's protective muscle splinting or muscle spasm.	Acute joint inflammation Bursitis Abscess Fracture Psychogenic disorder

ROM that is substantially less than normal values for that joint, given the subject's age and gender. The end-feel occurs earlier in the ROM and may be different in quality from what is expected. The limitation in passive ROM may be due to a variety of causes including abnormalities of the joint surfaces or passive shortening of joint capsules, ligaments, muscles, fascia, and skin, as well as inflammation of these structures. Hypomobility has been associated with many orthopedic conditions such as osteoarthritis, [28,29] adhesive capsulitis,[30,31] and spinal disorders.[32, 33] Decreased ROM is a common consequence of immobilization after fractures[34,35] and scar development after burns.[36, 37] Neurological conditions such as stroke, head trauma, and cerebral palsy can also result in hypomobility owing to loss of voluntary movement, increased muscle tone, and immobilization. In addition, metabolic conditions such as diabetes have been associated with limited joint motion.[38, 39]

Capsular Patterns of Restricted Motion

Cyriax[15] has proposed that pathological conditions involving the entire joint capsule cause a particular pattern of restriction involving all or most of the passive motions of the joint. This pattern of restriction is called a **capsular pattern**. The restrictions do not involve a fixed number of degrees for each motion, but rather, a fixed proportion of one motion relative to another motion.

EXAMPLE: The capsular pattern for the elbow joint is a greater limitation of flexion than of extension. The elbow joint normally has a passive flexion ROM of 0 to 150 degrees. If the capsular involvement is mild, the subject might lose the last 15 degrees of flexion and the last 5 degrees of extension so that the passive flexion ROM is 5 to 135 degrees. If the capsular involvement is more severe, the subject might lose the last 30 degrees of flexion and the first 10 degrees of extension so that the passive flexion ROM is 10 to 120 degrees.

Capsular patterns vary from joint to joint (Table 1–3). The capsular pattern for each joint, as presented by Cyriax[15] and Kaltenborn,[16] is listed at the beginning of Chapters 4 through 13. Studies are needed to test the hypotheses regarding the cause of capsular patterns and to determine the capsular pattern for each joint. Studies by Fritz and coworkers,[41] and Hayes and colleagues[42] have examined the construct validity of Cyriax's capsular pattern in patients with arthritis or arthrosis of the knee. Although differing opinions exist, the findings seem to support the concept of a capsular pattern of restriction for the knee but with more liberal interpretation of the proportions of limitation than suggested by Cyriax.[15]

TABLE 1–3 Capsular Patterns of Extremity Joints

Joints	Restricted Motions
Glenohumeral joint	Greatest loss of lateral rotation, moderate loss of abduction, minimal loss of medial rotation.
Elbow complex (humeroulnar, humeroradial, proximal radioulnar joints)	Loss of flexion greater than loss of extension. Rotations full and painless except in advanced cases.
Forearm (proximal and distal radioulnar joints)	Equal loss of supination and pronation, only occurring if elbow has marked restrictions of flexion and extension.
Wrist (radiocarpal and midcarpal joints)	Equal loss of flexion and extension, slight loss of ulnar and radial deviation (Cyriax). Equal loss of all motions (Kaltenborn).
Hand	
Carpometacarpal joint—digit 1	Loss of abduction (Cyriax). Loss of abduction greater than extension (Kaltenborn).
Carpometacarpal joint—digits 2–5	Equal loss of all motions.
Metacarpophalangeal and interphalangeal joints	Equal loss of flexion and extension (Cyriax). Restricted in all motions, but loss of flexion greater than loss of other motions (Kaltenborn).
Hip	Greatest loss of medial rotation and flexion, some loss of abduction, slight loss of extension. Little or no loss of adduction and lateral rotation (Cyriax). Greatest loss of medial rotation, followed by less restriction of extension, abduction, flexion, and lateral rotation (Kaltenborn).
Knee (tibiofemoral joint)	Loss of flexion greater than extension.
Ankle (talocrural joint)	Loss of plantarflexion greater than dorsiflexion.
Subtalar joint	Loss of inversion (varus).
Midtarsal joint	Loss of inversion (adduction and medial rotation); other motions full.
Foot	
Metatarsophalangeal joint—digit 1	Loss of extension greater than flexion.
Metatarsophalangeal joint—digits 2–5	Loss of flexion greater than extension.
Interphalangeal joints	Loss of extension greater than flexion.

Adapted from Cyriax,[15] Kaltenborn,[17] and Dyrek.[40]

Hertling and Kessler[43] have thoughtfully extended Cyriax's concepts on causes of capsular patterns. They suggest that conditions resulting in a capsular pattern of restriction can be classified into two general categories: "(1) conditions in which there is considerable joint effusion or synovial inflammation, and (2) conditions in which there is relative capsular fibrosis."[43]

Joint effusion and synovial inflammation accompany conditions such as traumatic arthritis, infectious arthritis, acute rheumatoid arthritis, and gout. In these conditions the joint capsule is distended by excessive intra-articular synovial fluid, causing the joint to maintain a position that allows the greatest intra-articular joint volume. Pain triggered by stretching the capsule and muscle spasms that protect the capsule from further insult inhibit movement and cause a capsular pattern of restriction.

Relative capsular fibrosis often occurs during chronic low-grade capsular inflammation, immobilization of a joint, and the resolution of acute capsular inflammation. These conditions increase the relative proportion of collagen compared with that of mucopolysaccharide in the joint capsule, or they change the structure of the collagen. The resulting decrease in extensibility of the entire capsule causes a capsular pattern of restriction.

Noncapsular Patterns of Restricted Motion

A limitation of passive motion that is not proportioned similarly to a capsular pattern is called a **noncapsular pattern** of restricted motion.[15,43] A noncapsular pattern is usually caused by a condition involving structures other than the entire joint capsule. Internal joint derangement, adhesion of a part of a joint capsule, ligament shortening, muscle strains, and muscle contractures are examples of conditions that typically result in noncapsular patterns of restriction. Noncapsular patterns usually involve only one or two motions of a joint, in contrast to capsular patterns, which involve all or most motions of a joint.

> **EXAMPLE:** A strain of the biceps muscle may result in pain and restriction at the end of the range of passive elbow extension. The passive motion of elbow flexion would not be affected.

Hypermobility

The term **hypermobility** refers to an increase in passive ROM that exceeds normal values for that joint, given the subject's age and gender. For example, in adults the normal ROM for extension at the elbow joint of the fingers is about 0 degrees.[8] An ROM measurement of 90 degrees or more of extension at the elbow is well beyond the average ROM and is indicative of a hypermobile joint in an adult. Children have some normally occurring specific instances of increased ROM as compared with adults. For example, neonates 6 to 72 hours old have been found to have a mean ankle dorsiflexion passive ROM of 59 degrees,[44] which contrasts with the mean adult ROM of between 12 [45] and 20[7] degrees. The increased motion that is present in these children is normal for their age. If the increased motion should persist beyond the expected age range, it would be considered abnormal and hypermobility would be present.

Hypermobility is due to the laxity of soft tissue structures such as ligaments, capsules, and muscles that normally prevent excessive motion at a joint. In some instances the hypermobility may be due to abnormalities of the joint surfaces. A frequent cause of hypermobility is trauma to a joint. Hypermobility also occurs in serious hereditary disorders of connective tissue such as Ehlers-Danlos syndrome, Marfan syndrome, rheumatoid arthritis, and osteogenesis imperfecta. One of the typical physical abnormalities of Down syndrome is hypermobility. In this instance generalized hypotonia is thought to be an important contributing factor to the hypermobility.

Hypermobility syndrome (HMS) or benign joint hypermobility syndrome (BJHS) is used to describe otherwise healthy individuals who have generalized hypermobility accompanied by musculoskeletal symptoms.[46,47] An inherited abnormality in collagen is thought to be responsible for the joint laxity in these individuals.[48] Traditionally, the diagnosis of HMS involves the exclusion of other conditions, a score of at least "4" on the Beighton scale (Table 1–4), and arthralgia for longer than 3 months in four or more joints.[49,50] Other criteria have also been proposed, which include additional joint motions and extra-articular signs.[47,48,50] According to Grahame[47] the following joint motions should also be considered: shoulder lateral rotation greater than 90 degrees, cervical spine lateral flexion greater than 60 degrees, distal interphalangeal joint hyperextension greater than 60 degrees, and first metatarsophalangeal joint extension greater than 90 degrees.

Factors Affecting Range of Motion

ROM varies among individuals and is influenced by factors such as age, gender, and whether the motion is performed actively or passively. A fairly extensive amount of research on the effects of age and gender on ROM has been conducted for the upper and lower extremities as well as the spine. Other factors relating to subject characteristics such as body mass index (BMI), occupational activities, and recreational activities may affect ROM but have not been as extensively researched as age and gender. In addition, factors relating to the testing process, such as the testing position, type of instru-

TABLE 1–4 **Beighton Hypermobility Score**	
The Ability to	*Points*
Passively appose thumb to forearm	
Right	1
Left	1
Passively extend fifth MCP joint more than 90°	
Right	1
Left	1
Hyperextend elbow more than 10°	
Right	1
Left	1
Hyperextend knee more than 10°	
Right	1
Left	1
Place palms on floor by flexing trunk with knees straight	1
Total Beighton Score = sum of points.	0–9

Adapted from Beighton.[49]

ment employed, experience of the examiner, and even time of day have been identified as affecting ROM measurements. A brief summary of research findings that examine age and gender effects on ROM is presented later in the chapter. To assist the examiner, more detailed information about the effects of age and gender on the featured joints is presented at the beginning of Chapters 4 through 13. Information on the effects of subject characteristics and the testing process is included if available.

Ideally, to determine whether an ROM is impaired, the value of the ROM of the joint under consideration should be compared with ROM values from people of the same age and gender and from studies that used the same method of measurement. Often such comparisons are not possible because age-related and gender-related norms have not been established for all groups. In such situations the ROM of the joint should be compared with the same joint of the individual's contralateral extremity, providing that the contralateral extremity is not impaired or used selectively in athletic or occupational activities. Most studies have found little difference between the ROM of the right and left extremities.[28, 45, 51–57] A few studies[58–60] have found slightly less ROM in some joints of the upper extremity on the dominant or right side as compared with the contralateral side, which Allender and coworkers[58] attribute to increased exposure to stress. If the contralateral extremity is inappropriate for comparison, the individual's ROM may be compared with average ROM values in the handbook of the American Academy of Orthopaedic Surgeons[7, 8] and other standard texts.[9, 61–65] However, in many of these texts, the populations from which the average values were derived, as well as the testing positions and type of measuring instruments used, are not identified.

Average ROM values published in several standard texts and studies are summarized in tables at the begin-

ning of Chapters 4 through 13 and in Appendix A. The average ROM values presented in these tables should serve as only a general guide to identifying normal versus impaired ROM. Considerable differences in average ROM values are noted between the various references.

Age

Numerous studies have been conducted to determine the effects of age on ROM of the extremities and spine. General agreement exists among investigators regarding the age-related effects on the ROM of the extremity joints of newborns, infants, and young children up to about 2 years of age.[44, 66–70] These effects are joint- and motion specific but do not seem to be affected by gender. In comparison with adults, the youngest age groups have more hip flexion, hip abduction, hip lateral rotation, ankle dorsiflexion, and elbow motion. Limitations in hip extension, knee extension, and plantar flexion are considered to be normal for these age groups. Mean values for these age groups differ by more than 2 standard deviations from adult mean values published by the American Academy of Orthopaedic Surgeons,[7] the American Medical Association,[9] and Boone and Azen.[45] Therefore, age-appropriate norms should be used whenever possible for newborns, infants, and young children up to 2 years of age.

Most investigators who have studied a wide range of age groups have found that older adult groups have somewhat less ROM of the extremities than younger adult groups. These age-related changes in the ROM of older adults also are joint and motion specific but may affect males and females differently. Allander and associates[58] found that wrist flexion-extension, hip rotation, and shoulder rotation ROM decreased with increasing age, whereas flexion ROM in the metacarpophalangeal (MCP) joint of the thumb showed no consistent loss of motion. Roach and Miles[71] generally found a small decrease (3 to 5 degrees) in mean active hip and knee motions between the youngest age group (25 to 39 years) and the oldest age group (60 to 74 years). Except for hip extension ROM, these decreases represented less than 15 percent of the arc of motion. Stubbs, Fernandez, and Glenn[59] found a decrease of between 4 percent and 30 percent in 11 of 23 joints studied in men between the ages of 25 and 54 years. James and Parker[13] found systematic decreases in 10 active and passive lower extremity motions in subjects who were between 70 and 92 years of age.

As with the extremities, age-related effects on spinal ROM appear to be motion specific. Investigators have reached varying conclusions regarding how large a decrease in ROM occurs with increasing age. Moll and Wright[72] found an initial increase in thoracolumbar spinal mobility (flexion, extension, lateral flexion) in subjects from 15 to 24 years of age through 25 to 34 years of age followed by a progressive decrease with increasing age. These authors concluded that age alone may decrease spinal mobility from 25 percent to 52 percent by the seventh decade, depending on the motion. Loebl[73] found that thoracolumbar spinal mobility (flexion-extension) decreases with age an average of 8 degrees per decade. Fitzgerald and colleagues[74] found a systematic decrease in lateral flexion and extension of the lumbar spine at 20-year intervals but no differences in rotation and forward flexion. Youdas and associates[75] concluded that with each decade both females and males lose approximately 5 degrees of active motion in neck extension and 3 degrees in lateral flexion and rotation.

Gender

The effects of gender on the ROM of the extremities and spine also appear to be joint and motion specific.

Bell and Hoshizaki[76] found that females across an age range of 18 to 88 years had more flexibility than males in 14 of 17 joint motions tested. Beighton, Solomon, and Soskoline,[49] in a study of an African population, found that females between 0 and 80 years of age were more mobile than their male counterparts. Walker and coworkers,[77] in a study of 28 joint motions in 60- to 84-year olds, reported that 8 motions were greater in females and 4 motions were greater in males. Looking at the spine, Moll and Wright[72] found that female thoracolumbar left lateral flexion exceeded male left lateral flexion by 11 percent. On the other hand, male mobility exceeded female mobility in thoracolumbar flexion and extension.

⬛ Muscle Length Testing

Muscle length is the greatest extensibility of a muscle-tendon unit.[2] It is the maximal distance between the proximal and the distal attachments of a muscle to bone. Clinically, muscle length is not measured directly but instead is measured indirectly by determining the end of the ROM of the joint(s) crossed by the muscle.[78,79] Muscle length, in addition to the integrity of the joint surfaces and the extensibility of the capsule, ligaments, fascia, and skin, affects the amount of passive ROM of a joint. The purpose of testing muscle length is to ascertain whether hypomobility or hypermobility is caused by the length of the inactive antagonist muscle or other structures. By ascertaining which structures are involved, the health professional can choose more specific and more effective treatment procedures.

Muscles can be categorized by the number of joints they cross from their proximal to their distal attachments. One-joint muscles cross and therefore influence the motion of only one joint. Two-joint muscles cross and influence the motion of two joints, whereas multijoint muscles cross and influence multiple joints.

No difference exists between the indirect measurement of the length of a one-joint muscle and the measurement of joint ROM in the direction opposite to the muscle's active motion. Usually, one-joint muscles have sufficient length to allow full passive ROM at the joint they cross. If a one-joint muscle is shorter than normal, passive ROM in the direction opposite to the muscle's action is decreased and the end-feel is firm owing to a muscular stretch. At the end of the ROM the examiner may be able to palpate tension within the musculotendinous unit if the structures are superficial. In addition, the subject may complain of pain in the region of the tight muscle and tendon. These signs and symptoms help to confirm muscle shortness as the cause of the joint limitation.

If a one-joint muscle is abnormally lax, passive tension in the capsule and ligaments may initially maintain a normal ROM. However, with time, these joint structures often lengthen as well and passive ROM at the joint increases. Because the indirect measurement of the length of one-joint muscles is the same as the measurement of joint ROM, we have not presented specific muscle length tests for one-joint muscles.

> **EXAMPLE:** The length of one-joint hip adductors such as the adductor longus, adductor magnus, and adductor brevis is assessed by measuring passive hip abduction ROM. The indirect measurement of the length of these hip adductor muscles is identical to the measurement of passive hip abduction ROM (Fig. 1–7).

In contrast to one-joint muscles, the length of two-joint and multijoint muscles is usually not sufficient to allow full passive ROM to occur simultaneously at all joints crossed by these muscles.[80] This inability of a muscle to lengthen and allow full ROM at all of the joints the muscle crosses is termed **passive insufficiency**. If a two-joint or multijoint muscle crosses a joint the examiner is assessing for ROM, the subject must be positioned so that passive tension in the muscle does not limit the joint's ROM. To allow full ROM at the joint under consideration and to ensure sufficient length in the muscle, the muscle must be put on slack at all of the joints the muscle crosses that are not being assessed. A muscle is put on slack by passively approximating the origin and insertion of the muscle.

> **EXAMPLE:** The triceps is a two-joint muscle that extends the elbow and shoulder. The triceps is passively insufficient during full shoulder flexion and full elbow flexion. When an examiner assesses elbow flexion ROM, the shoulder must be in a neutral position so there is sufficient length in the biceps to allow full extension at the elbow (Fig. 1–8).

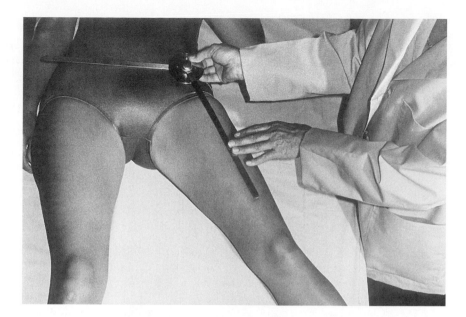

FIGURE 1–7 The indirect measurement of the muscle length of one-joint hip adductors is the same as measurement of passive hip abduction ROM.

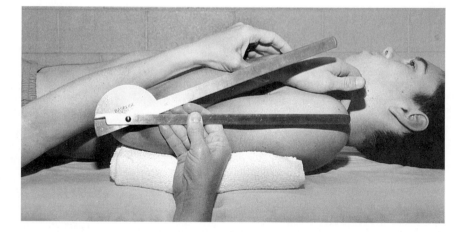

FIGURE 1–8 During the measurement of elbow flexion ROM, the shoulder must be in neutral to avoid passive insufficiency of the triceps, which would limit the ROM.

To assess the length of a two-joint muscle, the subject is positioned so that the muscle is lengthened over the proximal or distal joint that the muscle crosses. This joint is held in position while the examiner attempts to further lengthen the muscle by moving the second joint through full ROM. The end-feel in this situation is firm owing to the development of passive tension in the stretched muscle. The length of the two-joint muscle is indirectly assessed by measuring passive ROM in the direction opposite to the muscle's action at the second joint.

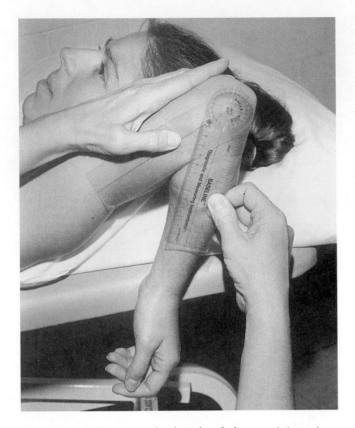

FIGURE 1–9 To assess the length of the two-joint triceps muscle, elbow flexion is measured while the shoulder is positioned in flexion.

EXAMPLE: To assess the length of a two-joint muscle such as the triceps, the shoulder is positioned and held in full flexion. The elbow is flexed until tension is felt in the triceps, creating a firm end-feel. The length of the triceps is determined by measuring passive ROM of elbow flexion with the shoulder in flexion (Fig. 1–9).

The length of multijoint muscles is assessed in a manner similar to that used in assessing the length of two-joint muscles. However, the subject is positioned and held so that the muscle is lengthened over all of the joints that the muscle crosses except for one last joint. The examiner attempts to further lengthen the muscle by moving the last joint through full ROM. Again, the end-feel is firm owing to tension in the stretched muscle. The length of the multijoint muscle is indirectly determined by measuring passive ROM in the direction opposite to the muscle's action at the last joint to be moved. Commonly used muscle length tests that indirectly assess two-joint and multijoint muscles have been included at the end of Chapters 4 through 13 as appropriate.

REFERENCES

1. MacConaill, MA, and Basmajian, JV: Muscles and Movement: A Basis For Human Kinesiology, ed 2. Robert E. Krieger, New York, 1977.
2. American Physical Therapy Association: Guide to Physical Therapist Practice, ed 2. Phys Ther 81:9, 2001.
3. Silver, D: Measurement of the range of motion in joints. J Bone Joint Surg 21:569, 1923.
4. Cave, EF, and Roberts, SM: A method for measuring and recording joint function. J Bone Joint Surg 18:455, 1936.
5. Moore, ML: The measurement of joint motion. Part II: The technic of goniometry. Phys Ther Rev 29:256, 1949.
6. Moore, ML: Clinical assessment of joint motion. In Basmajian, JV (ed): Therapeutic Exercise, ed 4. Williams & Wilkins, Baltimore, 1984.
7. American Academy of Orthopaedic Surgeons: Joint Motion: Methods of Measuring and Recording. AAOS, Chicago, 1965.
8. Greene, WB, and Heckman, JD (eds): The Clinical Measurement of Joint Motion. American Academy of Orthopaedic Surgeons, Rosemont, Ill., 1994.
9. American Medical Association: Guides to the Evaluation of Permanent Impairment, ed 3. AMA, Milwaukee, 1990.
10. Clark, WA: A system of joint measurement. J Orthop Surg 2:687, 1920.
11. West, CC: Measurement of joint motion. Arch Phys Med Rehabil 26:414, 1945.
12. Cole, TM, and Tobis, JS: Measurement of Musculoskeletal Function. In Kottke, FJ, and Lehmann, JF (eds): Krusenn's Handbook of Physical Medicine and Rehabilitation, ed 4. WB Saunders, Philadelphia, 1990.
13. James, B, and Parker, AW: Active and passive mobility of lower limb joints in elderly men and women. Am J Phys Med Rehabil 68:162, 1989.
14. Ball, P, and Johnson, GR: Reliability of hindfoot goniometry when using a flexible electrogoniometer. Clin Biomech 8:13, 1993.
15. Cyriax, J: Textbook of Orthopaedic Medicine: Diagnosis of Soft Tissue Lesions, ed 8. Bailliere Tindall, London, 1982.
16. Kaltenborn, FM: Manual Mobilization of the Extremity Joints, ed 4. Olaf Norlis Bokhandel, Oslo.
17. Paris, SV: Extremity Dysfunction and Mobilization. Institute Press, Atlanta, 1980.
18. Cookson, JC, and Kent, BE: Orthopedic manual therapy: An overview. Part I. Phys Ther 59:136, 1979.
19. Williams, P, et al: Gray's Anatomy of the Human Body, ed 38. Churchill Livingstone, New York, 1995.
20. Moore, KL, and Dalley, AF: Clinically Oriented Anatomy, ed 4. Williams & Wilkins, Baltimore, 1999.
21. Kapandji, IA: Physiology of the Joints, Vol 1, ed 2. Churchill Livingstone, London, 1970.
22. Kapandji, IA: Physiology of the Joints, Vol 2, ed 2. Williams & Wilkins, Baltimore, 1970.
23. Kapandji, IA: Physiology of the Joints, Vol 3, ed 2. Churchill Livingstone, London, 1970.
24. Steindler, A: Kinesiology of the Human Body. Charles C. Thomas, Springfield, Ill., 1955.
25. Gowitze, BA, and Milner, M: Understanding the Scientific Basis for Human Movement, ed 3. Williams & Wilkins, Baltimore, 1988.
26. Levangie, PK, and Norkin, CC: Joint Structure and Function, ed 3. FA Davis, Philadelphia, 2001.
27. Soderberg, GL: Kinesiology: Application to Pathological Motion. Williams & Wilkins, Baltimore, 1986.
28. Steultjens, MPM, et al: Range of joint motion and disability in patients with osteoarthritis of the knee or hip. Rheumatology 39:955, 2000.
29. Messier, SP, et al: Osteoarthritis of the knee: Effects on gait, strength, and flexibility. Arch Phys Med Rehabil 73:29, 1992.
30. Stam, HW: Frozen shoulder: A review of current concepts. Physiotherapy 80:588, 1994.
31. Roubal, PJ, Dobritt, D, and Placzek, JD: Glenohumeral gliding manipulation following interscalene brachial plexus block in patients with adhesive capsulitis. J Orthop Sports Phys Ther 24:66, 1996.

32. Hagen, KB, et al: Relationship between subjective neck disorders and cervical spine mobility and motion-related pain in male machine operators. Spine 22:1501, 1997.

33. Hermann, KM, and Reese, CS: Relationship among selected measures of impairment, functional limitation, and disability in patients with cervical spine disorders. Phys Ther 81:903, 2001.

34. MacKenzie, EJ, et al: Physical impairment and functional outcomes six months after severe lower extremity fractures. J Trauma 34:528, 1993.

35. Chesworth, BM, and Vandervoort, AA: Comparison of passive stiffness variables and range of motion in uninvolved and involved ankle joints of patients following ankle fractures. Phys Ther 75:254, 1995.

36. Staley, MJ, and Richard, RL: Burns. In O'Sullivan, SB and Schmitz, TJ (eds): Physical Rehabilitation: Assessment and Treatment, ed 4. FA Davis, Philadelphia, 2000.

37. Johnson, J, and Silverberg, R: Serial casting of the lower extremity to correct contractures during the acute phase of burn care. Phys Ther 75:262, 1995.

38. Schulte, L, et al: A quantitative assessment of limited joint mobility in patients with diabetes. Arthritis Rheum 10:1429, 1993.

39. Salsich, GB, Mueller, MJ, and Sahrmann, SA: Passive ankle stiffness in subjects with diabetes and peripheral neuropathy versus and age-matched comparison group. Phys Ther 80:352, 2000.

40. Dyrek, DA: Assessment and treatment planning strategies for musculoskeletal deficits. In O'Sullivan, SB, and Schmitz, TJ (eds): Physical Rehabilitation: Assessment and Treatment, ed 3. FA Davis, Philadelphia, 1994.

41. Fritz, JM, et al: An examination of the selective tissue tension scheme, with evidence for the concept of a capsular pattern of the knee. Phys Ther 78:1046, 1998.

42. Hayes, KW, Petersen, C, and Falconer, J: An examination of Cyriax's passive motion tests with patients having osteoarthritis of the knee. Phys Ther 74:697, 1994.

43. Hertling, DH, and Kessler, RM: Management of Common Musculoskeletal Disorders, ed 3. JB Lippincott, Philadelphia, 1996.

44. Waugh, KG, et al: Measurement of selected hip, knee and ankle joint motions in newborns. Phys Ther 63:1616, 1983.

45. Boone, DC, and Azen, SP: Normal range of motion of joints in male subjects. J Bone Joint Surg Am 61:756, 1979.

46. Everman, DB, and Robin, NH: Hypermobility syndrome. Pediatr Rev 19:111, 1998.

47. Grahame, R: Hypermobility not a circus act. Int J Clin Pract 54:314, 2000.

48. Russek, LN: Hypermobility syndrome. Phys Ther 79:59, 1999.

49. Beighton, P, Solomon, L, and Soskolne, CL: Articular mobility in an African population. Ann Rheum Dis 32:23, 1973.

50. Bird, HA: Joint hypermobility: Report from Special Interest Groups of the annual meeting of the British Society of Rheumatology. Br J Rheumatol 31:205, 1992.

51. Roaas, A, and Andersson, GB: Normal range of motion of the hip, knee and ankle joints in male subjects, 30–40 years of age. Acta Othop Scand 53:205, 1982.

52. Chang, DE, Buschbacher, LP, and Edlich, RF: Limited joint mobility in power lifters. Am J Sports Med 16:280, 1988.

53. Ahlberg, A, Moussa, M, and Al-Nahdi, M: On geographical variations in the normal range of joint motion. Clin Orthop Rel Res 234:229, 1988.

54. Schwarze, DJ, and Denton, JR: Normal values of neonatal limbs: An evaluation of 1000 neonates. J Res Pediatr Orthop 13:758, 1993.

55. Stefanyshyn, DJ, and Ensberg, JR: Right to left differences in the ankle joint complex range of motion. Med Sci Sports Exerc 26:551, 1993.

56. Mosley, AM, Crosbie, J, and Adams, R: Normative data for passive ankle plantarflexion-dorsiflexion flexibility. Clin Biomech 16:514, 2001.

57. Escalanate, A, et al: Determinants of hip and knee flexion range: Results from the San Antonio Longitudinal Study of Aging. Arthritis Care Res 12:8, 1999.

58. Allender, E, et al: Normal range of joint movements in shoulder, hip, wrist and thumb with special reference to side: A comparison between two populations. Int J Epidemiol 3:253, 1974.

59. Stubbs, NB, Fernandez, JE, and Glenn, WM: Normative data on joint ranges of motion for 25- to 54-year old males. Int J Ind Ergonomics 12:265, 1993.

60. Escalante, A, Lichtenstein, MJ, and Hazuda, HP: Determinants of shoulder and elbow flexion range: Results from the San Antonio longitudinal study of aging. Arthritis Care Res 12:277, 1999.

61. Kendall, FP, McCreary, EK, and Provance, PG: Muscles: Testing and Function, ed 4. Williams & Wilkins, Baltimore, 1993.

62. Hoppenfeld, S: Physical Examination of the Spine and Extremities. Appleton-Century-Crofts, New York, 1976.

63. Esch, D, and Lepley, M: Evaluation of Joint Motion: Methods of Measurement and Recording. University of Minnesota Press, Minneapolis, 1974.

64. Clarkson, HM: Musculoskeletal Assessment: Joint Range of Motion and Manual Muscle Strength, ed 2. Lippincott, Williams & Wilkins, Philadelphia, 2000.

65. Palmer, ML, and Epler, M: Fundamentals of Musculoskeletal Assessment Techniques. Lippincott, Williams & Wilkins, Philadelphia, 1998.

66. Drews, JE, Vraciu, JK, and Pellino, G: Range of motion of the joints of the lower extremities of newborns. Phys Occup Ther Pediatr 4:49, 1984.

67. Phelps, E, Smith, LJ, and Hallum, A: Normal range of hip motion of infants between nine and 24 months of age. Dev Med Child Neurol 27:785, 1985.

68. Wanatabe, H, et al: The range of joint motions of the extremities in healthy Japanese people: The differences according to age. Nippon Seikeigeka Gakkai Zasshi 53:275, 1979. Cited in Walker, JM: Musculoskeletal development: A review. Phys Ther 71:878, 1991.

69. Schwarze, DJ, and Denton, JR: Normal values of neonatal limbs: An evaluation of 1000 neonates. J Pediatr Orthop 13:758, 1993.

70. Broughton, NS, Wright, J, and Menelaus, MB: Range of knee motion in normal neonates. J Pediatr Orthop 13:263, 1993.

71. Roach, KE, and Miles, TP: Normal hip and knee active range of motion: The relationship to age. Phys Ther 71:656, 1991.

72. Moll, JMH, and Wright, V: Normal range of spinal mobility. Ann Rheum Dis 30:381, 1971.

73. Loebl, WY: Measurement of spinal posture and range of spinal movement. Ann Phys Med 9:103, 1967.

74. Fitzgerald, GK, et al: Objective assessment with establishment of normal values for lumbar spinal range of motion. Phys Ther 63:1776, 1983.

75. Youdas, JW, et al: Normal range of motion of the cervical spine: An initial goniometric study. Phys Ther 72:770, 1992.

76. Bell, RD, and Hoshizaki, TB: Relationship of age and sex with range of motion: Seventeen joint actions in humans. Can J Appl Sci 6:202, 1981.

77. Walker, JM, et al: Active mobility of the extremities older subjects. Phys Ther 64:919, 1984.

78. Gajdosik, RL, et al: Comparison of four clinical tests for assessing hamstring muscle length. J Orthop Sports Phys Ther 18:614, 1993.

79. Tardieu, G, Lespargot, A, and Tardieu, C: To what extent is the tibia-calcaneum angle a reliable measurement of the triceps surae length: Radiological correction of the torque-angle curve. Eur J Appl Physiol 37:163, 1977.

80. Gajdosik, RL, Hallett, JP, and Slaugher, LL: Passive insufficiency of two-joint shoulder muscles. Clin Biomech 9:377, 1994.

CHAPTER 2

Procedures

Competency in goniometry requires that the examiner acquire the following knowledge and develop the following skills.

The examiner must have knowledge of the following for each joint and motion:

1. Testing positions
2. Stabilization required
3. Joint structure and function
4. Normal end-feels
5. Anatomical bony landmarks
6. Instrument alignment

The examiner must have the skill to perform the following for each joint and motion:

1. Position and stabilize correctly
2. Move a body part through the appropriate range of motion
3. Determine the end of the range of motion (end-feel)
4. Palpate the appropriate bony landmarks
5. Align the measuring instrument with landmarks
6. Read the measuring instrument
7. Record measurements correctly

◗ Positioning

Positioning is an important part of goniometry because it is used to place the joints in a zero starting position and to help stabilize the proximal joint segment. Positioning affects the amount of tension in soft tissue structures (capsule, ligaments, muscles) surrounding a joint. A testing position in which one or more of these soft tissue structures become taut results in a more limited range of motion (ROM) than a position in which the same structures become lax. As can be seen in the following exam-

ple, the use of different testing positions alters the ROM obtained for hip flexion.

> **EXAMPLE:** A testing position in which the knee is flexed yields a greater hip flexion ROM than a testing position in which the knee is extended. When the knee is extended, hip flexion is prematurely limited by tension in the hamstring muscles.

If examiners use the same position during successive measurements of a joint ROM, the relative amounts of tension in the soft tissue structures should be the same as in previous measurements. Therefore, a comparison of ROM measurements taken in the same position should yield similar results. When different testing positions are used for successive measurements of a joint ROM, more variability is added to the measurement[1-4] and no basis for comparison exists.

Testing positions refer to the positions of the body that we recommend for obtaining goniometric measurements. The series of testing positions that are presented in this text are designed to:

1. Place the joint in a starting position of 0 degrees
2. Permit a complete ROM
3. Provide stabilization for the proximal joint segment

If a testing position cannot be attained because of restrictions imposed by the environment or limitations of the subject, the examiner must use creativity to decide how to obtain a particular joint measurement. The alternative testing position that is created must serve the same three functions as the recommended testing position. The examiner must describe the position precisely in the subject's records so that the same position can be used for all subsequent measurements.

Testing positions involve a variety of body positions such as supine, prone, sitting, and standing. When an examiner intends to test several joints and motions during one testing session, the goniometric examination should be planned to avoid moving the subject unnecessarily. For example, if the subject is prone, all possible measurements in this position should be taken before the subject is moved into another position. Table 2–1, which lists joint measurements by body position, has been designed to help the examiner plan a goniometric examination.

Stabilization

The testing position helps to stabilize the subject's body and proximal joint segment so that a motion can be isolated to the joint being examined. Isolating the motion to one joint helps to ensure that a true measurement of the motion is obtained rather than a measurement of combined motions that occur at a series of joints. Positional stabilization may be supplemented by manual stabilization provided by the examiner.

EXAMPLE: Measurement of medial rotation of the hip joint performed with the subject in a sitting position (Fig. 2–1A). The pelvis (proximal segment) is partially stabilized by the body weight, but the subject is moving her trunk and pelvis during hip rotation. Additional stabilization should be provided by the examiner and the subject (Fig. 2–1B). The examiner provides manual stabilization for the pelvis by exerting a downward pressure on the iliac crest of the side being tested. The subject is instructed to shift her body weight over the hip being tested to help keep the pelvis stabilized.

For most measurements, the amount of manual stabilization applied by an examiner must be sufficient to keep the proximal joint segment fixed during movement of the distal joint component. If both the distal and the proximal joint components are allowed to move during joint testing, the end of the ROM is difficult to determine. Learning how to stabilize requires practice because the examiner must stabilize with one hand while simul-

TABLE 2–1	**Joint Measurements by Body Position**			
	Prone	*Supine*	*Sitting*	*Standing*
Shoulder	Extension	Flexion Abduction Medial rotation Lateral rotation		
Elbow		Flexion		
Forearm			Pronation Supination	
Wrist			Flexion Extension Radial deviation Ulnar deviation All motions	
Hand			Medial rotation Lateral rotation	
Hip	Extension	Flexion Abduction Adduction		
Knee		Flexion		
Ankle and foot	Subtalar inversion Subtalar eversion	Dorsiflexion Plantar flexion Inversion Eversion Midtarsal inversion Midtarsal eversion	Dorsiflexion Plantar flexion Inversion Eversion Midtarsal inversion Midtarsal eversion	
Toes		All motions	All motions	
Cervical spine			Flexion Extension Lateral flexion Rotation	
Thoracolumbar spine			Rotation	Flexion Extension Lateral flexion
Temporomandibular joint			Depression Anterior protrusion Lateral deviation	

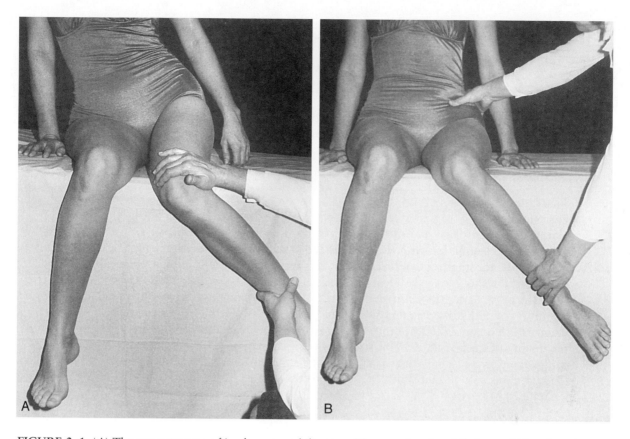

FIGURE 2–1 (*A*) The consequences of inadequate stabilization. The examiner has failed to stabilize the subject's pelvis and trunk; therefore, a lateral tilt of the pelvis and lateral flexion of the trunk accompany the motion of hip medial rotation. The range of medial rotation appears greater than it actually is because of the added motion from the pelvis and trunk. (*B*) The use of proper stabilization. The examiner uses her right hand to stabilize the pelvis (keeping the pelvis from raising off the table) during the passive range of motion (ROM). The subject assists in stabilizing the pelvis by placing her body weight on the left side. The subject keeps her trunk straight by placing both hands on the table.

taneously moving the distal joint segment with the other hand. The techniques of stabilizing the proximal joint segment and of determining the end of a ROM (end-feel) are basic to goniometry and must be mastered prior to learning how to use the goniometer. Exercise 1 is designed to help the examiner learn how to stabilize and determine the end of the ROM and end-feel.

EXERCISE 1

DETERMINING THE END OF THE RANGE OF MOTION AND END-FEEL

This exercise is designed to help the examiner determine the end of the ROM and to differentiate among the three normal end-feels: soft, firm, and hard.

ELBOW FLEXION: SOFT END-FEEL

Activities: See Figure 5–15 in Chapter 5.

1. Select a subject.
2. Position the subject supine with the arm placed close to the side of the body. A towel roll is placed under the distal end of the humerus to allow full elbow extension. The forearm is placed in full supination with the palm of the hand facing the ceiling.
3. With one hand, stabilize the distal end of the humerus (proximal joint segment) to prevent flexion of the shoulder.
4. With the other hand, slowly move the forearm through the full passive range of elbow flexion until you feel resistance limiting the motion.
5. Gently push against the resistance until no further flexion can be achieved. Carefully note the quality of the resistance. This soft end-feel is caused by compression of the muscle bulk of the anterior forearm with that of the anterior upper arm.
6. Compare this soft end-feel with the soft end-feel found in knee flexion (see knee flexion in Chapter 9).

ANKLE DORSIFLEXION: FIRM END-FEEL

Activities: See Figure 10–14 in Chapter 10.

1. Select a subject.
2. Place the subject sitting so that the lower leg is over the edge of the supporting surface and the knee is flexed at least 30 degrees.
3. With one hand, stabilize the distal end of the tibia and fibula to prevent knee extension and hip motions.
4. With the other hand on the plantar surface of the metatarsals, slowly move the foot through the full passive range of ankle dorsiflexion until you feel resistance limiting the motion.
5. Push against the resistance until no further dorsiflexion can be achieved. Carefully note the quality of the resistance. This firm end-feel is caused by tension in the Achilles tendon, the posterior portion of the deltoid ligament, the posterior talofibular ligament, the calcaneofibular ligament, the posterior joint capsule, and the wedging of the talus into the mortise formed by the tibia and fibula.
6. Compare this firm end-feel with the firm end-feel found in metacarpophalangeal (MCP) extension of the fingers (see Chapter 7).

ELBOW EXTENSION: HARD END-FEEL

Activities:

1. Select a subject.
2. Position the subject supine with the arm placed close to the side of the body. A small towel roll is placed under the distal end of the humerus to allow full elbow extension. The forearm is placed in full supination with the palm of the hand facing the ceiling.
3. With one hand resting on the towel roll and holding the posterior, distal end of the humerus, stabilize the humerus (proximal joint segment) to prevent extension of the shoulder.
4. With the other hand, slowly move the forearm through the full passive range of elbow extension until you feel resistance limiting the motion.
5. Gently push against the resistance until no further extension can be attained. Carefully note the quality of the resistance. When the end-feel is hard, it has no give to it. This hard end-feel is caused by contact between the olecranon process of the ulna and the olecranon fossa of the humerus.
6. Compare this hard end-feel with the hard end-feel usually found in radial deviation of the wrist (see radial deviation in Chapter 7).

Measurement Instruments

A variety of instruments are used to measure joint motion. These instruments range from simple paper tracings and tape measures to electrogoniometers and motion analysis systems. An examiner may choose to use a particular instrument based upon the purpose of the measurement (clinical versus research), the motion being measured, and the instrument's accuracy, availability, cost, ease of use, and size.

Universal Goniometer

The **universal goniometer** is the instrument most commonly used to measure joint position and motion in the clinical setting. Moore[5,6] designated this type of goniometer as "universal" because of its versatility. It can be used to measure joint position and ROM at almost all joints of the body. The majority of measurement techniques presented in this book demonstrate the use of the universal goniometer.

Universal goniometers may be constructed of plastic (Fig. 2–2) or metal (Fig. 2–3) and are produced in many sizes and shapes, but adhere to the same basic design. Typically the design includes a body and two thin extensions called arms—a stationary arm and a moving arm (Fig. 2–4).

The **body** of a universal goniometer resembles a protractor and may form a half circle or a full circle (Fig. 2–5). The scales on a half-circle goniometer read from 0 to 180 degrees and from 180 to 0 degrees. The scales on a full-circle instrument may read either from 0 to 180 degrees and from 180 to 0 degrees, or from 0 to 360 degrees and from 360 to 0 degrees. Sometimes full-circle instruments have both 180-degree and 360-degree scales. Increments on the scales may vary from 1 to 10 degrees, but 1- and 5-degree increments are the most common.

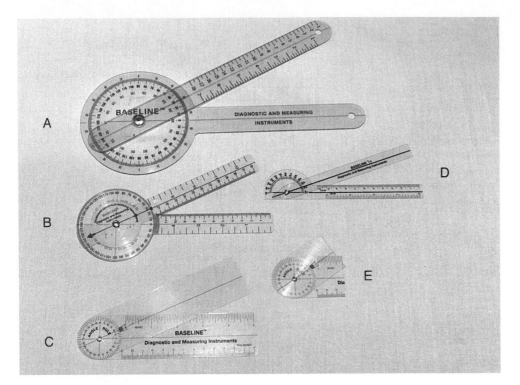

FIGURE 2–2 Plastic universal goniometers are available in different shapes and sizes. Some goniometers have full-circle bodies (A,B,C,E), whereas others have half-circle bodies (D). The 14-inch goniometer (A) is used to measure large joints such as the hip, knee, and shoulder. Six- to 8-inch goniometers (B,C,D) are used to assess midsized joints such as the wrist and ankle. The small goniometer (E) has been cut in length from a 6-inch goniometer (C) to make it easier to measure the fingers and toes.

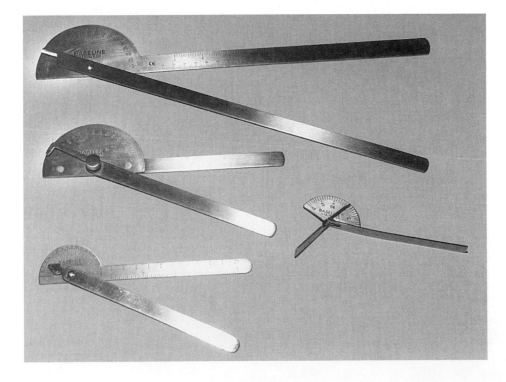

FIGURE 2–3 These metal goniometers are of different sizes but all have half-circle bodies. Metal goniometers with full-circle bodies are also available. The smallest goniometer is specifically designed to lie on the dorsal or ventral surface of the fingers and toes while measuring joint motion.

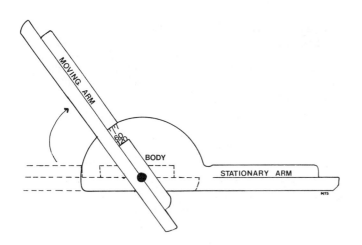

FIGURE 2–4 The body of this universal goniometer forms a half circle. The stationary arm is an integral part of the body of the goniometer. The moving arm is attached to the body by either a rivet or a screw so that it can be moved independently from the body. In this example, the moving arm has a cut-out portion sometimes referred to as a "window." The window permits the examiner to read the scale on the body of the instrument.

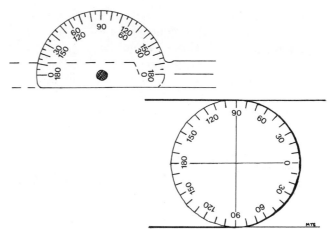

FIGURE 2–5 The body of the goniometer may be either a half circle (*top*) or a full circle (*bottom*).

Traditionally, the **arms** of a universal **goniometer** are designated as moving or stationary according to how they are attached to the body of the goniometer. The **stationary arm** is a structural part of the body of the goniometer and cannot be moved independently from the body. The **moving arm** is attached to the center of the body of most plastic goniometers by a rivet that permits the arm to move freely on the body. In some metal goniometers, a screwlike device (thumb knob) is used to attach the moving arm. Often the screwlike device may be tightened to hold the moving arm in a certain position

or loosened to allow free movement. The moving arm may have one or more of the following features: a pointed end, a black or white line extending the length of the arm, or a cut-out portion (window) (Fig. 2–6). Goniometers that are used to measure ROM on radiographs have an opaque white line extending the length of the arms and opaque markings on the body. These features help the examiner to read the scales.

The length of the arms varies among instruments from approximately 1 to 14 inches. These variations in length represent an attempt on the part of the manufacturers to adapt the size of the instrument to the size of the joints. The cost of the instruments also varies (See Appendix B: Features and Cost of Universal and Gravity-Based Goniometers).

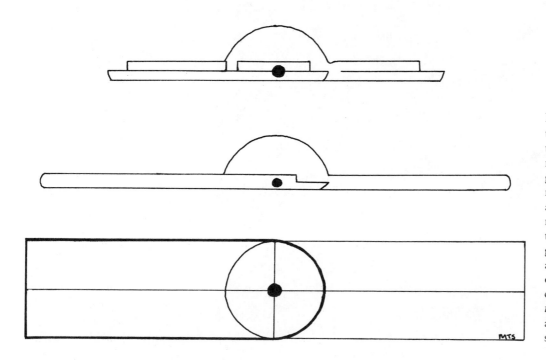

FIGURE 2–6 These goniometers have a number of features that make reading the instruments easier. The half-circle goniometer at the top has a moving arm with cut-out areas at both ends and in the middle, as well as a black center line. The half-circle goniometer in the middle has a cut-out area only at the end of its moving arm. The full-circle plastic goniometer (*bottom*) has a black center line along both the moving and the stationary arms.

EXAMPLE: A universal goniometer with 14-inch arms is appropriate for measuring motion at the knee joint because the arms are long enough to permit alignment with the greater trochanter of the femur and the lateral malleolus of the tibia (Fig. 2–7A). A universal goniometer with short arms would be difficult to use because the arms do not extend a sufficient distance along the femur and tibia to permit alignment with the bony landmarks (Fig. 2–7B). A goniometer with long arms would be awkward for measuring the MCP joints of the hand.

Gravity-Dependent Goniometers (Inclinometers)

Although not as common as the universal goniometer, several other types of manual goniometers may be found in the clinical setting. **Gravity-dependent goniometers** or **inclinometers** use gravity's effect on pointers and fluid levels to measure joint position and motion (Fig. 2–8). The **pendulum goniometer** consists of a 360-degree protractor with a weighted pointer hanging from the center of the protractor. This device was first described by Fox and Van Breemen[7] in 1934. The **fluid (bubble) goniometer**, which was developed by Schenkar[8] in 1956, has a

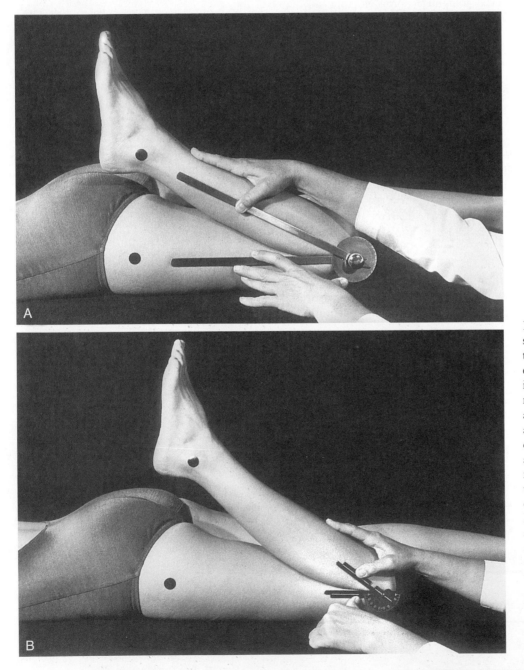

FIGURE 2–7 Selecting the right-sized goniometer makes it easier to measure joint motion. (*A*) The examiner is using a full-circle instrument with long arms to measure knee flexion ROM. The arms of the goniometer extend along the distal and proximal components of the joint to within a few inches of the bony landmarks (*black dots*) that are used to align the arms. The proximity of the ends of the arms to the landmarks makes alignment easy and helps ensure that the arms are aligned accurately. (*B*) The small half-circle metal goniometer is a poor choice for measuring knee flexion ROM because the landmarks are so far from the ends of the goniometer's arms that accurate alignment is difficult.

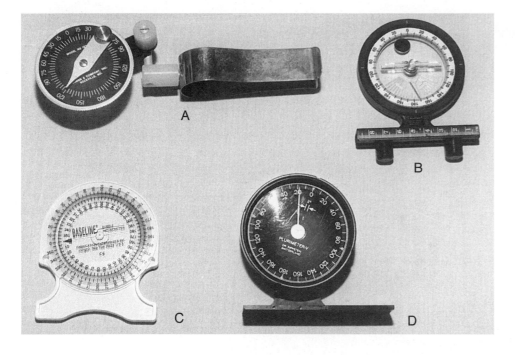

FIGURE 2–8 Each of these gravity-dependent goniometers uses a weighted pointer (*A*,*B*,*D*) or bubble (*C*) to indicate the position of the goniometer relative to the vertical pull of gravity. All of these inclinometers have a rotating dial so that the scale can be zeroed with the pointer or bubble in the starting position.

fluid-filled circular chamber containing an air bubble. It is similar to a carpenter's level but, being circular, has a 360-degree scale. Other inclinometers such as the Myrin OB Goniometer and the CROM (cervical range of motion) device use a pendulum needle that reacts to gravity to measure motions in the frontal and sagittal planes and use a compass needle that reacts to the earth's magnetic field to measure motions in the horizontal plane. A fairly large selection of manual inclinometers and a few digital inclinometers are commercially available. Generally these instruments are more expensive than universal goniometers (See Appendix B: Features and Cost of Universal and Gravity-Based Goniometers).

Inclinometers are attached to or held on the distal segment of the joint being measured. The angle between the long axis of the distal segment and the line of gravity is noted. Inclinometers may be easier to use in certain situations than universal goniometers because they do not have to be aligned with bony landmarks or centered over the axis of motion. However, it is critical that the proximal segment of the joint being measured be positioned vertically or horizontally to obtain accurate measurements; otherwise, adjustments must be made in determining the measurement.[6,9] Inclinometers are also difficult to use on small joints[10] and where there is soft tissue deformity or edema.[6,9]

Although universal and gravity-dependent goniometers may all be available within a clinical setting, they should not be used interchangeably.[11–14] For example, an examiner should not use a universal goniometer on Tuesday and an inclinometer on Wednesday to measure a subject's knee ROM. The goniometers may provide slightly different results, making comparisons for judging changes in ROM inappropriate.

Electrogoniometers

Electrogoniometers, introduced by Karpovich and Karpovich[15] in 1959, are used primarily in research to obtain dynamic joint measurements. Most devices have two arms, similar to those of the universal goniometer, which are attached to the proximal and distal segments of the joint being measured.[16–19] A potentiometer is connected to the two arms. Changes in joint position cause the resistance in the potentiometer to vary. The resulting change in voltage can be used to indicate the amount of joint motion. Potentiometers measuring angular displacement have also been integrated with strain gauges[20,21] and isokinetic dynamometers[22] for measuring resistive torque. Flexible electrogoniometers with two plastic end-blocks connected by a flexible strain gauge have been designed to measure angular displacement between the end-blocks in one or two planes of motion.[3,13]

Some electrogoniometers resemble pendulum goniometers.[23,24] Changes in joint position cause a change in contact between the pendulum and the small resistors. Contact with the resistors produces a change in electric current, which is used to indicate the amount of joint motion.

Electrogoniometers are expensive and take time to calibrate accurately and attach to the subject. Given these drawbacks, electrogoniometers are used more often in research than in clinical settings. Radiographs, photographs, film, videotapes, and computer-assisted video

EXERCISE 2

THE UNIVERSAL GONIOMETER

The following activities are designed to help the examiner become familiar with the universal goniometer.

Equipment: Full-circle and half-circle universal goniometers made of plastic and metal.

Activities:

1. Select a goniometer.
2. Identify the type of goniometer selected (full-circle or half-circle) by noting the shape of the body.
3. Differentiate between the moving and the stationary arms of the goniometer. (Remember that the stationary arm is an integral part of the body of the goniometer.)
4. Observe the moving arm to see if it has a cut-out portion.
5. Find the line in the middle of the moving arm and follow it to a number on the scale.
6. Study the body of the goniometer and answer the following questions:
   a. Is the scale located on one or both sides?
   b. Is it possible to read the scale through the body of the goniometer?
   c. What intervals are used?
   d. Does the face contain one or two scales?
7. Hold the goniometer in both hands. Position the arms so that they form a continuous straight line. When the arms are in this position, the goniometer is at 0 degrees.
8. Keep the stationary arm fixed in place and shift the moving arm while watching the numbers on the scale, either at the tip of the moving arm or in the cut-out portion. Shift the moving arm from 0 to 45, 90, 150, and 180 degrees.
9. Keep the stationary arm fixed and shift the moving arm from 0 degrees through an estimated 45-degree arc of motion. Compare the visual estimate with the actual arc of motion by reading the scale on the goniometer. Try to estimate other arcs of motion and compare the estimates with the actual arc of motion.
10. Keep the moving arm fixed in place and move the stationary arm through different arcs of motion.
11. Repeat steps 2 to 10 using different goniometers.

motion analysis systems are other joint measurement methods used more commonly in research settings.

Visual Estimation

Although some examiners make visual estimates of joint position and motion rather than use a measuring instrument, we do not recommend this practice. Several authors suggest the use of visual estimates in situations in which the subject has excessive soft tissue covering physical landmarks.[25,26] Most authorities report more accurate and reliable measurements with a goniometer than with visual estimates.[27–33] Even when produced by a skilled examiner, visual estimates yield only subjective information in contrast to goniometric measurements, which yield objective information. However, estimates are useful in the learning process. Visual estimates made prior to goniometric measurements help to reduce errors attributable to incorrect reading of the goniometer. If the goniometric measurement is not in the same quadrant as

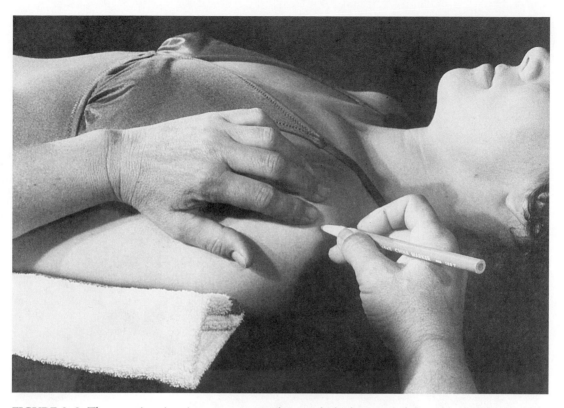

FIGURE 2–9 The examiner is using a grease pencil to mark the location of the subject's left acromion process. Note that the examiner is using the second and third digits of her left hand to palpate the bony landmark.

the estimate, the examiner is alerted to the possibility that the wrong scale is being read.

After the examiner has read and studied this section on measurement instruments, Exercise 2 should be completed. Given the adaptability and widespread use of the universal goniometer in the clinical setting, this book focuses on teaching the measurement of joint motion using a universal goniometer.

Alignment

Goniometer alignment refers to the alignment of the arms of the goniometer with the proximal and distal segments of the joint being evaluated. Instead of depending on soft tissue contour, the examiner uses bony **anatomical landmarks** to more accurately visualize the joint segments. These landmarks, which have been identified for all joint measurements, should be exposed so that they may be identified easily (Fig. 2–9). The landmarks should be learned and adhered to whenever possible. The stationary arm is often aligned parallel to the longitudinal axis of the proximal segment of the joint, and the moving arm is aligned parallel to the longitudinal axis of the distal segment of the joint (Fig. 2–10). In some situations,

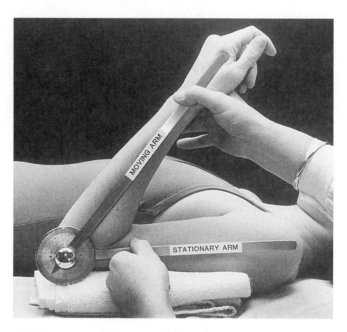

FIGURE 2–10 When using a full-circle goniometer to measure ROM of elbow flexion, align the stationary arm of the instrument parallel to the longitudinal axis of the proximal part (subject's humerus) and align the moving arm parallel to the longitudinal axis of the distal part (subject's forearm).

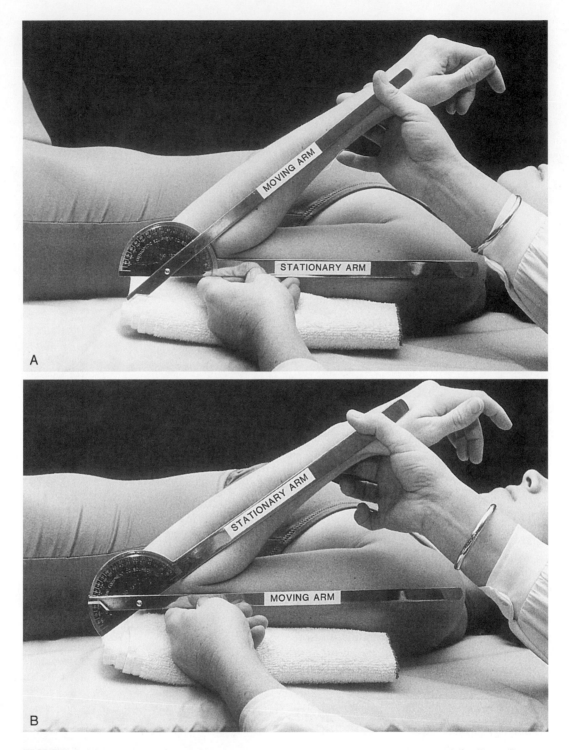

FIGURE 2–11 (*A*) When the examiner uses a half-circle goniometer to measure left elbow flexion, aligning the moving arm with the subject's forearm causes the pointer to move beyond the goniometer body, which makes it impossible to read the scale. (*B*) Reversing the arms of the instrument so that the stationary arm is aligned parallel to the distal part and the moving arm is aligned parallel to the proximal part causes the pointer to remain on the body of the goniometer, enabling the examiner to read the scale along the pointer.

because of limitations imposed by either the goniometer or the subject (Fig. 2–11*A*), it may be necessary to reverse the alignment of the two arms so that the moving arm is aligned with the proximal part and the stationary arm is aligned with the distal part (Fig. 2–11*B*). Therefore, we have decided to use the term **proximal arm** to refer to the arm of the goniometer that is aligned with the proximal segment of the joint. The term **distal arm** refers to the

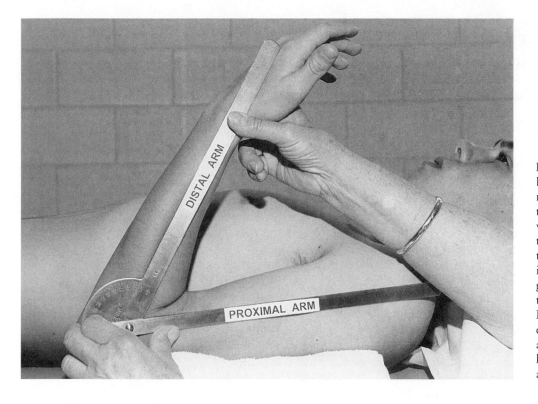

FIGURE 2–12 Throughout the book we use the term "proximal arm" to indicate the arm of the goniometer that is aligned with the proximal segment of the joint being examined. The term "distal arm" is used to indicate the arm of the goniometer that is aligned with the distal segment of the joint. During the measurement of elbow flexion, the proximal arm is aligned with the humerus, and the distal arm is aligned with the forearm.

arm aligned with the distal segment of the joint (Fig. 2–12). The anatomical landmarks provide reference points that help to ensure that the alignment of the arms is correct.

The **fulcrum** of the goniometer may be placed over the approximate location of the axis of motion of the joint being measured. However, because the axis of motion changes during movement, the location of the fulcrum must be adjusted accordingly. Moore[6] suggests that careful alignment of the proximal and distal arms ensures that the fulcrum of the goniometer is located at the approximate axis of motion. Therefore, alignment of the arms of the goniometer with the proximal and distal joint segments should be emphasized more than placement of the fulcrum over the approximate axis of motion.

Errors in measuring joint position and motion with a goniometer can occur if the examiner is not careful. When aligning the arms and reading the scale of the goniometer, the examiner must be at eye level with the goniometer to avoid parallax. If the examiner is higher or lower than the goniometer, the alignment and scales may be distorted. Often a goniometer will have several scales, one going from 0 to 180 degrees and another going from 180 to 0 degrees. Examiners must carefully determine which scale is correct for the measurement. If a visual estimate is made before the measurement is taken, gross errors caused by reading the wrong scale will be obvious. Another source of error is misinterpretation of the intervals on the scale. For example, the smallest interval of a particular goniometer may be 5 degrees, but an examin-

er may believe the interval represents 1 degree. In this case the examiner would incorrectly read 91 degrees instead of 95 degrees.

After the examiner has read this section on alignment, Exercise 3 should be completed.

Recording

Goniometric measurements are recorded in numerical tables, pictorial charts, or within the written text of an evaluation. Regardless of which method is used, recordings should provide enough information to permit an accurate interpretation of the measurement. The following items are recommended to be included in the recording:

1. Subject's name, age, and gender
2. Examiner's name
3. Date and time of measurement
4. Make and type of goniometer used
5. Side of the body, joint, and motion being measured; for example, left knee flexion
6. ROM, including the number of degrees at the beginning of the motion and the number of degrees at the end of the motion
7. Type of motion being measured; that is, passive or active motion
8. Any subjective information, such as discomfort or pain, that is reported by the subject during the testing

EXERCISE 3

GONIOMETER ALIGNMENT FOR ELBOW FLEXION

The following activities are designed to help the examiner learn how to align and read the goniometer.

Equipment: Full-circle and half-circle universal goniometers of plastic and metal in various sizes and a skin-marking pencil.

Activities: See Figures 5–15 to 5–17 in Chapter 5.

1. Select a goniometer and a subject.
2. Position the subject so that he or she is supine. The subject's right arm should be positioned so that it is close to the side of the body with the forearm in supination (palm of hand faces the ceiling). A towel roll placed under the distal humerus helps to ensure that the elbow is fully extended.
3. Locate and mark each of the following landmarks with the pencil: acromion process, lateral epicondyle of the humerus, radial head, and radial styloid process.
4. Align the proximal arm of the goniometer along the longitudinal axis of the humerus, using the acromion process and the lateral epicondyle as reference landmarks. Make sure that you are positioned so that the goniometer is at eye level during the alignment process.
5. Align the distal arm of the goniometer along the longitudinal axis of the radius, using the radial head and the radial styloid process as reference landmarks.
6. The fulcrum should be close to the lateral epicondyle. Check to make sure that the body of the goniometer is not being deflected by the supporting surface.
7. Recheck the alignment of the arms and readjust the alignment as necessary.
8. Read the scale on the goniometer.
9. Remove the goniometer from the subject's arm and place it nearby so it is handy for measuring the next joint position.
10. Move the subject's forearm into various positions in the flexion ROM, including the end of the flexion ROM. At each joint position, align and read the goniometer. Remember that you must support the subject's forearm while aligning the goniometer.
11. Repeat steps 3 to 10 on the subject's left upper extremity.
12. Repeat steps 4 to 10 using goniometers of different sizes and shapes.
13. Answer the following questions:
    a. Did the length of the goniometer arms affect the accuracy of the alignment? Explain.
    b. What length goniometer arms would you recommend as being the most appropriate for this measurement? Why?
    c. Did the type of goniometer used (full-circle or half-circle) affect either joint alignment or the reading of the scale? Explain.
    d. Did the side of the body that you were testing make a difference in your ability to align the goniometer? Why?

---

9. Any objective information obtained by the examiner during testing, such as a protective muscle spasm, crepitus, or capsular or noncapsular pattern of restriction
10. A complete description of any deviation from the recommended testing positions

If a subject has normal pain-free ROM during active or passive motion, the ROM may be recorded as normal (N) or within normal limits (WNL). To determine whether the ROM is normal, the examiner should compare the ROM of the joint being tested with ROM values from people of the same age and gender, and from studies that used the same method of measurement. Text and ROM tables that demonstrate mean values by age with information on gender and methods of measurement are presented at the beginning of Chapters 4 through 13. A selection of ROM values is also presented at the beginning of testing procedures for each motion and in Appendix A. The ROM of the joint being tested may also be compared with the same joint of the subject's contralateral extremity, provided that the contralateral extremity is neither impaired nor used selectively in athletic or occupational activities.

If passive ROM appears to be decreased or increased when compared with normal values, the ROM should be measured and recorded. Recordings should include both the starting and the ending positions to define the ROM. A recording that includes only the total ROM, such as 50 degrees of flexion, gives no information as to where a motion begins and ends. Likewise, a recording that lists –20 degrees (minus 20 degrees) of flexion is open to misinterpretation because the lack of flexion could occur at either the end or the beginning of the ROM.

A motion such as flexion that begins at 0 degrees and ends at 50 degrees of flexion is recorded as 0–50 degrees of flexion (Fig. 2–13A). A motion that begins with the joint flexed at 20 degrees and ends at 70 degrees of flexion is recorded as 20–70 degrees of flexion (Fig. 2–13B). The total ROM is the same (50 degrees) in both instances, but the arcs of motion are different.

Because both the starting and the ending positions have been recorded, the measurement can be interpreted correctly. If we assume that the normal ROM for this movement is 0 to 150 degrees, the subject who has a flexion ROM of 0–50 degrees lacks motion at the end of the flexion ROM. The subject with a flexion ROM of 20–70 degrees lacks motion at the beginning and at the end of the flexion ROM. The term hypomobile may be applied to both of these joints because both joints have a less-than-normal ROM.

Sometimes the opposite situation exists, in which a joint has a greater-than-normal range of motion and is hypermobile. If an elbow joint is hypermobile, the starting position for measuring elbow flexion may be in hyperextension rather than at 0 degrees. If the elbow was hyperextended 20 degrees in the starting position, the beginning of the flexion ROM would be recorded as 20 degrees of hyperextension (Fig. 2–14). To clarify that the 20 degrees represents hyperextension rather than limited flexion, a "0" representing the zero starting position, which is now within the ROM, is included. An ROM

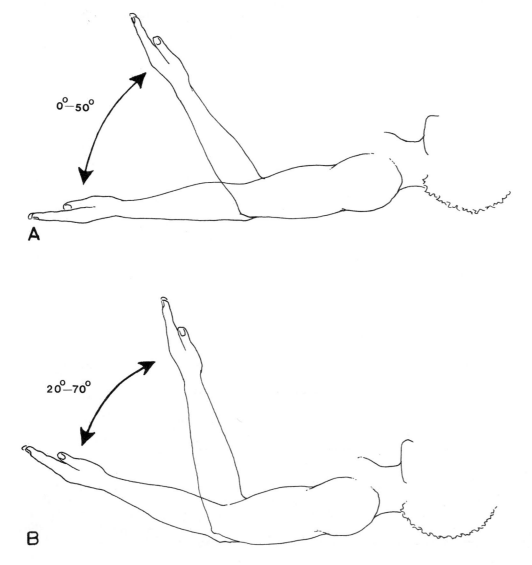

FIGURE 2–13 A recording of ROM should include the beginning of the range as well as the end. (A) In this illustration, the motion begins at 0 degrees and ends at 50 degrees so that the total ROM is 50 degrees. (B) In this illustration, the motion begins at 20 degrees of flexion and ends at 70 degrees, so that the total ROM is 50 degrees. For both subjects, the total ROM is the same, 50 degrees, even though the arcs of motion are different.

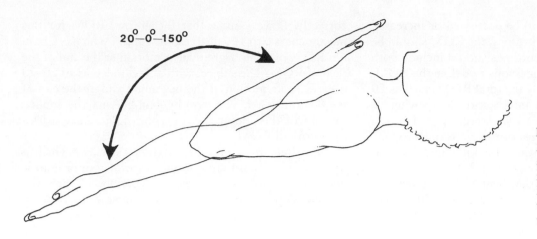

20°–0°–150°

FIGURE 2–14 This subject has 20 degrees of hyperextension at her elbow. In this case, motion begins at 20 degrees of hyperextension and proceeds through the 0-degree position to 150 degrees of flexion.

that begins at 20 degrees of hyperextension and ends at 150 degrees of flexion is recorded as 20–0–150 degrees of flexion.

Some authorities have suggested the use of plus (+) and minus (–) signs to indicate hypomobility and hypermobility. However, the use of these signs varies depending on the authority consulted. To avoid confusion, we have omitted the use of plus and minus signs. A ROM that does not start with 0 degrees or ends prematurely indicates hypomobility. The addition of zero, representing the usual starting position within the ROM indicates hypermobility.

Numerical Tables

Numerical tables typically list joint motions in a column down the center of the form (Fig. 2–15). Space to the left of the central column is reserved for measurements taken on the left side of the subject's body; space to the right is reserved for measurements taken on the right side of the body. The examiner's initials and the date of testing are noted at the top of the measurement columns. Subsequent measurements are recorded on the same form and identified by the examiner's initials and the date at the top of the appropriate measurement column. This format makes it easy to compare a series of measurements to identify problem motions and then to track rehabilitative response over time. Examples of numerical recording tables are included in Appendix C.

Pictorial Charts

Pictorial charts may be used in isolation or combined with numerical tables to record ROM measurements. Pictorial charts usually include a diagram of the normal starting and ending positions of the motion (Fig. 2–16).

Name	Paul Jones			Age 57		Gender	M		
	Left						Right		
		JW	JW	Examiner	JW				
		4/1/02	3/18/02	Date	3/18/02				
				Hip					
		0-98	0-73	Flexion	0-118				
		0-5	0-5	Extension	0-12				
		0-28	0-18	Abduction	0-32				
		0-12	0-6	Adduction	0-15				
		0-35	0-24	Medial Rotation	0-42				
		0-40	0-35	Lateral Rotation	0-44				
				Comments:					

FIGURE 2–15 This numerical table records the results of ROM measurements of a subject's left and right hips. The examiner has recorded her initials and the date of testing at the top of each column of ROM measurements. Note that the right hip was tested once, on March 18, 2002, and the left hip was tested twice, once on March 18, 2002, and again on April 1, 2002.

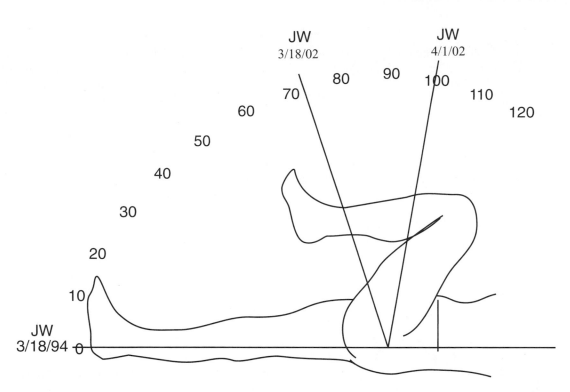

FIGURE 2–16 This pictorial chart records the results of flexion ROM measurements of a subject's left hip. For measurements taken on March 18, 2002, note the 0 to 73 degrees of left hip flexion; for measurements taken on April 1, 2002, note the 0 to 98 degrees of left hip flexion. (Adapted with permission from Range of Motion Test, New York University Medical Center, Rusk Institute of Rehabilitation Medicine.)

Sagittal-Frontal-Transverse-Rotation Method

Another method of recording, which may be included in a written text or formatted into a table, is the **sagittal-frontal-transverse-rotation (SFTR) recording method**, developed by Gerhardt and Russe.[34,35] Although it is rarely used in the United States, its advantages have been described by Miller.[9] In the SFTR method, three numbers are used to describe all motions in a given plane. The first and last numbers indicate the ends of the ROM in that plane. The middle number indicates the starting position, which would be 0 in normal motion.

In the sagittal plane, represented by S, the first number indicates the end of the extension ROM, the middle number the starting position, and the last number the end of the flexion ROM.

EXAMPLE: If a subject has 50 degrees of shoulder extension and 170 degrees of shoulder flexion, these motions would be recorded: Shoulder S: 50–0–170 degrees.

In the frontal plane, represented by F, the first number indicates the end of the abduction ROM, the middle number the starting position, and the last number the end of the adduction ROM. The ends of spinal ROM in the frontal plane (lateral flexion) are listed to the left first and to the right last.

EXAMPLE: If a subject has 45 degrees of hip abduction and 15 degrees of hip adduction, these motions would be recorded: Hip F: 45–0–15 degrees.

In the transverse plane, represented by T, the first number indicates the end of the horizontal abduction ROM, the middle number the starting position, and the last number the end of the horizontal adduction ROM.

EXAMPLE: If a subject has 30 degrees of shoulder horizontal abduction and 135 degrees of shoulder horizontal adduction, these motions would be recorded: Shoulder T: 30–0–135 degrees.

Rotation is represented by R. Lateral rotation ROM, including supination and eversion, is listed first; medial rotation ROM, including pronation and inversion, is listed last. Rotation ROM of the spine to the left is listed first; rotation ROM to the right is listed last. Limb position during measurement is noted if it varies from anatomical position. "F90" would indicate that a measurement was taken with the limb positioned in 90 degrees of flexion.

EXAMPLE: If a subject has 35 degrees of lateral rotation ROM of the hip and 45 degrees of medial rotation ROM of the hip, and these motions were measured with the hip in 90 degrees of flexion, these motions would be recorded: Hip R: (F90) 35–0–45 degrees.

Hypomobility is noted by the lack of 0 as the middle number or by less-than-normal values for the first and last numbers, which indicate the ends of the ROM.

EXAMPLE: If elbow flexion ROM was limited and a subject could move only between 20 and 90 degrees of flexion, it would be recorded: Elbow S: 0–20–90 degrees. The starting position is 20 degrees of flexion, and the end of the ROM is 90 degrees of flexion.

A fixed-joint limitation, ankylosis is indicated by the use of only two numbers. The zero starting position is included to clarify in which motion the fixed position occurs.

EXAMPLE: An elbow fixed in 40 degrees of flexion would be recorded: Elbow S: 0–40 degrees.

American Medical Association Guide to Evaluation Method

Another system of recording restricted motion has been described by the American Medical Association in the *Guides to the Evaluation of Permanent Impairment*.[36] This book provides ratings of permanent impairment for all major body systems, including the respiratory, cardiovascular, digestive, and visual systems. The longest chapter focuses on impairment evaluation of the extremities, spine, and pelvis. Restricted active motion, ankylosis, amputation, sensory loss, vascular changes, loss of strength, pain, joint crepitation, joint swelling, joint instability, and deformity are measured and converted to percentage of impairment for the body part. The total percentage of impairment for the body part is converted to the percentage of impairment for the extremity, and finally to a percentage of impairment for the entire body. Often these permanent impairment ratings are used, along with other information, to determine the patient's level of disability and the amount of monetary compensation to be expected from the employer or the insurer. Physicians and therapists working with patients with permanent impairments who are seeking compensation for their disabilities should refer to this book for more detail.

The system of recording restricted motion found in the *Guides to the Evaluation of Permanent Impairment* also uses the 0–to–180–degree notation method. The neutral starting position is recorded as 0 degrees; motions progress toward 180 degrees. However, the recording system proposed in the *Guides to the Evaluation of Permanent Impairment* does differ from other recording systems described in our text. In this system, when extension exceeds the neutral starting position, it is referred to as hyperextension and is expressed with the plus (+) symbol. For example, motion at the MCP joint of a finger from 15 degrees of hyperextension to 45 degrees of flexion would be recorded as +15 to 45 degrees. The plus (+) symbol is used to emphasize the fact that the joint has hyperextension.

In this system, the minus (–) symbol is used to emphasize the fact that a joint has an extension lag. When the neutral (zero) starting position cannot be attained, an extension lag exists and is expressed with the minus symbol. For example, motion at the MCP joint of a finger from 15 degrees of flexion to 45 degrees of flexion would be recorded as –15 to 45 degrees.

Procedures

Prior to beginning a goniometric evaluation, the examiner must:

- Determine which joints and motions need to be tested
- Organize the testing sequence by body position
- Gather the necessary equipment, such as goniometers, towel rolls, and recording forms
- Prepare an explanation of the procedure for the subject

Explanation Procedure

The listed steps and the example that follows provide the examiner with a suggested format for explaining goniometry to a subject.

Steps

1. Introduction and explanation of purpose
2. Explanation and demonstration of goniometer
3. Explanation and demonstration of anatomical landmarks
4. Explanation and demonstration of testing position
5. Explanation and demonstration of examiner's and subject's roles
6. Confirmation of subject's understanding

Lay rather than technical terms are used in the example so that the subject can understand the procedure. During the explanation, the examiner should try to establish a good rapport with the subject and enlist the subject's participation in the evaluation process. After reading the example, the examiner should practice Exercise 4.

EXAMPLE: Explanation of Goniometry

1. Introduction and Explanation of Purpose

   Introduction: My name is _____. I am a (occupational title).

   Explanation: I understand that you have been having some difficulty moving your elbow. I am going to measure the amount of motion that you have at your elbow joint to see if it is equal to, less than, or greater than normal. I will use this information to plan a treatment program and assess its effectiveness.

   Demonstration: The examiner flexes and extends his or her own elbow so that the subject is able to observe a joint motion.

2. Explanation and Demonstration of Goniometer

   Explanation: The instrument that I will be using to obtain the measurements is called a goniometer. It is similar to a protractor, but it has two extensions called arms.

   Demonstration: The examiner shows the goniometer to the subject and encourages the subject to ask questions. The examiner shows the subject how the goniometer is used by holding it next to his or her own elbow.

3. Explanation and Demonstration of Anatomical Landmarks

   Explanation: To obtain accurate measurements, I will need to identify some anatomical landmarks. These landmarks help me to align the arms of the goniometer. Because these landmarks are important, I may have to ask you to remove certain articles of clothing, such as your shirt or blouse. Also, to locate some of the landmarks, I may have to to press my fingers against your skin.

   Demonstration: The examiner shows the subject an easily identified anatomical landmark such as the ulnar styloid process.

4. Explanations and Demonstration of Recommended Testing Positions

   Explanation: Certain testing positions have been established to help make joint measurements easier and more accurate. Whenever possible, I would like you to assume these positions. I will be happy to help you get into a particular position. Please let me know if you need assistance.

   Demonstration: The sitting or supine positions.

5. Explanation and Demonstration of Examiner's and Subject's Roles During **Active Motion**

   Explanation: I will ask you to move your arm in exactly the same way that I move your arm.

   Demonstration: The examiner takes the subject's

arm through a passive ROM and then asks the subject to perform the same motion.

6. Explanation and Demonstration of Examiner's and Subjects Roles During **Passive Motion**

   Explanation: I will move your arm and take a measurement. You should relax and let me do all of the work. These measurements should not cause discomfort. Please let me know if you have any discomfort and I will stop moving your arm.

   Demonstration: The examiner moves the subject's arm gently and slowly through the range of elbow flexion.

7. Confirmation of Subject's Understanding

   Explanation: Do you have any questions? Are you ready to begin?

Testing Procedure

The testing process is initiated after the explanation of goniometry has been given and the examiner is assured that the subject understands the nature of the testing process. The testing procedure consists of the following 12-step sequence of activities.

Steps

1. Place the subject in the testing position.
2. Stabilize the proximal joint segment.
3. Move the distal joint segment to the zero starting position. If the joint cannot be moved to the zero starting position, it should be moved as close as possible to the zero starting position. Slowly move the distal joint segment to the end of the passive ROM and determine the end-feel. Ask the subject if there was any discomfort during the motion.
4. Make a visual estimate of the ROM.
5. Return the distal joint segment to the starting position.
6. Palpate the bony anatomical landmarks.
7. Align the goniometer.
8. Read and record the starting position. Remove the goniometer.
9. Stabilize the proximal joint segment.
10. Move the distal segment through the full ROM.
11. Replace and realign the goniometer. Palpate the anatomical landmarks again if necessary.
12. Read and record the ROM.

Exercise 5, which is based on the 12-step sequence, affords the examiner an opportunity to use the testing procedure for an evaluation of the elbow joint. This exercise should be practiced until the examiner is able to perform the activities sequentially without reference to the exercise.

EXERCISE 4

EXPLANATION OF GONIOMETRY

Equipment: A universal goniometer.

Activities: Practice the following six steps with a subject.

1. Introduce yourself and explain the purpose of goniometric testing. Demonstrate a joint ROM on yourself.
2. Show the goniometer to your subject and demonstrate how it is used to measure a joint ROM.
3. Explain why bony landmarks must be located and palpated. Demonstrate how you would locate a bony landmark on yourself, and explain why clothing may have to be removed.
4. Explain and demonstrate why changes in position may be required.
5. Explain the subject's role in the procedure. Explain and demonstrate your role in the procedure.
6. Obtain confirmation of the subject's understanding of your explanation.

EXERCISE 5

TESTING PROCEDURE FOR GONIOMETRIC EVALUATION OF ELBOW FLEXION

Equipment: A universal goniometer, skin-marking pencil, recording form, and pencil.

Activities: See Figures 5–15 to 5–17 in Chapter 5.

1. Place the subject in a supine position, with the arm to be tested positioned close to the side of the body. Place a towel roll under the distal end of the humerus to allow full elbow extension. Position the forearm in full supination, with the palm of the hand facing the ceiling.
2. Stabilize the distal end of the humerus to prevent flexion of the shoulder.
3. Move the forearm to the zero starting position and determine whether there is any motion (extension) beyond zero. Move to the end of the passive range of flexion. Evaluate the end-feel. Usually the end-feel is soft because of compression of the muscle bulk on the anterior forearm in conjunction with that on the anterior humerus. Ask the subject if there was any discomfort during the motion.
4. Make a visual estimate of the beginning and end of the ROM.
5. Return the forearm to the starting position.
6. Palpate the bony anatomical landmarks (acromion process, lateral epicondyle of the humerus, radial head, and radial styloid process) and mark with a skin pencil.
7. Align the arms and the fulcrum of the goniometer. Align the proximal arm with the lateral midline of the humerus, using the acromion process and lateral epicondyle for reference. Align the distal arm along the lateral midline of the radius, using the radial head and the radial styloid process for reference. The fulcrum should be close to the lateral epicondyle of the humerus.
8. Read the goniometer and record the starting position. Remove the goniometer.
9. Stabilize the proximal joint segment (humerus).
10. Perform the passive ROM, making sure that you complete the available range.
11. When the end of the ROM has been attained, replace and realign the goniometer. Palpate the anatomical landmarks again if necessary.
12. Read the goniometer and record your reading. Compare your reading with your visual estimate to make sure that you are reading the correct scale on the goniometer.

REFERENCES

1. Rothstein, JM, Miller, PJ, and Roettger, F: Goniometric reliability in a clinical setting. Phys Ther 63:1611, 1983.
2. Ekstrand, J, et al: Lower extremity goniometric measurements: A study to determine their reliability. Arch Phys Med Rehabil 63:171, 1982
3. Ball, P, and Johnson, GR: Reliability of hindfoot goniometry when using a flexible electrogoniometer. Clin Biomech 8:13, 1993
4. Sabar, JS, et al: Goniometric assessment of shoulder range of motion: Comparison of testing in supine and sitting positions. Arch Phys Med Rehabil 79:64,1998.
5. Moore, ML: The measurement of joint motion. Part II: The technic of goniometry. Phys Ther Rev 29:256, 1949.
6. Moore, ML: Clinical assessment of joint motion. In Basmajian, JV (ed): Therapeutic Exercise, ed 3. Williams & Wilkins, Baltimore, 1978.
7. Fox, RF, and Van Breemen, J: Chronic Rheumatism, Causation and Treatment. Churchill, London, 1934, p 327.
8. Schenkar, WW: Improved method of joint motion measurement. N Y J Med 56:539, 1956.
9. Miller, PJ: Assessment of joint motion. In Rothstein, JM (ed): Measurement in Physical Therapy. Churchill Livingstone, New York, 1985.
10. Clarkson, HM: Musculoskeletal Assessment: Joint Range of Motion and Manual Muscle Strength, ed. 2. Lippincott Williams & Wilkins, Philadelphia, 2000.
11. Petherick, M, et al: Concurrent validity and intertester reliability of universal and fluid-based goniometers for active elbow range of motion. Phys Ther 68:966, 1988.
12. Rheault, W, et al: Intertester reliability and concurrent validity of fluid-based and universal goniometers for active knee flexion. Phys Ther 68:1676, 1988.
13. Goodwin, J, et al: Clinical methods of goniometry: A comparative study. Disabil Rehabil 14:10, 1992.
14. Rome, K, and Cowieson, F: A reliability study of the universal goniometer, fluid goniometer, and electrogoniometer for the measurement of ankle dorsiflexion. Foot Ankle 17:28, 1996.
15. Karpovich, PV, and Karpovich, GP: Electrogoniometer: A new device for study of joints in action. Fed Proc 18:79, 1959.
16. Kettelkamp, DB, Johnson, RC, Smidt, GL, et al: An electrogoniometric study of knee motion in normal gait. J Bone Joint Surg Am 52:775, 1970.
17. Knutzen, KM, Bates, BT, and Hamill, J: Electrogoniometry of postsurgical knee bracing in running. Am J Phys Med Rehabil 62:172, 1983.
18. Carey, JR, Patterson, JR, and Hollenstein, PJ: Sensitivity and reliability of force tracking and joint-movement tracking scores in healthy subjects. Phys Ther 68:1087, 1988.
19. Torburn, L, Perry, J, and Gronley, JK: Assessment of rearfoot motion: Passive positioning, one-legged standing, gait. Foot Ankle 19:688:1998.
20. Vandervoort, AA, et al: Age and sex effects on mobility of the human ankle. J Gerontol 47:M17, 1992.
21. Chesworth, BM, and Vandervoort, AA: Comparison of passive stiffness variables and range of motion in uninvolved and involved ankle joints of patients following ankle fractures. Phys Ther 75:253, 1995
22. Gajdosik, RL, Vander Linden, DW, and Williams, AK: Influence of age on length and passive elastic stiffness characteristics of the calf muscles-tendon unit of woman. Phys Ther 79:827, 1999.
23. Clapper, MP, and Wolf, SL: Comparison of the reliability of the Orthoranger and the standard goniometer for assessing active lower extremity range of motion. Phys Ther 68:214, 1988.
24. Greene, BL, and Wolf, SL: Upper extremity joint movement: Comparison of two measurement devices. Arch Phys Med Rehabil 70:288, 1989.
25. American Academy of Orthopaedic Surgeons: Joint Motion: A Method of Measuring and Recording. AAOS, Chicago, 1965.
26. Rowe, CR: Joint measurement in disability evaluation. Clin Orthop 32:43, 1964.
27. Watkins, MA, et al: Reliability of goniometric measurements and visual estimates of knee range of motion obtained in a clinical setting. Phys Ther 71:90, 1991.
28. Youdas, JW, Carey, JR, and Garrett, TR: Reliability of measurements of cervical spine range of motion: Comparison of three methods. Phys Ther 71:98, 1991.
29. Low, JL: The reliability of joint measurement. Physiotherapy 62:227, 1976.
30. Moore, ML: The measurement of joint motion. Part I: Introductory review of the literature. Phys TherRev 29:195, 1949.
31. Salter, N: Methods of measurement of muscle and joint function. J Bone Joint Surg Br 34:474, 1955.
32. Minor, MA, and Minor, SD: Patient Evaluation Methods for the Health Professional. Reston, VA, 1985.
33. Greene, WB, and Heckman JD (eds): The Clinical Measurement of Joint Motion. AAOS, Rosemont, Ill., 1994.
34. Gerhardt, JJ, and Russe, OA: International SFTR Method of Measuring and Recording Joint Motion. Hans Huber, Bern, 1975.
35. Gerhardt, JJ: Clinical measurement of joint motion and position in the neutral-zero method and SFTR: Basic principles. Int Rehabil Med 5:161, 1983.
36. American Medical Association: Guides to the Evaluation of Permanent Impairment, ed 3. AMA, Milwaukee, 1990.

CHAPTER 3

Validity and Reliability

Validity

For goniometry to provide meaningful information, measurements must be valid and reliable. Currier[1] states that **validity** is "the degree to which an instrument measures what it is purported to measure; the extent to which it fulfills its purpose." Stated in another way, the validity of a measurement refers to how well the measurement represents the true value of the variable of interest. The purpose of goniometry is to measure the angle of joint position or range of joint motion. Therefore, a valid goniometric measurement is one that truly represents the actual joint angle or the total range of motion (ROM).

Face Validity

There are four main types of validity: face validity, content validity, criterion-related validity, and construct validity.[2–5] Most support for the validity of goniometry is in the form of face, content, and criterion-related validity. **Face validity** indicates that the instrument generally appears to measure what it proposes to measure—that it is plausible.[2–5] Much of the literature on goniometric measurement does not specifically address the issue of validity; rather, it assumes that the angle created by aligning the arms of a universal goniometer with bony landmarks truly represents the angle created by the proximal and distal bones composing the joint. One infers that changes in goniometer alignment reflect changes in joint angle and represent a range of joint motion. Portney and Watkins[3] report that face validity is easily established for some tests such as the measurement of ROM, because the instrument measures the variable of interest through direct observation.

Content Validity

Content validity is determined by judging whether or not an instrument adequately measures and represents the domain of content—the substance—of the variable of interest.[2–5] Both content and face validity are based on subjective opinion. However, face validity is the most basic and elementary form of validity, whereas content validity involves more rigorous and careful consideration. Gajdosik and Bohannon[6] state, "Physical therapists judge the validity of most ROM measurements based on their anatomical knowledge and their applied skills of visual inspection, palpation of bony landmarks, and accurate alignment of the goniometer. Generally, the accurate application of knowledge and skills, combined with interpreting the results as measurement of ROM only, provide sufficient evidence to ensure content validity."

Criterion-related Validity

Criterion-related validity justifies the validity of the measuring instrument by comparing measurements made with the instrument to a well-established gold standard of measurement—the criterion.[2–5] If the measurements made with the instrument and criterion are taken at approximately the same time, **concurrent validity** is tested. Concurrent validity is a type of criterion-related validity.[3,7] Criterion-related validity can be assessed objectively with statistical methods. In terms of goniometry, an examiner may question the construction of a particular goniometer on a very basic level and consider whether the degree units of the goniometer accurately represent the degree units of a circle. The angles of the goniometer can be compared with known angles of a protractor—the criterion. Usually the construction of goniometers is adequate, and the issue of validity focuses on whether the goniometer accurately measures the angle of joint position and ROM in a subject.

Criterion-related Validity Studies of Extremity Joints

The best gold standard used to establish criterion-related validity of goniometric measurements of joint position and ROM is radiography. Several studies have examined extremity joints for the concurrent validity of goniometric and radiographic measurements. Gogia and associates[8] measured the knee position of 30 subjects with radiography and with a universal goniometer. Knee positions ranged from 0 to 120 degrees. High correlation (correlation coefficient [r] = 0.97) and agreement (intraclass correlation coefficient [ICC] = 0.98) were found between the two types of measurements. Therefore goniometric measurement of knee joint position was considered to be valid. Enwemeka[9] studied the validity of measuring knee ROM with a universal goniometer by comparing the goniometric measurements taken on 10 subjects with radiographs. No significant differences were found between the two types of measurements when ROM was within 30 to 90 degrees of flexion (mean difference between the two measurements ranged from 0.5 to 3.8 degrees). However, a significant difference was found when ROM was within 0 to 15 degrees of flexion (mean difference 4.6 degrees). Ahlbach and Lindahl[10] found that a joint-specific goniometer used to measure hip flexion and extension in 14 subjects closely agreed with radiographic measurements.

Criterion-related Validity Studies of the Spine

Various instruments used to measure ROM of the spine have also been compared with a radiographic criterion, although some researchers question the use of radiographs as the gold standard given the variability of ROM measurement taken from spinal radiographs.[11] Three studies that contrasted cervical range of motion (cervical ROM) measurements taken with gravity-dependent goniometers with those recorded on radiographs found concurrent validity to be high. Herrmann,[12] in a study of 11 subjects, noted a high correlation (r = 0.97) and agreement (ICC = 0.98) between radiographic measures and pendulum goniometer measures of head and neck flexion-extension. Ordway and colleagues[13] simultaneously measured cervical flexion and extension in 20 healthy subjects with a cervical ROM goniometer, a computerized tracking system, and radiographs. There were no significant differences between measurements taken with the cervical ROM and radiographic angles determined by an occipital line and a vertical line, although there were differences between the cervical

ROM and the radiographic angles between the occiput and C-7. Tousignant and coworkers[14] measured cervical flexion and extension in 31 subjects with a cervical ROM goniometer and radiographs that included cervical and upper thoracic motion. They found a high correlation between the two measurements (r = 0.97).

Studies that compared clinical ROM measurement methods for the lumbar spine with radiographic results report high to low validity. Macrae and Wright[15] measured lumbar flexion in 342 subjects by using a tape measure, according to the Schober and modified Schober method, and compared these results with those shown in radiographs. Their findings support the validity of these measures: correlation coefficient values between the Schober method and the radiographic evidence were 0.90 (standard error = 6.2 degrees), and between the modified Schober and the radiographs were 0.97 (standard error = 3.3 degrees). Portek and associates,[16] in a study of 11 males, found no significant difference between lumbar flexion and extension ROM measurement taken with a skin distraction method and single inclinometer compared with radiographic evidence, but correlation coefficients were low (0.42 to 0.57). Comparisons may have been inappropriate because measurements were made sequentially rather than concurrently, with subjects in varying testing positions. Radiographs and skin distraction methods were performed on standing subjects, whereas inclinometer measurements were performed in subjects sitting for flexion and prone for extension. Burdett, Brown, and Fall,[17] in a study of 27 subjects, found a fair correlation between measurements taken with a single inclinometer and radiographs for lumbar flexion (r = 0.73), and a very poor correlation for lumbar extension (r = 0.15). Mayer and coworkers[18] measured lumbar flexion and extension in 12 patients with a single inclinometer, double inclinometer, and radiographs. No significant difference was noted between measurements. Saur and colleagues,[19] in a study of 54 patients, found lumbar flexion ROM measurement taken with two inclinometers correlated highly with radiographs (r = 0.98). Extension ROM measurement correlated with radiographs to a fair degree (r = 0.75). Samo and associates[20] used double inclinometers and radiographs to measure 30 subjects held in a position of flexion and extension. Radiographs resulted in flexion values that were 11 to 15 degrees greater than those found with inclinometers, and extension values that were 4 to 5 degrees less than those found with inclinometers.

Construct Validity

Construct validity is the ability of an instrument to measure an abstract concept (construct)[3] or to be used to make an inferred interpretation.[7] There is a movement within rehabilitative medicine to develop and validate measurement tools to identify functional limitations and predict disability.[21] Joint ROM may be one such measurement tool. In Chapters 4 through 13 on measurement procedures, we have included the results of research studies that report joint ROM observed during functional tasks. These findings begin to quantify the joint motion needed to avoid functional limitations. Several researchers have artificially restricted joint motion with splints or braces and examined the effect on function.[22–24] It appears that many functional tasks can be completed with severely restricted elbow or wrist ROM, providing other adjacent joints are able to compensate. A recent study by Hermann and Reese[25] examined the relationship between impairments, functional limitations, and disability in 80 patients with cervical spine disorders. The highest correlation (r = 0.82) occurred between impairment measures and functional limitation measures, with ROM contributing more to the relationship than the other two impairment measures of cervical muscle force and pain. Triffitt[26] found significant correlations between the amount of shoulder ROM and the ability to perform nine functional activities in 125 patients with shoulder symptoms. Wagner and colleagues[27] measured passive ROM of wrist flexion, extension, radial and ulnar deviation, and the strength of the wrist extensor and flexor muscles in 18 boys with Duchenne muscular dystrophy. A highly significant negative correlation was found between difficulty performing functional hand tasks and radial deviation ROM (r = –0.76 to –0.86) and between difficulty performing functional hand tasks and wrist extensor strength (r = –0.61 to –0.83).

Reliability

The **reliability** of a measurement refers to the amount of consistency between successive measurements of the same variable on the same subject under the same conditions. A goniometric measurement is highly reliable if successive measurements of a joint angle or ROM, on the same subject and under the same conditions yield the same results. A highly reliable measurement contains little measurement error. Assuming that a measurement is valid and highly reliable, an examiner can confidently use its results to determine a true absence, presence, or change in dysfunction. For example, a highly reliable goniometric measurement could be used to determine the presence of joint ROM limitation, to evaluate patient progress toward rehabilitative goals, and to assess the effectiveness of therapeutic interventions.

A measurement with poor reliability contains a large amount of measurement error. An unreliable measurement is inconsistent and does not produce the same results when the same variable is measured on the same subject under the same conditions. A measurement that has poor reliability is not dependable and should not be used in the clinical decision-making process.

Summary of Goniometric Reliability Studies

The reliability of goniometric measurement has been the focus of many research studies. Given the variety of study designs and measurement techniques, it is difficult to compare the results of many of these studies. However, some findings noted in several studies can be summarized. An overview of such findings is presented here. More information on reliability studies that pertain to the featured joint is reviewed in Chapters 4 through 13. Readers may also wish to refer to several review articles and book chapters on this topic. [6,28–30]

The measurement of joint position and ROM of the extremities with a universal goniometer has generally been found to have good-to-excellent reliability. Numerous reliability studies have been conducted on joints of the upper and lower extremities. Some studies have examined the reliability of measuring joints held in a fixed position, whereas others have examined the reliability of measuring passive or active ROM. Studies that measured a fixed joint position usually have reported higher reliability values than studies that measured ROM.[8,12,31,32] This finding is expected because more sources of variation and error are present in measuring ROM than in measuring a fixed joint position. Additional sources of error in measuring ROM include movement of the joint axis, variations in manual force applied by the examiner during passive ROM, and variations in a subject's effort during active ROM.

The reliability of goniometric ROM measurements varies somewhat depending on the joint and motion. ROM measurements of upper-extremity joints have been found by several researchers to be more reliable than ROM measurements of lower-extremity joints,[33,34] although opposing results have likewise been reported.[35] Even within the upper or lower extremities there are differences in reliability between joints and motions. For example, Hellebrandt, Duvall, and Moore,[36] in a study of upper-extremity joints, noted that measurements of wrist flexion, medial rotation of the shoulder, and abduction of the shoulder were less reliable than measurements of other motions of the upper extremity. Low[37] found ROM measurements of wrist extension to be less reliable than measurements of elbow flexion. Greene and Wolf[38] reported ROM measurements of shoulder rotation and wrist motions to be more variable than elbow motion and other shoulder motions. Reliability studies on ROM measurement of the cervical and thoracic spine in which a universal goniometer was used have generally reported lower reliability values than studies of the extremity joints.[17,39–42] Many devices and techniques have been developed to try to improve the reliability of measuring spinal motions. Gajdosik and Bohannon[6] suggested that the reliability of measuring certain joints and motions might be adversely affected by the complexity of the joint. Measurement of motions that are influenced by movement of adjacent joints or multijoint muscles may be less reliable than measurement of motions of simple hinge joints. Difficulty palpating bony landmarks and passively moving heavy body parts may also play a role in reducing the reliability of measuring ROM of the lower extremity and spine.[6,33]

Many studies of joint measurement methods have found intratester reliability to be higher than intertester reliability.[17,31–37,39,40,42–62] Reliability was higher when successive measurements were taken by the same examiner than when successive measurements were taken by different examiners. This is true for studies that measured joint position and ROM of the extremities and spine with universal goniometers and other devices such as joint-specific goniometers, pendulum goniometers, tape measures, and flexible rulers. Only a few studies found intertester reliability to be higher than intratester reliability.[63–66] In most of these studies, the time interval between repeated measurements by the same examiner was considerably greater than the time interval between measurements by different examiners.

The reliability of goniometric measurements is affected by the measurement procedure. Several studies found that intertester reliability improved when all the examiners used consistent, well-defined testing positions and measurement methods.[44,46,47,67] Intertester reliability was lower if examiners used a variety of positions and measurement methods.

Several investigators have examined the reliability of using the mean (average) of several goniometric measurements compared with using one measurement. Low[37] recommends using the mean of several measurements made with the goniometer to increase reliability over one measurement. Early studies by Cobe[68] and Hewitt[69] also used the mean of several measurements. However, Boone and associates[33] found no significant difference between repeated measurements made by the same examiner during one session and suggested that one measurement taken by an examiner is as reliable as the mean of repeated measurements. Rothstein, Miller, and Roettger,[47] in a study on knee and elbow ROM, found that intertester reliability determined from the means of two measurements improved only slightly from the intertester reliability determined from single measurements.

The authors of some texts on goniometric methods suggest the use of universal goniometers with longer arms to measure joints with large body segments such as the hip and shoulder.[28,70,71] Goniometers with shorter arms are recommended to measure joints with small body segments such as the wrist and fingers. Robson,[72] using a mathematical model, determined that goniometers with longer arms are more accurate in measuring an angle than goniometers with shorter arms. Goniometers with longer arms reduce the effects of errors in the placement of the goniometer axis. However, Rothstein, Miller, and Roettger[47] found no difference in reliability among large plastic, large metal, and small plastic universal goniometers used to measure knee and elbow ROM. Riddle, Rothstein, and Lamb[45] also reported no difference in reliability between large and small plastic universal goniometers used to measure shoulder ROM.

Numerous studies have compared the measurement values and reliability of different types of devices used to measure joint ROM. Universal, pendulum, and fluid goniometers, joint-specific devices, tape measures, and wire tracing are some of the devices that have been compared. Studies comparing clinical measurement devices have been conducted on the shoulder,[36,38] elbow,[31,36,38,56,73,74] wrist,[31,38] hand,[32,59,75,76] hip,[77,78] knee,[47,77,79,80] ankle,[77,81] cervical spine,[39,40,64,82] and thoracolumbar spine.[16,20,41,62,83–90] Many studies have found differences in values and reliability between measurement devices, whereas some studies have reported no differences.

In conclusion, on the basis of reliability studies and our clinical experience, we recommend the following procedures to improve the reliability of goniometric measurements (Table 3–1). Examiners should use consistent, well-defined testing positions and anatomical landmarks to align the arms of the goniometer. During successive measurements of passive ROM, examiners should strive to apply the same amount of manual force to move the subject's body. During successive measurements of active ROM, the subject should be urged to exert the same effort to perform a motion. To reduce measurement variability, it is prudent to take repeated measurements on a subject with the same type of measurement device. For example, an examiner should take all repeated measurements of an ROM with a universal goniometer, rather than taking the first measurement with a universal goniometer and the second measurement with an inclinometer. We believe most examiners find it easier and more accurate to use a large universal goniometer when measuring joints with large body segments, and a small goniometer when measuring joints with small body segments. Inexperienced examiners may wish to take several measurements and record the mean (average) of those measurements to improve reliability, but one measurement is usually sufficient for more experienced examiners using good technique. Finally, it is important to remember that successive measurements are more reliable if taken by the same examiner rather than by different examiners. The mean standard deviation of repeated ROM measurement of extremity joints taken by one examiner using a universal goniometer has been

TABLE 3–1	**Recommendations for Improving the Reliability of Goniometric Measurements**

- Use consistent, well-defined positions
- Use consistent, well-defined anatomical landmarks to align the goniometer
- Use the same amount of manual force to move subject's body part during successive measurements of passive ROM
- Urge subject to exert the same effort to move the body part during successive measurements of active ROM
- Use the same device to take successive measurements
- Use a goniometer that is suitable in size to the joint being measured
- If examiner is less experienced, record the mean of several measurements rather than a single measurement
- Have the *same* examiner take successive measurements, rather than a *different* examiner

found to range from 4 to 5 degrees.[33,35] Therefore, to show improvement or worsening of a joint motion measured by the same examiner, a difference of about 5 degrees (1 standard deviation) to 10 degrees (2 standard deviations) is necessary. The mean standard deviation increased to 5 to 6 degrees for repeated measurements taken by different examiners.[33,35] These values serve as a general guideline only, and will vary depending on the joint and motion being tested, the examiners and procedures used, and the individual being tested.

Statistical Methods of Evaluating Measurement Reliability

Clinical measurements are prone to three main sources of variation: (1) true biological variation, (2) temporal variation, and (3) measurement error.[91] **True biological variation** refers to variation in measurements from one individual to another, caused by factors such as age, sex, race, genetics, medical history, and condition. **Temporal variation** refers to variation in measurements made on the same individual at different times, caused by changes in factors such as a subject's medical (physical) condition, activity level, emotional state, and circadian rhythms. **Measurement error** refers to variation in measurements made on the same individual under the same conditions at different times, caused by factors such as the examiners (testers), measuring instruments, and procedural methods. For example, the skill level and experience of the examiners, the accuracy of the measurement instruments, and the standardization of the measurement methods affect the amount of measurement error. Reliability reflects the degree to which a measurement is free of measurement error; therefore, highly reliable measurements have little measurement error.

Statistics can be used to assess variation in numerical data and hence to assess measurement reliability.[91,92] A digression into statistical methods of testing and expressing reliability is included to assist the examiner in correctly interpreting goniometric measurements and in understanding the literature on joint measurement. Several statistics—the **standard deviation, coefficient of variation, Pearson product moment correlation coefficient, intraclass correlation coefficient, and standard error of measurement**—are discussed. Examples that show the calculation of these statistical tests are presented. For additional information, including the assumptions underlying the use of these statistical tests, the reader is referred to the cited references.

At the end of this chapter, two exercises are included for examiners to assess their reliability in obtaining goniometric measurements. Many authors recommend that clinicians conduct their own studies to determine reliability among their staff and patient population. Miller[29] has presented a step-by-step procedure for conducting such studies.

Standard Deviation

In the medical literature, the statistic most frequently used to indicate variation is the standard deviation.[91,92] The standard deviation is the square root of the mean of the squares of the deviations from the data mean. The standard deviation is symbolized as SD, s, or sd. If we denote each data observation as x and the number of observations as n, and the summation notation Σ is used, then the **mean** that is denoted by $\bar{x}$, is:

$$\text{mean} = \bar{x} = \frac{\Sigma x}{n}$$

Two formulas for the standard deviation are given below. The first is the definitional formula; the second is the computational formula. Both formulas give the same result. The definitional formula is easier to understand, but the computational formula is easier to calculate.

$$\text{Standard deviation} = SD = \sqrt{\frac{\Sigma (x - \bar{x})^2}{n - 1}}$$

$$SD = \sqrt{\frac{\Sigma (x)^2 - \frac{(\Sigma x)^2}{n}}{n - 1}}$$

The standard deviation has the same units as the original data observations. If the data observations have a normal (bell-shaped) frequency distribution, 1 standard deviation above and below the mean includes about 68 percent of all the observations, and 2 standard deviations above and below the mean include about 95 percent of the observations.

TABLE 3–2   Three Repeated ROM Measurements (in Degrees) Taken on Five Subjects

Subject	First Measurement	Second Measurement	Third Measurement	Total	Mean of Three Measurements ($\bar{x}$)
1	57	55	65	177	59
2	66	65	70	201	67
3	66	70	74	210	70
4	35	40	42	117	39
5	45	48	42	135	45

Grand mean $(\bar{X}) = \dfrac{(59+67+70+39+45)}{5} = 56$ degrees.

It is important to note that several standard deviations may be determined from a single study and represent different sources of variation.[91] Two of these standard deviations are discussed here. One standard deviation that can be determined represents mainly *inter*subject variation around the mean of measurements taken of a group of subjects, indicating biological variation. This standard deviation may be of interest in deciding whether a subject has an abnormal ROM in comparison with other people of the same age and gender. Another standard deviation that can be determined represents *intra*subject variation around the mean of measurements taken of an individual, indicating measurement error. This is the standard deviation of interest to indicate measurement reliability.

An example of how to determine these two standard deviations is provided. Table 3–2 presents ROM measurements taken on five subjects. Three repeated measurements (observations) were taken on each subject by the same examiner.

The **standard deviation indicating biological variation** (intersubject variation) is determined by first calculating the mean ROM measurement for each subject. The mean ROM measurement for each of the five subjects is found in the last column of Table 3–2. The grand mean of the mean ROM measurement for each of the five subjects equals 56 degrees. The grand mean is symbolized by $\bar{X}$. The standard deviation is determined by finding the differences between each of the five subjects' means and the grand mean. The differences are squared and added together. The sum is used in the definitional formula for the standard deviation. Calculation of the standard devi-

ation indicating biological variation is found in Table 3–3.

The standard deviation indicating biological variation equals 13.6 degrees. This standard deviation denotes primarily intersubject variation. Knowledge of intersubject variation may be helpful in deciding whether a subject has an abnormal ROM in comparison with other people of the same age and gender. If a normal distribution of the measurements is assumed, one way of interpreting this standard deviation is to predict that about 68 percent of all the subjects' mean ROM measurements would fall between 42.4 degrees and 69.6 degrees (plus or minus 1 standard deviation around the grand mean of 56 degrees). We would expect that about 95 percent of all the subjects' mean ROM measurements would fall between 28.8 degrees and 83.2 degrees (plus or minus 2 standard deviations around the grand mean of 56 degrees).

The **standard deviation indicating measurement error** (intrasubject variation) also is determined by first calculating the mean ROM measurement for each subject. However, this standard deviation is determined by finding the differences between each of the three repeated measurements taken on a subject and the mean of that subject's measurements. The differences are squared and added together. The sum is used in the definitional formula for the standard deviation. Calculation of the standard deviation indicating measurement error for subject 1 is found in Table 3–4.

Referring to Table 3–2 and using the same procedure as shown in Table 3–4 for each subject, the standard deviation for subject 1 = 5.3 degrees, the standard devi-

TABLE 3–3   Calculation of the Standard Deviation Indicating Biological Variation in Degrees

Subject	Mean of Three Measurements ($\bar{x}$)	Grand Mean ($\bar{X}$)	($\bar{x}-\bar{X}$)	($\bar{x}-\bar{X}$)^2
1	59	56	3	9
2	67	56	11	121
3	70	56	14	196
4	39	56	−17	289
5	45	56	−11	121

$\sum(\bar{x}-\bar{X})^2 = 9+121+196+289+121 = 736$ degrees; $SD = \sqrt{\dfrac{\sum(\bar{x}-\bar{X})^2}{(n-1)}} = \sqrt{\dfrac{736}{(5-1)}} = 13.6$ degrees.

ation for subject 2 = 2.6 degrees, the standard deviation for subject 3 = 4.0 degrees, the standard deviation for subject 4 = 3.6 degrees, and the standard deviation for subject 5 = 3.0 degrees. The mean standard deviation for all of the subjects combined is determined by summing the five subjects' standard deviations and dividing by the number of subjects, which is 5:

$$SD = \frac{5.3 + 2.6 + 4.0 + 3.6 + 3.0}{5} = \frac{18.5}{5} = 3.7 \text{ degrees}$$

TABLE 3–4 Calculation of the Standard Deviation Indicating Measurement Error in Degrees for Subject 1

Measurements (x)	Mean ($\bar{x}$)	($x-\bar{x}$)	($x-\bar{x}$)^2
57	59	−2	4
55	59	−4	16
65	59	6	36

$\sum(x-\bar{x})^2 = 4+16+36 = 56$ degrees.

$$SD = \sqrt{\frac{\sum(x-\bar{x})^2}{(n-1)}} = \sqrt{\frac{56}{2}} = 5.3 \text{ degrees}$$

The standard deviation indicating intrasubject variation equals 3.7 degrees. This standard deviation is appropriate for indicating measurement error, especially if the repeated measurements on each subject were taken within a short period of time. Note that in this example the standard deviation indicating measurement error (3.7 degrees) is much smaller than the standard deviation indicating biological variation (13.6 degrees). One way of interpreting the standard deviation for measurement error is to predict that about 68 percent of the repeated measurements on a subject would fall within 3.7 degrees (1 standard deviation) above and below the mean of the repeated measurements of a subject because of measurement error. We would expect that about 95 percent of the repeated measurements on a subject would fall within 7.4 degrees (2 standard deviations) above and below the mean of the repeated measurements of a subject, again because of measurement error. The smaller the standard deviation, the less the measurement error and the better the reliability.

Coefficient of Variation

Sometimes it is helpful to consider the percentage of variation rather than the standard deviation, which is expressed in the units of the data observation (measurement). The coefficient of variation is a measure of variation that is relative to the mean and standardized so that the variations of different variables can be compared. The coefficient of variation is the standard deviation divided by the mean and multiplied by 100 percent. It is

a percentage and is not expressed in the units of the original observation. The coefficient of variation is symbolized by CV and the formula is:

$$\text{coefficient of variation} = CV = \frac{SD}{\bar{x}}(100)\%$$

For the example presented in Table 3–2, the coefficient of variation indicating biological variation uses the standard deviation for biological variation (standard deviation = 13.6 degrees).

$$CV = \frac{SD}{\bar{x}}(100)\% = \frac{13.6}{56}(100)\% = 24.3\%$$

The coefficient of variation indicating measurement error uses the standard deviation for measurement error (standard deviation = 3.7 degrees)

$$CV = \frac{SD}{\bar{x}}(100)\% = \frac{3.7}{56}(100)\% = 6.6\%$$

In this example the coefficient of variation for measurement error (6.6 percent) is less than the coefficient of variation for biological variation (24.3 percent).

Another name for the coefficient of variation indicating measurement error is the **coefficient of variation of replication**.[93] The lower the coefficient of variation of replication, the lower the measurement error and the better the reliability. This statistic is especially useful in comparing the reliability of two or more variables that have different units of measurement; for example, comparing ROM measurement methods recorded in inches versus degrees.

Correlation Coefficients

Correlation coefficients are traditionally used to measure the relationship between two variables. They result in a number from −1 to +1, which indicates how well an equation can predict one variable from another variable.[2–4,91] A +1 describes a perfect positive linear (straight-line) relationship, whereas a −1 describes a perfect negative linear relationship. A correlation coefficient of 0 indicates that there is no linear relationship between the two variables. Correlation coefficients are used to indicate measurement reliability because it is assumed that two repeated measurements should be highly correlated and approach a +1. One interpretation of correlation coefficients used to indicate reliability is that 0.90 to 0.99 equals high reliability, 0.80 to 0.89 equals good reliability, 0.70 to 0.79 equals fair reliability, and 0.69 and below equals poor reliability.[94] Another interpretation offered by Portney and Watkins[3] states that correlation coefficients above 0.75 indicate good reliability, whereas those below 0.75 indicate poor to moderate reliability.

Because goniometric measurements produce ratio level data, the **Pearson product moment correlation coefficient** has been the correlation coefficient usually calculated to indicate the reliability of pairs of goniometric measurements. The Pearson product moment correlation coefficient is symbolized by r, and its formula is presented following this paragraph. If this statistic is used to indicate reliability, x symbolizes the first measurement and y symbolizes the second measurement.

$$r = \frac{\sum (x-\bar{x})(y-\bar{y})}{\sqrt{\sum (x-\bar{x})^2}\sqrt{\sum (y-\bar{y})^2}}$$

Referring to the example in Table 3–2, the Pearson correlation coefficient can be used to determine the relationship between the first and the second ROM measurements on the five subjects. Calculation of the Pearson product moment correlation coefficient for this example is found in Table 3–5. The resulting value of $r = 0.98$ indicates a highly positive linear relationship between the first and the second measurements. In other words, the two measurements are highly correlated.

$$r = \frac{\sum (x-\bar{x})(y-\bar{y})}{\sqrt{\sum (x-\bar{x})^2}\sqrt{\sum (y-\bar{y})^2}}$$

$$= \frac{650.6}{\sqrt{738.8}\sqrt{597.2}} = \frac{650.6}{(27.2)\,(24.4)} = 0.98$$

The Pearson product moment correlation coefficient indicates association between the pairs of measurements rather than agreement. Therefore, to decide whether the two measurements are identical, the equation of the straight line best representing the relationship should be determined. If the equation of the straight line representing the relationship includes a slope b equal to 1, and an intercept a equal to 0, then an r value that approaches +1 also indicates that the two measurements are identical. The equation of a straight line is $y = a + bx$, with x symbolizing the first measurement, y the second measurement, a the intercept, and b the slope. The equation for a slope is:

$$\text{slope} = b = \frac{\sum (x-\bar{x})(y-\bar{y})}{\sum (x-\bar{x})^2}$$

The equation for an intercept is: intercept $= a = \bar{y} - b\bar{x}$

For our example, the slope and intercept are calculated as follows:

$$b = \frac{\sum (x-\bar{x})(y-\bar{y})}{\sum (x-\bar{x})^2} = \frac{650.6}{738.8} = 0.88$$

$$a = \bar{y} - b\bar{x} = 55.6 - 0.88(53.8) = 8.26$$

The equation of the straight line best representing the relationship between the first and the second measurements in the example is $y = 8.26 + 0.88x$. Although the r value indicates high correlation, the two measurements are not identical given the linear equation.

One concern in interpreting correlation coefficients is that the value of the correlation coefficient is markedly influenced by the range of the measurements.[3,92,95] The greater the biological variation between individuals for the measurement, the more extreme the r value, so that r is closer to −1 or +1. Another limitation is the fact that the Pearson product moment correlation coefficient can evaluate the relationship between only two variables or measurements at a time.

To avoid the need for calculating and interpreting both the correlation coefficient and a linear equation, some investigators use the **intraclass correlation coefficient (ICC)** to evaluate reliability. The intraclass correlation coefficient is symbolized as ICC. The ICC also allows the comparison of two or more measurements at a time; one can think of it as an average correlation among all possible pairs of measurements.[95] This statistic is determined from an analysis of variance model, which compares different sources of variation. The ICC is conceptually expressed as the ratio of the variance

TABLE 3–5 Calculation of the Pearson Product Moment Correlation Coefficient for the first (x) and Second (y) ROM Measurements in Degrees

Subject	x	y	$(x-\bar{x})$	$(y-\bar{y})$	$(x-\bar{x})(y-\bar{y})$	$(x-\bar{x})^2$	$(y-\bar{y})^2$
1	57	55	3.2	−0.6	−1.92	10.24	0.36
2	66	65	12.2	9.4	114.68	148.84	88.36
3	66	70	12.2	14.4	175.68	148.84	207.36
4	35	40	−18.8	−15.6	293.28	353.44	243.36
5	45	48	−8.8	−7.6	68.88	77.44	57.76
					$\sum = 650.60$	$\sum = 738.80$	$\sum = 597.20$

$$\bar{x} = \frac{57 + 66 + 66 + 35 + 45}{5} = 53.8 \text{ degrees}; \quad \bar{y} = \frac{55 + 65 + 70 + 40 + 48}{5} = 55.6 \text{ degrees.}$$

associated with the subjects, divided by the sum of the variance associated with the subjects plus error variance.[96] The theoretical limits of the ICC are between 0 and +1; +1 indicates perfect agreement (no error variance), whereas 0 indicates no agreement (large amount of error variance).

There are six different formulas for determining ICC values based on the design of the study, the purpose of the study, and the type of measurement.[3,96,97] Three models have been described, each with two different forms. In Model l, each subject is tested by a different set of testers, and the testers are considered representative of a larger population of testers—to allow the results to be generalized to other testers. In Model 2, each subject is tested by the same set of testers, and again the testers are considered representative of a larger population of testers. In Model 3, each subject is tested by the same set of testers, but the testers are the only testers of interest— the results are not intended to be generalized to other testers. The first form of all three models is used when single measurements (1) are compared, whereas the second form is used when the means of multiple measurements (k) are compared. The different formulas for the ICC are identified by two numbers enclosed by parentheses. The first number indicates the model and the second number indicates the form. For further discussion, examples, and formulas, the reader is urged to refer to the following texts[3] and articles.[96-98]

In our example, a repeated measures analysis of variance was conducted and the ICC (3,1) was calculated as 0.94. This ICC model was used because each measurement was taken by the same tester, there was only an interest in applying the results to this tester, and single measurements were compared rather than the means of several measurements. This ICC value indicates a high reliability between the three repeated measurements. However, this value is slightly lower than the Pearson product moment correlation coefficient, perhaps due to the variability added by the third measurement on each subject.

Like the Pearson product moment correlation coefficient, the ICC is also influenced by the range of measurements between the subjects. As the group of subjects becomes more homogeneous, the ability of the ICC to detect agreement is reduced and the ICC can erroneously indicate poor reliability.[3,96,99] Because correlation coefficients are sensitive to the range of the measurements and do not provide an index of reliability in the units of the measurement, some experts prefer the use of the standard deviation of the repeated measurements (intrasubject standard deviation) or the standard error of measurement to assess reliability.[4,99,100]

Standard Error of Measurement

The **standard error of measurement** is the final statistic that we review here to evaluate reliability. It has received support because of its practical interpretation in estimating measurement error in the same units as the measurement. According to DuBois,[101] "the standard error of measurement is the likely standard deviation of the error made in predicting true scores when we have knowledge only of the obtained scores." The true scores (measurements) are forever unknown, but several formulas have been developed to estimate this statistic. The standard error of measurement is symbolized as SEM, SE_{meas}, or S_{meas}. If the standard deviation indicating biological variation is denoted SD_x, a correlation coefficient such as the intraclass correlation coefficient is denoted ICC, and the Pearson product moment correlation coefficient is denoted r, the formulas for the SEM are:

$$SEM = SD_x \sqrt{1-ICC}$$

or

$$SEM = SD_x \sqrt{1-r}$$

The SEM can also be determined from a repeated measures analysis of variance model. The SEM is equivalent to the square root of the mean square of the error.[102,103] Because the SEM is a special case of the standard deviation, 1 standard error of measurement above and below the observed measurement includes the true measurement 68 percent of the time. Two standard errors of measurement above and below the observed measurement include the true measurement 95 percent of the time.

It is important to note that another statistic, the standard error of the mean, is often confused with the standard error of measurement. The standard error of the mean is symbolized as SEM, SE_M, $SE_{\bar{x}}$, or $S_{\bar{x}}$.[2,4,91,92] The use of the same or similar symbols to represent different statistics has added much confusion to the reliability literature. These two statistics are not equivalent, nor do they have the same interpretation. The standard error of the mean is the standard deviation of a distribution of means taken from samples of a population.[1,2,92] It describes how much variation can be expected in the means from future samples of the same size. Because we are interested in the variation of individual measurements when evaluating reliability rather than the variation of means, the standard deviation of the repeated measurements or the standard error of measurement is the appropriate statistical tests to use.[104]

Let us return to the example and calculate the standard error of the measurement. The value for the intraclass correlation coefficient (ICC) is 0.94. The value for SD_x, the standard deviation indicating biological variation among the 5 subjects, is 13.6.

$$SEM = SD_x \sqrt{1-ICC}$$

$$13.6 \sqrt{1-0.94} = 13.6 \sqrt{0.06} = 3.3 \text{ degrees}$$

Likewise, if we use the results of the repeated measures analysis of variance to calculate the SEM, the SEM equals the square root of the mean square of the error = $\sqrt{10.9} = 3.3$ degrees.

In this example, about two thirds of the time the true measurement would be within 3.3 degrees of the observed measurement.

Exercises to Evaluate Reliability

The two exercises that follow (Exercises 6 and 7) have been included to help examiners assess their reliability in obtaining goniometric measurements. Calculations of the standard deviation and coefficient of variation are included in the belief that understanding is reinforced by practical application. Exercise 6 examines intratester reliability. **Intratester reliability** refers to the amount of agreement between repeated measurements of the same joint position or ROM by the same examiner (tester). An intratester reliability study answers the question: How accurately can an examiner reproduce his or her own measurements? Exercise 7 examines **intertester reliability**. Intertester reliability refers to the amount of agreement between repeated measurements of the same joint position or ROM by different examiners (testers). An intertester reliability study answers the question: How accurately can one examiner reproduce measurements taken by other examiners?

EXERCISE 6
INTRATESTER RELIABILITY

1. Select a subject and a universal goniometer.
2. Measure elbow flexion ROM on your subject three times, following the steps outlined in Chapter 2, Exercise 5.
3. Record each measurement on the recording form (see opposite page) in the column labeled x. A measurement is denoted by x.
4. Compare the measurements. If a discrepancy of more than 5 degrees exists between measurements, recheck each step in the procedure to make sure that you are performing the steps correctly, and then repeat this exercise.
5. Continue practicing until you have obtained three successive measurements that are within 5 degrees of each other.
6. To gain an understanding of several of the statistics used to evaluate reliability, calculate the standard deviation and coefficient of variation by completing the following steps.
   a. Add the three measurements together to determine the sum of the measurements. Σ is the symbol for summation. Record the sum at the bottom of the column labeled x.
   b. To determine the **mean**, divide this sum by 3, which is the number of measurements. The number of measurements is denoted by n. The mean is denoted by $\bar{x}$. Space to calculate the mean is provided on the recording form.
   c. Subtract the mean from each of the three measurements and record the results in the column labeled $x-\bar{x}$.
   d. Square each of the numbers in the column labeled $x-\bar{x}$, and record the results in the column labeled $(x-\bar{x})^2$.
   e. Add the three numbers in column $(x-\bar{x})^2$ to determine the sum of the squares. Record the results at the bottom of the column labeled $(x-\bar{x})^2$.
   f. To determine the **standard deviation**, divide this sum by 2, which is the number of measurements minus 1 ($n-1$). Then find the square root of this number. Space to calculate the standard deviation is provided on the recording form.
   g. To determine the **coefficient of variation**, divide the standard deviation by the mean. Multiply this number by 100 percent. Space to calculate the coefficient of variation is provided on the recording form.
7. Repeat this procedure with other joints and motions after you have learned the testing procedures.

RECORDING FORM FOR EXERCISE 6. INTRATESTER RELIABILITY

Follow the steps outlined in Exercise 6. Use this form to record your measurements and the result of your calculations.

Subject's Name _____ Date _____

Examiner's Name _____

Joint and Motion _____ Right or Left Side _____

Passive or Active Motion _____ Type of Goniometer _____

Measurement	x	$x-\bar{x}$	$(x-\bar{x})^2$	x^2
1				
2				
3				
$n=3$	$\Sigma x=$		$\Sigma(x-\bar{x})^2 =$	$\Sigma x^2=$

$$\text{Mean of the three measurements} = \bar{x} = \frac{\Sigma x}{n} =$$

$$\text{Standard deviation} = \sqrt{\frac{\Sigma (x-\bar{x})^2}{n}} =$$

$$\text{or use SD} = \sqrt{\frac{\Sigma x^2 - \frac{(\Sigma x)^2}{n}}{n-1}}$$

$$\text{Coefficient of variation} = \frac{\text{SD}}{\bar{x}}(100)\% =$$

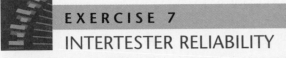

EXERCISE 7
INTERTESTER RELIABILITY

1. Select a subject and a universal goniometer.
2. Measure elbow flexion ROM on your subject once, following the steps outlined in Chapter 2, Exercise 5.
3. Ask two other examiners to measure the same elbow flexion ROM on your subject, using your goniometer and following the steps outlined in Chapter 2, Exercise 5.
4. Record each measurement on the recording form (see opposite page) in the column labeled x. A measurement is denoted by x.
5. Compare the measurements. If a discrepancy of more than 5 degrees exists between measurements, repeat this exercise. The examiners should observe one another's measurements to discover differences in technique that might account for variability, such as faulty alignment, lack of stabilization, or reading the wrong scale.
6. To gain an understanding of several of the statistics used to evaluate reliability, calculate the mean deviation, standard deviation, and coefficient of variation by completing the following steps.
   a. Add the three measurements together to determine the sum of the measurements. Σ is the symbol for summation. Record the sum at the bottom of the column labeled x.
   b. To determine the **mean**, divide this sum by 3, which is the number of measurements. The number of measurements is denoted by n. The mean is denoted by $\bar{x}$. Space to calculate the mean is provided on the recording form.
   c. Subtract the mean from each of the three measurements, and record the results in the column labeled $x-\bar{x}$.
   d. Square each of the numbers in the column labeled $x-\bar{x}$ and record the results in the column labeled $(x-\bar{x})^2$.
   e. Add the three numbers in column $(x-\bar{x})^2$ to determine the sum of the squares. Record the results at the bottom of column $(x-\bar{x})^2$.
   f. To determine the **standard deviation**, divide this sum by 2, which is the number of measurements minus 1 ($n-1$). Then find the square root of this number. Space to calculate the standard deviation is provided on the recording form.
   g. To determine the **coefficient of variation**, divide the standard deviation by the mean. Multiply this number by 100 percent. Space to calculate the coefficient of variation is provided on the recording form.
7. Repeat this exercise with other joints and motions after you have learned the testing procedures.

RECORDING FORM FOR EXERCISE 7. INTRATESTER RELIABILITY

Follow the steps outlined in Exercise 7. Use this form to record your measurements and the results of your calculations.

Subject's Name _____   Date _____

Examiner 1. Name _____

Examiner 2. Name _____   Joint and Motion _____

Examiner 3. Name_____   Right or Left Side _____

Passive or Active Motion _____   Type of Goniometer _____

Measurement	x	$x-\bar{x}$	$(x-\bar{x})^2$	x^2
1				
2				
3				
$n = 3$	$\sum x =$		$\sum(x-\bar{x})^2 =$	$\sum x^2 =$

$$\text{Mean of the three measurements} = \bar{x} = \frac{\sum x}{n} =$$

$$\text{Standard deviation} = \sqrt{\frac{\sum (x-\bar{x})^2}{(n-1)}} =$$

$$\text{or use SD} = \sqrt{\frac{\sum x^2 - \frac{(\sum x)^2}{n}}{n-1}}$$

$$\text{Coefficient of variation} = \frac{\text{SD}}{\bar{x}}(100)\% =$$

REFERENCES

1. Currier, DP: Elements of Research in Physical Therapy, ed 3. Williams & Wilkins, Baltimore, 1990, p 171.
2. Kerlinger, FN: Foundations of Behavioral Research, ed 2. Holt, Rinehart, & Winston, New York, 1973.
3. Portney, LG, and Watkins, MP: Foundations of Clinical Research: Applications to Practice, ed 2. Prentice-Hall, Upper Saddle River, NJ, 2000.
4. Rothstein, JM: Measurement and clinical practice: Theory and application. In Rothstein, JM (ed): Measurement in Physical Therapy. Churchill Livingstone, New York, 1985.
5. Sims, J, and Arnell, P: Measurement validity in physical therapy research. Phys Ther 73:102, 1993.
6. Gajdosik, RL, and Bohannon, RW: Clinical measurement of range of motion: Review of goniometry emphasizing reliability and validity. Phys Ther 67:1867, 1987.
7. American Physical Therapy Association: Standards for tests and measurements in physical therapy practice. Phys Ther 71:589, 1991.
8. Gogia, PP, et al: Reliability and validity of goniometric measurements at the knee. Phys Ther 67:192, 1987.
9. Enwemeka, CS: Radiographic verification of knee goniometry. Scand J Rehabil Med 18:47, 1986.
10. Ahlback, SO, and Lindahl, O: Sagittal mobility of the hip-joint. Acta Orthop Scand 34:310, 1964.
11. Chen, J, et al: Meta-analysis of normative cervical motion. Spine 24:1571, 1999.
12. Herrmann, DB: Validity study of head and neck flexion-extension motion comparing measurements of a pendulum goniometer and roentgenograms. J Orthop Sports Phys Ther 11:414, 1990.
13. Orway, NR, et al: Cervical sagittal range-of-motion analysis using three methods. Spine 22:501, 1997.
14. Tousignant, M, et al: Criterion validity of the cervical range of motion (CROM) goniometer for cervical flexion and extension. Spine 25:324, 2000.
15. Macrae, JF, and Wright, V: Measurement of back movement. Ann Rheum Dis 28:584, 1969.
16. Portek, I, et al: Correlation between radiographic and clinical measurement of lumbar spine movement. Br J Rheumatol 22:197, 1983.
17. Burdett, RG, Brown, KE, and Fall, MP: Reliability and validity of four instruments for measuring lumbar spine and pelvic positions. Phys Ther 66:677, 1986.
18. Mayer, TG, et al: Use of noninvasive techniques for quantification of spinal range-of-motion in normal subjects and chronic low-back dysfunction patients. Spine 9:588, 1984.

19. Saur, PM, et al: Lumbar range of motion: Reliability and validity of the inclinometer technique in the clinical measurement of trunk flexibility. Spine 21:1332, 1996.

20. Samo, DG, et al: Validity of three lumbar sagittal motion measurement methods: Surface inclinometers compared with radiographs. J Occup Environ Med 39:209, 1997.

21. Campbell, SK: Commentary: Measurement validity in physical therapy research. Phys Ther 73:110, 1993.

22. Vasen, AP, et al: Functional range of motion of the elbow. J Hand Surg 20A:288, 1995.

23. Cooper, JE, et al: Elbow joint restriction: Effect on functional upper limb motion during performance of three feeding activities. Arch Phys Med Rehabil 74:805, 1993.

24. Nelson, DL: Functional wrist motion. Hand Clin 13:83, 1997.

25. Hermann, KM, and Reese, CS: Relationships among selected measures of impairment, functional limitation, and disability in patients with cervical spine disorder. Phys Ther 81:903, 2001.

26. Triffitt, PD: The relationship between motion of the shoulder and the stated ability to perform activities of daily living. J Bone Joint Surg 80:41, 1998.

27. Wagner, MB, et al: Assessment of hand function in Duchenne muscular dystrophy. Arch Phys Med Rehabil 74:801, 1993.

28. Moore, ML: Clinical assessment of joint motion. In Basmajian, JV (ed): Therapeutic Exercise, ed 3. Williams & Wilkins, Baltimore, 1978.

29. Miller, PJ: Assessment of joint motion. In Rothstein, JM (ed): Measurement in Physical Therapy. Churchill Livingstone, New York, 1985.

30. Lea, RD, and Gerhardt, JJ: Current concepts review: Range-of-motion measurements. J Bone Joint Surg Am 77:784, 1995.

31. Grohmann, JEL: Comparison of two methods of goniometry. Phys Ther 63:922, 1983.

32. Hamilton, GF, and Lachenbruch, PA: Reliability of goniometers in assessing finger joint angle. Phys Ther 49:465, 1969.

33. Boone, DC, et al: Reliability of goniometric measurements. Phys Ther 58:1355, 1978.

34. Pandya, S, et al: Reliability of goniometric measurements in patients with Duchenne muscular dystrophy. Phys Ther 65:1339, 1985.

35. Bovens, AMP, et al: Variability and reliability of joint measurements. Am J Sport Med 18:58, 1990.

36. Hellebrandt, FA, Duvall, EN, and Moore, ML: The measurement of joint motion. Part III: Reliability of goniometry. Phys Ther Rev 29:302, 1949. 65:1339, 1985.

37. Low, JL: The reliability of joint measurement. Physiotherapy 62:227, 1976.

38. Greene, BL, and Wolf, SL: Upper extremity joint movement: Comparison of two measurement devices. Arch Phys Med Rehabil 70:299, 1989.

39. Tucci, SM, et al: Cervical motion assessment: A new, simple and accurate method. Arch Phys Med Rehabil 67:225, 1986.

40. Youdas, JW, Carey, JR, and Garrett, TR: Reliability of measurements of cervical spine range of motion: Comparison of three methods. Phys Ther 71:2, 1991.

41. Fitzgerald, GK, et al: Objective assessment with establishment of normal values for lumbar spine range of motion. Phys Ther 63:1776, 1983.

42. Nitschke, JE, et al: Reliability of the American Medical Association Guides' model for measuring spinal range of motion. Spine 24:262, 1999.

43. Mayerson, NH, and Milano, RA: Goniometric measurement reliability in physical medicine. Arch Phys Med Rehabil 65:92, 1984.

44. Watkins, MA, et al: Reliability of goniometric measurements and visual estimates of knee range of motion obtained in a clinical setting. Phys Ther 71:90, 1991.

45. Riddle, DL, Rothstein, JM, and Lamb, RL: Goniometric reliability in a clinical setting: Shoulder measurements. Phys Ther 67:668, 1987.

46. Ekstrand, J, et al: Lower extremity goniometric measurements: A study to determine their reliability. Arch Phys Med Rehabil 63:171, 1982.

47. Rothstein, JM, Miller, PJ, and Roettger, RF: Goniometric relia-

bility in a clinical setting: Elbow and knee measurements. Phys Ther 63:1611, 1983.

48. Solgaard, S, et al: Reproducibility of goniometry of the wrist. Scand J Rehabil Med 18:5, 1986.

49. Patel, RS: Intratester and intertester reliability of the inclinometer in measuring lumbar flexion [abstract]. Phys Ther 72:S44, 1992.

50. Lovell, FW, Rothstein, JM, and Personius, WJ: Reliability of clinical measurements of lumbar lordosis taken with a flexible rule. Phys Ther 69:96, 1989.

51. Bartlett, JD, et al: Hip flexion contractures: A comparison of measurement methods. Arch Phys Med Rehabil 66:620, 1985.

52. Jonson, SR, and Gross, MT: Intraexaminer reliability, interexaminer reliability, and mean values for nine lower extremity skeletal measures in healthy naval midshipmen. J Orthop Sports Phys Ther 25:253, 1997

53. Elveru, RA, Rothstein, JM, and Lamb, RL: Goniometric reliability in a clinical setting. Phys Ther 68:672, 1988.

54. Diamond, JE, et al: Reliability of a diabetic foot evaluation. Phys Ther 69:797, 1989.

55. MacDermid, JC, et al: Intratester and intertester reliability of goniometric measurement of passive lateral shoulder rotation. J Hand Ther 12:187, 1999.

56. Armstrong, AD, et al: Reliability of range-of-motion measurement in the elbow and forearm. J Shoulder Elbow Surg 7:573, 1998.

57. Boon, AJ, and Smith, J: Manual scapular stabilization: Its effect on shoulder rotational range of motion Arch Phys Med Rehabil 81:978, 2000.

58. Horger, MM: The reliability of goniometric measurements of active and passive wrist motions. Am J Occup Ther 44:342, 1990.

59. Ellis, B, Bruton, A, and Goddard, JR: Joint angle measurement: A comparative study of the reliability of goniometry and wire tracing for the hand. Clin Rehabil 11:314, 1997.

60. Pellecchia, GL, and Bohannon, RW: Active lateral neck flexion range of motion measurements obtained with a modified goniometer. Reliability and estimates of normal. J Manipulative Physiol Ther 21:443, 1998.

61. Nilsson, N: Measuring passive cervical motion: A study of reliability. J Manipulative Physiol Ther 18:293, 1995.

62. Williams, R, et al: Reliability of the modified-modified Schober and double inclinometer methods for measuring lumbar flexion and extension. Phys Ther 73:26, 1993.

63. Defibaugh, JJ: Measurement of head motion. Part II: An experimental study of head motion in adult males. Phys Ther 44:163, 1964.

64. Balogun, JA, et al: Inter- and intratester reliability of measuring neck motions with tape measure and Myrin Gravity-Reference Goniometer. J Orthop Sports Phys Ther 10:248, 1989.

65. Capuano-Pucci, D, et al: Intratester and intertester reliability of the cervical range of motion. Arch Phys Med Rehabil 72:338, 1991.

66. LaStayo, PC, and Wheeler, DL: Reliability of passive wrist flexion and extension goniometric measurements: A multicenter study. Phys Ther 74:162, 1994.

67. Mayer, TG, et al: Spinal range of motion. Spine 22:1976, 1997.

68. Cobe, HM: The range of active motion at the wrist of white adults. J Bone Joint Surg Br 10:763, 1928.

69. Hewitt, D: The range of active motion at the wrist of women. J Bone Joint Surg Br 10:775, 1928.

70. Palmer, ML, and Epler, M: Clinical Assessment Procedures in Physical Therapy, ed 2. JB Lippincott, Philadelphia, 1998.

71. Clarkson, HM: Musculoskeletal Assessment: Joint Range of Motion and Manual Muscle Strength, ed 2. Williams & Wilkins, Baltimore, 2000.

72. Robson, P: A method to reduce the variable error in joint range measurement. Ann Phys Med 8:262, 1966.

73. Goodwin, J, et al: Clinical methods of goniometry: A comparative study. Disabil Rehabil 14:10, 1992.

74. Petherick, M, et al: Concurrent validity and intertester reliability of universal and fluid-based goniometers for active elbow range of motion. Phys Ther 68:966, 1988.

75. Brown, A, et al: Validity and reliability of the Dexter hand eval-

uation and therapy system in hand-injured patients. J Hand Ther 13:37, 2000.

76. Weiss, PL, et al: Using the Exos Handmaster to measure digital range of motion: Reliability and validity. Med Eng Phys 16:323, 1994.

77. Clapper, MP, and Wolf, SL: Comparison of the reliability of the Orthoranger and the standard goniometer for assessing active lower extremity range of motion. Phys Ther 68:214, 1988.

78. Ellison, JB, Rose, SJ, and Sahrman, SA: Patterns of hip rotation: A comparison between healthy subjects and patients with low back pain. Phys Ther 70:537, 1990.

79. Rheault, W, et al: Intertester reliability and concurrent validity of fluid-based and universal goniometers for active knee flexion. Phys Ther 68:1676, 1988.

80. Bartholomy, JK, Chandler, RF, and Kaplan, SE: Validity analysis of fluid goniometer measurements of knee flexion [abstract]. Phys Ther 80:S46, 2000.

81. Rome, K, and Cowieson, F: A reliability study of the universal goniometer, fluid goniometer, and electrogoniometer for the measurement of ankle dorsiflexion. Foot Ankle Int 17:28, 1996.

82. White, DJ, et al: Reliability of three methods of measuring cervical motion [abstract]. Phys Ther 66:771, 1986.

83. Reynolds, PMG: Measurement of spinal mobility: A comparison of three methods. Rheumatolo Rehabil 14:180, 1975.

84. Miller, MH, et al: Measurement of spinal mobility in the sagittal plane: New skin distraction technique compared with established methods. J Rheumatol 11:4, 1984.

85. Gill, K, et al: Repeatability of four clinical methods for assessment of lumbar spinal motion. Spine 13:50, 1988.

86. Lindahl, O: Determination of the sagittal mobility of the lumbar spine. Acta Orthop Scand 37:241, 1966.

87. White, DJ, et al: Reliability of three clinical methods of measuring lateral flexion in the thoracolumbar pine [abstract]. Phys Ther 67:759, 1987.

88. Mayer, RS, et al: Variance in the measurement of sagittal lumbar range of motion among examiners, subjects, and instruments. Spine 20:1489, 1995.

89. Chen, SP, et al: Reliability of the lumbar sagittal motion measurement methods: Surface inclinometers. J Occup Environ Med 39:217, 1997.

90. Breum, J, Wilberg, J, and Bolton, JE: Reliability and concurrent validity of the BROM II for measuring lumbar mobility. J Manipulative Physiol Ther 18:497, 1995.

91. Colton, T: Statistics in Medicine. Little, Brown, Boston, 1974.

92. Dawson-Saunders, B, and Trapp, RG: Basic and Clinical Biostatistics. Appleton & Lange, Norwalk, CT, 1990.

93. Francis, K: Computer communication: Reliability. Phys Ther 66:1140, 1986.

94. Blesh, TE: Measurement in Physical Education, ed 2. Ronald Press, New York, 1974. Cited by Currier, DP: Elements of Research in Physical Therapy, ed 3. Williams & Wilkins, Baltimore, 1990.

95. Bland, JM, and Altman, DG: Measurement error and correlation coefficients. [statistics notes]. BMJ 313:41, 1996.

96. Lahey, MA, Downey, RG, and Saal, FE: Intraclass correlations: There's more there than meets the eye. Psychol Bull 93:586, 1983.

97. Shout, PE, and Fleiss, JL: Intraclass correlations: Uses in assessing rater reliability. Psychol Bull 86:420, 1979.

98. Krebs, DE: Computer communication: Intraclass correlation coefficients. Phys Ther 64:1581, 1984.

99. Stratford, P: Reliability: Consistency or differentiating among subjects? [letters to the editor]. Phys Ther 69:299, 1989.

100. Bland, JM, and Altman, DG: Measurement error. [statistics notes]. BMJ 312:1654, 1996.

101. DuBois, PH: An Introduction to Psychological Statistics. Harper & Row, New York, 1965, p 401.

102. Stratford, P: Use of the standard error as a reliability index of interest: An applied example using elbow flexor strength data. Phys Ther 77:745, 1997.

103. Eliasziw, M, et al: Statistical methodology for the concurrent assessment of interrater and intrarater reliability: Using goniometric measurement as an example. Phys Ther 74:777, 1994.

104. Bartko, JJ: Rationale for reporting standard deviations rather than standard errors of the mean. Am J Psychiatry 142:1060, 1985.

PART II

Upper-Extremity Testing

Objectives

ON COMPLETION OF PART II THE READER WILL BE ABLE TO:

1. **Identify:**
   Appropriate planes and axes for each upper-extremity joint motion
   Structures that limit the end of the range of motion
   Expected normal end-feels

2. **Describe:**
   Testing positions used for each upper-extremity joint motion and muscle length test
   Goniometer alignment
   Capsular pattern of restricted motion
   Range of motion necessary for selected functional activities

3. **Explain:**
   How age, gender, and other factors can affect the range of motion
   How sources of error in measurement can affect testing results

4. **Perform a goniometric measurement of any upper-extremity joint including:**
   A clear explanation of the testing procedure
   Proper positioning of the subject
   Adequate stabilization of the proximal joint component

   Correct determination of the end of the range of motion
   Correct identification of the end-feel
   Palpation of the appropriate bony landmarks
   Accurate alignment of the goniometer and correct reading and recording

5. **Plan goniometric measurements of the shoulder, elbow, wrist, and hand that are organized by body position**

6. **Assess intratester and intertester reliability of goniometric measurements of the upper-extremity joints using methods described in Chapter 3.**

7. **Perform tests of muscle length at the shoulder, elbow, wrist, and hand including:**
   A clear explanation of the testing procedure
   Proper positioning of the subject in the starting position
   Adequate stabilization
   Use of appropriate testing motion
   Correct identification of the end-feel
   Accurate alignment of the goniometer and correct reading and recording

The testing positions, stabilization techniques, end-feels, and goniometer alignment for the joints of the upper extremities are presented in Chapters 4 through 7. The goniometric evaluation should follow the 12-step sequence presented in Exercise 5 in Chapter 2.

CHAPTER 4

The Shoulder

Structure and Function

Glenohumeral Joint

Anatomy

The glenohumeral joint is a synovial ball-and-socket joint. The ball is the convex head of the humerus, which faces medially, superiorly, and posteriorly with respect to the shaft of the humerus (Fig. 4–1). The socket is formed by the concave glenoid fossa of the scapula. The socket is shallow and smaller than the humeral head but is deepened and enlarged by the fibrocartilaginous glenoid labrum. The joint capsule is thin and lax, blends with the glenoid labrum, and is reinforced by the tendons of the rotator cuff muscles and by the glenohumeral (superior, middle, inferior) and coracohumeral ligaments (Fig. 4–2).

Osteokinematics

The glenohumeral joint has 3 degrees of freedom. The motions permitted at the joint are flexion-extension, abduction-adduction, and medial-lateral rotation. In addition, horizontal abduction and horizontal adduction are functional motions performed at the level of the shoulder and are created by combining abduction and extension, and adduction and flexion, respectively. Full range of motion (ROM) of the shoulder requires humeral, scapular, and clavicular motion at the glenohumeral, sternoclavicular, acromioclavicular, and scapulothoracic joints.

Arthrokinematics

Motion at the glenohumeral joint occurs as a rolling and sliding of the head of the humerus on the glenoid fossa.

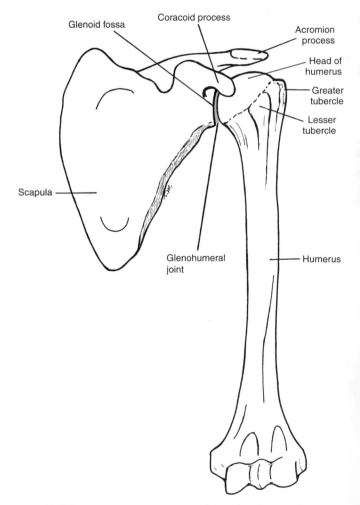

FIGURE 4–1 An anterior view of the glenohumeral joint.

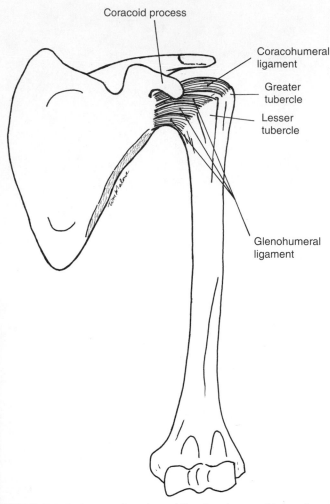

FIGURE 4–2 An anterior view of the glenohumeral joint showing the coracohumeral and glenohumeral ligaments.

The direction of the sliding is opposite to the movement of the shaft of the humerus. The humeral head slides posteriorly and inferiorly in flexion, anteriorly and superiorly in extension, inferiorly in abduction, and superiorly in adduction. In lateral rotation, the humeral head slides anteriorly on the glenoid fossa. In medial rotation, the humeral head slides posteriorly. The sliding motions help to maintain contact between the head of the humerus and the glenoid fossa of the scapular during the rolling motions.

Capsular Pattern

The greatest restriction of passive motion is in lateral rotation, followed by some restriction in abduction and less restriction in medial rotation.[1]

Sternoclavicular Joint

Anatomy

The sternoclavicular (SC) joint is a synovial joint linking the medial end of the clavicle with the sternum and the

cartilage of the first rib (Fig. 4–3A). The joint surfaces are saddle-shaped. The clavicular joint surface is convex cephalocaudally and concave anteroposteriorly. The opposing joint surface, located at the notch formed by the manubrium of the sternum and the first costal cartilage, is concave cephalocaudally and convex anteroposteriorly. An articular disc divides the joint into two separate compartments.

The associated joint capsule is strong and reinforced by anterior and posterior SC ligaments (Fig. 4–3B). These ligaments limit anterior-posterior movement of the medial end of the clavicle. The costoclavicular ligament, which extends from the inferior surface of the medial end of the clavicle to the first rib, limits clavicular elevation and protraction. The interclavicular ligament extends from one clavicle to another and limits excessive inferior movement of the clavicle.[2]

Osteokinematics

The SC joint has 3 degrees of freedom, and motion consists of movement of the clavicle on the sternum. These motions are described by the movement at the lateral end of the clavicle. Clavicular motions include elevation-depression, protraction-retraction, and anterior-posterior rotation.[2,3]

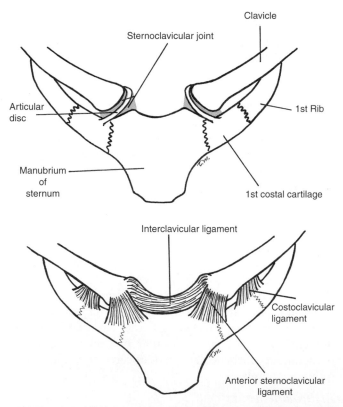

FIGURE 4–3 (A) An anterior view of the sternoclavicular (SC) joint showing the bone structures and articular disc. (B) An anterior view of the SC joint showing the interclavicular, SC, and costoclavicular ligaments.

Arthrokinematics

During clavicular elevation and depression, the convex surface of the clavicle slides on the concave manubrium in a direction opposite the movement of the lateral end of the clavicle. In protraction and retraction, the concave portion of the clavicular joint surface slides on the convex surface of the manubrium in the same direction as the lateral end of the clavicle. In rotation, the clavicular joint surface spins on the opposing joint surface. In summary, the clavicle slides inferiorly in elevation, superiorly in depression, anteriorly in protraction, and posteriorly in retraction.

Acromioclavicular Joint

Anatomy

The acromioclavicular (AC) joint is a synovial joint linking the scapula and the clavicle. The scapular joint surface is a concave facet located on the acromion of the scapula (Fig. 4–4). The clavicular joint surface is a convex facet located on the lateral end of the clavicle. The joint contains a fibrocartilaginous disc and is surrounded by a weak joint capsule. The superior and inferior AC ligaments reinforce the capsule (Fig. 4–5). The coracoclavicular ligament, which extends between

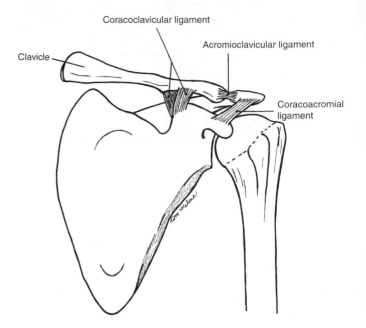

FIGURE 4–5   An anterior view of the acromioclavicular (AC) joint showing the coracoclavicular, acromioclavicular, and coracoacromial ligaments.

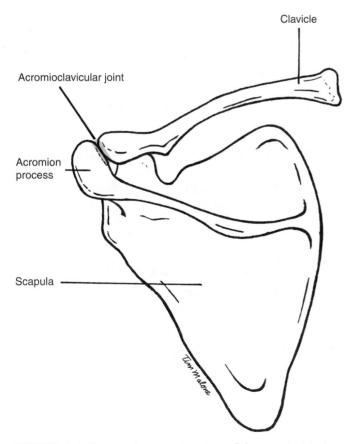

FIGURE 4–4   A posterior-superior view of the acromioclavicular joint.

the clavicle and the scapular coracoid process, provides additional stability.

Osteokinematics

The AC joint has 3 degrees of freedom and permits movement of the scapula on the clavicle in three planes.[3] Numerous terms have been used to describe these motions. Tilting (tipping) is movement of the scapula in the sagittal plane around a coronal axis. During anterior tilting the superior border of the scapula and glenoid fossa moves anteriorly, whereas the inferior angle moves posteriorly. During posterior tilting (tipping) the superior border of the scapula and glenoid fossa moves posteriorly, whereas the inferior angle moves anteriorly.

Upward and downward rotations of the scapula occur in the frontal plane around an anterior-posterior axis. During upward rotation the glenoid fossa moves cranially, whereas during downward rotation the glenoid fossa moves caudally.

Protraction and retraction of the scapula occur in the transverse plane around a vertical axis. During protraction (also termed medial rotation, or winging) the glenoid fossa moves medially and anteriorly, whereas the vertebral border of the scapula moves away from the spine. During retraction (also termed lateral rotation) the glenoid fossa moves laterally and posteriorly, whereas the vertebral border of the scapula moves toward the spine. The terms abduction-adduction have been used by various authors to indicate the motions of upward

TABLE 4–1	Shoulder Complex Motion: Mean Values in Degrees from Selected Sources			
	AAOS[5]	AMA[6]	Boone and Azen[7] n = 109*	Greene and Wolf[8] n = 20†
Motion			Mean (SD)	Mean (SD)
Flexion	180	150	166.7 (4.7)	155.8 (1.4)
Extension	60	50	62.3 (9.5)	
Abduction	180	180	184.0 (7.0)	167.6 (1.8)
Medial rotation	70	90	68.8 (4.6)	48.7 (2.8)
Lateral rotation	90	90	103.7 (8.5)	83.6 (3.0)

* Values are for male subjects 18 months to 54 years of age.
† Values are for male and female subjects 18 to 55 years of age.

rotation-downward rotation as well as protraction-retraction.[2,4]

Arthrokinematics

Motion of the joint surfaces consists of a sliding of the concave acromial facet on the convex clavicular facet. Acromial sliding on the clavicle occurs in the same direction as movement of the scapula.

Scapulothoracic Joint

Anatomy

The scapulothoracic joint is considered to be a functional rather than an anatomical joint. The joint surfaces are the anterior surface of the scapula and the posterior surface of the thorax.

Osteokinematics

The motions that occur at the scapulothoracic joint are caused by the independent or combined motions of the sternoclavicular and acromioclavicular joints. These motions include scapular elevation-depression, upward-downward rotation, anterior-posterior tilting, and protraction-retraction (also called medial-lateral rotation).

Arthrokinematics

Motion consists of a sliding of the scapula on the thorax.

⬤ Research Findings

Effects of Age, Gender, and Other Factors

Table 4–1 shows the mean values of shoulder complex ROM measurements obtained from various sources. The data on age, gender, and number of subjects that were measured to obtain the values reported for the American Academy of Orthopaedic Surgeons (AAOS)[5] in 1965, and for the American Medical Association (AMA)[6] were not noted. Boone and Azen[7] measured active ROM using a universal goniometer in 109 males between 18 months and 54 years of age. Greene and Wolf[8] measured active ROM with a universal goniometer in 10 males and 10 females aged 18 to 55 years. Unless otherwise noted, the reader should assume that shoulder ROM refers to shoulder complex ROM.

Few studies have specifically measured glenohumeral ROM using clinical tools such as a universal goniometer. The glenohumeral joint is generally considered to contribute about 120 degrees of flexion and between 90 and 120 degrees of abduction to shoulder complex motions.[3] In general, the overall ratio of glenohumeral to

TABLE 4–2	Glenohumeral Motion: Mean Values in Degrees from Selected Sources			
	Lannan et al[12] n = 60*	Boon & Smith[13] n = 50†	Ellenbecker et al[14] Males n = 113‡	Ellenbecker et al[14] Females n = 90‡
Motion	Mean (SD)	Mean (SD)	Mean (SD)	Mean (SD)
Flexion	106.2 (10.2)			
Extension	20.1 (5.8)			
Abduction	128.9 (9.1)			
Medial rotation	49.2 (9.0)	62.8 (12.7)	50.9 (12.6)	56.3 (10.3)
Lateral rotation	94.2 (12.2)	108.1 (14.1)	102.8 (10.9)	104.6 (10.3)

* Values are for male and female subjects 21 to 40 years of age.
† Values are for male and female subjects 12 to 18 years of age.
‡ Values are for subjects who were elite tennis players 11 to 17 years of age.

TABLE 4-3 Effects of Age on Shoulder Complex Motions for Newborns through Adolescents: Mean Values in Degrees

| | Wanatabe et al[15] | Boone[16] | | |
| | 0–2 yrs n = 45 | 1–5 yrs n = 19 | 6–12 yrs n = 17 | 13–19 yrs n = 17 |
Motion	Range of Means	Mean (SD)	Mean (SD)	Mean (SD)
Flexion	172–180	168.8 (3.7)	169.0 (3.5)	167.4 (3.9)
Extension	79–89	68.9 (6.6)	69.6 (7.0)	64.0 (9.3)
Medial rotation	72–90	71.2 (3.6)	70.0 (4.7)	70.3 (5.3)
Lateral rotation	118–134	110.0 (10.0)	107.4 (3.6)	106.3 (6.1)
Abduction	177–187	186.3 (2.6)	184.7 (3.8)	185.1 (4.3)

scapulothoracic motion during flexion and abduction is given as 2:1.[3,9–11] Therefore, about two-thirds of shoulder complex motion is attributed to the glenohumeral joint. Table 4–2 shows the mean values of glenohumeral ROM obtained from three sources. Lannan, Lehman, and Toland[12] measured passive ROM using a universal goniometer in 20 males and 40 females aged 21 to 40 years. Boon and Smith[13] examined 50 high school athletes (32 females and 18 males) for passive medial and lateral glenohumeral rotation. Ellenbecker and colleagues[14] measured active rotation in 113 male and 90 female elite tennis players between the ages of 11 and 17 years. These three studies used manual stabilization of the scapula and universal goniometers to obtain glenohumeral measurements. More studies are needed to establish normative values for glenohumeral ROM, especially in older adults.

Age

A review of shoulder complex ROM values presented in Table 4–3 shows very slight differences among children from birth through adolescence. Values from the study by Wanatabe and coworkers[15] were derived from measurements of passive ROM of Japanese males and females. The mean values listed from Boone[16] were derived from measurements of active ROM taken with a universal goniometer on Caucasian males. Although the values obtained from Wanatabe and coworkers[15] for infants are greater than those obtained from Boone[16] for children between the ages of 1 and 19 years, it is difficult to compare values across studies. Within one study, Boone[16] and Boone and Azen[7] found that shoulder ROM varied little in boys between 1 and 19 years of age.

There is some indication that children have greater values than adults for certain shoulder complex motions. Wanatabe and coworkers[15] found that the ROM in shoulder extension and lateral rotation was greater in Japanese infants than the average values typically reported for adults. Boone and Azen[7] found significantly greater active ROM in shoulder flexion, extension, lateral rotation, and medial rotation in male children between 1 and 19 years of age compared with findings in male adults between 20 and 54 years of age. However, they found no significant differences in shoulder abduction owing to age.

Table 4–4 summarizes the effects of age on shoulder complex ROM in adults. There appears to be a trend for older adults (between 60 and 93 years of age) to have lower mean values than younger adults (between 20 and 39 years of age) for the motions of extension, lateral rotation, and abduction. Values cited from Boone[16] were obtained from measurements made with a universal

TABLE 4-4 Effects of Age on Shoulder Complex Motion in Adults 20 to 93 Years of Age: Mean Values in Degrees

| | Boone[16] | | | Walker et al[17] | Downey et al[18] |
| | 20–29 yrs n = 19 | 30–39 yrs n = 18 | 40–54 yrs n = 19 | 60–85 yrs n = 30 | 61–93 yrs n = 106 |
Motion	Mean (SD)	Mean (SD)	Mean (SD)	Mean (SD)	Mean (SD)
Flexion	164.5 (5.9)	165.4 (3.8)	165.1 (5.2)	160.0 (11.0)	165.0 (10.7)
Extension	58.3 (8.3)	57.5 (8.5)	56.1 (7.9)	38.0 (11.0)	
Medial rotation	65.9 (4.0)	67.1 (4.2)	68.3 (3.8)	59.0 (16.0)	65.0 (11.7)
Lateral rotation	100.0 (7.2)	101.5 (6.9)	97.5 (8.5)	76.0 (13.0)	80.6 (11.0)
Abduction	182.6 (9.8)	182.8 (7.7)	182.6 (9.8)	155.0 (22.0)	157.9 (17.4)

goniometer of active ROM in male subjects. The values from Walker and associates[17] were obtained from measurements of active ROM in 30 male subjects using a universal goniometer. The values from Downey, Fiebert, and Stackpole-Brown[18] were obtained from measurements of active ROM made with a universal goniometer in 140 female and 60 male shoulders. It is interesting to note that the standard deviations for the older groups are much larger than the values reported for the younger groups. The larger standard deviations appear to indicate that ROM is more variable in the older groups than in the younger groups. However, the fact that the measurements of the two oldest groups were obtained by different investigators should be considered when drawing conclusions from this information.

In addition to the evidence for age-related changes presented in Tables 4–3 and 4–4, West,[19] Clarke and coworkers,[20] and Allander and associates[21] have also identified age-related trends. West[19] found that older subjects had between 15 and 20 degrees less shoulder complex flexion ROM and 10 degrees less extension ROM than younger subjects. Subjects ranged in age from the first decade to the eighth decade. Clarke and coworkers[20] found significant decreases with age in passive glenohumeral lateral rotation, total rotation, and abduction in a study that included 60 normal males and females ranging in age from 21 to 80 years. Mean reduction in these three glenohumeral ROMs in those aged 71 to 80 years compared with those aged 21 to 30 years, ranged from 7 to 29 degrees. Allander and associates,[21] in a study of 517 females and 203 males aged 33 to 70 years, also found that passive shoulder complex rotation ROM significantly decreased with increasing age.

Gender

Several studies have noted that females have greater shoulder complex ROM than males. Walker and coworkers,[17] in a study of 30 men and 30 women between 60 and 84 years of age, found that women had statistically significant greater ROM than their male counterparts in all shoulder motions studied except for medial rotation. The mean differences for women were 20 degrees greater than those of males for shoulder abduction, 11 degrees greater for shoulder extension, and 9 degrees greater for shoulder flexion and lateral rotation. Allander and associates,[21] in a study of passive shoulder rotation in 208 Swedish women and 203 men aged 45 to 70 years, likewise found that women had a greater ROM in total shoulder rotation than men. Escalante, Lichenstein, and Hazuda[22] studied shoulder flexion in 687 community-dwelling adults aged 65 to 74 years and found that women had 3 degrees more flexion than men.

Gender differences have also been noted in glenohumeral ROM. Clarke and associates,[20] in a study that included 60 males and 60 females, found that females

had greater glenohumeral ROM for shoulder abduction as well as lateral and total rotation. Six age groups with subjects between 20 and 40 years of age were included in the study. These gender differences were present in all age groups. Males had, on average, 92 percent of the ROM of their female counterparts, the difference being most marked in abduction. Lannan, Lehman, and Toland,[12] in a study of 40 women and 20 men aged 21 to 40 years, found that women had statistically significant greater amounts of glenohumeral flexion, extension, abduction, medial and lateral rotation than men. The mean differences typically varied between 3 and 8 degrees. Boon and Smith,[13] in a study of 32 females and 18 males aged 12 to 18 years, reported that females had significantly more lateral and total rotation than males. The mean difference in lateral and total rotation was 4.5 and 9.1 degrees, respectively. Ellenbecker and colleagues[14] studied 113 male and 90 female elite tennis players aged 11 to 17 years (see Table 4–2). Their data seem to indicate that the females had greater ROM than males for glenohumeral medial and lateral rotation, although no statistical tests focused on the effect of gender on ROM.

Testing Position

A subject's posture and testing position have been shown to affect certain shoulder complex motions. Kebaetse, McClure, and Pratt,[23] in a study of 34 healthy adults, measured active shoulder abduction and scapula ROM while subjects were sitting in both erect and slouched trunk postures. There was significantly less active shoulder abduction ROM in the slouched than in the erect postures (mean difference = 23.6 degrees). The slouched posture also resulted in more scapula elevation during 0 to 90 degrees of abduction and less scapula posterior tilting in the interval between 90-degree and maximal abduction.

Sabari and associates[24] studied 30 adult subjects and noted greater amounts of active and passive shoulder abduction measured in the supine than in the sitting position. The mean differences in abduction ranged from 3.0 to 7.1 degrees. On visual inspection of the data there were also greater amounts of shoulder flexion in the supine versus the sitting position; however, these differences did not attain significance.

Body-Mass Index

Escalante, Lichenstein, and Hazuda[22] studied shoulder complex flexion ROM in 695 community-dwelling subjects, aged 65 to 74 years, who participated in the San Antonio Longitudinal Study of Aging. They found no relationship between shoulder flexion and body-mass index.

Sports

Several studies of professional and collegiate baseball players have found a significant increase in lateral rotation ROM and a decrease in medial rotation ROM of the shoulder complex in the dominant shoulder compared with the nondominant shoulder. These differences have been found in position players as well as in pitchers. Bigliani and coworkers[25] studied 148 professional baseball players (72 pitchers and 76 position players) with no history of shoulder problems. Mean lateral rotation ROM measured with the shoulder in 90 degrees of abduction was 113.5 degrees in the dominant arm and 99.9 degrees in the nondominant arm. Mean medial rotation ROM, recorded as the highest vertebral level reached behind the back and converted to a numerical value, was significantly less in the dominant arm. There were no significant differences between the dominant and the nondominant arms in shoulder flexion and shoulder lateral rotation measured with the arm at the side of the body. A study by Baltaci, Johnson, and Kohl[26] of 15 collegiate pitchers and 23 position players had similar findings. Pitchers had an average of 14 degrees more lateral rotation, and 11 degrees less medial rotation in the dominant versus nondominant shoulders. Position players had an average of 8 degrees more lateral rotation and 10 degrees less medial rotation in the dominant shoulder. All measurements of rotation were taken with the shoulder in 90 degrees of abduction.

Decreases in shoulder medial rotation ROM have also been noted in the dominant (playing) compared with the nondominant (nonplaying) arms of tennis players. Chinn, Priest, and Kent,[27] in a study of 83 national and international men and women tennis players aged 14 to 50 years, found a significant decrease in active medial rotation ROM of the shoulder complex in the playing versus the nonplaying arm (mean difference = 6.8 degrees in males, 11.9 degrees in females). Men also had a significant increase in lateral rotation ROM in the playing compared with the nonplaying arm. A study by Kibler and colleagues[28] of 39 members of the U. S. Tennis Association National Tennis Team and touring professional program found a decrease in passive glenohumeral medial rotation ROM, an increase in glenohumeral lateral rotation ROM, and a decrease in total rotation ROM in the playing versus the nonplaying arm. The differences in medial rotation ROM increased with age and years of tournament play. A study by Ellenbecker and associates[14] of 203 junior elite tennis players aged 11 to 17 years reported a significant decrease in active medial rotation ROM and total rotation ROM of the glenohumeral joint in the playing versus the nonplaying arm. The average differences in medial rotation ROM were 11 degrees in the 113 males and 8 degrees in the 90 females. There were no significant differences in glenohumeral lateral rotation ROM between playing and nonplaying arms.

Power lifters were found to have decreased ROM in shoulder complex flexion, extension, and medial and lateral rotation compared with nonlifters in a study by Chang, Buschbacker, and Edlich.[29] Ten male power lifters and 10 aged-matched male nonlifters were included in the study. The authors suggest that athletic training programs that emphasize muscle strengthening exercise without stretching exercise may cause progressive loss of ROM.

Functional Range of Motion

Numerous activities of daily living (ADL) require adequate shoulder ROM. Tiffitt,[30] in a study of 25 patients, found a significant correlation between the amount of specific shoulder complex motions and the ability to perform activities such as combing the hair, putting on a coat, washing the back, washing the contralateral axilla, using the toilet, reaching a high shelf, lifting above the shoulder level, pulling, and sleeping on the affected side. Flexion and adduction ROM correlated best with the ability to comb the hair, whereas medial and lateral rotation ROM correlated best with the ability to wash the back.

Several studies[31,32] have examined the ROM that occurs during certain functional tasks (Table 4–5). A large amount of abduction (112 degrees) and lateral rotation is required to reach behind the head for activities such as grooming the hair (Fig 4–6), positioning a necktie, and fastening a dress zipper. Maximal flexion (148 degrees) is needed to reach a high shelf (Fig. 4–7), whereas less flexion (36 to 52 degrees) is needed for self-feeding tasks (Fig 4–8). Thirty-eight to 56 degrees of extension and considerable medial rotation and horizontal abduction are necessary for reaching behind the back for tasks such as fastening a bra (Fig 4–9), tucking in a shirt, and reaching the perineum to perform hygiene activities. Horizontal adduction is needed for activities performed in front of the body such as washing the contralateral axilla (104 degrees) and eating (87 degrees). If patients have difficulty performing certain functional activities, evaluation and treatment procedures need to focus on the shoulder motions necessary for the activity. Likewise, if patients have known limitations in shoulder ROM, therapists and physicians should anticipate patient difficulty in performing these tasks, and adaptations should be suggested.

Reliability and Validity

The intratester and intertester reliability of measurements of shoulder motions with a universal goniometer have been studied by many researchers. Most of these studies have presented evidence that intratester reliability is better than intertester reliability. Reliability varied according to the motion being measured. In other words, the reliability of measuring certain shoulder motions was better than the reliability of measuring other motions.

Hellebrandt, Duvall, and Moore,[33] in a study of 77

TABLE 4–5   Maximal Shoulder Complex Motion Necessary for Functional Activities: Mean Values in Degrees

Activity	Motion	Mean	(SD)	Source
Eating	Flexion	52	(8)	Matsen*[31]
	Flexion	36	(14)	Safaee-Rad et al[†32]
	Abduction	22	(7)	Safaee-Rad et al
	Medial rotation	18	(10)	Safaee-Rad et al
	Horizontal adduction‡	87	(29)	Matsen
Drinking with a cup	Flexion	43	(16)	Safaee-Rad et al
	Abduction	31	(9)	Safaee-Rad et al
	Medial rotation	23	(12)	Safaee-Rad et al
Washing axilla	Flexion	52	(14)	Matsen
	Horizontal adduction	104	(12)	Matsen
Combing hair	Abduction	112	(10)	Matsen
	Horizontal adduction	54	(27)	Matsen
Maximal elevation	Flexion/abduction	148	(11)	Matsen
	Horizontal adduction	55	(17)	Matsen
Maximal reaching up back	Extension	56	(13)	Matsen
	Horizontal abduction‡	69	(11)	Matsen
Reaching perineum	Extension	38	(10)	Matsen
	Horizontal abduction	86	(13)	Matsen

* Eight normal subjects were assessed with electromagnetic sensors on the humerus.
† Ten normal male subjects were assessed with a three-dimensional video recording system.
‡ The 0 degree starting position for measuring horizontal adduction and horizontal abduction was in 90 degrees of abduction.

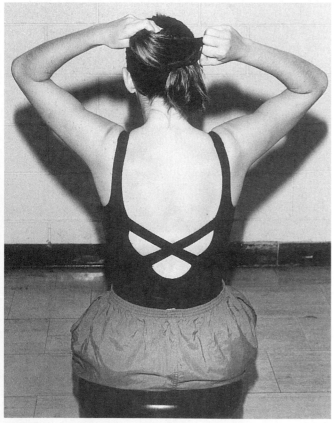

FIGURE 4–6 Reaching behind the head requires a large amount of abduction (112 degrees)[31] and lateral rotation of the shoulder.

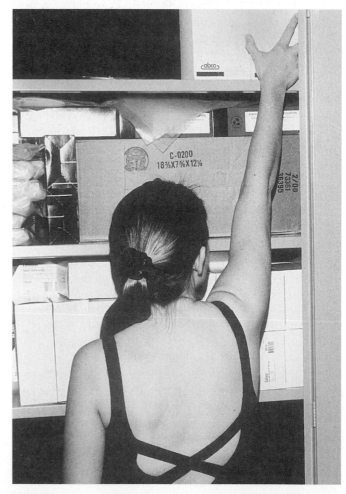

FIGURE 4–7 Reaching objects on a high shelf requires 148 degrees of shoulder flexion.[31]

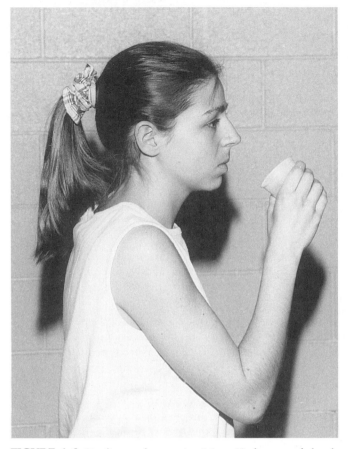

FIGURE 4–8 Feeding tasks require 36 to 52 degrees of shoulder flexion.[31,32]

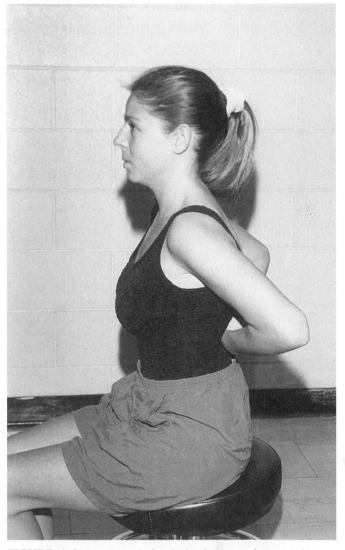

FIGURE 4–9 Reaching behind the back to fasten a bra or bathing suit requires 56 degrees of extension, 69 degrees of horizontal abduction,[31] and a large amount of medial rotation of the shoulder.

patients, found the intratester reliability of measurements of active ROM of shoulder complex abduction and medial rotation to be less than the intratester reliability of shoulder flexion, extension, and lateral rotation. The mean difference between the repeated measurements ranged from 0.2 to 1.5 degrees. Measurements were taken with a universal goniometer and devices designed by the U.S. Army for specific joints. For most ROM measurements taken throughout the body, the universal goniometer was a more dependable tool than the special devices.

Boone and coworkers[34] examined the reliability of measuring passive ROM for lateral rotation of the shoulder complex, elbow extension-flexion, wrist ulnar deviation, hip abduction, knee extension-flexion, and foot inversion. Four physical therapists used universal goniometers to measure these motions in 12 normal males once a week for 4 weeks. Measurement of lateral rotation ROM of the shoulder was found to be more reliable than that of the other motions tested. For all motions except lateral rotation of the shoulder, intratester reliability was noted to be greater than intertester reliability. Intratester and intertester reliability was simi-lar (r = 0.96 and 0.97, respectively) for lateral rotation ROM.

Pandya and associates,[35] in a study in which five testers measured the range of shoulder complex abduction of 150 children and young adults with Duchenne muscular dystrophy, found that the intratester intraclass correlation coefficient (ICC) for measurements of shoulder abduction was 0.84. The intertester reliability for measuring shoulder abduction was lower (ICC=0.67). In comparison with measurements of elbow and wrist extension, the measurement of shoulder abduction was less reliable.

Riddle, Rothstein, and Lamb[36] conducted a study to determine intratester and intertester reliability for passive ROM measurements of the shoulder complex. Sixteen physical therapists, assessing in pairs, used two different sized universal goniometers (large and small) for their measurements on 50 patients. Patient position and goniometer placement during measurements were not controlled. ICC values for intratester reliability for all motions ranged from 0.87 to 0.99. ICC values for intertester reliability for flexion, abduction, and lateral rotation ranged from 0.84 to 0.90. Intertester reliability was considerably lower for measurements of horizontal abduction, horizontal adduction, extension, and medial rotation, with ICC values ranging from 0.26 to 0.55. The authors concluded that passive ROM measurements for all shoulder motions can be reliable when taken by the same physical therapist, regardless of whether large or small goniometers are used. Measurements of flexion, abduction, and lateral rotation can be reliable when assessed by different therapists. However, because repeated measurements of horizontal abduction, horizontal adduction, extension, and medial rotation were unreliable when taken by more than one tester, these measurements should be taken by the same therapist.

Greene and Wolf[8] compared the reliability of the Ortho Ranger, an electronic pendulum goniometer, with that of a standard universal goniometer for active upper extremity motions in 20 healthy adults. Shoulder complex motions were measured three times with each instrument during three sessions that occurred over a 2-week period. Both instruments demonstrated high intra-session correlations (ICCs ranged from 0.98 to 0.87), but correlations were higher and 95 percent confidence levels were much lower for the universal goniometer. Measurements of medial rotation and lateral rotation were less reliable than measurements of flexion, extension, abduction, and adduction. There were significant differences between measurements taken with the Ortho Ranger and the universal goniometer. Interestingly, there were significant differences in measurements between sessions for both instruments. The authors noted that the daily variations that were found might have been caused by normal fluctuation in ROM as suggested by Boone and colleagues,[34] or by daily differences in subjects' efforts while performing active ROM.

Bovens and associates,[37] in a study of the variability and reliability of nine joint motions throughout the body, used a universal goniometer to examine active lateral rotation ROM of the shoulder complex with the arm at the side. Three physician testers and eight healthy subjects participated in the study. Intratester reliability coefficients for lateral rotation of the shoulder ranged from 0.76 to 0.83, whereas the intertester reliability coefficient was 0.63. Mean intratester standard deviations for the measurements taken on each subject ranged from 5.0 to 6.6 degrees, whereas the mean intertester standard deviation was 7.4 degrees. The measurement of lateral rotation ROM of the shoulder was more reliable than ROM measurements of the forearm and wrist. Mean standard deviations between repeated measurement of shoulder lateral rotation ROM were similar to those of the forearm and larger than those of the wrist.

Sabari and associates[24] examined intrarater reliability in the measurement of active and passive shoulder complex flexion and abduction ROM when 30 adults were positioned in supine and sitting positions. The ICCs between two trials by the same tester for each procedure ranged in value from 0.94 to 0.99, indicating high intratester reliability, regardless of whether the measurements were active or passive, or whether they were taken with the subject in the supine or the sitting position. ICCs between measurements taken in supine compared with taken in sitting positions ranged from 0.64 to 0.81. There were no significant differences between comparable flexion measurements taken in supine and sitting positions. However, significantly greater abduction ROM was found in the supine than in the sitting position.

In a study by MacDermid and colleagues,[38] two experienced physical therapists measured passive shoulder complex rotation ROM in 34 patients with a variety of shoulder pathologies. A universal goniometer was used to measure lateral rotation with the shoulder in 20 to 30 degrees of abduction. Intratester ICCs (0.88 and 0.93) and intertester ICCs (0.85 and 0.80) were high. Intratester standard errors of measurement (SEMs) (4.9 and 7.0 degrees) and intertester SEMs (7.5 and 8.0 degrees) also indicated good reliability. The SEMs indicate that differences of 5 to 7 degrees could be attributed to measurement error when the same tester repeats a measurement, and about 8 degrees could be attributed to measurement error when different testers take a measurement.

Boon and Smith[13] studied 50 high school athletes to determine the reliability of measuring passive shoulder rotation ROM with and without manual stabilization of the scapula. Four experienced physical therapists working in pairs took goniometric measurements with the shoulder in 90 degrees of abduction and repeated those measurements 5 days later. Scapular stabilization, which resulted in more isolated glenohumeral motion, produced significantly smaller ROM values than when the scapula was not stabilized. According to the authors, intratester reliability for medial rotation was poor for nonstabilized motion (ICC = 0.23, SEM = 20.2 degrees), and good for stabilized motion (ICC = 0.60, SEM = 8.0). The authors state that intratester reliability for lateral rotation was good for both nonstabilized (ICC = 0.79, SEM = 5.6) and stabilized motion (ICC = 0.53, SEM = 9.1). Intertester reliability for medial rotation improved from nonstabilized motion (ICC = 0.13, SEM = 21.5) to stabilized motion (ICC = 0.38, SEM = 10.0), and was comparable for both nonstabilized and stabilized lateral rotation (ICC = 0.84, SEM = 4.9 and ICC = 0.78, SEM = 6.6), respectively.

The reliability of measurement devices other than a universal goniometer for assessing shoulder ROM has also been studied and is briefly mentioned here. Intratester and intertester reliability for the different motions and methods varied widely. Green and associates[39] investigated the reliability of measuring active shoulder complex ROM with a plurimeter-V inclinometer in six patients with shoulder pain and stiffness. Tiffitt, Wildin, and Hajioff[40] studied the reliability of using an inclinometer to measure active shoulder complex motions in 36 patients with shoulder disorders. Bower[41] and Clarke and coworkers[20] examined the reliability of measuring passive glenohumeral motions with a hydrogoniometer. Croft and colleagues[42] investigated the reliability of observing shoulder complex flexion and lateral rotation, and sketching the ROMs onto diagrams that were then measured with a protractor.

Range of Motion Testing Procedures: The Shoulder

Full ROM of the shoulder requires movement at the glenohumeral, SC, AC, and scapulothoracic joints. To make measurements more informative, we suggest using two methods of measuring the ROM of the shoulder. One method measures passive motion primarily at the glenohumeral joint. The other method measures passive ROM at all the joints included in the shoulder complex.

We have found the method that measures primarily glenohumeral motion is helpful in identifying glenohumeral joint problems within the shoulder complex. The ability to differentiate and quantify ROM at the glenohumeral joint from other joints in the shoulder complex is important in diagnosing and treating many shoulder conditions. This method of measuring glenohumeral motion requires the use of passive motion and careful stabilization of the scapula. Active motion is avoided because it results in synchronous motion throughout the shoulder complex, making isolation of glenohumeral motion difficult. Certain studies have begun establishing some normative values (Table 4–2) and assessing the reliability of this measurement method.

The second method measures full motion of the shoulder complex and is useful in evaluating the functional ROM of the shoulder. This more traditional method of assessing shoulder motion incorporates the stabilization of the thoracic spine and rib cage. Tissue resistance to further motion is typically due to the stretch of structures connecting the clavicle to the sternum, and the scapula to the ribs and spine. ROM values for shoulder complex motion are presented in Tables 4–1, 4–3, and 4–4. Both methods of measuring the ROM of the shoulder are presented in the following discussions of stabilization techniques and end-feels. However, the alignment of the goniometer is the same for measuring glenohumeral and shoulder complex motions.

Landmarks for Goniometer Alignment

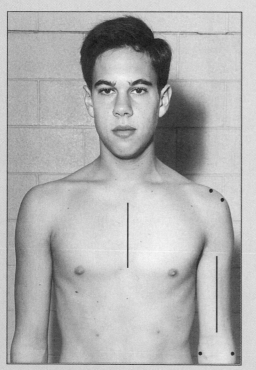

FIGURE 4–10 An anterior view of the humerus, clavicle, sternum, and scapula showing surface anatomy landmarks for aligning the goniometer.

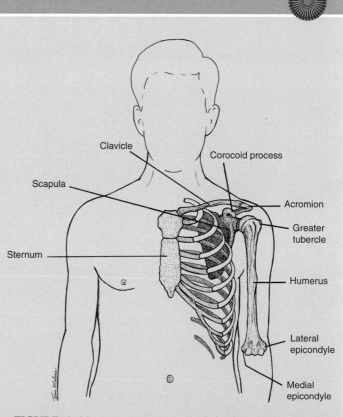

FIGURE 4–11 An anterior view of the humerus, clavicle, sternum, and scapula showing bony anatomical landmarks for aligning the goniometer.

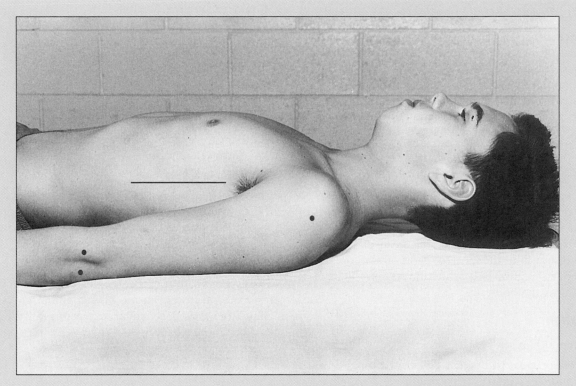

FIGURE 4–12 A lateral view of the upper arm showing surface anatomy landmarks for aligning the goniometer.

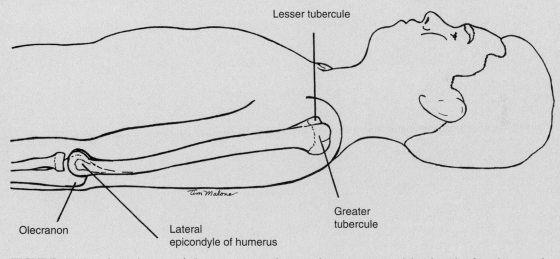

FIGURE 4–13 A lateral view of the upper arm showing bony anatomical landmarks for aligning the goniometer.

FLEXION

Motion occurs in the sagittal plane around a medial-lateral axis. Mean shoulder complex flexion ROM is 180 degrees according to the AAOS,[5] 167 degrees according to Boone and Azen,[7] and 150 degrees according to the AMA.[6] Mean glenohumeral flexion ROM is 106 degrees according to Lannan, Lehman, and Toland[12] and 120 degrees according to Levangie and Norkin.[3] See Tables 4–1 to 4–4 for additional information.

Testing Position

Place the subject supine, with the knees flexed to flatten the lumbar spine. Position the shoulder in 0 degrees of abduction, adduction, and rotation. Place the elbow in extension so that tension in the long head of the triceps muscle does not limit the motion. Position the forearm in 0 degrees of supination and pronation so that the palm of the hand faces the body.

Stabilization

Glenohumeral Flexion

Stabilize the scapula to prevent posterior tilting, upward rotation, and elevation of the scapula.

Shoulder Complex Flexion

Stabilize the thorax to prevent extension of the spine and movement of the ribs. The weight of the trunk may assist stabilization.

Testing Motion

Flex the shoulder by lifting the humerus off the examining table, bringing the hand up over the subject's head. Maintain the extremity in neutral abduction and adduction during the motion.

Glenohumeral Flexion

The end of glenohumeral flexion ROM occurs when resistance to further motion is felt and attempts to overcome the resistance cause upward rotation, posterior tilting, or elevation of the scapula (Fig. 4–14).

Shoulder Complex Flexion

The end of shoulder complex flexion ROM occurs when resistance to further motion is felt and attempts to overcome the resistance cause extension of the spine or motion of the ribs (Fig. 4–15).

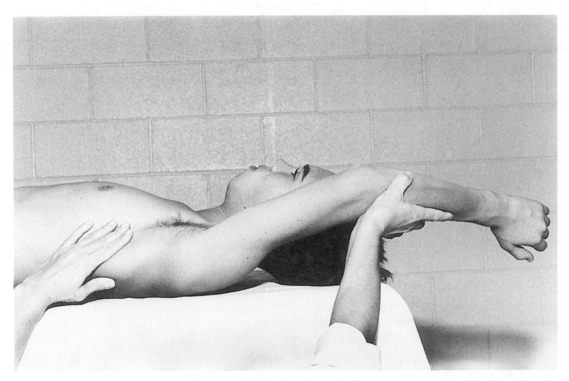

FIGURE 4–14 The end of the ROM of glenohumeral flexion. The examiner stabilizes the lateral border of the scapula with her hand. The examiner is able to determine that the end of the ROM has been reached because any attempt to move the extremity into additional flexion causes the lateral border of the scapula to move anteriorly and laterally.

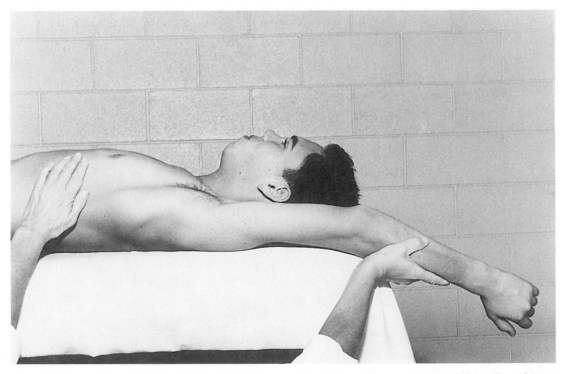

FIGURE 4–15 The end of the ROM of shoulder complex flexion. The examiner stabilizes the subject's trunk and ribs with her hand. The examiner is able to determine that the end of the ROM has been reached because any attempt to move the extremity into additional flexion causes extension of the spine and movement of the ribs.

Normal End-feel

Glenohumeral Flexion

The end-feel is firm because of tension in the posterior band of the coracohumeral ligament and in the posterior joint capsule, and the and in the posterior deltoid, teres minor, teres major, and infraspinatus muscles.

Shoulder Complex Flexion

The end-feel is firm because of tension in the costoclavicular ligament and SC capsule and ligaments, and the latissimus dorsi, sternocostal fibers of the pectoralis major and pectoralis minor, and rhomboid major and minor muscles.

Goniometer Alignment

This goniometer alignment is used for measuring glenohumeral and shoulder complex flexion (Figs. 4–16 through 4–18).

1. Center the fulcrum of the goniometer over the lateral aspect of the greater tubercle.
2. Align the proximal arm parallel to the midaxillary line of the thorax.
3. Align the distal arm with the lateral midline of the humerus. Depending on how much flexion and medial rotation occur, the lateral epicondyle of the humerus or the olecranon process of the ulnar may be helpful references.

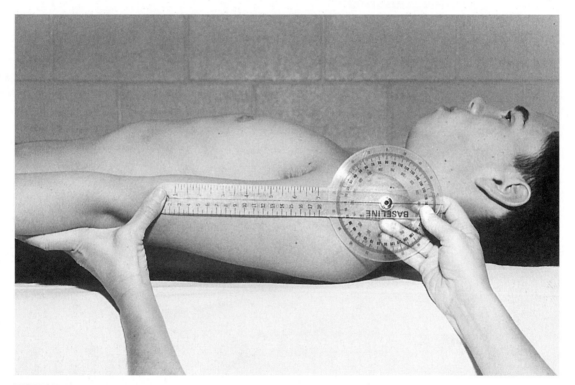

FIGURE 4–16   The alignment of the goniometer at the beginning of the ROM of glenohumeral and shoulder complex flexion.

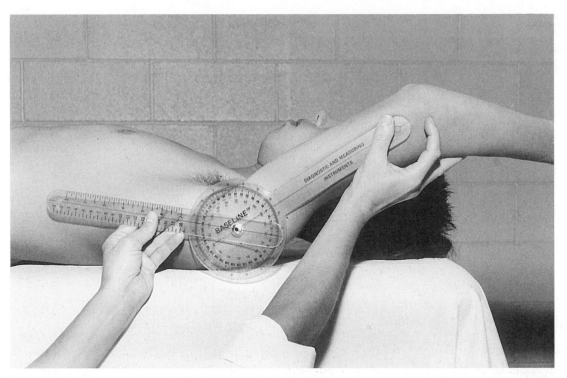

FIGURE 4–17 The alignment of the goniometer at the end of the ROM of glenohumeral flexion. The examiner's hand supports the subject's extremity and maintains the goniometer's distal arm in correct alignment over the lateral epicondyle. The examiner's other hand releases its stabilization and aligns the goniometer's proximal arm with the lateral midline of the thorax.

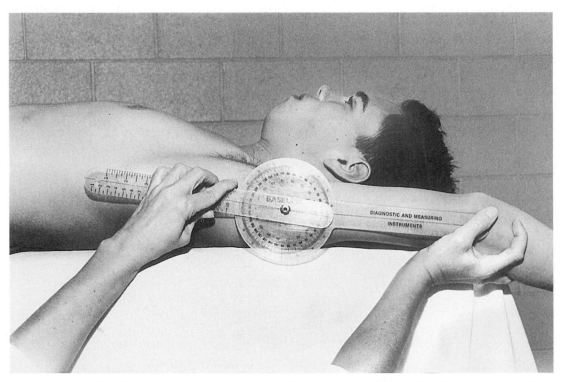

FIGURE 4–18 The alignment of the goniometer at the end of the ROM of shoulder complex flexion. More ROM is noted during shoulder complex flexion than in glenohumeral flexion.

EXTENSION

Motion occurs in the sagittal plane around a medial-lateral axis. Mean shoulder complex extension ROM is 62 degrees according to Boone and Azen,[7] 60 degrees according to the AAOS,[5] and 50 degrees according to the AMA.[6] Mean glenohumeral extension ROM is 20 degrees as cited by Lannan, Lehman, and Toland.[12] See Tables 4–1 to 4–4 for additional information.

Testing Position

Position the subject prone, with the face turned away from the shoulder being tested. A pillow is not used under the head. Place the shoulder in 0 degrees of abduction, adduction, and rotation. Position the elbow in slight flexion so that tension in the long head of the biceps brachii muscle will not restrict the motion. Place the forearm in 0 degrees of supination and pronation so that the palm of the hand faces the body.

Stabilization

Glenohumeral Extension

Stabilize the scapula at the inferior angle or at the acromion and coracoid processes to prevent elevation and anterior tilting (inferior angle moves posteriorly) of the scapula.

Shoulder Complex Extension

The examining table and the weight of the trunk stabilize the thorax to prevent forward flexion of the spine. The examiner can also stabilize the trunk to prevent rotation of the spine.

Testing Motion

Extend the shoulder by lifting the humerus off the examining table. Maintain the extremity in neutral abduction and adduction during the motion.

Glenohumeral Extension

The end of ROM occurs when resistance to further motion is felt and attempts to overcome the resistance cause anterior tilting or elevation of the scapula (Fig. 4–19).

Shoulder Complex Extension

The end of ROM occurs when resistance to further motion is felt and attempts to overcome the resistance cause forward flexion or rotation of the spine (Fig. 4–20).

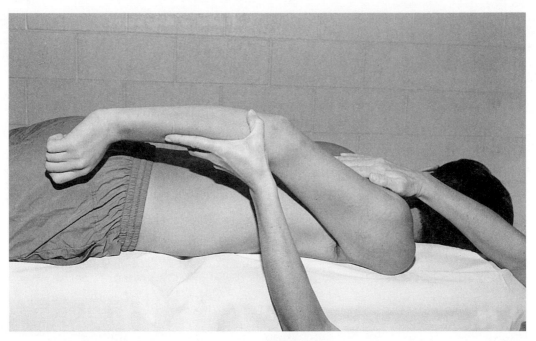

FIGURE 4–19 The end of the ROM of glenohumeral extension. The examiner is stabilizing the inferior angle of the scapula with her hand. The examiner is able to determine that the end of the ROM in extension has been reached because any attempt to move the humerus into additional extension causes scapula to tilt anteriorly and to elevate, causing the inferior angle of the scapula to move posteriorly. Alternatively, the examiner may stabilize the acromion and coracoid processes of the scapula.

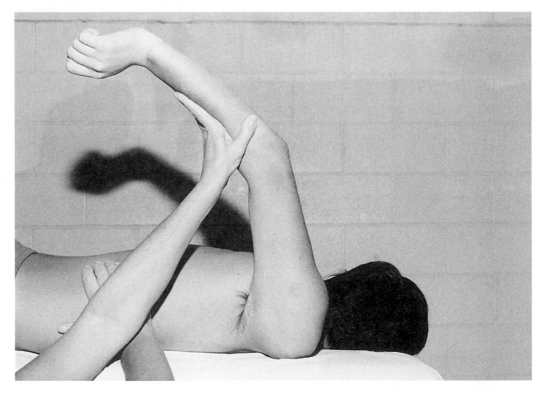

FIGURE 4–20 The end of the ROM of shoulder complex extension. The examiner stabilizes the subject's trunk and ribs with her hand. The examiner is able to determine that the end of the ROM has been reached because any attempt to move the extremity into additional extension causes flexion and rotation of the spine.

Normal End-feel

Glenohumeral Extension

The end-feel is firm because of tension in the anterior band of the coracohumeral ligament, anterior joint capsule, and clavicular fibers of the pectoralis major, coracobrachialis, and anterior deltoid muscles.

Shoulder Complex Extension

The end-feel is firm because of tension in the SC capsule and ligaments, and in the serratus anterior muscle.

Goniometer Alignment

This goniometer alignment is used for measuring glenohumeral and shoulder complex extension (Figs. 4–21 to 4–23).

1. Center the fulcrum of the goniometer over the lateral aspect of the greater tubercle.
2. Align the proximal arm parallel to the midaxillary line of the thorax.
3. Align the distal arm with the lateral midline of the humerus, using the lateral epicondyle of the humerus for reference.

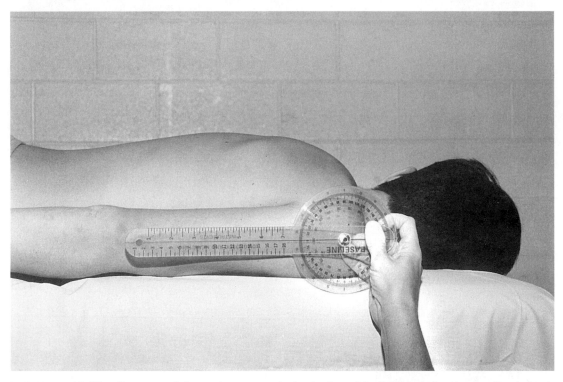

FIGURE 4–21 The alignment of the goniometer at the beginning of the ROM of glenohumeral and shoulder complex extension.

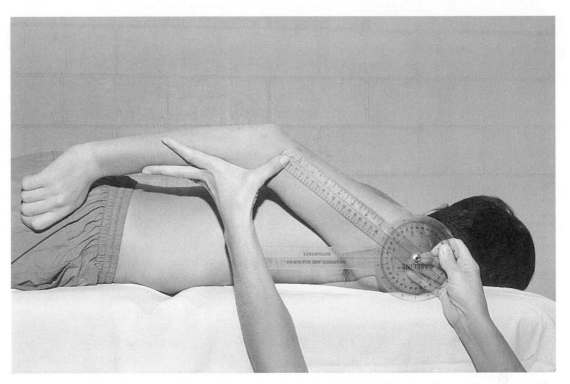

FIGURE 4–22 The alignment of the goniometer at the end of the ROM in glenohumeral extension. The examiner's left hand supports the subject's extremity and holds the distal arm of the goniometer in correct alignment over the lateral epicondyle of the humerus.

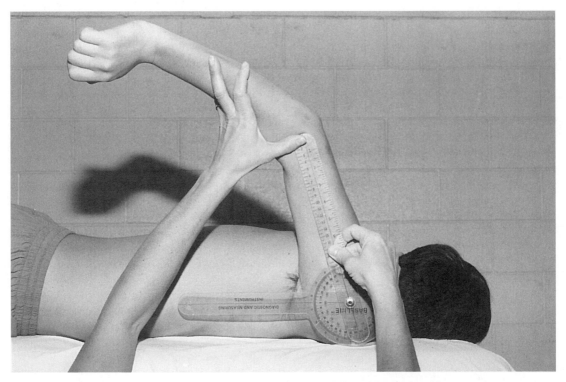

FIGURE 4–23 The alignment of the goniometer at the end of the ROM in shoulder complex extension. The examiner's hand that formerly stabilized the subject's trunk now positions the goniometer

ABDUCTION

Motion occurs in the frontal plane around an anterior-posterior axis. Mean shoulder complex abduction ROM is 180 degrees according to the AAOS[5] and AMA,[6] and 184 degrees according to Boone and Azen.[7] Glenohumeral abduction ROM is 129 degrees as noted by Lannan, Lehman, and Toland,[12] and 90 or 120 degrees according to Levangie and Norkin.[3] See Tables 4–1 to 4–4 for additional information.

Testing Position

Position the subject supine, with the shoulder in lateral rotation and 0 degrees of flexion and extension so that the palm of the hand faces anteriorly. If the humerus is not laterally rotated, contact between the greater tubercle of the humerus and the upper portion of the glenoid fossa or the acromion process will restrict the motion. The elbow should be extended so that tension in the long head of the triceps does not restrict the motion.

Stabilization

Glenohumeral Abduction

Stabilize the scapula to prevent upward rotation and elevation of the scapula.

Shoulder Complex Abduction

Stabilize the thorax to prevent lateral flexion of the spine. The weight of the trunk may assist stabilization.

Testing Motion

Abduct the shoulder by moving the humerus laterally away from the subject's trunk. Maintain the upper extremity in lateral rotation and neutral flexion and extension during the motion.

Glenohumeral Abduction

The end of ROM occurs when resistance to further motion is felt and attempts to overcome the resistance cause upward rotation or elevation of the scapula (Fig. 4–24).

Shoulder Complex Abduction

The end of ROM occurs when resistance to further motion is felt and attempts to overcome the resistance cause lateral flexion of the spine (Fig. 4–25).

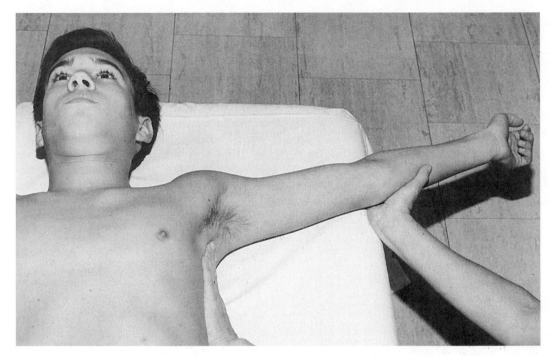

FIGURE 4–24 The end of the ROM of glenohumeral abduction. The examiner stabilizes the lateral border of the scapula with her hand to detect upward rotation of the scapula. Alternatively, the examiner may stabilize the acromion and coracoid processes of the scapula to detect elevation of the scapula.

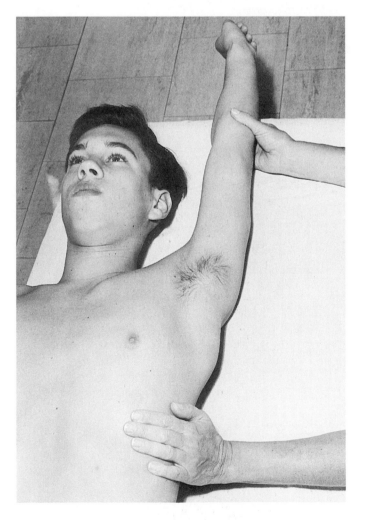

FIGURE 4–25 The end of the ROM of shoulder complex abduction. The examiner stabilizes the subject's trunk and ribs with her hand to detect lateral flexion of the spine and movement of the ribs.

Normal End-feel

Glenohumeral Abduction

The end-feel is usually firm because of tension in the middle and inferior bands of the glenohumeral ligament, inferior joint capsule, and the teres major, and clavicular fibers of the pectoralis major muscles.

Shoulder Complex Abduction

The end-feel is firm because of tension in the costoclavicular ligament, sternoclavicular capsule and ligaments, and latissimus dorsi, sternocostal fibers of the pectoralis major, and major and minor rhomboid muscles.

Goniometer Alignment

This goniometer alignment is used for measuring glenohumeral and shoulder complex abduction (Figs. 4–26 to 4–28).

1. Center the fulcrum of the goniometer close to the anterior aspect of the acromial process.
2. Align the proximal arm so that it is parallel to the midline of the anterior aspect of the sternum.
3. Align the distal arm with the anterior midline of the humerus. Depending on the amount of abduction and lateral rotation that has occurred, the medial epicondyle may be a helpful reference.

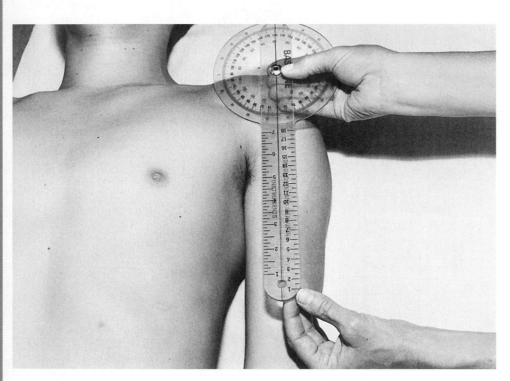

FIGURE 4–26 The alignment of the goniometer at the beginning of the ROM in glenohumeral and shoulder complex abduction.

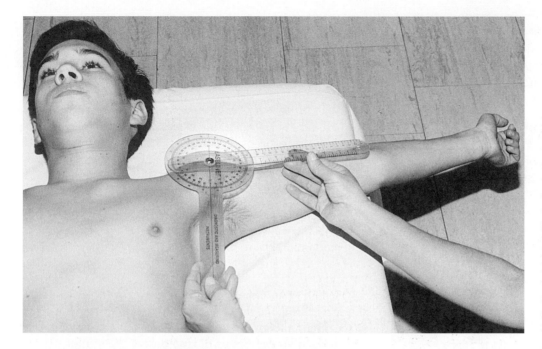

FIGURE 4–27 The alignment of the goniometer at the end of the ROM in glenohumeral abduction. The examining table or the examiner's hand can support the subject's extremity and align the goniometer's distal arm with the anterior midline of the humerus. The examiner's other hand has released its stabilization of the scapula and is holding the proximal arm of the goniometer parallel to the sternum.

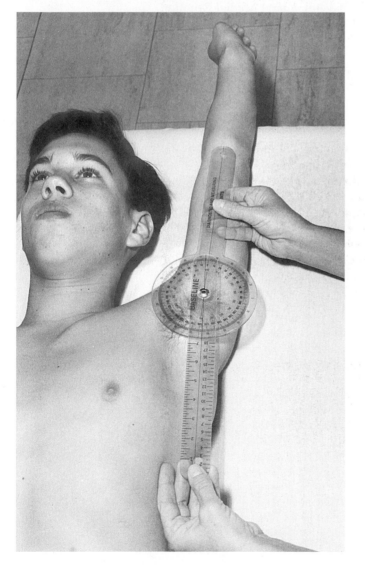

FIGURE 4–28 The alignment of the goniometer at the end of the ROM in shoulder complex abduction. Note that the humerus is laterally rotated and the medial epicondyle is a helpful anatomical landmark for aligning the distal arm of the goniometer.

ADDUCTION

Motion occurs in the frontal plane around an antero-posterior axis. Adduction is not usually measured and recorded because it is the return to the zero starting position from full abduction.

MEDIAL (INTERNAL) ROTATION

When the subject is in anatomical position, the motion occurs in the transverse plane around a vertical axis. When the subject is in the testing position, the motion occurs in the sagittal plane around a coronal axis. Mean shoulder complex medial rotation is 69 degrees according to Boone and Azen,[7] 70 degrees according to the AAOS,[5] and 90 degrees according to the AMA.[5] Mean glenohumeral medial rotation is 49 degrees according to Lannan, Lehman, and Toland,[12] 54 degrees according to Ellenbecker,[14] and 63 degrees according to Boon and Smith.[13] See Tables 4–1 to 4–4 for additional information.

Testing Position

Position the subject supine, with the arm being tested in 90 degrees of shoulder abduction. Place the forearm perpendicular to the supporting surface and in 0 degrees of supination and pronation so that the palm of the hand faces the feet. Rest the full length of the humerus on the examining table. The elbow is not supported by the examining table. Place a pad under the humerus so that the humerus is level with the acromion process.

Stabilization

Glenohumeral Medial Rotation

In the beginning of the ROM, stabilization is often needed at the distal end of the humerus to keep the shoulder in 90 degrees of abduction. Toward the end of the ROM, the clavicle and corocoid and acromion processes of the scapula are stabilized to prevent anterior tilting and protraction of the scapula.

Shoulder Complex Medial Rotation

Stabilization is often needed at the distal end of the humerus to keep the shoulder in 90 degrees of abduction. The thorax may be stabilized by the weight of the subject's trunk or with the examiner's hand to prevent flexion or rotation of the spine.

Testing Motion

Medially rotate the shoulder by moving the forearm anteriorly, bringing the palm of the hand toward the floor. Maintain the shoulder in 90 degrees of abduction and the elbow in 90 degrees of flexion during the motion.

Glenohumeral Medial Rotation

The end of ROM occurs when resistance to further motion is felt and attempts to overcome the resistance cause an anterior tilt or protraction of the scapula (Fig. 4–29).

Shoulder Complex Medial Rotation

The end of ROM occurs when resistance to further motion is felt and attempts to overcome the resistance cause flexion or rotation of the spine (Fig. 4–30).

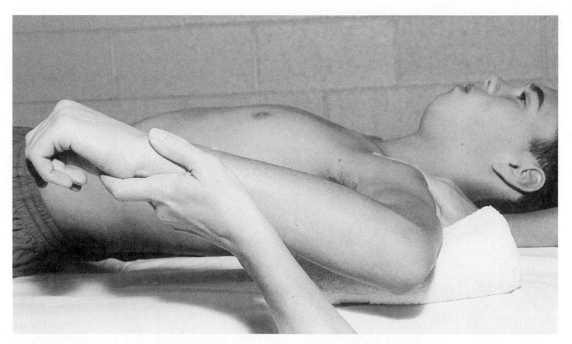

FIGURE 4–29 The end of the ROM of glenohumeral medial (internal) rotation. The examiner stabilizes the acromion and coracoid pro-cesses of the scapula. The examiner is able to determine that the end of the ROM has been reached because any attempt to move the extremity into additional medial rotation causes the scapula to tilt anteriorly or protract. The examiner should also maintain the shoulder in 90 degrees of abduction and the elbow in 90 degrees of flexion during the motion.

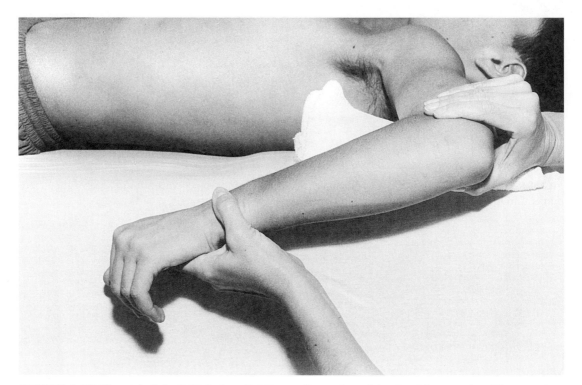

FIGURE 4–30 The end of the ROM of medial (internal) rotation of the shoulder complex. The examiner stabilizes the distal end of the humerus to maintain the shoulder in 90 degrees of abduction and the elbow in 90 degrees of flexion during the motion. Resistance is noted at the end of medial rotation of the shoulder complex because attempts to move the extremity into further motion cause the spine to flex or rotate. The clavicle and scapula are allowed to move as they participate in shoulder complex motions.

Normal End-Feel

Glenohumeral Medial Rotation

The end-feel is firm because of tension in the posterior joint capsule and the infraspinatus and teres minor muscles.

Shoulder Complex Medial Rotation

The end-feel is firm because of tension in the sternoclavicular capsule and ligaments, the costoclavicular ligament, and the major and minor rhomboid and trapezius muscles.

Goniometer Alignment

This goniometer alignment is used for measuring glenohumeral and shoulder complex medial rotation (Figs. 4–31 to 4–33).

1. Center the fulcrum of the goniometer over the olecranon process.
2. Align the proximal arm so that it is either perpendicular to or parallel with the floor.
3. Align the distal arm with the ulna, using the olecranon process and ulnar styloid for reference.

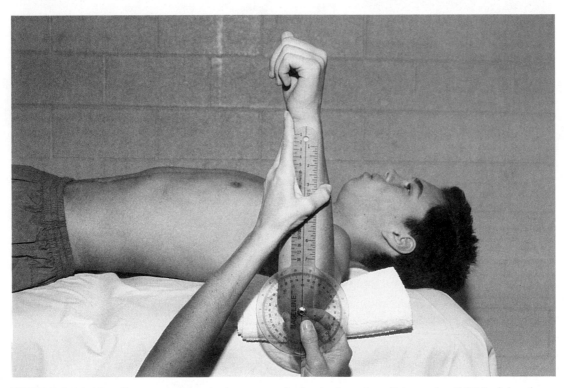

FIGURE 4–31 The alignment of the goniometer at the beginning of medial rotation ROM of the glenohumeral joint and shoulder complex.

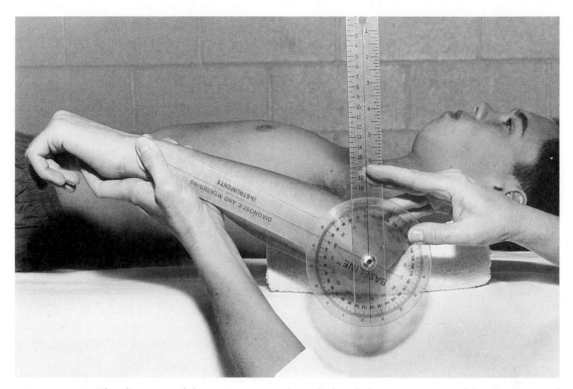

FIGURE 4–32 The alignment of the goniometer at the end of medial rotation ROM of the glenohumeral joint. The examiner uses one hand to support the subject's forearm and the distal arm of the goniometer. The examiner's other hand holds the body and the proximal arm of the goniometer.

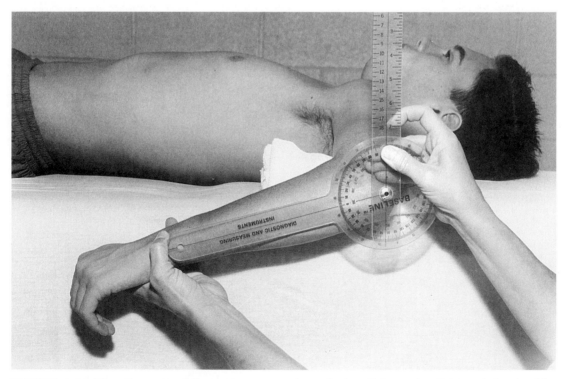

FIGURE 4–33 The alignment of the goniometer at the end of medial rotation ROM of the shoulder complex.

LATERAL (EXTERNAL) ROTATION

When the subject is in anatomical position, the motion occurs in the transverse plane around a vertical axis. When the subject is in the testing position, the motion occurs in the sagittal plane around a coronal axis. Mean shoulder complex lateral rotation is 90 degrees according to the AAOS[5] and AMA[6] and 104 degrees according to Boone and Azen.[7] Mean glenohumeral medial rotation is 94 degrees according to Lannan, Lehman, and Toland,[12] 104 degrees according to Ellenbecker,[14] and 108 degrees according to Boon and Smith.[13] See Tables 4–1 to 4–4 for additional information.

Testing Position

Position the subject supine, with the arm being tested in 90 degrees of shoulder abduction. Place the forearm perpendicular to the supporting surface and in 0 degrees of supination and pronation so that the palm of the hand faces the feet. Rest the full length of the humerus on the examining table. The elbow is not supported by the examining table. Place a pad under the humerus so that the humerus is level with the acromion process.

Stabilization

Glenohumeral Lateral Rotation

At the beginning of the ROM, stabilization is often needed at the distal end of the humerus to keep the shoulder in 90 degrees of abduction. Toward the end of the ROM, the spine of the scapula is stabilized to prevent posterior tilting and retraction.

Shoulder Complex Lateral Rotation

Stabilization is often needed at the distal end of the humerus to keep the shoulder in 90 degrees of abduction. To prevent extension or rotation of the spine, the thorax may be stabilized by the weight of the subject's trunk or by the examiner's hand.

Testing Motion

Rotate the shoulder laterally by moving the forearm posteriorly, bringing the dorsal surface of the palm of the hand toward the floor. Maintain the shoulder in 90 degrees of abduction and the elbow in 90 degrees of flexion during the motion.

Glenohumeral Lateral Rotation

The end of ROM occurs when resistance to further motion is felt and attempts to overcome the resistance cause a posterior tilt or retraction of the scapula (Fig. 4–34).

Shoulder Complex Lateral Rotation

The end of ROM occurs when resistance to further motion is felt and attempts to overcome the resistance cause extension or rotation of the spine (Fig. 4–35).

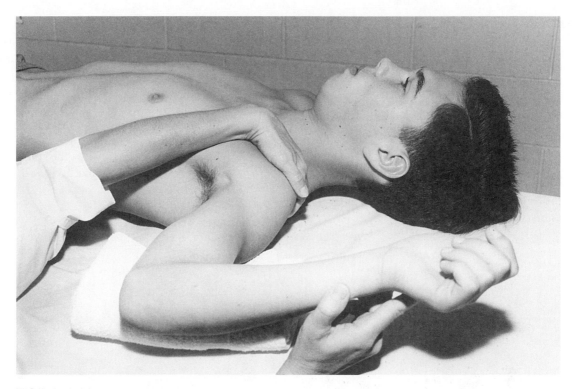

FIGURE 4–34 The end of lateral rotation ROM of the glenohumeral joint. The examiner's hand stabilizes the spine of the scapula. The end of the ROM in lateral rotation is reached when additional motion causes the scapula to posteriorly tilt or retract and push against the examiner's hand.

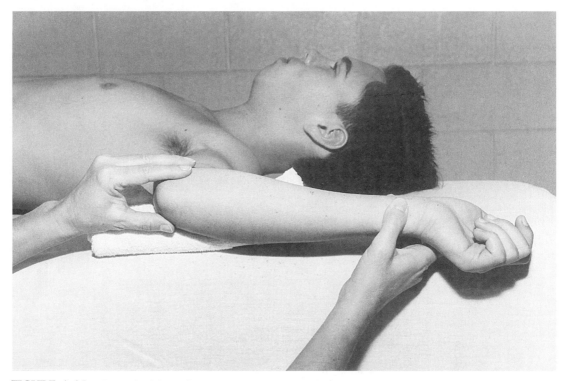

FIGURE 4–35 The end of lateral rotation ROM of the shoulder complex. The examiner stabilizes the distal humerus to prevent shoulder abduction beyond 90 degrees. The elbow is maintained in 90 degrees of flexion during the motion.

Normal End-feel

Glenohumeral Lateral Rotation

The end-feel is firm because of tension in the anterior joint capsule, the three bands of the glenohumeral ligament, and the coracohumeral ligament, as well as in the subscapularis, the teres major, and the clavicular fibers of the pectoralis major muscles.

Shoulder Complex Lateral Rotation

The end-feel is firm because of tension in the SC capsule and ligaments and in the latissimus dorsi, sternocostal fibers of the pectoralis major, pectoralis minor, and serratus anterior muscles.

Goniometer Alignment

This goniometer alignment is used for measuring glenohumeral and shoulder complex lateral rotation (Figs. 4–36 to 4–38).

1. Center the fulcrum of the goniometer over the olecranon process.
2. Align the proximal arm so that it is either parallel to or perpendicular to the floor.
3. Align the distal arm with the ulna, using the olecranon process and ulnar styloid for reference.

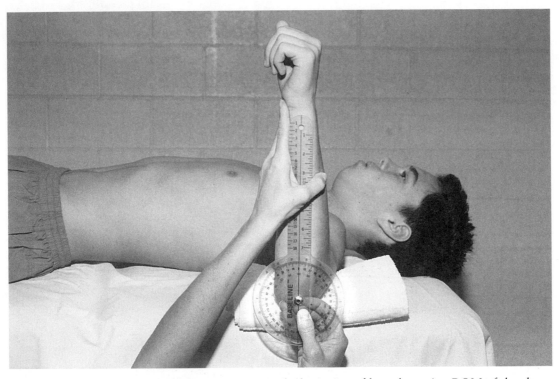

FIGURE 4–36 The alignment of the goniometer at the beginning of lateral rotation ROM of the glenohumeral joint and shoulder complex.

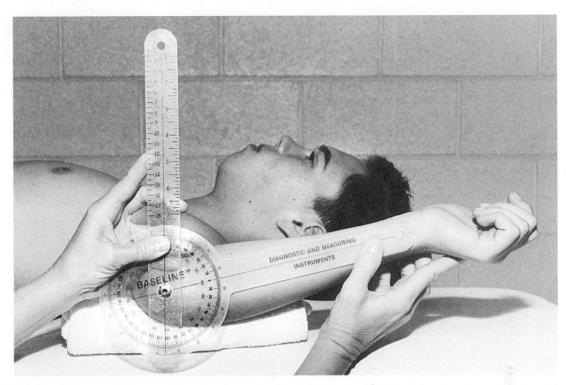

FIGURE 4–37 The alignment of the goniometer at the end of lateral rotation ROM of the glenohumeral joint. The examiner's hand supports the subject's forearm and the distal arm of the goniometer. The examiner's other hand holds the body and proximal arm of the goniometer. The placement of the examiner's hands would be reversed if the subject's right shoulder were being tested.

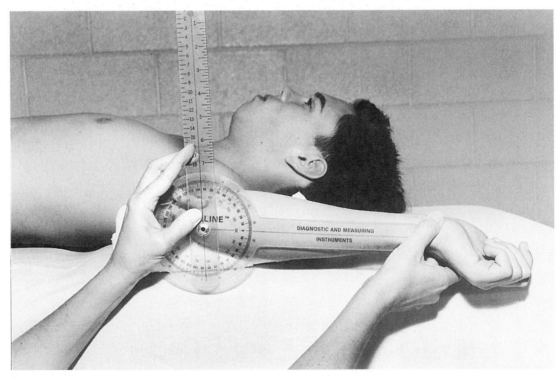

FIGURE 4–38 The alignment of the goniometer at the end of lateral rotation ROM of the shoulder complex.

REFERENCES

1. Cyriax, JH, and Cyriax, PJ: Illustrated Manual of Orthopaedic Medicine. Butterworths, London, 1983.
2. Culham, E, and Peat, M: Functional anatomy of the shoulder complex. J Orthop Sports Phys Ther 18:342, 1993.
3. Levangie, P, and Norkin, C: Joint Structure and Function: A Comprehensive Analysis, ed 3. FA Davis, Philadelphia, 2001.
4. Kaltenborn, FM: Manual Mobilization of the Extremity Joints, ed 5. Olaf Norlis Bokhandel, Oslo,1999.
5. American Academy of Orthopaedic Surgeons: Joint Motion: Method of Measuring and Recording. AAOS, Chicago, 1965.
6. American Medical Association: Guides to the Evaluation of Permanent Impairment, ed 3. AMA, Chicago, 1988.
7. Boone, DC, and Azen, SP: Normal range of motion in male subjects. J Bone Joint Surg Am 61:756, 1979.
8. Greene, BL, and Wolf, SL: Upper extremity joint movement: Comparison of two measurement devices. Arch Phys Med Rehabil 70:288, 1989.
9. Soderberg, GL: Kinesiology: Application to Pathological Motion. Williams & Wilkins, Baltimore, 1986.
10. Doody, SG, Freedman, L, and Waterland, JC: Shoulder movements during abduction in the scapular plane. Arch Phys Med Rehabil 51:595, 1970.
11. Poppen, NK, and Walker, PS: Forces at the glenohumeral joint in abduction. Clin Orthop 135:165, 1978.
12. Lannan, D, Lehman, T, and Toland, M: Establishment of normative data for the range of motion of the glenohumeral joint. Master of Science Thesis, University of Massachusetts Lowell, 1996.
13. Boon, AJ, and Smith, J: Manual scapular stabilization: Its effect on shoulder rotational range of motion. Arch Phys Med Rehabil 81:978, 2000.
14. Ellenbecker, TS, et al: Glenohumeral joint internal and external rotation range of motion in elite junior tennis players. J Orthop Sports Phys Ther 24:336, 1996.
15. Wanatabe, H, et al: The range of joint motions of the extremities in healthy Japanese people: The difference according to age. Nippon Seikeigeka Gakkai Zasshi 53:275, 1979. Cited by Walker, JM: Musculoskeletal development: A review. Phys Ther 71:878, 1991.
16. Boone, DC: Techniques of measurement of joint motion. (Unpublished supplement to Boone, DC, and Azen, SP: Normal range of motion in male subjects. J Bone Joint Surg Am 61:756, 1979.)
17. Walker, JM, et al: Active mobility of the extremities in older subjects. Phys Ther 64:919, 1984.
18. Downey, PA, Fiebert, I, and Stackpole-Brown, JB: Shoulder range of motion in persons aged sixty and older [abstract]. Phys Ther 71:S75, 1991.
19. West, CC: Measurement of joint motion. Arch Phys Med Rehabil 26:414, 1945.
20. Clarke, GR, et al: Preliminary studies in measuring range of motion in normal and painful stiff shoulders. Rheumatol Rehabil 14:39, 1975.
21. Allander, E, et al: Normal range of joint movement in shoulder, hip, wrist and thumb with special reference to side: A comparison between two populations. Int J Epidemiol 3:253, 1974.
22. Escalante, A, Lichenstein, MJ, and Hazuda, HP: Determinants of shoulder and elbow flexion range: Results from the San Antonio longitudinal study of aging. Arthritis Care Res 12:277, 1999.
23. Kebaetse, M, McClure, P, and Pratt, NA: Thoracic position effect on shoulder range of motion, strength, and three-dimensional scapular kinematics. Arch Phys Med Rehabil 80:945, 1999.
24. Sabari, JS, et al: Goniometric assessment of shoulder range of motion: Comparison of testing in supine and sitting positions. Arch Phys Med Rehabil 79:64, 1998.
25. Bigliani, LU, et al: Shoulder motion and laxity in the professional baseball player. Am J Sports Med 25:609, 1997.
26. Baltaci, G, Johnson, R, and Kohl H: Shoulder range of motion characteristics in collegiate baseball players. J Sports Med Phys Fitness 41:236, 2001.
27. Chinn, CJ, Priest, JD, and Kent, BA: Upper extremity range of motion, grip strength and girth in highly skilled tennis players. Phys Ther 54:474, 1974.
28. Kibler, WB, et al: Shoulder range of motion in elite tennis players: Effect of age and years of tournament play. Am J Sports Med 24:279, 1996.
29. Chang, DE, Buschbacker, LP, and Edlich, RF: Limited joint mobility in power lifters. Am J Sports Med 16:280, 1988.
30. Tiffitt, PD: The relationship between motion of the shoulder and the stated ability to perform activities of daily living. J Bone Joint Surg 80:41, 1998.
31. Matsen, FA, et al: Practical Evaluation and Management of the Shoulder. WB Saunders, Philadelphia, 1994.
32. Safaee-Rad, R, et al: Normal functional range of motion of upper limb joints during performance of three feeding activities. Arch Phys Med Rehabil 71:505, 1990.
33. Hellebrandt, FA, Duvall, EN, and Moore, ML: The measurement of joint motion. Part III: Reliability of goniometry. Phys Ther Rev 29:302, 1949.
34. Boone, DC, et al: Reliability of goniometric measurements. Phys Ther 58:1355, 1978.
35. Pandya, S, et al: Reliability of goniometric measurements in patients with Duchenne muscular dystrophy. Phys Ther 65:1339, 1985.
36. Riddle, DL, Rothstein, JM, and Lamb, RL: Goniometric reliability in a clinical setting: Shoulder measurements. Phys Ther 67:668, 1987.
37. Bovens, AMP, et al: Variability and reliability of joint measurements. Am J Sports Med 18:58, 1990.
38. MacDermid, JC, et al: Intratester and intertester reliability of goniometric measurement of passive lateral shoulder rotation. J Hand Ther 12:187, 1999.
39. Green, A, et al: A standardized protocol for measurement of range of movement of the shoulder using the Plurimeter-V inclinometer and assessment of its intrarater and interrater reliability. Arthritis Care Res 11:43, 1998.
40. Tiffitt, PD, Wildin, C, and Hajioff, D: The reproducibility of measurement of shoulder movement. Acta Orthop Scand 70:322, 1999.
41. Bower, KD: The hydrogoniometer and assessment of glenohumeral joint motion. Aust J Physiother 28:12, 1982.
42. Croft, P, et al: Observer variability in measuring elevation and external rotation of the shoulder. Br J Rheumatol 33:942, 1994.

CHAPTER 5

The Elbow and Forearm

⬤ Structure and Function

Humeroulnar and Humeroradial Joints

Anatomy

The humeroulnar and humeroradial joints between the upper arm and the forearm are considered to be a hinged compound synovial joint (Figs. 5–1 and 5–2). The proximal joint surface of the humeroulnar joint consists of the convex trochlea located on the anterior medial surface of the distal humerus. The distal joint surface is the concave trochlear notch on the proximal ulna.

The proximal joint surface of the humeroradial joint is the convex capitulum located on the anterior lateral surface of the distal humerus. The concave radial head on the proximal end of the radius is the opposing joint surface.

The joints are enclosed in a large, loose, weak joint capsule that also encloses the superior radioulnar joint. Medial and lateral collateral ligaments reinforce the sides of the capsule and help to provide medial-lateral stability (Figs. 5–3 and 5–4).[1]

When the arm is in the anatomical position, the long axes of the humerus and the forearm form an acute angle

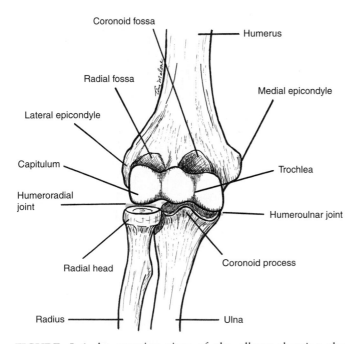

FIGURE 5–1 An anterior view of the elbow showing the humeroulnar and humeroradial joints.

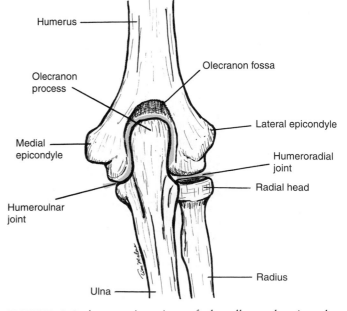

FIGURE 5–2 A posterior view of the elbow showing the humeroulnar and humeroradial joints.

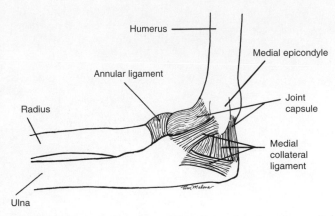

FIGURE 5–3 A medial view of the elbow showing the medial (ulnar) collateral ligament, annular ligament, and joint capsule.

at the elbow. The angle is called the "carrying angle." This angle is about 5 degrees in men and approximately 10 to 15 degrees in women.[2] An angle that is greater (more acute) than average is called "cubitus valgus." An angle that is less than average is called "cubitus varus."

Osteokinematics

The humeroulnar and humeroradial joints have 1 degree of freedom; flexion-extension occurs in the sagittal plane around a medial-lateral (coronal) axis. In elbow flexion and extension, the axis of rotation lies approximately through the center of the trochlea.[3]

Arthrokinematics

At the humeroulnar joint, posterior sliding of the concave trochlear notch of the ulna on the convex trochlea of the humerus continues during extension until the ulnar olecranon process enters the humeral olecranon fossa. In flexion, the ulna slides anteriorly along the humerus until the coronoid process of the ulna reaches the floor of the

coronoid fossa of the humerus or until soft tissue in the anterior aspect of the elbow blocks further flexion.

At the humeroradial joint, the concave radial head slides posteriorly on the convex surface of the capitulum during extension. In flexion, the radial head slides anteriorly until the rim of the radial head enters the radial fossa of the humerus.

Capsular Pattern

The capsular pattern is variable, but usually the range of motion (ROM) in flexion is more limited than in extension. For example, 30 degrees of limitation in flexion would correspond to 10 degrees of limitation in extension.[4]

Superior and Inferior Radioulnar Joints

Anatomy

The ulnar portion of the superior radioulnar joint includes both the radial notch located on the lateral aspect of the proximal ulna and the annular ligament (Fig. 5–5). The radial notch and the annular ligament

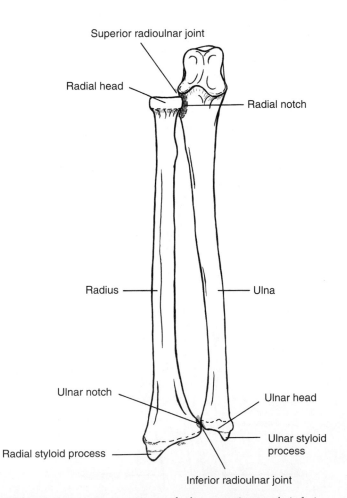

FIGURE 5–5 Anterior view of the superior and inferior radioulnar joints.

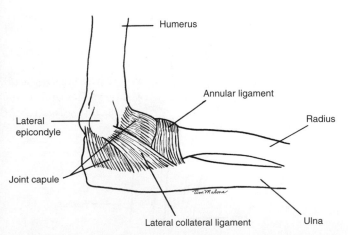

FIGURE 5–4 A lateral view of the elbow showing the lateral (radial) collateral ligament, annular ligament, and joint capsule.

form a concave joint surface. The radial aspect of the joint is the convex head of the radius.

The ulnar component of the inferior radioulnar joint is the convex ulnar head (see Fig. 5–5). The opposing articular surface is the ulnar notch of the radius.

The interosseous membrane, a broad sheet of collagenous tissue linking the radius and ulna, provides stability for both joints (Fig. 5–6). The following three structures provide stability for the superior radioulnar joint: the annular and quadrate ligaments and the oblique cord. Stability of the inferior radioulnar joint is provided by the articular disc and the anterior and posterior radioulnar ligaments (Fig. 5–7).[1]

Osteokinematics

The superior and inferior radioulnar joints are mechanically linked. Therefore, motion at one joint is always accompanied by motion at the other joint. The axis for motion is a longitudinal axis extending from the radial

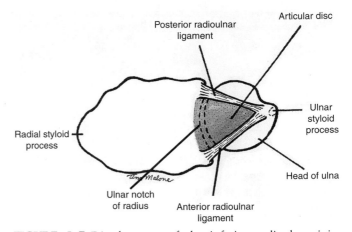

FIGURE 5–7 Distal aspect of the inferior radioulnar joint showing the\ articular disc and radioulnar ligaments.

head to the ulnar head. The mechanically linked joint is a synovial pivot joint with 1 degree of freedom. The motions permitted are pronation and supination. In pronation the radius crosses over the ulna, whereas in supination the radius and ulna lie parallel to one another.

Arthrokinematics

At the superior radioulnar joint the convex rim of the head of the radius spins within the annular ligament and the concave radial notch during pronation and supination. The articular surface on the head of the radius spins posteriorly during pronation and anteriorly during supination.

At the inferior radioulnar joint the concave surface of the ulnar notch on the radius slides over the ulnar head. The concave articular surface of the radius slides anteriorly (in the same direction as the hand) during pronation and slides posteriorly (in the same direction as the hand) during supination.

Capsular Pattern

According to Cyriax and Cyriax,[4] Kaltenborn,[5] and Magee,[6] the capsular pattern is equal limitation of pronation and supination.

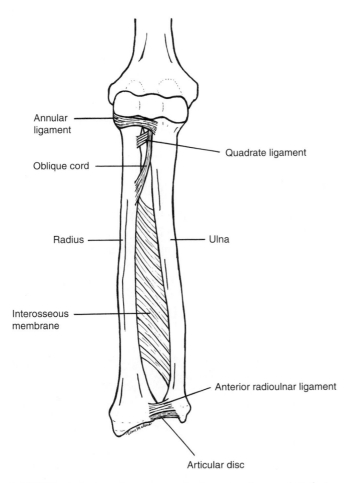

FIGURE 5–6 Anterior view of the superior and inferior radioulnar joints showing the annular ligament, quadrate ligament, oblique cord, interosseous membrane, anterior radioulnar ligament, and articular disc.

TABLE 5–1	Elbow and Forearm Motion: Mean Values in Degrees from Selected Sources				
	AAOS[7,8]	AMA[9]	Boone & Azen[10] $n = 109$*	Greene & Wolf[11] $n = 20$†	Petherick et al[12] $n = 30$‡
Motion			Mean (SD)	Mean (SD)	Mean (SD)
Flexion	150	140	142.9 (5.6)	145.3 (1.2)	145.8 (6.3)
Extension	0	0	0.6 (3.1)		
Pronation	80	80	75.8 (5.1)	84.4 (2.2)	
Supination	80	80	82.1 (3.8)	76.9 (2.1)	

* Values are for males 18 months to 54 years of age.

† Values are for 10 males and 10 females, 18 to 55 years of age.

‡ Values are for 10 males and 20 females, with a mean age of 24.0 years.

◗ Research Findings

Effects of Age, Gender, and Other Factors

Table 5–1 shows the mean values of ROM for various motions at the elbow. The age, gender, and number of subjects that were measured to obtain the values reported by the American Academy of Orthopaedic Surgeons (AAOS)[7,8] and the American Medical Association (AMA)[9] in Table 5–1 were not noted. Boone and Azen,[10] using a universal goniometer, measured active ROM in 109 males between the ages of 18 months and 54 years. Greene and Wolf[11] measured active ROM with a universal goniometer in 10 males and 10 females aged 18 to 55 years. Petherick and associates[12] measured active ROM with a universal goniometer in 10 males and 20 females with a mean age of 24.0 years. In addition to the sources listed in Table 5–1, Goodwin and coworkers[13] found mean active elbow flexion to be 148.9 degrees when measured with a universal goniometer in 23 females between 18 and 31 years of age.

Age

A comparison of cross-sectional studies of normative ROM values for various age groups suggests that elbow and forearm ROM decreases slightly with age. Tables 5–2 and 5–3 summarize the effects of age on ROM of the elbow and forearm. The male and female infants reported in the study by Wanatabe and colleagues[14] had more ROM in flexion, pronation, and supination than the older males in studies by Boone[15] and by Walker and coworkers.[16] However, it can be difficult to compare values obtained from various studies because subject selection and measurement methods can differ.

Within one study of 109 males ranging in age from 18 months to 54 years, Boone and Azen[10] noted a significant difference in elbow flexion and supination between subjects less than or equal to 19 years of age and those greater than 19 years of age. Further analyses found that the group between 6 and 12 years of age had more elbow flexion and extension than other age groups. The youngest group (between 18 months and 5 years) had a significantly greater amount of pronation and supination than other age groups. However, the greatest differences between the age groups were small: 6.8 degrees of flexion, 4.4 degrees of supination, 3.9 degrees of pronation, and 2.5 degrees of extension.[15]

Older persons appear to have difficulty fully extending their elbows to 0 degrees. Walker and associates[16] found that the older men and women (between 60 and 84 years of age) in their study were unable to extend their elbows to 0 degrees to attain a neutral starting position for flexion. The mean value for the starting position was 6 degrees in men and 1 degree in women. Boone and

TABLE 5–2	Effects of Age on Elbow and Forearm Motion: Mean Values in Degrees for Newborns, Children, and Adolescents 2 Weeks to 19 Years of Age			
	Wanatabe et al[14]	Boone[15]		
	2 wks–2 yrs $n = 45$	18 mos–5 yrs $n = 19$	6–12 yrs $n = 17$	13–19 yrs $n = 17$
Motion	Range of Means	Mean (SD)	Mean (SD)	Mean (SD)
Flexion	148–158	144.9 (5.7)	146.5 (4.0)	144.9 (6.0)
Extension		0.4 (3.4)	2.1 (3.2)	0.1 (3.8)
Pronation	90–96	78.9 (4.4)	76.9 (3.6)	74.1 (5.3)
Supination	81–93	84.5 (3.8)	82.9 (2.7)	81.8 (3.2)

TABLE 5–3 Effects of Age on Elbow and Forearm Motion: Mean Values in Degrees for Adults 20 to 85 Years of Age				
	Boone[15]			Walker et al[16]
	20–29 yrs n = 19	30–39 yrs n = 18	40–54 yrs n = 19	60–85 yrs n = 30
Motion	Mean (SD)	Mean (SD)	Mean (SD)	Mean (SD)
Flexion	140.1 (5.2)	141.7 (3.2)	139.7 (5.8)	139.0 (14.0)
Extension	0.7 (3.2)	0.7 (1.7)	−0.4* (3.0)	−6.0* (5.0)
Pronation	76.2 (3.9)	73.6 (4.3)	75.0 (7.0)	68.0 (9.0)
Supination	80.1 (3.7)	81.7 (4.2)	81.4 (4.0)	83.0 (11.0)

* The minus sign indicates flexion.

Azen[10] also found that the oldest subjects in their study (between 40 and 54 years of age) had lost elbow extension and began flexion from a slightly flexed position. Bergstrom and colleagues,[17] in a study of 52 women and 37 men aged 79 years, found that 11 percent had flexion contractures of the right elbow greater than 5 degrees, and 7 percent had bilateral flexion contractures.

Gender

Studies seem to concur that gender differences exist for elbow flexion and extension ROM but these studies are unclear concerning forearm supination and pronation ROM. Bell and Hoshizaki,[18] using a Leighton Flexometer, studied the ROM of 124 females and 66 males between the ages of 18 and 88 years. Females had significantly more elbow flexion than males. Extrapolating from a graph, the mean differences between males and females ranged from 14 degrees in subjects aged 32 to 44 years, to 2 degrees in subjects older than 75 years. Although females had greater supination-pronation ROM than males, this increase was not significant. Fairbanks, Pynsent, and Phillips,[19] in a study of 446 normal adolescents, found that females had significantly more elbow extension (8 degrees) than males (5 degrees) when measured on the extensor aspect with a universal goniometer. It is unclear from the method used whether hyperextension of the elbow or the carrying angle was measured. Salter and Darcus,[20] measuring forearm supination-pronation with a specialized arthrometer in 20 males and 5 females between the ages of 16 and 29 years, found that the females had an average of 8 degrees more forearm rotation than males, although the difference was not statistically significant. Thirty older females and 30 older males, aged 60 to 84 years, were included in a study by Walker and coworkers.[16] Females had significantly more flexion ROM (1 to 148 degrees) than males (5 to 139 degrees), but males had significantly more supination (83 degrees) than females (65 degrees). Females had more pronation ROM than males, but the difference was not significant.

Escalante, Lichenstein, and Hazuda,[21] in a study of 695 community-dwelling older subjects between 65 and 74 years of age, found that females had an average of 4 degrees more elbow flexion than males.

Body-Mass Index

Body-mass index (BMI) was found by Escalante, Lichenstein, and Hazuda[21] to be inversely associated with elbow flexion in 695 older subjects. Each unit increase in BMI (kg/m²) was significantly associated with a 0.22 decrease in degrees of elbow flexion.

Right versus Left Side

Comparisons between the right and the left or between the dominant and the nondominant limbs have found no clinically relevant differences in elbow and forearm ROM. Boone and Azen[10] studied 109 males between the ages of 18 months and 54 years, who were subdivided into six age groups. They found no significant differences between right and left elbow flexion, extension, supination, and pronation, except for the age group of subjects between 20 and 29 years of age, whose flexion ROM was greater on the left than on the right. This one significant finding was attributed to chance. Escalante, Lichenstein, and Hazudal,[21] in a study of 695 older subjects, found significantly greater elbow flexion on the left than on the right, but the difference averaged only 2 degrees. Chang, Buschbacher, and Edlich[22] studied 10 power lifters and 10 age-matched nonlifters, all of whom were right handed, and found no differences between sides in elbow and forearm ROM.

Sports

It appears that the frequent use of the upper extremities in sport activities may reduce elbow and forearm ROM. Possible causes for this association include muscle hypertrophy, muscle tightness, and joint trauma from overuse. Chinn, Priest, and Kent,[23] in a study of 53 male and 30 female national and international tennis players, found significantly less active pronation and supination ROM in the playing arms of all subjects. Male players also

TABLE 5–4   Elbow and Forearm Motion During Functional Activities: Mean Values in Degrees

Activity	Flexion			Pronation	Supination		Source
	Min	Max	Arc	Max	Max	Arc	
Use telephone	42.8	135.6	92.8	40.9	22.6	63.5	Morrey[24]
	75	140	65				Packer[25]
Rise from chair	20.3	94.5	74.2	33.8	−9.5*	24.3	Morrey
	15	100	85				Packer
Open door	24.0	57.4	33.4	35.4	23.4	58.8	Morrey
Read newspaper	77.9	104.3	26.4	48.8	−7.3*	41.5	Morrey
Pour pitcher	35.6	58.3	22.7	42.9	21.9	64.8	Morrey
Put glass to mouth	44.8	130.0	85.2	10.1	13.4	23.5	Morrey
Drink from cup	71.5	129.2	57.7	−3.4†	31.2	27.8	Safaee-Rad[26]
Cut with knife	89.2	106.7	17.5	41.9	−26.9*	15.0	Morrey
Eat with fork	85.1	128.3	43.2	10.4	51.8	62.2	Morrey
	93.8	122.3	28.5	38.2	58.8	97.0	Safaee-Rad
Eat with spoon	101.2	123.2	22.0	22.9	58.7	81.6	Safaee-Rad
	70	115	45				Packer

* The minus sign indicates pronation.
† The minus sign indicates supination.

demonstrated a significant decrease (4.1 degrees) in elbow extension in the playing arm versus the nonplaying arm. Chang, Buschbacher, and Edlich[22] studied 10 power lifters and 10 age-matched nonlifters and found significantly less active elbow flexion in the power lifters than in the nonlifters. No significant differences were found between the two groups for supination and pronation ROM.

Functional Range of Motion

The amount of elbow and forearm motion that occurs during activities of daily living has been studied by several investigators. Table 5–4 has been adapted from the works of Morrey and associates,[24] Packer and colleagues,[25] and Safaee-Rad and coworkers.[26] Morrey and associates[24] used a triaxial electrogoniometer to measure elbow and forearm motion in 33 normal subjects during performance of 15 activities. They concluded that most of activities of daily living that were studied required a total arc of about 100 degrees of elbow flexion (between 30 and 130 degrees) and 100 degrees of rotation (50 degrees of supination and 50 degrees of pronation). Using a telephone necessitated the greatest total ROM. The greatest amount of flexion was required to reach the back of the head (144 degrees), whereas feeding tasks such as drinking from a cup (Fig. 5–8) and eating with a fork required about 130 degrees of flexion. Reaching the shoes and rising from a chair (Fig. 5–9) required the greatest amount of extension (between 16 and 20 degrees of elbow flexion). Among the tasks studied, the greatest amount of supination was needed for eating with a fork. Reading a newspaper (Fig. 5–10), pouring from a pitcher, and cutting with a knife required the most pronation.

Five healthy subjects participated in a study by Packer and colleagues,[25] which examined elbow ROM during three functional tasks. A uniaxial electrogoniometer was used to determine ROM required for using a telephone, for rising from a chair to a standing position, and for eating with a spoon. A range of 15 to 140 degrees of flexion was needed for these three activities. This ROM is slightly greater than the arc reported by Morrey and associates, but the activities that required the minimal and maximal flexion angles did not differ. The authors suggest that the height of the chair, the type of chair arms, and the positioning of the telephone could account for the different ranges found in the studies.

Safaee-Rad and coworkers[26] used a three-dimensional video system to measure ROM during three feeding activities: eating with a spoon, eating with a fork, and drinking from a handled cup. Ten healthy males participated in the study. The feeding activities required approximately 70 to 130 degrees of elbow flexion, 40 degrees of pronation, and 60 degrees of supination. Drinking with a cup required the greatest arc of elbow flexion (58 degrees) of the three activities, whereas eating with a spoon required the least (22 degrees). Eating with a fork required the greatest arc of pronation-supination (97 degrees), whereas drinking from a cup required the least (28 degrees). Maximum ROM values during feeding tasks were comparable with those reported by Morrey and associates. However, minimum values varied, possibly owing to the different chair and table heights used in the two studies.

Several investigators have taken a different approach in determining the amount of elbow and forearm motion needed for activities of daily living. Vasen and associates[27] studied the ability of 50 healthy adults to comfortably complete 12 activities of daily living while their

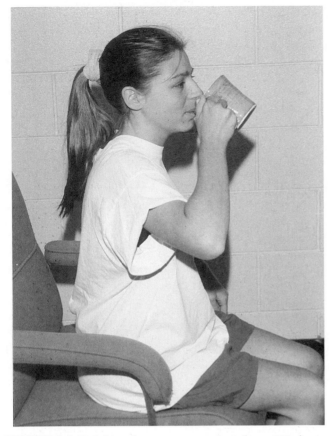

FIGURE 5–8 Drinking from a cup requires about 130 degrees of elbow flexion.

In a study published in 1949 by Hellebrandt, Duvall, and Moore,[29] one therapist repeatedly measured 13 active upper extremity motions, including elbow flexion and extension and forearm pronation and supination, in 77 patients. The differences between the means of two trials ranged from 0.10 degrees for elbow extension to 1.53 degrees for supination. A significant difference between the measurements was noted for elbow flexion, although the difference between the means was only 1.0 degrees. Significant differences were also noted between measurements taken with a universal goniometer and those obtained by means of specialized devices, leading the author to conclude that different measuring devices could not be used interchangeably. The universal goniometer was generally found to be the more reliable device.

Boone and colleagues[30] examined the reliability of measuring six passive motions, including elbow extension-flexion. Four physical therapists used universal goniometers to measure these motions in 12 normal males weekly for 4 weeks. They found that intratester reliability (r=0.94) was slightly higher than intertester reliability (r=0.88).

Rothstein, Miller, and Roettger[31] found high intra-tester and intertester reliability for passive ROM of

elbows were restricted in an adjustable Bledsoe brace. Forty-nine subjects were able to complete all of the tasks with the elbow motion limited to between 75 and 120 degrees of flexion. Subjects used compensatory motions at adjacent normal joints to complete the activities. Cooper and colleagues[28] studied upper extremity motion in subjects during three feeding tasks, with the elbow unrestricted and then fixed in 110 degrees of flexion with a splint. The 19 subjects were assessed with a video-based, 3-dimensional motion analysis system while they were drinking with a handled cup, eating with a fork, and eating with a spoon. Compensatory motions to accommodate the fixed elbow occurred to a large extent at the shoulder and to a lesser extent at the wrist.

Reliability and Validity

Many studies have focused on the reliability of goniometric measurement of elbow ROM. Most researchers have found intratester and intertester reliability of measuring elbow motions with a universal goniometer to be high. Comparisons between ROM measurement taken with different devices have also been conducted. Fewer studies have examined the reliability and concurrent validity of measuring forearm supination and pronation ROM.

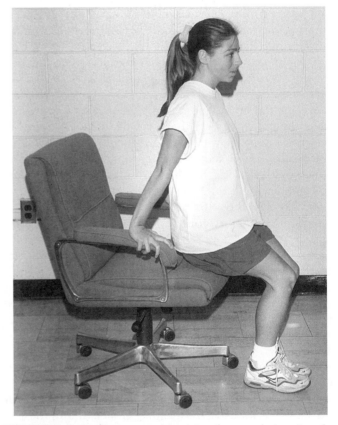

FIGURE 5–9 Studies report that rising from a chair using the upper extremities requires a large amount of elbow and wrist extension.

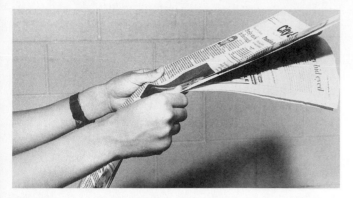

FIGURE 5–10 Approximately 50 degrees of pronation occur during the action of reading a newspaper.

elbow flexion and extension. Their study involved 12 testers who used three different commonly used universal goniometers (large plastic, small plastic, and large metal) to measure 24 patients. Pearson product-moment correlation values ranged from 0.89 to 0.97 for elbow flexion and extension ROM, whereas intraclass correlation coefficient (ICC) values ranged from 0.85 to 0.95.

Fish and Wingate[32] found that the standard deviation of passive elbow ROM goniometric measurements (2.4 to 3.4 degrees) was larger than the standard deviation from photographic measurements (0.7 to 1.1 degrees). These authors postulated that measurement error was due to improper identification of bony landmarks, inaccurate alignment of the goniometer, and variations in the amount of torque applied by the tester.

Grohmann,[33] in a study involving 40 testers and one subject, found that no significant differences existed between elbow measurements obtained by an over-the-joint method for goniometer alignment and the traditional lateral method. Differences between the means of the measurements were less than 2 degrees. The elbow was held in two fixed positions (an acute and an obtuse angle) by a plywood stabilizing device.

Petherick and associates,[12] in a study in which two testers measured 30 healthy subjects, found that intertester reliability for measuring active elbow ROM with a fluid-based goniometer was higher than with a universal goniometer. The Pearson product moment correlation between the two devices was 0.83. A significant difference was found between the two devices. The authors concluded that no concurrent validity existed between the fluid-based and the universal goniometers and that these instruments could not be used interchangeably.

Greene and Wolf[11] compared the reliability of the Ortho Ranger, an electronic pendulum goniometer, with the reliability of a universal goniometer for active upper extremity motions in 20 healthy adults. Elbow flexion and extension were measured three times for each instrument during each session. The three sessions were conducted by one physical therapist during a 2-week period. Within-session reliability was higher for the universal goniometer, as indicated by ICC values and 95 percent confidence intervals. Measurements taken with the Ortho Ranger correlated poorly with those taken with the universal goniometer (r = 0.11 to 0.21), and there was a significant difference in measurements between the two devices.

Goodwin and coworkers[13] evaluated the reliability of a universal goniometer, a fluid goniometer, and an electrogoniometer for measuring active elbow ROM in 23 healthy women. Three testers took three consecutive readings using each type of goniometer on two occasions that were 4 weeks apart. Significant differences were found between types of goniometers, testers, and replications. Measurements taken with the universal and fluid goniometers correlated the best (r = 0.90), whereas the electrogoniometer correlated poorly with the universal goniometer (r = 0.51) and fluid goniometer (r = 0.33). Intratester and intertester reliability was high during each occasion, with correlation coefficients greater than 0.98 and 0.90, respectively. Intratester reliability between occasions was highest for the universal goniometer. ICC values ranged from 0.61 to 0.92 for the universal goniometer, 0.53 to 0.85 for the fluid goniometer, and 0.00 to 0.61 for the electrogoniometer. Similar to other researchers, the authors do not advise the interchangeable use of different types of goniometers in the clinical setting.

Armstrong and associates[34] examined the intratester, intertester, and interdevice reliability of active ROM measurements of the elbow and forearm in 38 patients. Five testers measured each motion twice with each of the three devices: a universal goniometer, an electrogoniometer, and a mechanical rotation measuring device. Intratester reliability was high (r values generally greater than 0.90) for all three devices and all motions. Intertester reliability was high for pronation and supination with all three devices. Intertester reliability for elbow flexion and extension was high for the electrogoniometer and moderate for the universal goniometer. Measurements taken with different devices varied widely, with 95 percent confidence intervals for mean device differences of more than 30 degrees for most measures. The authors concluded that meaningful changes in intratester ROM taken with a universal goniometer occur with 95 percent confidence if they are greater than 6 degrees for flexion, 7 degrees for extension, and 8 degrees for pronation and supination. Meaningful changes in intertester ROM taken with a universal goniometer occur if they are greater than 10 degrees for flexion, extension, and pronation, and greater than 11 degrees for supination.

Range of Motion Testing Procedures: Elbow and Forearm

Landmarks for Goniometer Alignment: Elbow and Forearm

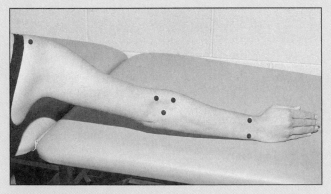

FIGURE 5–11 Anterior view of the right upper extremity showing surface anatomy landmarks for goniometer alignment during the measurement of elbow and forearm ROM.

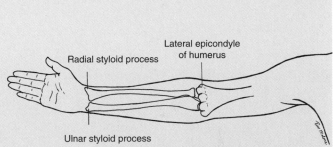

FIGURE 5–12 Anterior view of the right upper extremity showing bony anatomical landmarks for goniometer alignment during the measurement of elbow and forearm ROM.

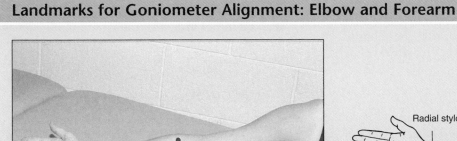

FIGURE 5–13 Posterior view of the right upper extremity showing surface anatomy landmarks for goniometer alignment during the measurement of elbow and forearm ROM.

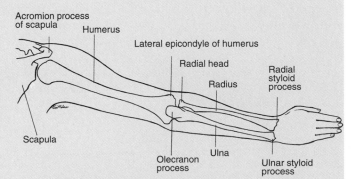

FIGURE 5–14 Posterior view of the right upper extremity showing anatomical landmarks for goniometer alignment during the measurement of elbow and forearm ROM.

FLEXION

Motion occurs in the sagittal plane around a medial-lateral axis. Mean elbow flexion ROM ranges from 140 degrees according to the AMA[9] to 150 degrees according to the AAOS.[7,8] See Tables 5–1 to 5–3 for additional information. See Figures 5–11 to 5–14.

Testing Position

Position the subject supine, with the shoulder in 0 degrees of flexion, extension, and abduction so that the arm is close to the side of the body. Place a pad under the distal end of the humerus to allow full elbow extension. Position the forearm in full supination with the palm of the hand facing the ceiling.

Stabilization

Stabilize the humerus to prevent flexion of the shoulder. The pad under the distal humerus and the examining table prevent extension of the shoulder.

Testing Motion

Flex the elbow by moving the hand toward the shoulder. Maintain the forearm in supination during the motion (Fig. 5–15). The end of flexion ROM occurs when resistance to further motion is felt and attempts to overcome the resistance cause flexion of the shoulder.

Normal End-feel

Usually the end-feel is soft because of compression of the muscle bulk of the anterior forearm with that of the anterior upper arm. If the muscle bulk is small, the end-feel may be hard because of contact between the coronoid process of the ulna and the coronoid fossa of the humerus and because of contact between the head of the radius and the radial fossa of the humerus. The end-feel may be firm because of tension in the posterior joint capsule, the lateral and medial heads of the triceps muscle, and the anconeus muscle.

Goniometer Alignment

See Figures 5–16 and 5–17.

1. Center the fulcrum of the goniometer over the lateral epicondyle of the humerus.
2. Align the proximal arm with the lateral midline of the humerus, using the center of the acromion process for reference.
3. Align the distal arm with the lateral midline of the radius, using the radial head and radial styloid process for reference.

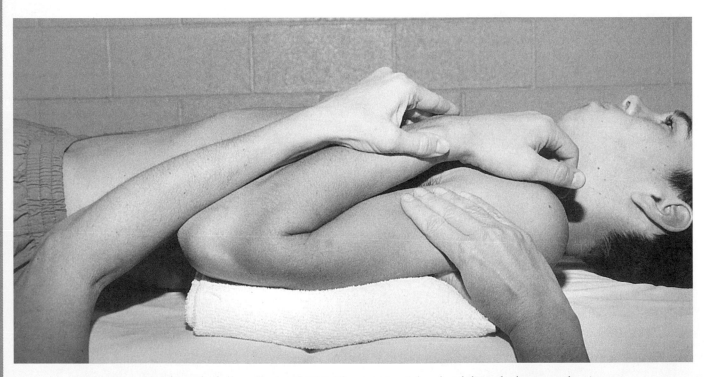

FIGURE 5–15 The end of elbow flexion ROM. The examiner's hand stabilizes the humerus, but it must be positioned so it does not limit the motion.

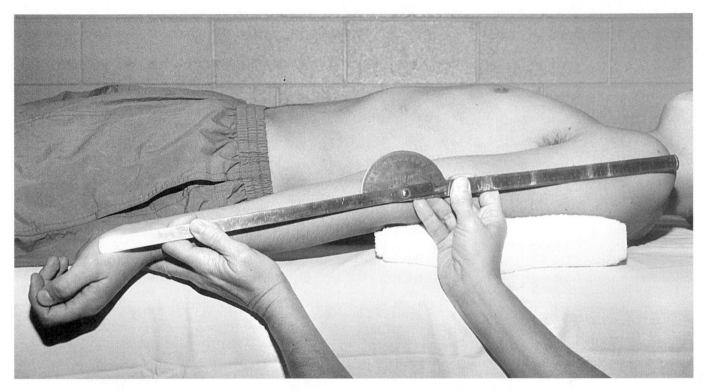

FIGURE 5–16 The alignment of the goniometer at the beginning of elbow flexion ROM. A towel is placed under the distal humerus to ensure that the supporting surface does not prevent full elbow extension. As can be seen in this photograph, the subject's elbow is in about 5 degrees of hyperextension.

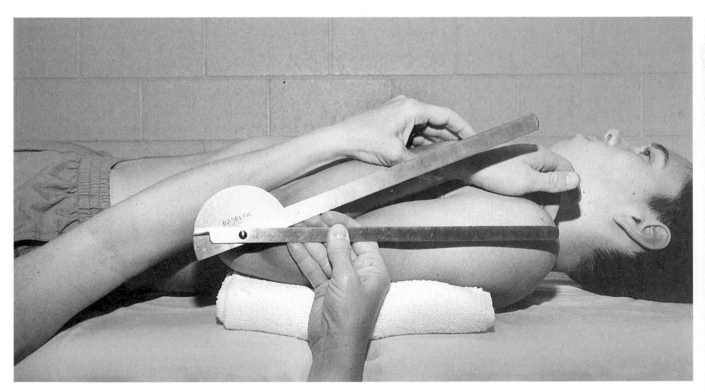

FIGURE 5–17 The alignment of the goniometer at the end of elbow flexion ROM. The proximal and distal arms of the goniometer have been switched from the starting position so that the ROM can be read from the pointer on the body of this 180-degree goniometer.

EXTENSION

Motion occurs in the sagittal plane around a medial-lateral axis. Elbow extension ROM is not usually measured and recorded separately because it is the return to the starting position from the end of elbow flexion ROM.

Testing Position, Stabilization, and Goniometer Alignment

The testing position, stabilization, and alignment are the same as those used for elbow flexion.

Testing Motion

Extend the elbow by moving the hand dorsally toward the examining table. Maintain the forearm in supination during the motion. The end of extension ROM occurs when resistance to further motion is felt and attempts to overcome the resistance cause extension of the shoulder.

Normal End-feel

Usually the end-feel is hard because of contact between the olecranon process of the ulna and the olecranon fossa of the humerus. Sometimes the end-feel is firm because of tension in the anterior joint capsule, the collateral ligaments, and the brachialis muscle.

PRONATION

Motion occurs in the transverse plane around a vertical axis when the subject is in the anatomical position. When the subject is in the testing position, the motion occurs in the frontal plane around an anterior-posterior axis. Mean pronation ROM is 76 degrees according to Boone and Azen,[10] and 84 degrees according to Greene and Wolf.[11] Both the AMA[9] and the AAOS[7,8] state that pronation ROM is 80 degrees. See Tables 5–1 to 5–3 for additional ROM information.

Testing Position

Position the subject sitting, with the shoulder in 0 degrees of flexion, extension, abduction, adduction, and rotation so that the upper arm is close to the side of the body. Flex the elbow to 90 degrees, and support the forearm. Initially position the forearm midway between supination and pronation so that the thumb points toward the ceiling.

Stabilization

Stabilize the distal end of the humerus to prevent medial rotation and abduction of the shoulder.

Testing Motion

Pronate the forearm by moving the distal radius in a volar direction so that the palm of the hand faces the floor. See Figure 5–18. The end of pronation ROM occurs when resistance to further motion is felt and attempts to overcome the resistance cause medial rotation and abduction of the shoulder.

Normal End-feel

The end-feel may be hard because of contact between the ulna and the radius, or it may be firm because of tension in the dorsal radioulnar ligament of the inferior radioulnar joint, the interosseous membrane, and the supinator muscle.

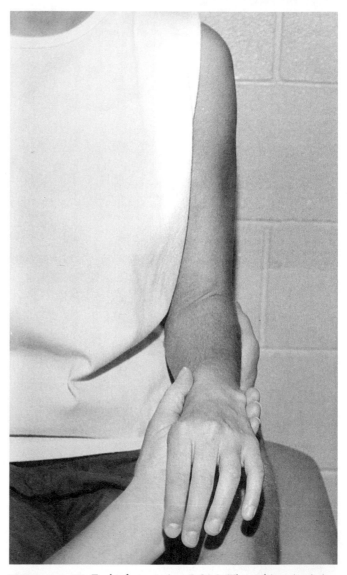

FIGURE 5–18 End of pronation ROM. The subject is sitting on the edge of a table and the examiner is standing facing the subject. The examiner uses one hand to hold the elbow close to the subject's body and in 90 degrees of elbow flexion, helping to prevent both medial rotation and abduction of the shoulder. The examiner's other hand pushes on the radius rather than on the subject's hand. If the examiner pushes on the subject's hand, movement of the wrist may be mistaken for movement at the radioulnar joints.

Goniometer Alignment

See Figures 5–19 and 5–20.

1. Center the fulcrum of the goniometer laterally and proximally to the ulnar styloid process.
2. Align the proximal arm parallel to the anterior midline of the humerus.
3. Place the distal arm across the dorsal aspect of the forearm, just proximal to the styloid processes of the radius and ulna, where the forearm is most level and free of muscle bulk. The distal arm of the goniometer should be parallel to the styloid processes of the radius and ulna.

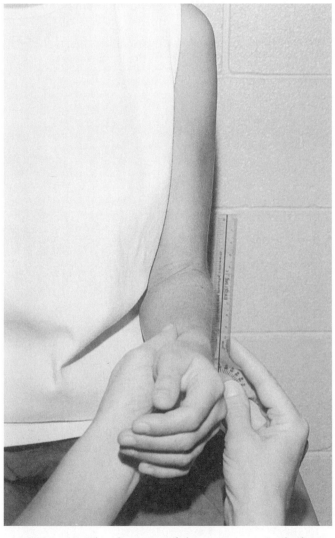

FIGURE 5–19 The alignment of the goniometer in the beginning of pronation ROM. The goniometer is placed laterally to the distal radioulnar joint. The arms of the goniometer are aligned parallel to the anterior midline of the humerus.

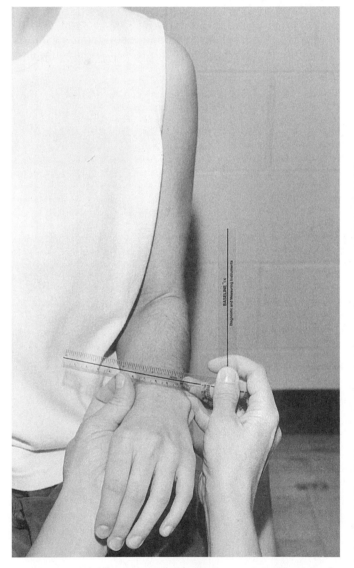

FIGURE 5–20 Alignment of the goniometer at the end of pronation ROM. The examiner uses one hand to hold the proximal arm of the goniometer parallel to the anterior midline of the humerus. The examiner's other hand supports the forearm and assists in placing the distal arm of the goniometer across the dorsum of the forearm just proximal to the radial and ulnar styloid process. The fulcrum of the goniometer is proximal and lateral to the ulnar styloid process.

SUPINATION

Motion occurs in the transverse plane around a longitudinal axis when the subject is in the anatomical position. When the subject is in the testing position, the motion occurs in the frontal plane around an anterior-posterior axis. Mean supination ROM is 82 degrees according to Boone and Azen,[10] and 77 degrees according to Greene and Wolf.[11] Both the AMA[9] and the AAOS[7,8] state that supination ROM is 80 degrees. See Tables 5–1 to 5–3 for additional ROM information.

Testing Position

Position the subject sitting, with the shoulder in 0 degrees of flexion, extension, abduction, adduction, and rotation so that the upper arm is close to the side of the body. Flex the elbow to 90 degrees, and support the forearm. Initially position the forearm midway between supination and pronation so that the thumb points toward the ceiling.

Stabilization

Stabilize the distal end of the humerus to prevent lateral rotation and adduction of the shoulder.

Testing Motion

Supinate the forearm by moving the distal radius in a dorsal direction so that the palm of the hand faces the ceiling. See Figure 5–21. The end of supination ROM occurs when resistance to further motion is felt and attempts to overcome the resistance cause lateral rotation and adduction of the shoulder.

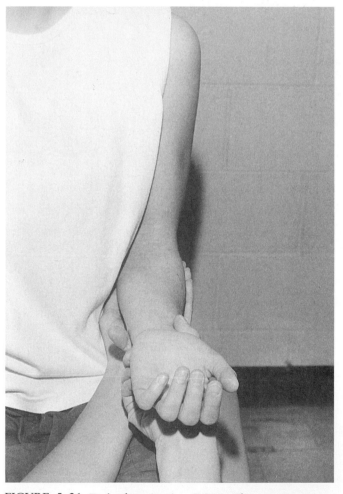

FIGURE 5–21 End of supination ROM. The examiner uses one hand to hold the elbow close to the subject's body and in 90 degrees of elbow flexion, preventing lateral rotation and adduction of the shoulder. The examiner's other hand pushes on the distal radius while supporting the forearm.

Normal End-feel

The end-feel is firm because of tension in the palmar radioulnar ligament of the inferior radioulnar joint, oblique cord, interosseous membrane, and pronator teres and pronator quadratus muscles.

Goniometer Alignment

See Figures 5–22 and 5–23.

1. Center the goniometer medially and proximally to the ulnar styloid process.

2. Align the proximal arm parallel to the anterior midline of the humerus.

3. Place the distal arm across the ventral aspect of the forearm, just proximal to the styloid processes, where the forearm is most level and free of muscle bulk. The distal arm of the goniometer should be parallel to the styloid processes of the radius and ulna.

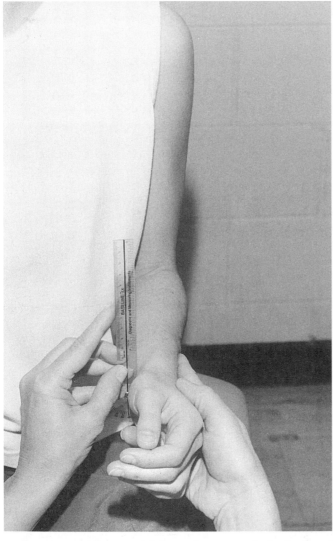

FIGURE 5–22 Alignment of the goniometer at the beginning of supination ROM. The body of the goniometer is medial to the distal radioulnar joint, and the arms of the goniometer are parallel to the anterior midline of the humerus.

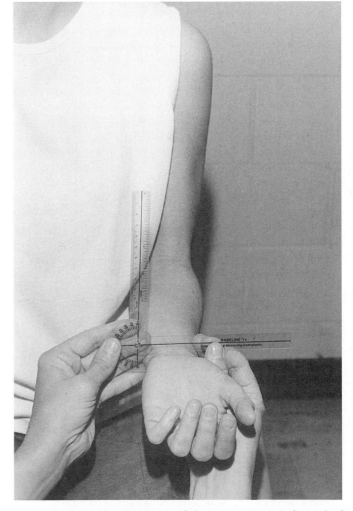

FIGURE 5–23 The alignment of the goniometer at the end of supination ROM. The examiner uses one hand to hold the proximal arm of the goniometer parallel to the anterior midline of the humerus. The examiner's other hand supports the forearm while holding the distal arm of the goniometer across the volar surface of the forearm just proximal to the radial and ulnar styloid process. The fulcrum of the goniometer is proximal and medial to the ulnar styloid process.

Muscle Length Testing Procedures: Elbow and Forearm

BICEPS BRACHII

The biceps brachii muscle crosses the glenohumeral, humeroulnar, humeroradial, and superior radioulnar joints. The short head of the biceps brachii originates proximally from the coracoid process of the scapula (Fig. 5–24). The long head originates from the supraglenoid tubercle of the scapula. The biceps brachii attaches distally to the radial tuberosity.

When it contracts it flexes the elbow and shoulder and supinates the forearm. The muscle is passively lengthened by placing the shoulder and elbow in full extension and the forearm in pronation. If the biceps brachii is short, it limits elbow extension when the shoulder is positioned in full extension.

If elbow extension is limited regardless of shoulder position, the limitation is caused by abnormalities of the joint surfaces, shortening of the anterior joint capsule, and collateral ligaments, or by muscles that cross only the elbow, such as the brachialis and brachioradialis.

Starting Position

Position the subject supine at the edge of the examining table. See Figure 5–25. Flex the elbow and position the shoulder in full extension and 0 degrees of abduction, adduction, and rotation.

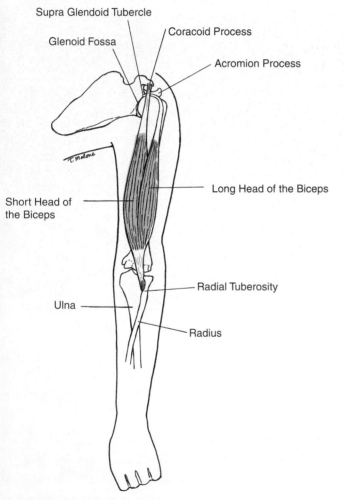

FIGURE 5–24 A lateral view of the upper extremity showing the origins and insertion of the biceps brachii while being stretched over the glenohumeral, elbow, and superior radioulnar joints.

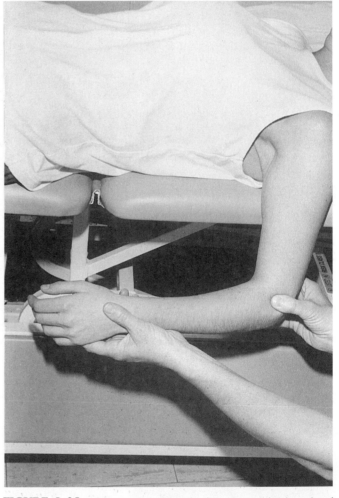

FIGURE 5–25 The starting position for testing the length of the biceps brachii.

Stabilization

The examiner stabilizes the subject's humerus. The examining table and passive tension in the serratus anterior muscle help to stabilize the scapula.

Testing motion

Extend the elbow while holding the forearm in pronation. See Figures 5–26 and 5–25. The end of the testing motion occurs when resistance is felt and additional elbow extension causes shoulder flexion.

Normal End-feel

The end-feel is firm because of tension in the biceps brachii muscle.

Goniometer Alignment

See Figure 5–27.

1. Center the fulcrum of the goniometer over the lateral epicondyle of the humerus.
2. Align the proximal arm with the lateral midline of the humerus, using the center of the acromion process for reference.
3. Align the distal arm with the lateral midline of the ulna, using the ulna styloid process for reference.

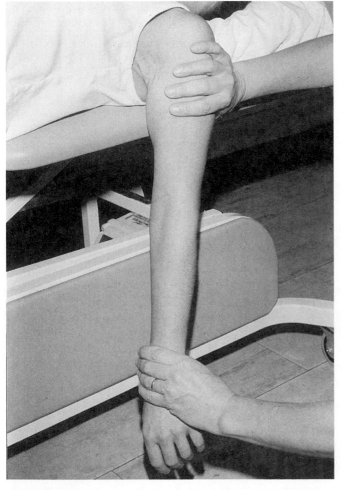

FIGURE 5–26 The end of the testing motion for the length of the biceps brachii. The examiner uses one hand to stabilize the humerus in full shoulder extension while the other hand holds the forearm in pronation and moves the elbow into extension.

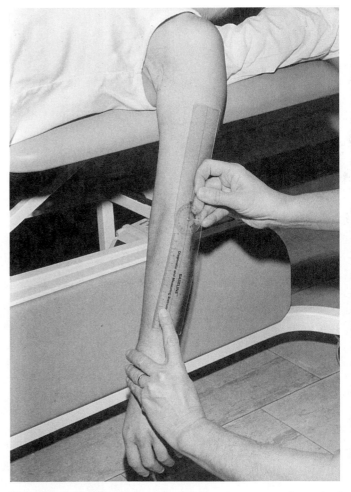

FIGURE 5–27 The alignment of the goniometer at the end of testing the length of the biceps brachii. The examiner releases the stabilization of the humerus and now uses her hand to position the goniometer.

TRICEPS BRACHII

The triceps brachii muscle crosses the glenohumeral and humeroulnar joints. The long head of the triceps brachii muscle originates proximally from the infraglenoid tubercle of the scapula (Fig. 5–28). The lateral head of the triceps brachii originates from the posterior and lateral surfaces of the humerus, whereas the medial head originates from the posterior and medial surfaces of the humerus. All parts of the triceps brachii insert distally on the olecranon process of the ulna. When this muscle contracts, it extends the shoulder and elbow. The long head of the triceps brachii is passively lengthened by placing the shoulder and elbow in full flexion. If the long head of the triceps brachii is short, it limits elbow flexion when the shoulder is positioned in full flexion.

If elbow flexion is limited regardless of shoulder position, the limitation is due to abnormalities of the joint surfaces, shortening of the posterior capsule or muscles that cross only the elbow, such as the anconeus and the lateral and medial heads of the triceps brachii.

Starting Position

Position the subject supine, close to the edge of the examining table. Extend the elbow and position the shoulder in full flexion and 0 degrees of abduction, adduction, and rotation. Supinate the forearm (Fig. 5–29).

Stabilization

The examiner stabilizes the subject's humerus. The weight of the subject's trunk on the examining table and the passive tension in the latissumus dorsi, pectoralis minor, and rhomboid major and minor muscles help to stabilize the scapula.

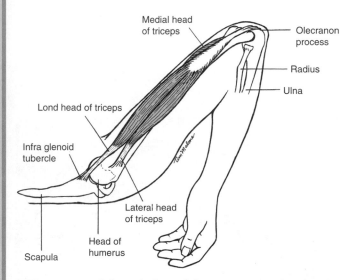

Medial head of triceps

Olecranon process

Radius

Ulna

Lond head of triceps

Infra glenoid tubercle

Lateral head of triceps

Head of humerus

Scapula

FIGURE 5–28 A lateral view of the upper extremity showing the origins and insertions of the triceps brachii while being stretched over the glenohumeral and elbow joints.

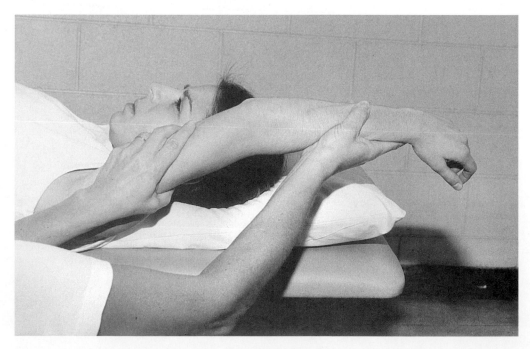

FIGURE 5–29 The starting position for testing the length of the triceps brachii.

Testing Motion

Flex the elbow by moving the hand closer to the shoulder. See Figures 5–30 and 5–28. The end of the testing motion occurs when resistance is felt and additional elbow flexion causes shoulder extension.

Normal End-feel

The end-feel is firm because of tension in the long head of the triceps brachii muscle.

Goniometer Alignment

See Figure 5–31.

1. Center the fulcrum of the goniometer over the lateral epicondyle of the humerus.
2. Align the proximal arm with the lateral midline of the humerus, using the center of the acromion process for reference.
3. Align the distal arm with the lateral midline of the radius, using the radial styloid process for reference.

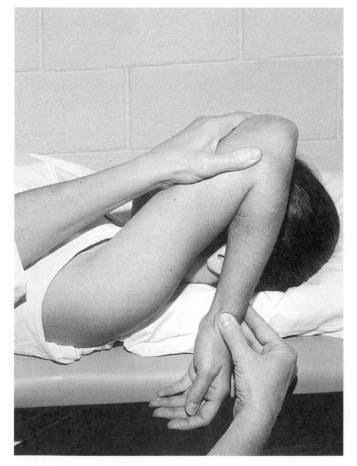

FIGURE 5–30 The end of the testing motion for the length of the triceps brachii. The examiner uses one hand to stabilize the humerus in full shoulder flexion and the other hand to move the elbow into flexion.

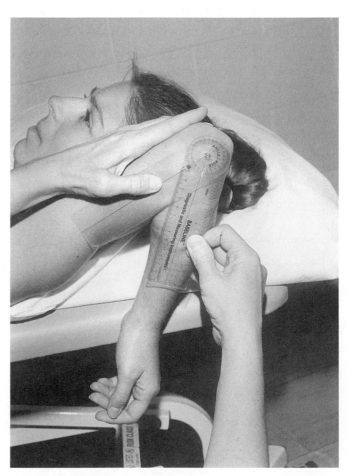

FIGURE 5–31 The alignment of the goniometer at the end of testing the length of the triceps brachii. The examiner uses one hand to continue to stabilize the humerus and align the proximal arm of the goniometer. The examiner's other hand holds the elbow in flexion and aligns the distal arm of the goniometer with the radius.

REFERENCES

1. Levangie, PK, and Norkin, CC: Joint Structure and Function: A Comprehensive Analysis, ed 3. FA Davis, Philadelphia, 2001.
2. Hoppenfeld, S: Physical Examination of the Spine and Extremities. Appleton-Century-Crofts, New York, 1977.
3. Morrey, BF, and Chao, EYS: Passive motion of the elbow joint. J Bone Joint Surg Am 58:50, 1976.
4. Cyriax, JH, and Cyriax, PJ: Illustrated Manual of Orthopaedic Medicine. Butterworths, London, 1983.
5. Kaltenborn, FM: Manual Mobilization of the Extremity Joints, ed 5. Olaf Norlis Bokhandel, Oslo, 1999.
6. Magee, DJ: Orthopedic Physical Assessment, ed. 2. WB Saunders, Philadelphia, 1992.
7. American Academy of Orthopaedic Surgeons: Joint Motion: Methods of Measuring and Recording. AAOS, Chicago, 1965.
8. Green, WB, and Heckman, JD (eds): The Clinical Measurement of Joint Motion. American Academy of Orthopaedic Surgeons, Rosemont, Ill., 1994.
9. American Medical Association: Guides to the Evaluation of Permanent Impairment, ed 3. AMA, Chicago, 1988.
10. Boone, DC, and Azen, SP: Normal range of motion in male subjects. J Bone Joint Surg Am 61:756, 1979.
11. Greene, BL, and Wolf, SL: Upper extremity joint movement: Comparison of two measurement devices. Arch Phys Med Rehabil 70:288, 1989.
12. Petherick, M, et al: Concurrent validity and intertester reliability of universal and fluid-based goniometers for active elbow range of motion. Phys Ther 68:966, 1988.
13. Goodwin, J, et al: Clinical methods of goniometry: A comparative study. Disabil Rehabil, 14:10, 1992.
14. Wanatabe, H, et al: The range of joint motions of the extremities in healthy Japanese people: The difference according to age. Nippon Seikeigeka Gakkai Zasshi 53:275, 1999. (Cited in Walker, JM: Musculoskeletal development: A review. Phys Ther 71:878, 1991.)
15. Boone, DC: Techniques of measurement of joint motion. (Unpublished supplement to Boone, DC, and Azen, SP: Normal range of motion in male subjects. J Bone Joint Surg Am 61:756, 1979.)
16. Walker, JM, et al: Active mobility of the extremities in older subjects. Phys Ther 64:919, 1984.
17. Bergstrom, G, et al: Prevalence of symptoms and signs of joint impairment. Scand J Rehabil Med 17:173, 1985.
18. Bell, RD, and Hoshizaki, TB: Relationships of age and sex with range of motion of seventeen joint actions in humans. Can J Appl Spt Sci 6:202, 1981.
19. Fairbanks, JC, Pynsent, PB, and Phillips, H: Quantitative measurements of joint mobility in adolescents. Ann Rheum Dis 43:288, 1984.
20. Salter, N, and Darcus, HD: The amplitude of forearm and of humeral rotation. J Anat 87:407, 1953.
21. Escalante, A, Lichenstein, MJ, and Hazuda, HP: Determinants of shoulder and elbow flexion range: Results from the San Antonio Longitudinal Study of Aging. Arthritis Care Res 12:277, 1999.
22. Chang, DE, Buschbacher, LP, and Edlich, RF: Limited joint mobility in power lifters. Am J Sports Med 16:280, 1988.
23. Chinn, CJ, Priest, JD, and Kent, BA: Upper extremity range of motion, grip strength and girth in highly skilled tennis players, Phys Ther 54:474, 1974.
24. Morrey, BF, Askew, KN, and Chao, EYS: A biomechanical study of normal functional elbow motion. J Bone Joint Surg Am 63:872, 1981.
25. Packer, TL, et al: Examining the elbow during functional activities. Occup Ther JRes. 10:323, 1990.
26. Safaee-Rad, R, et al: Normal functional range of motion of upper limb joints during performance of three feeding activities. Arch Phys Med Rehabil 71:505, 1990.
27. Vasen, AP, et al: Functional range of motion of the elbow. J Hand Surg 20A: 288, 1995.
28. Cooper, JE, et al: Elbow joint restriction: Effect on functional upper limb motion during performance of three feeding activities. Arch Phys Med Rehabil 74:805, 1993.
29. Hellebrandt, FA, Duvall, EN, and Moore, ML: The measurement of joint motion. Part III: Reliability of Goniometry. Phys Ther Rev 29:302, 1949.
30. Boone, DC, et al: Reliability of goniometric measurements. Phys Ther 58:1355, 1978.
31. Rothstein, JM, Miller, PJ, and Roettger, RF: Goniometric reliability in a clinical setting: Elbow and knee measurements. Phys Ther 63:1611, 1983.
32. Fish, DR, and Wingate, L: Sources of goniometric error at the elbow. Phys Ther 65:1666, 1985.
33. Grohmann, JEL: Comparison of two methods of goniometry. Phys Ther 63:922, 1983.
34. Armstrong, AD, et al: Reliability of range-of-motion measurement in the elbow and forearm. J Shoulder Elbow Surg 7:573, 1998.

CHAPTER 6

The Wrist

Structure and Function

Radiocarpal and Midcarpal Joints

Anatomy

The radiocarpal joint attaches the hand to the forearm. The proximal joint surface consists of the lateral and medial facets on the distal radius and radioulnar articu-

lar disc (Fig. 6–1; see also Fig. 5–7).[1] The disc connects the medial aspect of the distal radius to the distal ulna. The radial facets and the disc form a continuous concave surface.[2,3] The distal joint surface includes three bones from the proximal carpal row: the scaphoid, lunate, and triquetrium (Fig. 6–1). The carpal bones, which are connected by interosseous ligaments, form a convex surface. The lateral radial facet articulates with the scaphoid, and the medial radial facet with the lunate. The radioulnar disc articulates with the triquetrium and, to a lesser extent, the lunate. The pisiform, although found in the proximal row of carpal bones, does not participate in the radiocarpal joint. The joint is enclosed by a strong capsule and reinforced by the palmar radiocarpal, ulnocarpal, dorsal radiocarpal, ulnar collateral, and radial collateral ligaments, as well as numerous intercarpal ligaments (Figs. 6–2 and 6–3).

The midcarpal joint is considered to be a functional

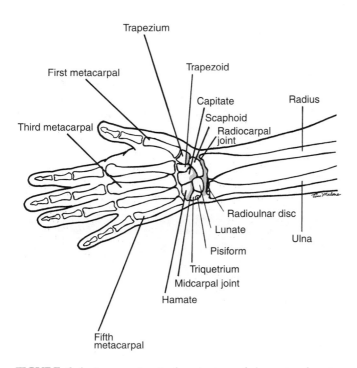

FIGURE 6–1 An anterior (palmar) view of the wrist showing the radiocarpal and midcarpal joints.

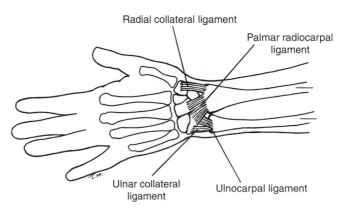

FIGURE 6–2 An anterior (palmar) view of the wrist showing the palmar radiocarpal, ulnocarpal, and collateral ligaments.

111

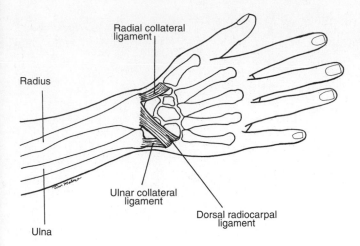

FIGURE 6–3 A posterior view of the wrist showing the dorsal radiocarpal and collateral ligaments.

rather than an anatomical joint. It has a joint capsule that is continuous with each intercarpal joint and some carpometacarpal and intermetacarpal joints. The joint surfaces are reciprocally convex and concave and consist of the scaphoid, lunate, and triquetrum proximally, and the trapezium, trapezoid, capitate, and hamate bones distally (Fig. 6–1). Many of the ligaments that reinforce the radiocarpal joint also support the midcarpal joint (Figs. 6–2 and 6–3).

Osteokinematics

The radiocarpal and midcarpal joints are of the condyloid type, with 2 degrees of freedom.[2] The wrist complex (radiocarpal and midcarpal joints) permits flexion-extension in the sagittal plane around a medial-lateral axis, and radial-ulnar deviation in the frontal plane around an anterior-posterior axis. Both joints contribute to these motions.[4–6] Some sources also report that a small amount of supination-pronation occurs at the wrist complex,[7] but this rotation is not usually measured in the clinical setting.

Arthrokinematics

Motion at the radiocarpal joint occurs because the convex surfaces of the proximal row of carpals slide on the concave surfaces of the radius and radioulnar disc. The proximal row of carpals slides in a direction opposite to the movement of the hand.[3,8] The carpals move dorsally on the radius and disc during wrist flexion, and ventrally toward the palm during wrist extension. During ulnar deviation, the carpals slide in a radial direction. During radial deviation, they slide in an ulnar direction.

Motion at the midcarpal joint occurs because the distal row of carpals slides on the proximal row. During flexion, the convex surfaces of the capitate and hamate slide dorsally on the concave surfaces of portions of the scaphoid, lunate, and triquetrum.[3,8] The surfaces of the trapezium and trapezoid are concave and slide volarly on the convex surface of the scaphoid. During extension, the capitate and hamate slide volarly on the scaphoid, lunate, and triquetrum; the trapezium and the trapezoid slide dorsally on the scaphoid. During radial deviation, the capitate and hamate slide ulnarly, and the trapezium and trapezoid slide dorsally. In ulnar deviation, the capitate and hamate slide radially; the trapezium and trapezoid slide volarly.

Capsular Pattern

Cyriax and Cyriax[9] report that the capsular pattern at the wrist is an equal limitation of flexion and extension and a slight limitation of radial and ulnar deviation. Kaltenborn[3] notes that the capsular pattern is an equal restriction in all motions.

◗ Research Findings

Effects of Age, Gender, and Other Factors

Table 6–1 provides range of motion (ROM) information for all wrist motions. The age, gender, and number of subjects that were measured to obtain the values reported by the American Academy of Orthopaedic Surgeons

TABLE 6–1 Wrist Motion: Mean Values in Degrees from Selected Sources					
	AAOS[10,11]	AMA[12]	Boone & Azen[13] n = 109*	Greene & Wolf[14] n = 20†	Ryu et al[15] n = 40‡
Motion			Mean (SD)	Mean (SD)	Mean
Flexion	80	60	76.4 (6.3)	73.3 (2.1)	79.1
Extension	70	60	74.9 (6.4)	64.9 (2.2)	59.3
Radial deviation	20	20	21.5 (4.0)	25.4 (2.0)	21.1
Ulnar deviation	30	30	36.0 (3.8)	39.2 (2.1)	37.7

* Values are for males 18 months to 54 years of age.
† Values are for 10 males and 10 females, 18 to 55 years of age.
‡ Values are for 20 males and 20 females (ages unknown).

TABLE 6–2   Effects of Age on Wrist Motion: Mean Values in Degrees for Newborns, Children, and Adolescents

| | Wanatabe et al[21] | Boone[22] | | |
| | 2 wks–2 yrs
n = 45 | 18 mos–5 yrs
n = 19 | 6–12 yrs
n = 17 | 13–19 yrs
n = 17 |
Motion	Range of Means	Mean (SD)	Mean (SD)	Mean (SD)
Flexion	88–96	82.2 (3.8)	76.3 (5.6)	75.4 (4.5)
Extension	82–89	76.1 (4.9)	78.4 (5.9)	72.9 (6.4)
Radial deviation		24.2 (3.7)	21.3 (4.1)	19.7 (3.0)
Ulnar deviation		38.7 (3.6)	35.4 (2.4)	35.7 (4.2)

(AAOS)[10,11] and the American Medical Association (AMA)[12] were not noted. Boone and Azen,[13] using a universal goniometer, measured active ROM in 109 healthy male subjects aged 18 months to 54 years. Greene and Wolf,[14] using a universal goniometer, measured active ROM in 10 males and 10 females aged 18 to 55 years. The values presented in Table 6–1 for Ryu and associates[15] were obtained with a hand goniometer from 20 males and 20 females (ages unknown). Other studies which provide normative wrist ROM data for various age and gender groups include Slogaard and colleagues,[16] Solveborn and Olerud,[17] Stubbs and coworkers,[18] Walker and associates,[19] and Chaparro and colleagues.[20]

Age

Table 6–2 provides wrist ROM values for newborns and children. Although caution must be used in drawing conclusions from comparisons between values obtained by different researchers, the mean flexion and extension values for infants from Wanatabe and coworkers[21] are larger than values reported for males aged 18 months to 19 years reported by Boone.[22] The ROM values for both ulnar and radial deviation for the youngest age group (18 months to 5 years) were significantly larger than the values for other age groups reported by Boone[22] and presented in Tables 6–2 and 6–3. Boone and Azen[13] noted that wrist extension ROM values were significantly

larger for males 6 to 12 years of age than for those in other age groups.

Table 6–3 provides wrist ROM values obtained with universal goniometers from male adults. Boone and Azen[13] found a significant difference in wrist flexion and extension ROM between males less than or equal to 19 years of age and those who were older. However, the effects of age on wrist motion in adults from 20 to 54 years of age appear to be very slight. Values for flexion and extension in adults 60 years of age and older, as presented by Walker and associates[19] and Chaparro and colleagues,[20] are less than values for other age groups presented by Boone.[22] Chaparro and colleagues[20] further divided the 62 male subjects in their study into four age groups: 60 to 69 years of age, 70 to 79 years of age, 80 to 89 years of age, and older than 90 years of age. They found a trend of decreasing ROM with increasing age, with the oldest group having significantly lower wrist flexion and ulnar deviation values than the two youngest groups.

Four other studies offer additional information on the effects of age on wrist motion. Hewitt,[23] in a study of 112 females between 11 and 45 years of age, found slight differences in the average amount of active motion in different age groups. A group of 17 individuals ranging in age from 11 to 15 years had slightly less flexion and radial deviation but more ulnar deviation and extension than the general average. Allander and coworkers,[24] in a

TABLE 6–3   Effects of Age on Wrist Motion: Mean Values in Degrees for Men

| | Boone[22] | | | Walker et al[19] | Chaparro et al[20] |
| | 20–29 yrs
n = 19 | 30–39 yrs
n = 18 | 40–54 yrs
n = 19 | 60–85 yrs
n = 30 | 60–90+ yrs
n = 62 |
Motion	Mean (SD)	Mean (SD)	Mean (SD)	Mean (SD)	Mean (SD)
Flexion	76.8 (5.5)	74.9 (4.0)	72.8 (8.9)	62.0 (12.0)	50.8 (13.8)
Extension	77.5 (5.1)	72.8 (6.9)	71.6 (6.3)	61.0 (6.0)	44.0 (9.9)
Radial deviation	21.4 (3.6)	20.3 (3.1)	21.6 (5.1)	20.0 (6.0)	
Ulnar deviation	35.1 (3.8)	36.1 (2.9)	34.7 (4.5)	28.0 (7.0)	35.0 (9.5)

study of 309 Icelandic females, 208 Swedish females, and 203 Swedish males ranging in age from 33 to 70 years, found that with increasing age there was a decrease in flexion and extension ROM at both wrists. Males lost an average of 2.2 degrees of motion every 5 years. Bell and Hoshizaki[25] studied 124 females and 66 males ranging in age from 18 to 88 years. A significant negative correlation was noted between range of motion and age for wrist flexion-extension and radial-ulnar deviation in females, and for wrist flexion-extension in males. As age increased, wrist motions generally decreased. There was a significant difference among the five age groups of females for all wrist motions, although the difference was not significant for males. Stubbs, Fernandez, and Glenn[18] placed 55 male subjects between the ages of 25 and 54 years into three age groups. There was no significant difference among the age groups for wrist flexion, extension, and radial deviation ROM. A significant difference in ulnar deviation (7 degrees) was found between the oldest and the youngest age groups, with the oldest group having less motion.

Gender

The following four studies offer evidence of gender effects on the wrist joint, with most supporting the belief that women have slightly more wrist ROM than men. Cobe,[26] in a study of 100 college men and 15 women ranging in age from 20 to 30 years, found that women had a greater active ROM in all motions at the wrist than men. Allander and coworkers[24] compared wrist flexion and extension ROM in 203 Swedish men and 208 Swedish women between the ages of 45 and more than 70 years of age, and noted that women had significantly greater motion than men. Both studies measured active motion with joint-specific mechanical devices. Walker and associates,[19] in a study of 30 men and 30 women aged 60 to 84 years found that the women had more active wrist extension and flexion than the men, whereas the men had more ulnar and radial deviation than the women. These differences were statistically significant for wrist extension (4 degrees) and ulnar deviation (5 degrees). Chaparro and colleagues[20] examined wrist flexion, extension, and ulnar deviation ROM in 62 men and 85 women from 60 to more than 90 years of age. Women had significantly greater wrist extension (6.4 degrees) and ulnar deviation (3.0 degrees) than men.

Right versus Left Sides

Study results vary as to whether there is a difference between left and right wrist ROM. Boone and Azen,[13] in a study of 109 normal males between 18 months and 54 years of age, found no significant difference in wrist flexion, extension, or radial and ulnar deviation between sides. Likewise, Chang, Buschbacher, and Edlich[27] found no significant difference between right and left wrist flexion and extension in the 10 power lifters and 10

nonlifters who were their subjects. Solgaard and coworkers[16] studied 8 males and 23 females aged 24 to 65 years. Right and left wrist extension and radial deviation differed significantly, but the differences were small and not significant when the total range (i.e., flexion and extension) was assessed. The authors stated that the opposite wrist could be satisfactorily used as a reference.

In contrast, several studies have found the left wrist to have greater ROM than the right wrist. Cobe[26] measured wrist motions in the positions of pronation and supination in 100 men and 15 women. He found that men had greater ROM in their left wrist than in their right for all motions except ulnar deviation measured in pronation. However, he reported that the women had greater wrist motion on the right except for extension in pronation and radial deviation in supination. No statistical tests were conducted in the 1928 study, but Allander and associates[24] reported that a recalculation of the original data collected by Cobe found a significantly greater ROM on the left. Cobe[26] suggests that the heavy work that men performed using their right extremities may account for the decrease in right-side motion in comparison with left-side motion.

Allander and associates,[24] in a study subgroup of 309 Icelandic women aged 34 to 61 years found no significant difference between the right and the left wrists. However, a subgroup of 208 women and 203 Swedish men in the study showed significantly smaller ranges of wrist flexion and extension on the right than on the left, independent of gender. The authors state that these differences may be due to a higher level of exposure to trauma of the right hand in a predominantly right-handed society. Solveborn and Olerud[17] measured wrist ROM in 16 healthy subjects in addition to 123 patients with unilateral tennis elbow. Among the healthy subjects a significantly greater ROM was found for wrist flexion and extension on the left compared with the right. However, mean differences between sides were only 2 degrees. The authors concurred with Boone and Azen[13] that a patient's healthy limb can be used to establish a norm for comparing with the affected side.

Testing Position

Several studies have reported differences in wrist ROM depending on the testing position used during measurement. Cobe,[26] in a study of 100 men and 15 women, found that ulnar deviation ROM was greater in supination, whereas radial deviation was greater in pronation. Interestingly, the total amount of ulnar and radial deviation combined was similar between the two positions. Hewitt[23] measured wrist ROM in 112 females in supination and pronation and found that ulnar deviation was greater in supination, whereas radial deviation, flexion, and extension were greater in pronation. Werner and Plancher,[6] in a review article, also stated that ulnar deviation has a greater ROM when the forearm is supinated than when the forearm is pronated. They noted that radial and ulnar deviation ROMs become minimal when the wrist is fully flexed or extended. No specific references for these observations were cited.

Spilman and Pinkston[28] examined the effect of three frequently used goniometric testing positions on active wrist radial and ulnar deviation ROM in 100 subjects (63 males, 37 females). In Position One the subject's arm was at the side, with the elbow flexed to 90 degrees and the forearm fully pronated. In Position Two the shoulder was in 90 degrees of flexion, with the elbow extended and the hand prone. In Position Three the subject's shoulder was in 90 degrees of abduction, with the elbow in 90 degrees of flexion and the hand prone (in this position the forearm is in neutral pronation). Ulnar deviation and the total range of radial and ulnar deviation were significantly greater when measured in Position Three. Radial deviation was significantly greater when the subject was in Position Three or Position Two than in Position One. The difference between the means for the three positions was approximately 3 degrees.

Marshall, Morzall, and Shealy[29] evaluated 35 men and 19 women for wrist ROM in one plane of motion while the subjects were fixed in secondary wrist and forearm positions. For example, during the measurement of radial and ulnar deviation, the wrist was alternatively positioned in 0 degrees, 40 degrees of flexion, and 40 degrees of extension. These three wrist positions were repeated with the forearm in 45 degrees of pronation and 90 degrees of pronation. The effects of the secondary wrist and forearm postures, although statistically significant, were small (less than 5 degrees), except for the effect of wrist flexion and extension on radial deviation. Radial deviation ROM was greatest when performed in wrist extension and lowest in wrist flexion, with a decrease of over 30 percent. The authors believed that the changes that occur in wrist ROM with positional alterations might have been due to changes in contact between articular surfaces and tautness of ligaments that span the wrist region.

Functional Range of Motion

Several investigators have examined the range of motion that occurs at the wrist during activities of daily living (ADLs) and during the placement of the hand on the body areas necessary for personal care. Tables 6–4 and 6–5 are adapted from the works of Brumfield and Champoux,[30] Ryu and associates,[15] Safaee-Rad and colleagues,[31] and Cooper and coworkers.[32] Differences in ROM values reported for certain functional tasks were most likely the result of variations in task definitions, measurement methods, and subject selection. However, in spite of the range of values reported, certain trends are evident.

A review of Table 6–4 shows that the majority of ADLs required wrist extension and ulnar deviation. Drinking activities generally required the least amount of extension (6 to 24 degrees) and the smallest arc of motion (13 to 20 degrees). Using the telephone (Fig. 6–4), turning a steering wheel or a doorknob, and rising from a chair (see Fig. 5–9) required the greatest amounts of

TABLE 6–4   Wrist Motions During Functional Activities: Mean Values in Degrees

Activity	Extension*			Ulnar Deviation†			Source
	Min	Max	Arc	Min	Max	Arc	
Put glass to mouth	11.2	24.0	12.8				Brumfield[30]
Drink from glass	2	22	20	5	20	15	Ryu[‡15]
Drink from handled cup	−7.5*	5.9	13.4	8.3	16.1	7.8	Safaee-Rad[31]
Eat with fork	9.3	36.5	27.7				Brumfield
	3.3	17.7	14.4	3.2	−4.9†	8.1	Safaee-Rad
Feeding tasks: fork, spoon, cup	−6.8*	20.9	27.2	18.7	−2.4†	21.1	Cooper (males)[32]
Cut with knife	−3.5*	20.2	23.7				Brumfield
	−30*	−5	25	12	27	15	Ryu
Pour from pitcher	8.7	29.7	21.0				Brumfield
	−20*	22	42	12	32	20	Ryu
Turn doorknob	−40*	45	85	−2†	32	34	Ryu
Use telephone	−0.1*	42.6	42.7				Brumfield
	−15*	40	55	−10†	12	22	Ryu
Turn steering wheel	−15*	45	60	−17†	27	44	Ryu
Rise from chair	0.6	63.4	62.8				Brumfield
	−10*	60	70	5	30	25	Ryu

* The minus sign denotes flexion.
† The minus sign denotes radial deviation.
‡ Values from Ryu et al were extrapolated from graphs.

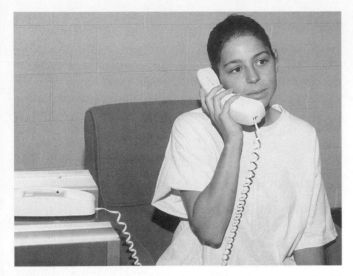

FIGURE 6–4 Using a telephone requires approximately 40 degrees of wrist extension.

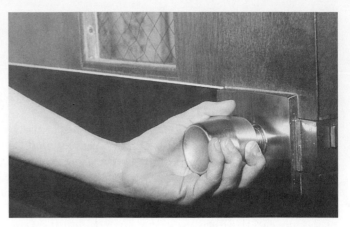

FIGURE 6–5 Turning a doorknob requires 40 degrees of wrist flexion and 45 degrees of wrist extension.

extension (40 to 64 degrees) and arc of motion (43 to 85 degrees). Turning a doorknob (Fig. 6–5) involved the greatest amount of flexion (40 degrees). The greatest amounts of ulnar deviation (27 to 32 degrees) were noted while rising from a chair, turning a door knob and steering wheel, and pouring from a pitcher.

Table 6–5 provides information on wrist position during the placement of the hand on the body areas commonly touched during personal care. The majority of positions required wrist flexion, and less overall wrist motion than the activities of daily living presented in Table 6–4. Among the positions studied, placing the palm to the front of the chest consistently required the greatest amount of wrist flexion, whereas placing the palm to the sacrum required the greatest amount of ulnar deviation.

Brumfield and Champoux[30] used a uniaxial electrogo-

niometer to determine the range wrist flexion and extension during 15 ADL performed by 12 men and 7 women ranging from 25 to 60 years of age. They determined that ADLs such as eating, drinking and using a telephone were accomplished with 5 degrees of flexion to 35 degrees of extension. Personal care activities that involved placing the hand on the body required 20 degrees of flexion to 15 degrees of extension. The authors concluded that an arc of wrist motion of 45 degrees (10 degrees of flexion to 35 degrees of extension) is sufficient to perform most of the activities studied.

Palmer and coworkers[33] used a triaxial electrogoniometer to study 10 normal subjects while they performed 52 tasks. A range of 32.5 degrees of flexion, 58.6 degrees of extension, 23.0 degrees of radial deviation, and 21.5 degrees of ulnar deviation was used in performing ADLs and personal hygiene. During these tasks the average amount of motion was about 5 degrees of flexion, 30 degrees of extension, 10 degrees of radial

TABLE 6–5 Wrist Motions During Hand Placement Needed for Personal Care Activities: Mean Values in Degrees					
	Extension	Flexion	Ulnar Dev	Radial Dev	
Activity	Mean (SD)	Mean (SD)	Mean (SD)	Mean (SD)	Source
Hand to top of head		2.3 (12.5)			Brumfield[30]
		20.9 (13.9)	16.1 (12.7)		Ryu[15]
Hand to occiput	12.7 (9.9)				Brumfield
		0.9 (17.6)	9.7 (11.9)		Ryu
Hand to front of chest		18.9 (8.9)			Brumfield
		24.5 (16.7)		5.1 (10.3)	Ryu
Hand to sacrum		0.6 (9.8)			Brumfield
		19.5 (19.3)	47.8 (16.8)		Ryu
Hand to foot	14.2 (10.6)				Brumfield
	0.8 (14.6)		8.7 (12.2)		Ryu

deviation, and 15 degrees of ulnar deviation. ROM values for individual tasks were not presented in the study.

Ryu and associates[15] found that 31 examined tasks could be performed with 54 degrees of flexion, 60 degrees of extension, 17 degrees of radial deviation, and 40 degrees of ulnar deviation. The 40 normal subjects (20 men and 20 women) were evaluated with a biaxial electrogoniometer during performance of palm placement activities, personal care and hygiene, diet and food preparation, and miscellaneous ADLs.

Studies by Safaee-Rad and coworkers[31] and Cooper and coworkers[32] examined wrist ROM with a video-based three-dimensional motion analysis system during three feeding tasks: drinking from a cup, eating with a fork, and eating with a spoon. The 10 males studied by Safaee-Rad and coworkers used from 10 degrees of wrist flexion to 25 degrees of extension, and from 20 degrees of ulnar deviation to 5 degrees of radial deviation during the tasks. Cooper and coworkers examined 10 males and 9 females during feeding tasks, with the elbow unrestricted and then fixed in 110 degrees of flexion. With the elbow unrestricted, males used from 7 degrees of wrist flexion to 21 degrees of extension, and from 19 degrees of ulnar deviation to 2 degrees of radial deviation. Females had similar values for flexion and extension but used from 3 degrees of ulnar deviation to 18 degrees of radial deviation. Both studies found that drinking from a cup required less of an arc of wrist motion than eating with a fork or spoon.

Nelson[34] took a different approach to determining the amount of wrist motion necessary for carrying out functional tasks. He evaluated the ability of 12 healthy subjects (9 males and 3 females) to perform 123 ADLs with a splint on the dominant wrist that limited motion to 5 degrees of flexion, 6 degrees of extension, 7 degrees of radial deviation, and 6 degrees of ulnar deviation. All 123 activities could be completed with the splint in place, with 9 activities having a mean difficulty rating of greater than or equal to 2 (could be done with minimal difficulty or frustration and with satisfactory outcome). The most difficult activities included: putting on/taking off a brassiere (Fig. 6–6), washing legs/back, writing, dusting low surfaces, cutting vegetables, handling a sharp knife, cutting meat, using a can opener, and using a manual eggbeater. It should be noted that these subjects were pain free and had normal shoulders and elbows to compensate for the restricted wrist motions. The ability to generalize these results to a patient population with pain and multiply involved joints may be limited.

Repetitive trauma disorders such as carpal tunnel syndrome and wrist/hand tendinitis have been noted to occur more frequently in performing certain types of work, sports, and artistic endeavors. To elucidate the cause of these higher incidences of injury, studies have been conducted on the wrist positions used, the amount

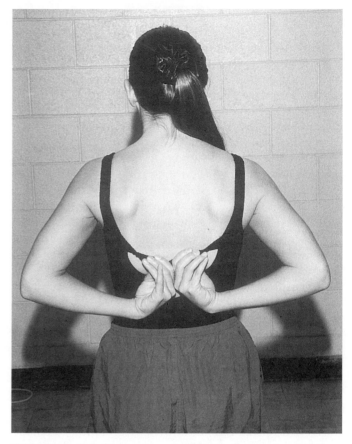

FIGURE 6–6 A large amount of wrist flexion is needed to fasten a bra or bathing suit. This is one of the most difficult activities to perform if wrist motion is limited.

and frequency of wrist motions required during grocery bagging,[35] grocery scanning,[36] piano playing,[37] industrial work,[38] handrim wheelchair propulsion,[39,40] and in playing sports such as basketball, baseball pitching, and golf.[6,41] The reader is advised to refer directly to these studies to gain information about the amount of wrist ROM that occurs during these activities. In general, an association has been noted between activities that require extreme wrist postures and the prevalence of hand/wrist tendinitis.[42] Tasks that involve repeated wrist flexion and extreme wrist extension, repetitive work with the hands, and repeated force applied to the base of the palm and wrist have been associated with carpal tunnel syndrome.[43]

Reliability and Validity

In early studies of wrist motion conducted by Hewitt[23] and Cobe,[26] both authors observed considerable differences in repeated measurements of active wrist motions. These differences were attributed to a lack of motor control on the part of the subjects in expending maximal effort. Cobe suggested that only average values have much validity and that changes in ROM should exceed 5 degrees to be considered clinically significant.

Later studies of intratester and intertester reliability were conducted by numerous researchers. The majority of these investigators found that intratester reliability was greater than intertester reliability, that reliability varied according to the motion being tested, and that different instruments should not be used interchangeably during joint measurement.

Hellebrandt, Duvall, and Moore[44] found that wrist motions measured with a universal goniometer were more reliable than those measured with a joint-specific device. Measurements of wrist flexion and extension were less reliable than measurements of radial and ulnar deviation, although mean differences between successive measurements taken with a universal goniometer by a skilled tester were 1.1 degrees for flexion and 0.9 degrees for extension. The mean differences between successive measurements increased to 5.4 degrees for flexion and 5.7 degrees for extension when successive measurements were taken with different instruments.

In a study by Low,[45] 50 testers using a universal goniometer visually estimated and then measured the author's active wrist extension and elbow flexion. Five testers also took 10 repeated measurements over the course of 5 to 10 days. Mean error improved from 12.8 degrees for visual estimates to 7.8 degrees for goniometric measurement. Intraobserver error was less than interobserver error. The measurement of wrist extension was less reliable than the measurement of elbow flexion, with mean errors of 7.8 and 5.0 degrees respectively.

Boone et al[46] conducted a study in which four testers using a universal goniometer measured ulnar deviation on 12 male volunteers. Measurements were repeated over a period of 4 weeks. Intratester reliability was found to be greater than intertester reliability. The authors concluded that to determine true change when more than one tester measures the same motion, differences in motion should exceed 5 degrees.

In a study by Bird and Stowe,[47] two observers repeatedly measured active and passive wrist ROM in three subjects. They concluded that interobserver error was greatest for extension (±8 degrees), and least for radial and ulnar deviation (±2 to 3 degrees). Error during passive ROM measurements was slightly greater than during active ROM measurements.

Greene and Wolf[14] compared the reliability of the OrthoRanger, an electronic pendulum goniometer, with a universal goniometer for active upper-extremity motions in 20 healthy adults. Wrist ROM was measured by one therapist three times with each instrument during each of three sessions over a 2-week period. There was a significant difference between instruments for wrist extension and ulnar deviation. Within-session reliability was slightly higher for the universal goniometer (intraclass correlation coefficient [ICC] 0.91 to 0.96) than for the

OrthoRanger (ICC 0.88 to 0.92). The 95 percent confidence level, which represents the variability around the mean, ranged from 7.6 to 9.3 degrees for the goniometer, and from 18.2 to 25.6 degrees for the OrthoRanger. The authors concluded that the OrthoRanger provided no advantages over the universal goniometer.

Solgaard and coworkers[16] found intratester standard deviations of 5 to 8 degrees and intertester standard deviations of 6 to 10 degrees in a study of wrist and forearm motions involving 31 healthy subjects. Measurements were taken with a universal goniometer by four testers on three different occasions. The coefficients of variation (percent variation) between testers were greater for ulnar and radial deviation than for flexion, extension, pronation, and supination.

Horger[48] conducted a study in which 13 randomly paired therapists performed repeated measurements of active and passive wrist motions on 48 patients. Therapists were free to select their own method of measurement with a universal goniometer. The six specialized hand therapists used an ulnar alignment for flexion and extension, whereas the nonspecialized therapists used a radial goniometer alignment. Intratester reliability of both active and passive wrist motions were highly reliable (all ICCs above 0.90) for all motions. Intratester reliability was consistently higher than intertester reliability (ICC 0.66 to 0.91). Standard errors of measurements (SEM) ranged from 2.6 to 4.4 for intratester values and from 3.0 to 8.2 for intertester values. Agreement between measures was better for flexion and extension than for radial and ulnar deviation. Intertester reliability coefficients for measurements of active motion (ICC 0.78 to 0.91) were slightly higher than coefficients for passive motion (ICC 0.66 to 0.86) except for radial deviation. Generally, reliability was higher for the specialized therapists than for the nonspecialized therapists. The author determined that the presence of pain reduced the reliability of both active and passive measurements, but active measurements were affected more than passive measurements.

LaStayo and Wheeler[49] studied the intratester and intertester reliability of passive ROM measurements of wrist flexion and extension in 120 patients as measured by 32 randomly paired therapists, who used three goniometric alignments (ulnar, radial, and dorsal-volar). The reliability of measuring wrist flexion ROM was consistently higher than that of measuring extension ROM. Mean intratester ICCs for wrist flexion were 0.86 for radial, 0.87 for ulnar, and 0.92 for dorsal alignment. Mean intratester ICCs for wrist extension were 0.80 for radial, 0.80 for ulnar, and 0.84 for volar alignment. The authors recommended that these three alignments, although generally having good reliability, should not be used interchangeably because there were some significant differences between the measurements taken with the three alignments. The authors suggested that the dorsal-volar alignment should be the technique of choice for measuring passive wrist flexion and extension, given its higher reliability. In an invited commentary on this study, Flower[50] suggested using the fifth metacarpal, which is easier to visualise and align with the distal arm of the goniometer in the ulnar technique, rather than the third metacarpal, which was used in the study. Flower noted that the presence and fluctuation of edema on the dorsal surface of the hand may reduce the reliability of the dorsal alignment and necessitate the use of the ulnar (fifth metacarpal) alignment in the clinical setting.

Range of Motion Testing Procedures: Wrist

Landmarks for Goniometer Alignment: The Wrist

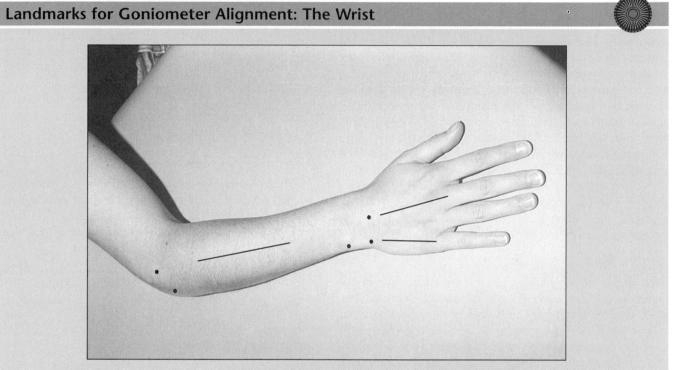

FIGURE 6–7 Posterior view of the upper extremity showing surface anatomy landmarks for goniometer alignment during the measurement of wrist ROM.

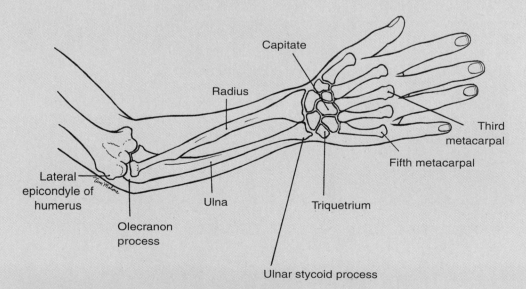

FIGURE 6–8 Posterior view of the upper extremity showing bony anatomical landmarks for goniometer alignment during the measurement of wrist ROM.

FLEXION

This motion occurs in the sagittal plane around a medial-lateral axis. Wrist flexion is sometimes referred to as volar or palmar flexion. Mean wrist flexion ROM values are 60 degrees according to the AMA[12] and 76 degrees according to Boone and Azen.[13] See Tables 6–1 to 6–3 for additional information.

Testing Position

Position the subject so that he or she is sitting next to a supporting surface with the shoulder abducted to 90 degrees and the elbow flexed to 90 degrees. Place the forearm midway between supination and pronation so that the palm of the hand faces the ground. Rest the forearm on the supporting surface, but leave the hand free to move. Avoid radial or ulnar deviation of the wrist and flexion of the fingers. If the fingers are flexed, tension in the extensor digitorum communis, extensor indicis, and extensor digiti minimi muscles will restrict the motion.

Stabilization

Stabilize the radius and ulna to prevent supination or pronation of the forearm and motion of the elbow.

Testing Motion

Flex the wrist by pushing on the dorsal surface of the third metacarpal, moving the hand toward the floor (Fig. 6–9). Maintain the wrist in 0 degrees of radial and ulnar deviation. The end of flexion ROM occurs when resistance to further motion is felt and attempts to overcome the resistance cause the forearm to lift off the supporting surface.

Normal End-feel

The end-feel is firm because of tension in the dorsal radiocarpal ligament and the dorsal joint capsule. Tension in the extensor carpi radialis brevis and longus and extensor carpi ulnaris muscles may also contribute to the firm end-feel.

Goniometer Alignment

See Figures 6–10 and 6–11.

1. Center the fulcrum of the goniometer on the lateral aspect of the wrist over the triquetrum.
2. Align the proximal arm with the lateral midline of the ulna, using the olecranon and ulnar styloid processes for reference.
3. Align the distal arm with the lateral midline of the fifth metacarpal. Do not use the soft tissue of the hypothenar eminence for reference.

Alternative Goniometer Alignment

This alternative goniometer alignment is recommended by the AMA *Guides to the Evaluation of Permanent Impairment*[12] and LaStoya and Wheeler,[49] although edema may make accurate alignment over the dorsal surfaces of the forearm and hand difficult.

1. Center the fulcrum of the goniometer over the capitate on the dorsal aspect of the wrist joint.
2. Align the proximal arm along the dorsal midline of the forearm.
3. Align the distal arm with the dorsal aspect of the third metacarpal.

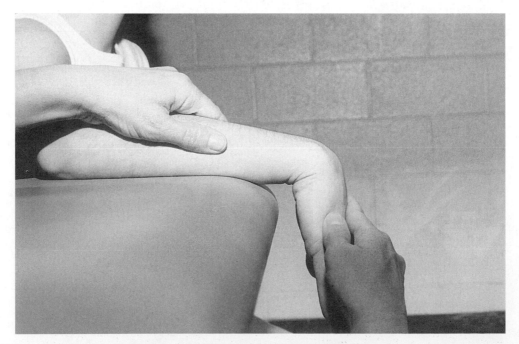

FIGURE 6–9 The end of wrist flexion ROM. Only about three-quarters of the subject's forearm is supported by the examining table, so that there is sufficient space for the hand to complete the motion.

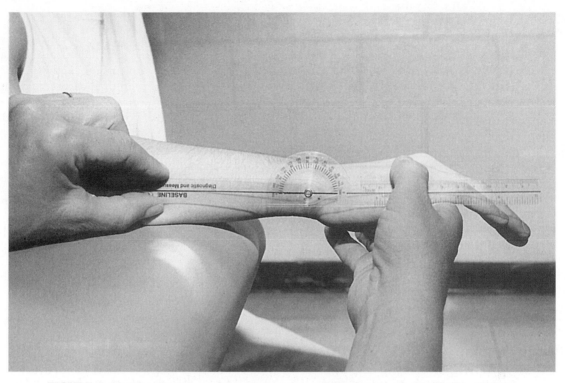

FIGURE 6–10 The alignment of the goniometer at the beginning of wrist flexion ROM.

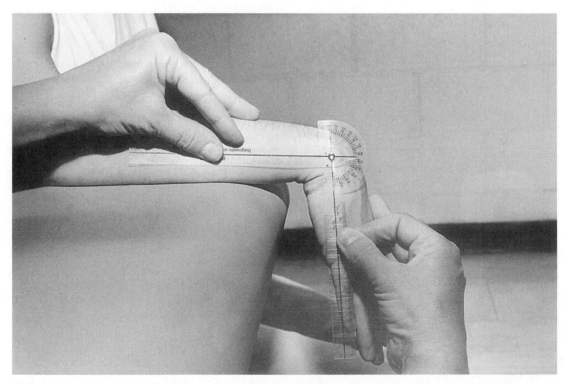

FIGURE 6–11 At the end of wrist flexion ROM the examiner uses one hand to align the distal arm of the goniometer with the fifth metacarpal while maintaining the wrist in flexion. The examiner exerts pressure on the middle of the dorsum of the subject's hand and avoids exerting pressure directly on the fifth metacarpal because such pressure will distort the goniometer alignment. The examiner uses her other hand to stabilize the forearm and hold the proximal arm of the goniometer.

EXTENSION

Motion occurs in the sagittal plane around a medial-lateral axis. Wrist extension is sometimes referred to as dorsal flexion. Mean wrist extension ROM values are 60 degrees according to the AMA[12] and 75 degrees according to Boone and Azen.[13] See Tables 6–1 to 6–3 for additional information.

Testing Position

Position the subject sitting next to a supporting surface with the shoulder abducted to 90 degrees and the elbow flexed to 90 degrees. Place the forearm midway between supination and pronation so that the palm of the hand faces the ground. Rest the forearm on the supporting surface, but leave the hand free to move. Avoid radial or ulnar deviation of the wrist, and extension of the fingers. If the fingers are held in extension tension in the flexor digitorum superficialis and profundus muscles will restrict the motion.

Stabilization

Stabilize the radius and ulna to prevent supination or pronation of the forearm, and motion of the elbow.

Testing Motion

Extend the wrist by pushing evenly across the palmar surface of the metacarpals, moving the hand in a dorsal direction toward the ceiling (Fig. 6–12). Maintain the wrist in 0 degrees of radial and ulnar deviation. The end of extension ROM occurs when resistance to further motion is felt and attempts to overcome the resistance cause the forearm to lift off of the supporting surface.

Normal End-feel

Usually the end-feel is firm because of tension in the palmar radiocarpal ligament, ulnocarpal ligament, and palmar joint capsule. Tension in the palmaris longus, flexor carpi radialis, and flexor carpi ulnaris muscles may also contribute to the firm end-feel. Sometimes the end-feel is hard because of contact between the radius and the carpal bones.

Goniometer Alignment

See Figures 6–13 and 6–14.

1. Center the fulcrum of the goniometer on the lateral aspect of the wrist over the triquetrum.
2. Align the proximal arm with the lateral midline of the ulna, using the olecranon and ulnar styloid process for reference.
3. Align the distal arm with the lateral midline of the fifth metacarpal. Do not use the soft tissue of the hypothenar eminence for reference.

Alternative Goniometer Alignment

This alternative alignment is recommended by the AMA *Guides to the Evaluation of Permanent Impairment*[12] and LaStayo and Wheeler,[49] although edema may make accurate alignment over the palmar surfaces of the forearm and hand difficult.

1. Center the fulcrum over the wrist joint at the level of the capitate.
2. Align the proximal arm with the palmar midline of the forearm.
3. Align the distal arm with the palmar midline of the third metacarpal.

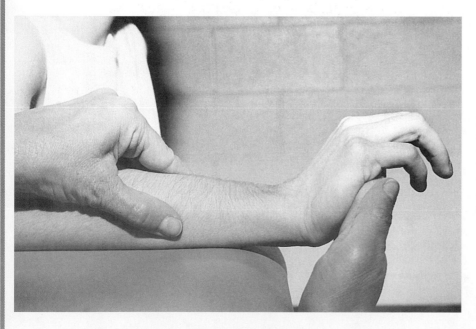

FIGURE 6–12 At the end of the wrist extension ROM, the examiner stabilizes the subject's forearm with one hand and uses her other hand to hold the subject's wrist in extension. The examiner is careful to distribute pressure equally across the subject's metacarpals.

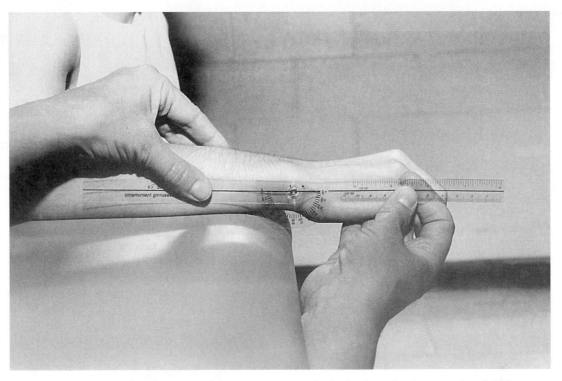

FIGURE 6–13 The alignment of the goniometer at the beginning of wrist extension ROM.

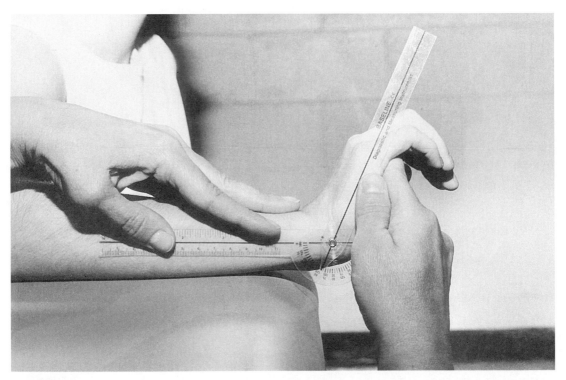

FIGURE 6–14 At the end of the ROM of wrist extension, the examiner aligns the distal goniometer arm with the fifth metacarpal while holding the wrist in extension. The examiner avoids exerting excessive pressure on the fifth metacarpal.

RADIAL DEVIATION

Motion occurs in the frontal plane around an anterior-posterior axis. Radial deviation is sometimes referred to as radial flexion or abduction. Mean radial deviation ROM is 20 degrees according to the AMA[12] and 25 degrees according to Greene and Wolf.[14] See Tables 6–1 to 6–3 for additional information.

Testing Position

Position the subject sitting next to a supporting surface with the shoulder abducted to 90 degrees and the elbow flexed to 90 degrees. Place the forearm midway between supination and pronation so that the palm of the hand faces the ground. Rest the forearm and hand on the supporting surface.

Stabilization

Stabilize the radius and ulna to prevent pronation or supination of the forearm and elbow flexion beyond 90 degrees.

Testing Motion

Radially deviate the wrist by moving the hand toward the thumb (Fig. 6–15). Maintain the wrist in 0 degrees of flexion and extension.[12] The end of radial deviation ROM occurs when resistance to further motion is felt and attempts to overcome the resistance cause the elbow to flex.

Normal End-feel

Usually the end-feel is hard because of contact between the radial styloid process and the scaphoid, but it may be firm because of tension in the ulnar collateral ligament, the ulnocarpal ligament, and the ulnar portion of the joint capsule. Tension in the extensor carpi ulnaris and flexor carpi ulnaris muscles may also contribute to the firm end-feel.

Goniometer Alignment

See Figures 6–16 and 6–17.

1. Center the fulcrum of the goniometer on the dorsal aspect of the wrist over the capitate.
2. Align the proximal arm with the dorsal midline of the forearm. If the shoulder is in 90 degrees of abduction and the elbow is in 90 of flexion, the lateral epicondyle of the humerus can be used for reference.
3. Align the distal arm with the dorsal midline of the third metacarpal. Do not use the third phalanx for reference.

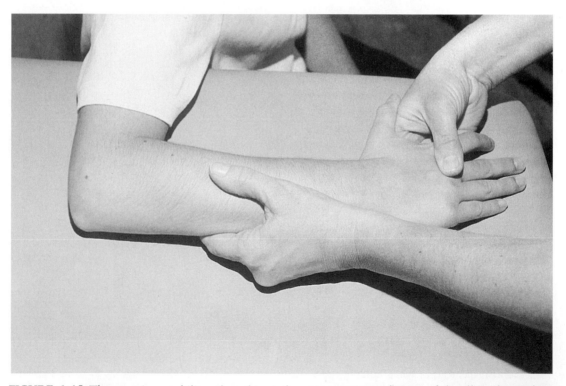

FIGURE 6–15 The examiner stabilizes the subject's forearm to prevent flexion of the elbow beyond 90 degrees when the wrist is moved into radial deviation. The examiner avoids moving the wrist into either flexion or extension.

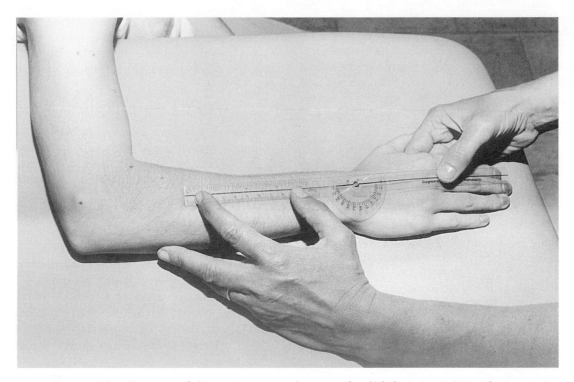

FIGURE 6–16 The alignment of the goniometer at the start of radial deviation ROM. The examining table can be used to support the hand.

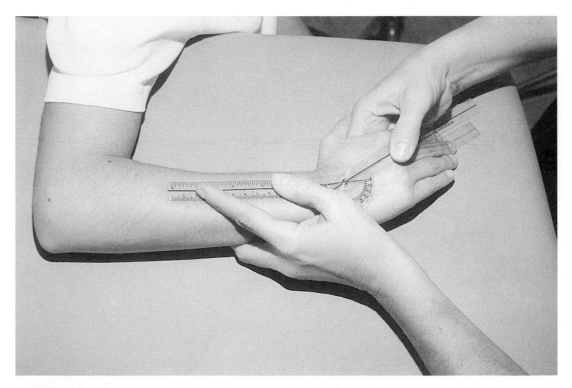

FIGURE 6–17 The alignment of the goniometer at the end of the radial deviation ROM. The examiner must center the fulcrum over the dorsal surface of the capitate. If the fulcrum shifts to the ulnar side of the wrist, there will be an incorrect measurement of excessive radial deviation.

ULNAR DEVIATION

Motion occurs in the frontal plane around an anterior-posterior axis. Ulnar deviation is sometimes referred to as ulnar flexion or adduction. Mean ulnar deviation ROM is 30 degrees according to the AMA[12] and 39 degrees according to Greene and Wolf.[14] See Tables 6–1 to 6–3 for additional information.

Testing Position

Position the subject sitting next to a supporting surface with the shoulder abducted to 90 degrees and the elbow flexed to 90 degrees. Place the forearm midway between supination and pronation so that the palm of the hand faces the ground. Rest the forearm and hand on the supporting surface.

Stabilization

Stabilize the radius and ulna to prevent pronation or supination of the forearm and less than 90 degrees of elbow flexion.

Testing Motion

Deviate the wrist in the ulnar direction by moving the hand toward the little finger (Fig. 6–18). Maintain the wrist in 0 degrees of flexion and extension, and avoid rotating the hand. The end of ulnar deviation ROM occurs when resistance to further motion is felt and attempts to overcome the resistance cause the elbow to extend.

Normal End-feel

The end-feel is firm because of tension in the radial collateral ligament and the radial portion of the joint capsule. Tension in the extensor pollicis brevis and abductor pollicis longus muscles may contribute to the firm end-feel.

Goniometer Alignment

See Figures 6–19 and 6–20.

1. Center the fulcrum of the goniometer on the dorsal aspect of the wrist over the capitate.
2. Align the proximal arm with the dorsal midline of the forearm. If the shoulder is in 90 degrees of abduction and the elbow is in 90 degrees of flexion, the lateral epicondyle of the humerus can be used for reference.
3. Align the distal arm with the dorsal midline of the third metacarpal. Do not use the third phalanx for reference.

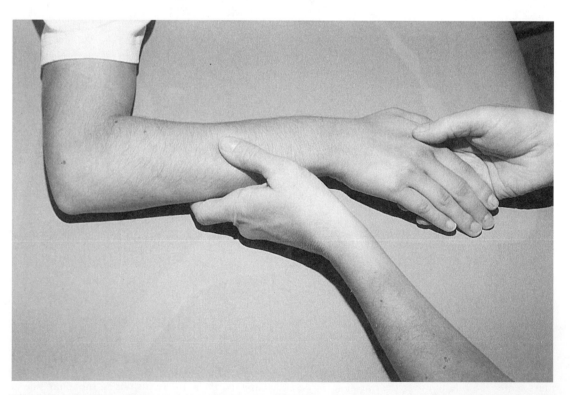

FIGURE 6–18 The examiner uses one hand to stabilize the subject's forearm and maintain the elbow in 90 degrees of flexion. The examiner's other hand moves the wrist into ulnar deviation, being careful not to flex or extend the wrist.

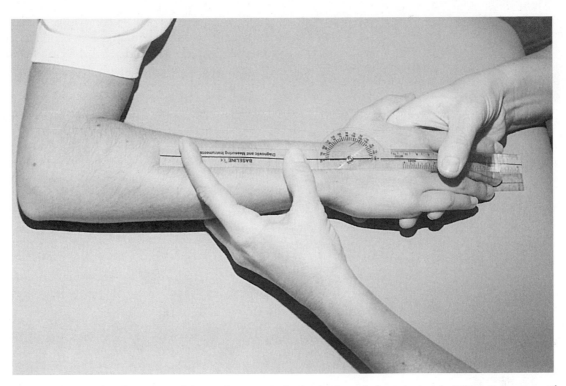

FIGURE 6–19 The alignment of the goniometer at the beginning of ulnar deviation ROM. Sometimes if a half-circle goniometer is used, the proximal and distal arms of the goniometer will have to be reversed so that the pointer remains on the body of the goniometer at the end of the ROM.

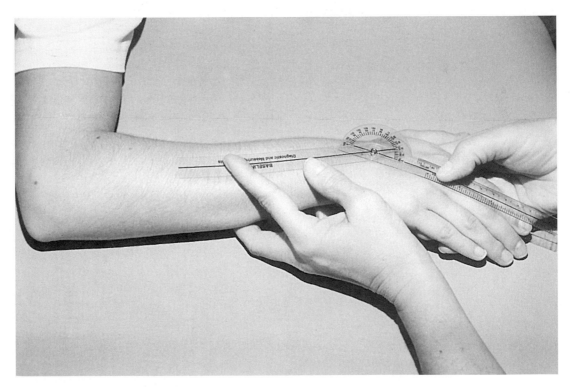

FIGURE 6–20 The alignment of the goniometer at the end of the ulnar deviation ROM. The examiner must center the fulcrum over the dorsal surface of the capitate. If the fulcrum shifts to the radial side of the wrist, there will be an incorrect measurement of excessive ulnar deviation.

Muscle Length Testing Procedures: Wrist

FLEXOR DIGITORUM PROFUNDUS AND FLEXOR DIGITORUM SUPERFICIALIS

The flexor digitorum profundus crosses the elbow, wrist, metacarpophalangeal (MCP), proximal interphalangeal (PIP), and distal interphalangeal (DIP) joints. The **flexor digitorum profundus** originates proximally from the upper three-fourths of the ulna, the coronoid process of the ulna, and the interosseus membrane (Fig. 6–21). This muscle inserts distally onto the palmar surface of the bases of the distal phalanges of the fingers. When it contracts, it flexes the MCP, PIP, and DIP joints of the fingers and flexes the wrist. The flexor digitorum profundus is passively lengthened by placing the elbow, wrist, MCP, PIP, and DIP joints in extension.

The **flexor digitorum superficialis** crosses the elbow, wrist, MCP, and PIP joints. The humeroulnar head of the flexor digitorum superficialis muscle originates proxi-

mally from the medial epicondyle of the humerus, the ulnar collateral ligament, and the coronoid process of the ulna (Fig. 6–22). The radial head of the flexor digitorum superficialis muscle originates proximally from the anterior surface of the radius. It inserts distally via two slips into the sides of the bases of the middle phalanges of the fingers. When the flexor digitoroum superficialis contracts, it flexes the MCP and PIP joints of the fingers and flexes the wrist. The muscle is passively lengthened by placing the elbow, wrist, MCP, and PIP joints in extension.

If the flexor digitorum profundus and flexor digitorum superficialis muscles are short, they will limit wrist extension when the elbow, MCP, PIP, and DIP joints are positioned in extension. If passive wrist extension is limited regardless of the position of the MCP, PIP, and DIP joints, the limitation is due to abnormalities of wrist joint surfaces or shortening of the palmar joint capsule, palmar radiocarpal ligament, ulnocarpal ligament, palmaris longus, flexor carpi radialis, or flexor carpi ulnaris muscles.

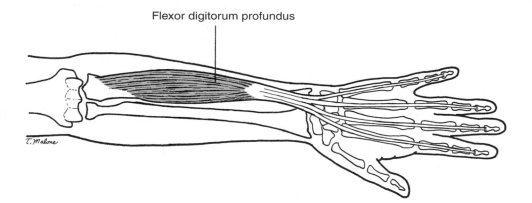

FIGURE 6–21   An anterior view of the forearm showing the attachments of the flexor digitorum profundus muscle.

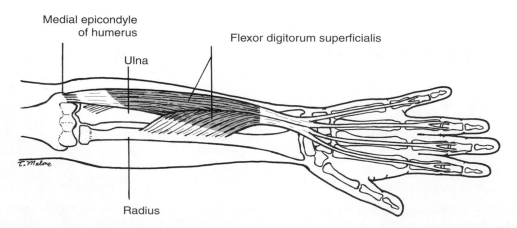

FIGURE 6–22   An anterior view of the forearm and hand showing the attachments of the flexor digitorum superficialis muscle.

Starting Position

Position the subject sitting next to a supporting surface with the upper extremity resting on the surface. Place the elbow, MCP, PIP, and DIP joints in extension (Fig. 6–23). Pronate the forearm and place the wrist in neutral.

Stabilization

Stabilize the forearm to prevent elbow flexion.

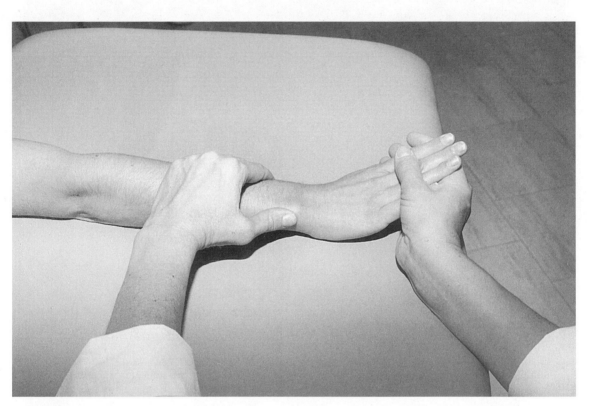

FIGURE 6–23 The starting position for testing the length of the flexor digitorum profundus and flexor digitorum superficialis muscles.

Testing Motion

Hold the MCP, PIP, and DIP joints in extension while extending the wrist (Figs. 6–24 and 6–25). The end of the testing motion occurs when resistance is felt and additional wrist extension causes the fingers or elbow to flex.

End-feel

The end-feel is firm because of tension in the flexor digitorum profundus and flexor digitorum superficialis muscles.

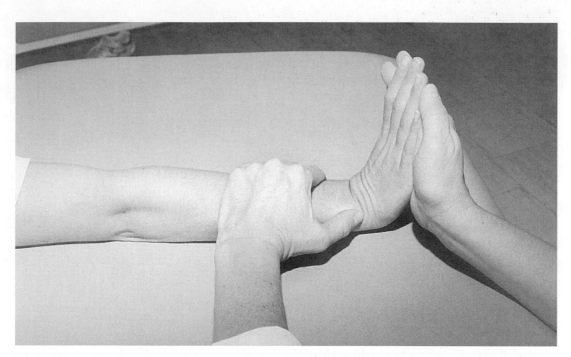

FIGURE 6–24 The end of the testing motion for the length of the flexor digitorum profundus and flexor digitorum superficialis muscles. The examiner uses one hand to stabilize the forearm, while the other hand holds the fingers in extension and moves the wrist into extension. The examiner has moved her right thumb from the dorsal surface of the fingers to allow a clearer photograph, but keeping the thumb placed on the dorsal surface would help to prevent the fingers from flexing at the PIP joints.

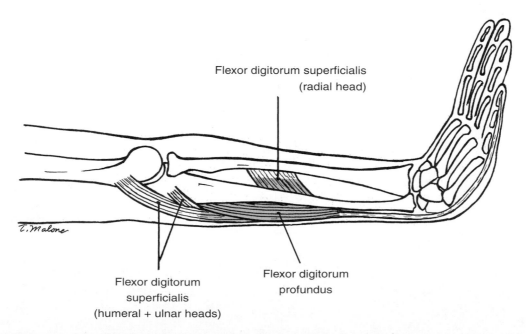

Flexor digitorum superficialis (radial head)

Flexor digitorum superficialis (humeral + ulnar heads)

Flexor digitorum profundus

FIGURE 6–25 A lateral view of the forearm and hand showing the flexor digitorum profundus and flexor digitorum superficialis being stretched over the elbow, wrist, MCP, PIP, and DIP joints.

Goniometer Alignment

See Figure 6–26.

1. Center the fulcrum of the goniometer on the lateral aspect of the wrist over the triquetrum.
2. Align the proximal arm with the lateral midline of the ulna, using the olecranon and ulnar styloid process for reference.
3. Align the distal arm with the lateral midline of the fifth metacarpal. Do not use the soft tissue of the hypothenar eminence for reference.

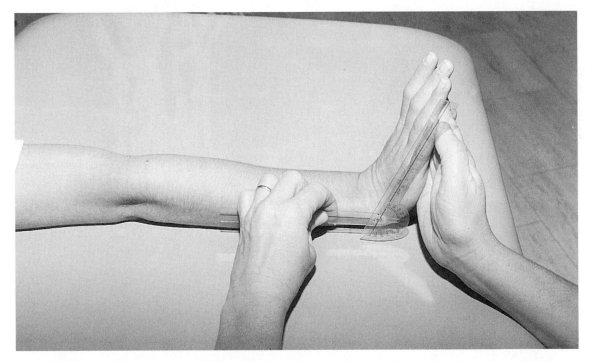

FIGURE 6–26 The alignment of the goniometer at the end of testing the length of the flexor digitorum profundus and flexor digitorum superficialis muscles.

EXTENSOR DIGITORUM, EXTENSOR INDICIS, AND EXTENSOR DIGITI MINIMI

The extensor digitorum, extensor indicis, and extensor digiti minimi muscles cross the elbow, wrist, and MCP, PIP, and DIP joints. When these muscles contract, they extend the MCP, PIP, and DIP joints of the fingers and extend the wrist. These muscles are passively lengthened by placing the elbow in extension, and the wrist, MCP, PIP, and DIP joints in full flexion.

The **extensor digitorum** originates proximally from the lateral epicondyle of the humerus and inserts distally onto the middle and distal phalanges of the fingers via the extensor hood (Fig. 6–27). The **extensor indicis** originates proximally from the posterior surface of the ulna and the interosseous membrane. This muscle inserts distally onto the extensor hood of the index finger. The **extensor digiti minimi** also originates proximally from the lateral epicondyle of the humerus but inserts distally onto the extensor hood of the little finger.

If the extensor digitorum, extensor indicis, and extensor digiti minimi muscles are short, they will limit wrist flexion when the elbow is positioned in extension and the MCP, PIP, and DIP joints are positioned in full flexion. If wrist flexion is limited regardless of the position of the MCP, PIP, and DIP joints, the limitation is due to abnormalities of joint surfaces of the wrist or shortening of the dorsal joint capsule, dorsal radiocarpal ligament, extensor carpi radialis longus, extensor carpi radialis brevis, or extensor carpi ulnaris muscles.

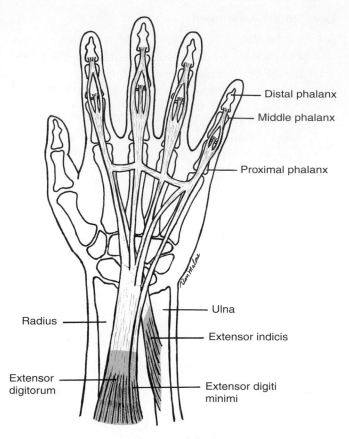

Distal phalanx

Middle phalanx

Proximal phalanx

Ulna

Radius

Extensor indicis

Extensor digitorum

Extensor digiti minimi

FIGURE 6–27 A posterior view of the forearm and hand showing the distal attachments of the extensor digitorum, extensor indicis, and extensor digit minimi muscles.

Starting Position

Position the subject sitting next to a supporting surface. Ideally, the upper arm and the forearm should rest on the supporting surface, but the hand should be free to move into flexion. Place the elbow in extension and the MCP, PIP, and DIP joints in full flexion (Fig. 6–28). Place the forearm in pronation and the wrist in neutral.

Stabilization

Stabilize the forearm to prevent elbow flexion.

Testing Motion

Hold the MCP, PIP, and DIP joints in full flexion while flexing the wrist (Figs. 6–29 and 6–30). The end of the testing motion occurs when resistance is felt and additional wrist flexion causes the fingers to extend or the elbow to flex.

Normal End-feel

The end-feel is firm because of tension in the extensor digitorum, extensor indicis, and extensor digiti minimi muscles.

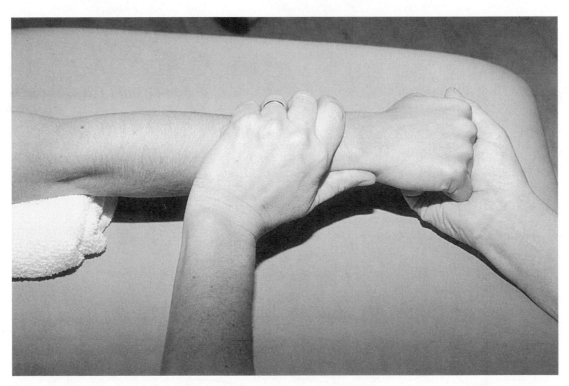

FIGURE 6–28 The starting position for testing the length of the extensor digitorum, extensor indicis, and extensor digit minimi muscles. The forearm must be elevated or the hand positioned off the end of the examining table to allow room for finger and wrist flexion.

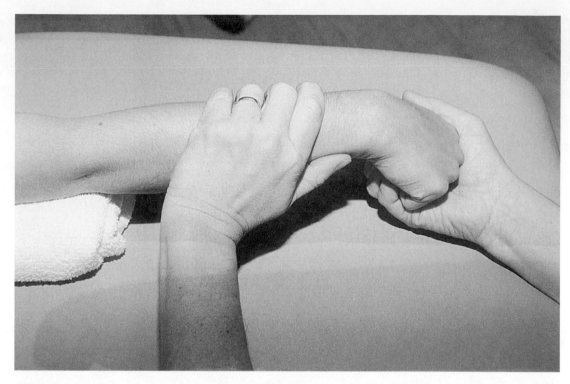

FIGURE 6–29 The end of the testing motion for the length of the extensor digitorum, extensor indicis, and extensor digit minimi muscles. One of the examiner's hands stabilizes the forearm, while the other hand holds the fingers in full flexion and moves the wrist into flexion.

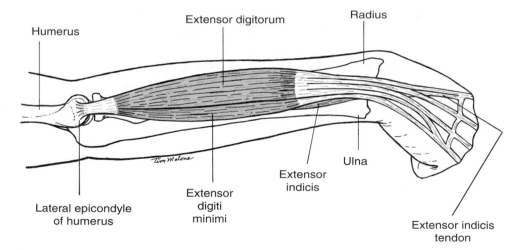

FIGURE 6–30 A posterior view of the forearm and hand showing the extensor digitorum, extensor indicis, and extensor digit minimi muscles stretched over the elbow, wrist, MCP, PIP, and DIP joints.

Goniometer Alignment

See Figure 6–31.

1. Center the fulcrum of the goniometer on the lateral aspect of the wrist over the triquetrum.
2. Align the proximal arm with the lateral midline of the ulna, using the olecranon and ulnar styloid process for reference.
3. Align the distal arm with the lateral midline of the fifth metacarpal. Do not use the soft tissue of the hypothenar eminence for reference.

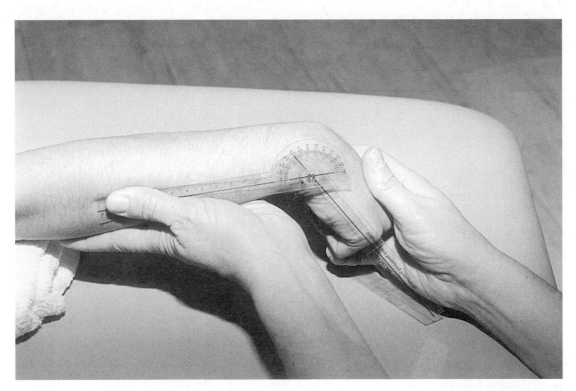

FIGURE 6–31 The alignment of the goniometer at the end of testing the length of the extensor digitorum, extensor indicis, and extensor digit minimi muscles.

REFERENCES

1. Linscheid, RL: Kinematic considerations of the wrist. Clin Orthop 202:27, 1986.
2. Levangie, PK, and Norkin, CC: Joint Structure and Function: A Comprehensive Analysis, ed 3. FA Davis, Philadelphia, 2001.
3. Kaltenborn, FM: Manual Mobilization of the Joints, Vol l: The Extremities, ed 5. Olaf Norlis Bokhandel, Oslo, Norway, 1999.
4. Sarrafian, SH, Melamed, JL, and Goshgarian, GM: Study of wrist motion in flexion and extension. Clin Orthop 126:153, 1977.
5. Youm, Y, et al: Kinematics of the wrist: I. An experimental study of radial-ulnar deviation and flexion-extension. J Bone Joint Surg (Am) 60:423, 1978.
6. Werner, SL, and Plancher, KD: Biomechanics of wrist injuries in sports. Clin Sports Med 17:407, 1998.
7. Ritt, M, et al: Rotational stability of the carpus relative to the forearm. J Hand Surg 20A:305, 1995.
8. Kisner, C, and Colby, LA: Therapeutic Exercise: Foundations and Techniques, ed 4. FA Davis, Philadelphia, 2002.
9. Cyriax, JH, and Cyriax, PJ: Illustrated Manual of Orthopaedic Medicine. Butterworths, London, 1983.
10. American Academy of Orthopaedic Surgeons: Joint Motion: Methods of Measuring and Recording. AAOS, Chicago, 1965.
11. Greene, WB, and Heckman, JD (eds):The Clinical Measurement of Joint Motion. American Academy of Orthopaedic Surgeons, Rosemont, Ill., 1994.
12. American Medical Association: Guides to the Evaluation of Permanent Impairment, ed 3. AMA, Chicago, 1990.
13. Boone, DC, and Azen, SP: Normal range of motion in male subjects. J Bone Joint Surg (Am) 61:756, 1979.
14. Greene, BL, and Wolf, SL: Upper extremity joint movement: Comparison of two measurement devices. Arch Phys Med Rehabil 70:288, 1989.
15. Ryu, J, et al: Functional ranges of motion of the wrist joint. J Hand Surg 16A:409, 1991.
16. Solgaard, S, et al: Reproducibility of goniometry of the wrist. Scand J Rehabil Med 18:5, 1986.
17. Solveborn, SA, and Olerud, C: Radial epicondylalgia (tennis elbow): Measurement of range of motion of the wrist and the elbow. J Orthop Sports Phys Ther 23:251, 1996.
18. Stubbs, NB, Fernandez, JE, and Glenn, WM: Normative data on joint ranges of motion of 25- to 54-year-old males. International Journal of Industrial Ergonomics 12; 265, 1993.
19. Walker, JM, et al: Active mobility of the extremities in older subjects. Phys Ther 64:919, 1984.
20. Chaparro, A, et al: Range of motion of the wrist: Implications for designing computer input devices for the elderly. Disabil Rehabil 22:633:2000.
21. Wanatabe, H, et al: The range of joint motions of the extremities in healthy Japanese people: The difference according to age. Nippon Seikeigeka Gokkai Zasshi 53:275, 1979. (Cited in Walker, JM: Musculoskeletal development: A review. Phys Ther 71:878, 1991.)
22. Boone, DC: Techniques of measurement of joint motion. (Unpublished supplement to Boone, DC, and Azen, SP: Normal range of motion in male subjects. J Bone Joint Surg (Am) 61:756, 1979.)
23. Hewitt, D: The range of active motion at the wrist of women. J Bone Joint Surg (Br) 26:775, 1928.
24. Allander, E, et al: Normal range of joint movements in shoulder, hip, wrist and thumb with special reference to side: A comparison between two populations. Int J Epidemiol 3:253, 1974.
25. Bell, RD, and Hoshizaki, TB: Relationships of age and sex with range of motion of seventeen joint actions in humans. Can J Appl Spt Sci 6:202, 1981.
26. Cobe, HM: The range of active motion of the wrist of white adults. J Bone Joint Surg (Br) 26:763, 1928.
27. Chang, DE, Buschbacher, LP, and Edlich, RF: Limited joint mobility in power lifters. Am J Sports Med 16:280, 1988.
28. Spilman, HW, and Pinkston, D: Relation of test positions to radial and ulnar deviation. Phys Ther 49:837, 1969.
29. Marshall, MM, Morzall, JR, and Shealy, JE: The effects of complex wrist and forearm posture on wrist range of motion. Human Factors, 41:205, 1999.
30. Brumfield, RH, and Champoux, JA: A biomechanical study of normal functional wrist motion. Clin Orthop 187:23, 1984.
31. Safaee-Rad, R, et al: Normal functional range of motion of upper limb joints during perfromance of three feeding tasks. Arch Phys Med Rehabil 71:505, 1990.
32. Cooper, JE, et al: Elbow joint restriction: Effect on functional upper limb motion during performance of three feeding tasks. Arch Phys Med Rehabil 74:805, 1993.
33. Palmer, AK, et al: Functional wrist motion: A biomechanical study. J Hand Surg 10A:39, 1985.
34. Nelson, DL: Functional wrist motion. Hand Clin 13:83, 1997.
35. Estill, CF, and Kroemer, KH: Evaluation of supermarket bagging using a wrist motion monitor. Hum Factors 40:624, 1998.
36. Marras, WS, et al: Quantification of wrist motion during scanning. Hum Factors 37:412, 1995.
37. Wagner, CH: The pianist's hand: Anthropometry and biomechanics. Ergonomics 31:97, 1988.
38. Marras, WS, and Schoenmarklin, RW: Wrist motions in industry. Ergonomics 36:341, 1995.
39. Veeger, DHEJ, et al: Wrist motion in handrim wheelchair propulsion. J Rehabil Res Dev 35:305, 1998.
40. Boninger, ML, et al: Wrist biomechanics during two speeds of wheelchair propulsion: An analysis using a local coordinate system. Arch Phys Med Rehabil 78:364, 1997.
41. Ohinishi, N, et al: Analysis of wrist motion during basketball shooting. In Nakamura, RL, Linscheid, RL, and Miura, T (eds): Wrist Disorder: Current Concepts and Challenges. New York, Springer-Verlag, 1992.
42. Bernard, BP (ed): Musculoskeletal disorders and workplace factors. Cincinnati, Oh.: National Institute of Occupational Safety and Health. 1997.
43. Armstrong, TJ, et al: Ergonomic considerations in hand and wrist tendinitis. J Hand Surg. 12A: 830, 1982.
44. Hellebrandt, FA, Duvall, EN, and Moore, ML: The measurement of joint motion. Part III: Reliability of goniometry. Physical Therapy Review 29:302, 1949.
45. Low, JL: The reliability of joint measurement. Physiotherapy 62:227, 1976.
46. Boone, DC, et al: Reliability of goniometric measurements. Phys Ther 58:1355, 1978.
47. Bird, HA, and Stowe, J: The wrist. Clinics in Rheumatic Disease 8:559, 1982.
48. Horger, MM: The reliability of goniometric measurements of active and passive wrist motions. Am J Occup Ther 44:342, 1990.
49. LaStayo, PC, and Wheeler, DL: Reliability of passive wrist flexion and extension measurements: A multicenter study. Phys Ther 74:162, 1994
50. Flower, KR: Invited Commentary. Phys Ther 74:174, 1994.

CHAPTER 7

The Hand

Structure and Function

Fingers: Metacarpophalangeal Joints

Anatomy

The metacarpophalangeal (MCP) joints of the fingers are composed of the convex distal end of each metacarpal and the concave base of each proximal phalanx (Fig. 7–1). The joints are enclosed in fibrous capsules (Figs. 7–2 and 7–3). The anterior portion of each capsule has a fibrocartilaginous thickening called the palmar plate (palmar ligament), which is firmly attached to the proximal phalanx.[1] Ligamentous support is provided by collateral and deep transverse metacarpal ligaments.

Osteokinematics

The MCP joints are biaxial condyloid joints that have 2 degrees of freedom, allowing flexion-extension in the sagittal plane and abduction-adduction in the frontal plane. Abduction-adduction is possible with the MCP joints positioned in extension, but limited with the MCP

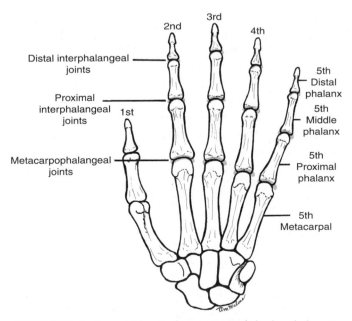

FIGURE 7–1 An anterior (palmar) view of the hand showing metacarpophalangeal, proximal interphalangeal, and distal interphalangeal joints.

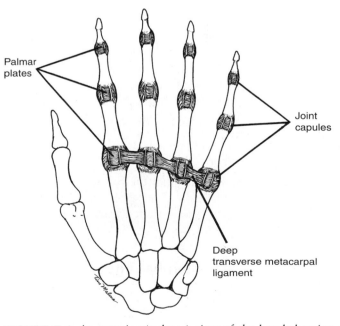

FIGURE 7–2 An anterior (palmar) view of the hand showing joint capsules and palmar plates of the metacarpophalangeal, proximal interphalangeal, and distal interphalangeal joints, as well as the deep transverse metacarpal ligament.

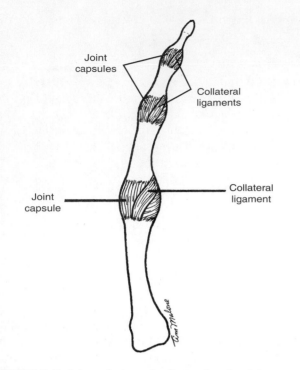

Joint capsules

Collateral ligaments

Joint capsule

Collateral ligament

FIGURE 7–3 A lateral view of a finger showing joint capsules and collateral ligaments of the metacarpophalangeal, proximal interphalangeal, and distal interphalangeal joints.

joints in flexion because of tightening of the collateral ligaments.[2] A small amount of passive axial rotation has been reported at the MCP joints,[2,3] but this motion is not usually measured in the clinical setting.

Arthrokinematics

The concave base of the phalanx glides over the convex head of the metacarpal in the same direction as the shaft of the phalanx. In flexion, the base of the phalanx glides toward the palm, whereas, in extension, the base glides dorsally on the metacarpal head. In abduction, the base of the phalanx glides in the same direction as the movement of the finger.

Capsular Pattern

Cyriax and Cyriax[4] report that the capsular pattern is an equal restriction of flexion and extension. Kaltenborn[5] notes that all motions are restricted with more limitation in flexion.

Fingers: Proximal Interphalangeal and Distal Interphalangeal Joints

Anatomy

The structure of both the proximal interphalangeal (PIP) and the distal interphalangeal (DIP) joints is very similar (see Fig. 7–1). Each phalanx has a concave base and a convex head. The joint surfaces comprise the head of the

more proximal phalanx and the base of the adjacent, more distal phalanx. Each joint is supported by a joint capsule, a palmar plate, and two collateral ligaments (see Figs. 7–2 and 7–3).

Osteokinematics

The PIP and DIP joints of the fingers are classified as synovial hinge joints with 1 degree of freedom: flexion-extension in the sagittal plane.

Arthrokinematics

Motion of the joint surfaces includes a sliding of the concave base of the more distal phalanx on the convex head of the proximal phalanx. Sliding of the base of the moving phalanx occurs in the same direction as the movement of the shaft. For example, in PIP flexion, the base of the middle phalanx slides toward the palm. In PIP extension, the base of the middle phalanx slides toward the dorsum of the hand.

Capsular Pattern

The capsular pattern is an equal restriction of both flexion and extension, according to Cyriax and Cyriax. Kaltenborn[5] notes that all motions are restricted with more limitation in flexion.

Thumb: Carpometacarpal Joint

Anatomy

The carpometacarpal (CMC) joint of the thumb is the articulation between the trapezium and the base of the first metacarpal (Fig. 7–4). The saddle-shaped trapezium is concave in the sagittal plane and convex in the frontal plane. The base of the first metacarpal has a reciprocal shape that conforms to that of the trapezium. The joint capsule is thick but lax and is reinforced by radial, ulnar, palmar, and dorsal ligaments (Fig. 7–5).

Osteokinematics

The first CMC joint is a saddle joint with 2 degrees of freedom: flexion-extension in the frontal plane parallel to the palm and abduction-adduction in the sagittal plane perpendicular to the palm.[1] The laxity of the joint capsule also permits some axial rotation. This rotation allows the thumb to move into position for contact with the fingers during opposition. The sequence of motions that combines with rotation and results in opposition is as follows: abduction, flexion, and adduction. Reposition returns the thumb to the starting position.

Arthrokinematics

The concave portion of the first metacarpal slides on the convex portion of the trapezium in the same direction as the metacarpal shaft to produce flexion-extension. During flexion, the base of the metacarpal slides in an ulnar direction. During extension, it slides in a radial

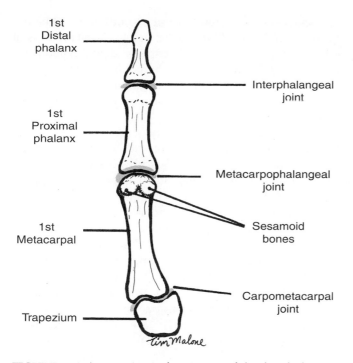

FIGURE 7–4 An anterior (palmar) view of the thumb showing carpometacarpal, metacarpophalangeal, and interphalangal joints

1st Distal phalanx

Interphalangeal joint

1st Proximal phalanx

Metacarpophalangeal joint

1st Metacarpal

Sesamoid bones

Trapezium

Carpometacarpal joint

direction. The convex portion of the first metacarpal base slides on the concave portion of the trapezium in a direction opposite to the shaft of the metacarpal to produce abduction-adduction. The base of the first metacarpal slides toward the dorsal surface of the hand in abduction and toward the palmar surface of the hand in adduction.

Capsular Pattern

The capsular pattern is a limitation of abduction according to Cyriax and Cyriax.[4] Kaltenborn[5] reports limitation in abduction and extension.

Thumb: Metacarpophalangeal Joint

Anatomy

The MCP joint of the thumb is the articulation between the convex head of the first metacarpal and the concave base of the first proximal phalanx (see Fig. 7–4). The joint is reinforced by a joint capsule, palmar plate, two sesamoid bones on the palmar surface, two intersesamoid ligaments (cruciate ligaments), and two collateral ligaments (see Fig. 7–5).

Osteokinematics

The MCP joint is a condyloid joint with 2 degrees of freedom.[1,6] The motions permitted are flexion-extension and a minimal amount of abduction-adduction. Motions at this joint are more restricted than at the MCP joints of

the fingers. Extension beyond neutral is not usually present.

Arthrokinematics

At the MCP joint the concave base of the first phalanx glides on the convex head of the first metacarpal in the same direction as the shaft. The base of the proximal phalanx moves toward the palmar surface of the thumb in flexion and toward the dorsal surface of the thumb in extension.

Capsular Pattern

The capsular pattern for the MCP joint is a restriction of motion in all directions, but flexion is more limited than extension.[4,5]

Thumb: Interphalangeal Joint

Anatomy

The interphalangeal joint of the thumb is identical in structure to the IP joints of the fingers. The head of the proximal phalanx is convex and the base of the distal phalanx is concave (see Fig. 7–4). The joint is supported by a joint capsule, a palmar plate, and two lateral collateral ligaments (see Fig. 7–5).

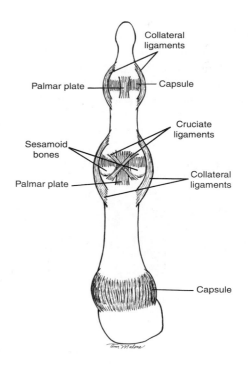

Collateral ligaments

Palmar plate

Capsule

Cruciate ligaments

Sesamoid bones

Collateral ligaments

Palmar plate

Capsule

FIGURE 7–5 An anterior (palmar) view of the thumb showing joint capsules, collateral ligaments, palmar plates, and cruciate (intersesamoid) ligaments.

Osteokinematics

The IP joint is a synovial hinge joint with 1 degree of freedom: flexion-extension in the sagittal plane.

Arthrokinematics

At the IP joint the concave base of the distal phalanx glides on the convex head of the proximal phalanx, in the same direction as the shaft of the bone. The base of the distal phalanx moves toward the palmar surface of the thumb in flexion and toward the dorsal surface of the thumb in extension.

Capsular Pattern

The capsular pattern is an equal restriction in both flexion and extension according to Cyriax.[4] Kaltenborn[5] notes that all motions are restricted with more limitation in flexion.

Research Findings

Effects of Age, Gender, and Other Factors

Table 7–1 provides a summary of range of motion (ROM) values for the MCP, PIP, and DIP joints of the fingers. Although the values reported by the different sources in Table 7–1 vary, certain trends are evident. The PIP joints, followed by the MCP and DIP joints, have the greatest amount of flexion. The MCP joints have the greatest amount of extension, whereas the PIP joints have the least amount of extension. Total active motion (TAM) is the sum of flexion and extension ROM of the MCP, PIP, and DIP joints of a digit. The mean TAM varies from 290 to 310 degrees for the fingers.

The age, gender, and number of subjects used to obtain the values reported by the AAOS[7] and the AMA[8] in Table 7–1 are not noted. Hume and coworkers[9] measured active finger motions in 35 men by means of a goniometer on the lateral aspect of both hands. Mallon, Brown, and Nunley[10] measured active finger motions in 60 men and 60 women with a special digital goniometer on the dorsal surface of both hands. Skvarilova and Plevkova[11] used a metallic slide goniometer to measure active finger motions on the dorsal aspect of both hands of 100 men and 100 women.

Mallon, Brown, and Nunley[10] and Skvarilova and Plevkova[11] also assessed passive and active joint motion in individual fingers. Table 7–2 presents passive ROM values for the joints of individual fingers. Some differences in ROM values are noted between the fingers. Flexion ROM at the MCP joints increases linearly in an ulnar direction from the index finger to the little finger.[10,11] Mallon, Brown, and Nunley[10] report that extension at the MCP joints is approximately equal for all fingers. However, Skvarilova and Plevkova[11] note that the little finger has the greatest amount of MCP extension. PIP flexion and extension and DIP flexion are generally equal for all fingers.[10] Some passive extension beyond neutral is possible at the DIP joints, with a minor increase in a radial direction from the little finger toward the index finger.[10]

Only the MCP joints of the fingers have a considerable amount of abduction-adduction. The amount of abduction-adduction varies with the position of the MCP joint. Abduction-adduction ROM is greatest in extension and least in full flexion. The collateral ligaments of the MCP joints are slack and allow full abduction in extension. However, the collateral ligaments tighten and restrict abduction in the fully flexed position.[1,2,12] The index and little fingers have a greater ROM in abduction-adduction than the middle and ring fingers.[1]

Table 7–3 presents ROM values for the CMC, MCP, and IP joints of the thumb. Flexion is greatest at the IP joint and least at the CMC joint. The greatest amount of extension is reported at the IP and CMC joints. The age,

---

TABLE 7–1.   Finger Motion: Mean Values in Degrees from Selected Sources

Joint	Motion	AAOS[7]	AMA[8]	Hume*[9] (active)	Mallon†[10] (active)	Skvarilova‡[11] (active) Mean (SD)
MCP	Flexion	90	90	100	95	91.0 (6.2)
	Extension	45	20	0	20	25.8 (6.7)
PIP	Flexion	100	100	105	105	107.9 (5.6)
	Extension	0	0	0	7	
DIP	Flexion	90	70	85	68	84.5 (7.9)
	Extension	0	0	0	8	
Total active motion				290	303	309.2 (6.6)

AAOS = American Association of Orthopaedic Surgeons; AMA = American Medical Association; DIP = distal interphalangeal; MCP = metacarpophalangeal; PIP = proximal interphalangeal; (SD) = standard deviation.

* Values are for 35 males aged 26 to 28 years.

† Values are for 60 males and 60 females, aged 18 to 35 years. Values were recalculated to include both genders and all fingers.

‡ Values are for 100 males and 100 females, aged 20 to 25 years. Values were recalculated to include both genders, both hands, all fingers, and converted from a 360-degree to a 180-degree recording system.

TABLE 7–2 Individual Passive Finger Motion: Mean Values in Degrees from Selected Sources

Finger	Joint	Motion	Mallon*[10]		Skvarilova†[11]	
			Male	Female	Male	Female
Index	MCP	Flexion	94	95	97	97
		Extension	29	56	55	56
	PIP	Flexion	106	107	115	117
		Extension	11	19		
	DIP	Flexion	75	75	87	95
		Extension	22	24		
Middle	MCP	Flexion	98	100	102	104
		Extension	34	54	48	48
	PIP	Flexion	110	112	115	118
		Extension	10	20		
	DIP	Flexion	80	79	87	98
		Extension	19	23		
Ring	MCP	Flexion	102	103	104	102
		Extension	29	60	48	49
	PIP	Flexion	110	108	115	119
		Extension	14	20		
	DIP	Flexion	74	76	83	92
		Extension	17	18		
Little	MCP	Flexion	107	107	107	104
		Extension	48	62	63	65
	PIP	Flexion	111	110	111	113
		Extension	13	21		
	DIP	Flexion	72	72	89	102
		Extension	15	21		

DIP = Distal interphalangeal; MCP = metacarpophalangeal; PIP = proximal interphalangeal.
* Values are for 60 males and 60 females, aged 18 to 35 years. Flexion values were measured with the contiguous proximal joint extended, except for DIP flexion in which the PIP joint was flexed. Extension values were measured with the contiguous proximal joint flexed. These contiguous proximal joint positions resulted in the greatest ROM values in the measured joint.
† Values are for 100 males and 100 females, aged 20 to 25. Values were converted from a 360-degree to a 180-degree recording system.

gender, and number of subjects used to obtain the values reported by the AAOS[7] and the AMA[8] are not noted. Jenkins and associates[13] measured active motions of both thumbs in 69 females and 50 males by means of a computerized Greenleaf goniometer. DeSmet and colleagues[14] measured ROM with a goniometer applied to the dorsal aspect of both thumbs in 58 females and 43 males. Skvarilova and Plevkova[11] used a metallic slide goniometer to measure active and passive motions on the dorsal aspect of both thumbs of 100 men and 100 women.

TABLE 7–3   Thumb Motion: Mean Values in Degrees from Selected Sources

		AAOS[7]	AMA[8]	Jenkins*[13] (active)	DeSmet†[14]	Skvarilova‡[11] (active)	(passive)
Joint	Motion			Mean (SD)	Mean (SD)	Mean (SD)	Mean (SD)
CMC	Abduction	70					
	Flexion	15					
	Extension	20	50				
MCP	Flexion	50	60	59 (11)	54.0 (13.7)	57.0 (10.7)	67.0 (9.0)
	Extension	0				13.7 (10.5)	22.6 (10.9)
IP	Flexion	80	80	67 (11)	79.8 (10.2)	79.1 (8.7)	85.8 (8.3)
	Extension	20				23.2 (13.3)	34.7 (13.3)

CMC = Carpometacarpal; IP = interphalangeal; MCP = metacarpophalangeal; (SD) = standard deviation.
* Values are for active ROM in 69 females and 50 males, aged 16 to 72 years.
† Values are for 58 females and 43 males, aged 16 to 83 years.
‡ Values are for 100 males and 100 females, aged 20 to 25 years. Values were recalculated to include both thumbs for both genders and converted from a 360-degree to a 180-degree recording system.

Age

Goniometric studies focusing on the effects of age on ROM typically exclude the joints of the fingers and thumb; therefore, not much information is available on these joints. DeSmet and colleagues[14] found a significant correlation between decreasing MCP and IP flexion of the thumb and increasing age. The 58 females and 43 males who were included in the study ranged in age from 16 to 83 years. Beighton, Solomon, and Soskolne[15] used passive opposition of the thumb (with wrist flexion) to the anterior aspect of the forearm and passive hyperextension of the MCP joint of the fifth finger beyond 90 degrees as indicators of hypermobility in a study of 456 men and 625 women in an African village. They found that joint laxity decreased with age. However, Allander and associates[16] found that active flexion and passive extension of the MCP joint of the thumb demonstrated no consistent pattern of age-related effects in a study of 517 women and 208 men (between 33 and 70 years of age). These authors stated that the typical reduction in mobility with age resulting from degenerative arthritis found in other joints may be exceeded by an accumulation of ligamentous ruptures that lessen the stability of the first MCP joint.

Gender

Studies that examined the effect of gender on the ROM of the fingers reported varying results. Mallon, Brown, and Nunley[10] found no significant effect of gender on the amount of flexion in any joints of the fingers. However, in this study women generally had more extension at all joints of the fingers than men. Skvarilova and Plevkova[11] found that PIP flexion, DIP flexion, and MCP extension of the fingers were greater in women than in men, whereas MCP flexion of the fingers was greater in men.

Several studies have found no significant differences between males and females in the ROM of the thumb, whereas other studies have reported more mobility in females. Joseph[17] used radiographs to examine MCP and IP flexion ROM of the thumb in 90 males and 54 females; no significant differences were found between the two groups. He found two general shapes of MCP joints, round and flat, with the round MCP joints having greater range of flexion. Shaw and Morris[18] noted no differences in MCP and IP flexion ROM between 199 males and 149 females aged 16 to 86 years. Likewise, DeSmet and colleagues,[14] as well as Jenkins and associates,[13] found no differences in MCP and IP flexion of the thumb owing to gender.

Allander and associates[16] found that, in some age groups, females showed more mobility in the MCP joint of the thumb than their male counterparts. Skvarilova and Plevkova[11] noted that MCP flexion and extension of the thumb were greater in females, whereas differences owing to gender were small and unimportant at the IP joint. Beighton, Solomon, and Soskolne,[15] in a study of 456 men and 625 women of an African village, and Fairbank, Pynsett, and Phillips,[19] in a study of 227 male and 219 female adolescents, measured passive opposition of the thumb toward the anterior surface of the forearm and hyperextension of the MCP joints of the fifth or middle fingers. Both studies reported an increase in laxity in females compared with males.

Right versus Left Sides

The few studies that have compared ROM in the right and left joints of the fingers have generally found no significant difference between sides. Mallon, Brown, and Nunley,[10] in a study in which half of the 120 subjects were right-handed and the other half left-handed, noted no difference between sides in finger motions at the MCP, PIP, and DIP joints. Skvarilova and Plevkova[11] reported only small right-left differences in the majority of the joints of the fingers and thumb in 200 subjects. Only MCP extension of the fingers and thumb and IP flexion of the thumb seemed to have greater ROM values on the left.

Similar to findings in studies of the fingers, most studies have reported no difference in ROM between the right and left thumbs. Joseph[17] and Shaw and Morris,[18] in a study of 144 and 248 subjects, respectively, found no significant difference between sides in MCP and IP flexion ROM of the thumb. DeSmet and colleagues[14] examined 101 healthy subjects and reported no difference between sides for the MCP and IP joints of the thumb. No difference between sides in IP flexion of the thumb was found by Jenkins and associates[13] in a study of 119 subjects. A statistically significant greater amount of MCP flexion was reported for the right thumb than for the left; however, this difference was only 2 degrees. Allander and associates[16] also found no differences attributed to side in MCP motions of the thumb in 720 subjects.

Testing Position

Mallon, Brown, and Nunley,[10] in addition to establishing normative ROM values for the fingers, also studied passive joint ROM while positioning the next most proximal joint in maximal flexion and extension. The DIP joint had significantly more flexion (18 degrees) when the PIP joint was flexed than when the PIP joint was extended. This finding has been cited as an indication of abnormal tightness of the oblique retinacular ligament (Landsmeer's Ligament).[20] However, the results of Mallon, Brown, and Nunley's study suggest that this finding is normal. The MCP joint had about 6 degrees more flexion when the wrist was extended than when the wrist was flexed, although this difference was not statistically significant. The extensor digitorum, extensor indicis, and extensor digiti minimi were more slack to allow greater flexion of the MCP joint when the wrist was extended than when flexed. There was no effect on PIP motion with changes in MCP joint position.

Knutson and associates[21] examined eight subjects to study the effect of seven wrist positions on the torque required to passively move the MCP joint of the index finger. The findings indicated that in many wrist positions, extrinsic tissues (those that cross more than one joint) such as the extensor digitorum, extensor indicis, flexor digitorum superficialis, and flexor digitorum profundus muscles offered greater restraint to MCP flexion and extension than intrinsic tissues (those that cross only one joint). Intrinsic tissues offered greater resistance to passive moment at the MCP joint when the wrist was flexed or extended enough to slacken the extrinsic tissues.

Functional Range of Motion

Joint motion, muscular strength and control, sensation, adequate finger length, and sufficient palm width and depth are necessary for a hand that is capable of performing functional, occupational, and recreational activities. Numerous classification systems and terms for describing functional hand patterns have been proposed.[2,22-25] Some common patterns include (1) finger-thumb prehension such as tip (Fig. 7–6), pulp, lateral, and three-point pinch (Fig. 7–7); (2) full-hand prehension, also called a power grip or cylindrical grip (Fig. 7–8); (3) nonprehension, which requires parts of the hand to be used as an extension of the upper extremity; and (4) bilateral prehension, which requires use of the palmar surfaces of both hands.[23] Texts by Stanley and Tribuzi,[26] Hunter and coworkers,[27] and the American Society of Hand Therapists[28] have reviewed many functional patterns and tests for the hand.

Table 7–4 summarizes the active ROM of the dominant fingers and thumb during 11 activities of daily living

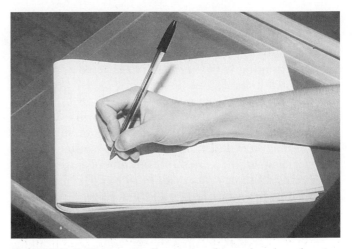

FIGURE 7–7 Writing usually requires finger-thumb prehension in the form of a three-point pinch.

that require various types of finger-thumb prehension or full-hand prehension. Hume and coworkers[9] used an electrogoniometer and a universal goniometer to study 35 right-handed men aged 26 to 28 years during performance of these 11 tasks. Of the tasks that were included, holding a soda can required the least amount of

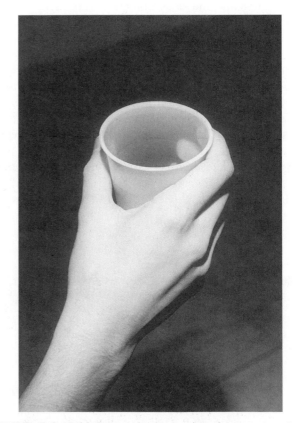

FIGURE 7–8 Holding a cylinder such as a cup requires full-hand prehension (power grip). The amount of metacarpophalangeal and proximal interphalangeal flexion varies, depending on the diameter of the cylinder.

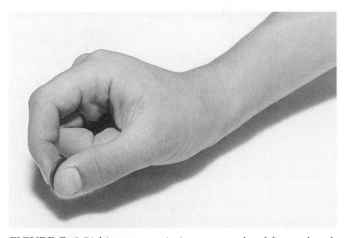

FIGURE 7–6 Picking up a coin is an example of finger-thumb prehension that requires use of the tips or pulps of the digits. In this photograph the pulp of the thumb and the tip of the index finger are being employed.

finger and thumb motion, whereas holding a toothbrush required the most motion. Joint ROM during other tasks, such as holding a telephone, holding a fork, turning a key, and printing with a pen, were clustered around the means listed in Table 7–4.

Lee and Rim[29] examined the amount of motion required at the joints of the fingers to grip five different-size cylinders. Data were collected from four subjects by means of markers and multi-camera photogrammetry. As cylinder diameter decreased, the amount of flexion of the MCP and PIP joints increased. However, DIP joint flexion remained constant with all cylinder sizes.

Sperling and Jacobson-Sollerman[30] used movie film in their study of the grip pattern of 15 men and 15 women aged 19 to 56 years during serving, eating, and drinking activities. The use of different digits, types of grips, contact surfaces of the hand, and relative position of the digits was reported; however, ROM values were not included.

Reliability and Validity

Several studies have been conducted to assess the reliability and validity of goniometric measurements in the hand. Most studies found that ROM measurements of the fingers and thumb that were taken with universal goniometers and finger goniometers were highly reliable. Measurements taken over the dorsal surface of the digits appear to be similar to those taken laterally. Consistent with other regions of the body, measurements of finger and thumb ROM taken by one examiner are more reliable than measurements taken by several examiners. Research studies support the opinions of Bear-Lehman and Abreu[31] and Adams, Greene, and Topoozian,[32] that the margin of error is generally accepted to be 5 degrees for goniometric measurement of joints in the hand, provided that measurements are taken by the same examiner and that standardized techniques are employed.

Hamilton and Lachenbruch[33] had seven testers take measurements of MCP, PIP, and DIP flexion in one subject whose fingers were held in a fixed position. The daily measurements were taken for 4 days with three types of goniometers. These authors found intertester reliability was lower than intratester reliability. No significant differences existed between measurements taken with a dorsal (over-the-joint) finger goniometer, a universal goniometer, or a pendulum goniometer.

Groth and coworkers[34] had 39 therapists measure the PIP and DIP joints of the index and middle fingers of one patient, both dorsally and laterally, using either a six-inch plastic universal goniometer or a DeVore metal finger goniometer. No significant difference in measurements was found between the two instruments. No differences were found between the dorsal and lateral measurement methods for seven of the eight joint motions, with mean differences ranging from 2 to 0 degrees. In a subset of six therapists, intertester reliability was high for both methods, with intraclass correlation coefficients (ICCs) ranging from 0.86 for lateral methods to 0.99 for dorsal methods. In terms of concurrent validity, there were significant differences in measurements obtained from radiographs versus those from goniometers excepting laterally measured index PIP extension and flexion. Differences between radiographic and goniometric measurements ranged from 1 to 10 degrees, but these differences may have been due to variations in procedures and positioning.

Weiss and associates[35] compared measurements of index finger MCP, PIP, and DIP joint positions taken by a dorsal metal finger goniometer with those taken by the Exos Handmaster, a Hall-effect instrumented exoskeleton. Twelve subjects were measured with each device during one session by one examiner, and again within 2 weeks of the initial session. Test-retest reliability was high for both devices, with ICCs ranging from 0.98 to 0.99. Mean differences between sessions for each instrument were statistically significant but less than 1 degree. Measurements taken by the finger goniometer and those taken by the Exos Handmaster were significantly different (mean difference = 7 degrees) but highly correlated (r = 0.89 to 0.94).

Ellis, Bruton, and Goddard[36] placed one subject in two splints while a total of 40 therapists measured the MCP, PIP, and DIP joints of the middle finger by means of a dorsal finger goniometer and a wire tracing. Each therapist measured each joint three times with each device. The goniometer consistently produced smaller ranges and smaller standard deviations than the wire tracing, indicating better reliability for the goniometer. The 95 percent confidence limit for the difference between measurements ranged from 3.8 to 9.9 degrees for the goniometer and 8.9 to 13.2 degrees for the wire tracing. Both methods had more variability when distal joints were measured, possibly because of the shorter levers used to align the goniometer or wire. Intratester reliability was always higher than intertester reliability.

TABLE 7–4   Finger and Thumb Motions During 11 Functional Activities: Values in Degrees[9]

Motion	Range	Mean	SD
Finger MCP flexion	33–73	61	12
PIP flexion	36–86	60	12
IP flexion	20–61	39	14
Thumb MCP flexion	10–32	21	5
IP flexion	2–43	18	5

IP = Interphalangeal; MCP = metacarpophalangeal; PIP = proximal interphalangeal; (SD) = standard deviation.
The 11 functional activities include: holding a telephone, can, fork, scissors, toothbrush, and hammer; using a zipper and comb; turning a key; printing with a pen; and unscrewing a jar.

Brown and colleagues[37] evaluated the ROM of the MCP, PIP, and DIP joints of two fingers in 30 patients to calculate total active motion (TAM) by means of the dorsal finger goniometer and the computerized Dexter Hand Evaluation and Treatment System. Three therapists measured each finger three times with each device during one session. Intratester and intertester reliability was high for both methods, with ICCs ranging from 0.97 to 0.99. The mean difference between methods ranged from 0.1 degrees to 2.4 degrees.

The distance between the fingertip pulp and distal palmar crease has been suggested as a simple and quick method of estimating total finger flexion ROM at the MCP, PIP, and DIP joints.[32, 38] MacDermid and coworkers[39] studied the validity of using the pulp-to-palm distance versus total finger flexion to predict disability as measured by an upper extremity disability score (DASH). active MCP, PIP, and DIP flexion was measured in 50 patients by one examiner who used a dorsally placed electrogoniometer NK Hand Assessment System. A ruler was used to measure pulp-to-palm distance in the same patients. The correlation between pulp-to-palm distance and total active flexion was -0.46 to -0.51, indicating that the measures were not interchangeable. The relationship between DASH scores and total active flexion was stronger (r = 0.45) than the relationship between DASH scores and pulp-to-palm distances (r = 0.21 to 0.30). The authors suggested that total active motion is a more functional measure than pulp-to-palm distance, and that pulp-to-palm distance "should only be used to monitor individual patient progress and not to compare outcomes between patients or groups of patients."

Range of Motion Testing Procedures: Fingers

Included in this section are the common clinical techniques for measuring motions of the fingers and thumb. These techniques are appropriate for evaluating these motions in the majority of people. However, swelling and bony deformities sometimes require that the examiner either measure the MCP and IP joints from the lateral aspect or create alternative evaluation techniques. Photocopies, photographs, and tracings of the hand at the beginning and end of the ROM may be helpful.

Landmarks for Goniometer Alignment

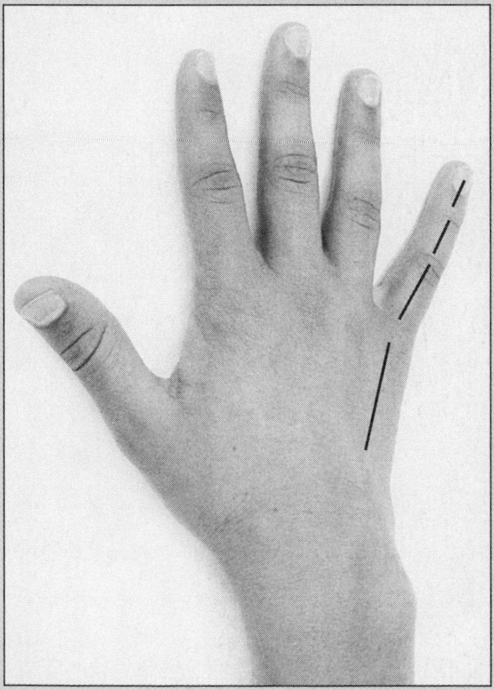

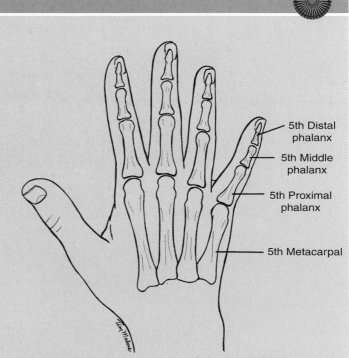

FIGURE 7–9 Posterior view of the hand showing surface anatomy landmarks for goniometer alignment during measurement of finger range of motion.

FIGURE 7–10 Posterior view of the hand showing bony anatomical landmarks for goniometer alignment during the measurement of finger range of motion. The index, middle, ring, and little fingers each have a metacarpal and a proximal, middle, and distal phalanx.

METACARPOPHALANGEAL FLEXION

Motion occurs in the sagittal plane around a medial-lateral axis. Mean finger flexion ROM values are 90 degrees according to the AAOS[7] and the AMA,[8] and 100 degrees according to Hume and coworkers.[9] MCP flexion appears to increase slightly in an ulnar direction from the index finger to the little finger. See Tables 7–1 and 7–2 for additional information.

Testing Position

Place the subject sitting, with the forearm and hand resting on a supporting surface. Place the forearm midway between pronation and supination, the wrist in 0 degrees of flexion, extension, and radial and ulnar deviation; and the MCP joint in a neutral position relative to abduction and adduction. Avoid extreme flexion of the PIP and DIP joints of the finger being examined.

Stabilization

Stabilize the metacarpal to prevent wrist motion. Do not hold the MCP joints of the other fingers in extension because tension in the transverse metacarpal ligament will restrict the motion.

Testing Motion

Flex the MCP joint by pushing on the dorsal surface of the proximal phalanx, moving the finger toward the palm (Fig. 7–11). Maintain the MCP joint in a neutral position relative to abduction and adduction. The end of flexion ROM occurs when resistance to further motion is felt and attempts to overcome the resistance cause the wrist to flex.

Normal End-feel

The end-feel may be hard because of contact between the palmar aspect of the proximal phalanx and the metacarpal, or it may be firm because of tension in the dorsal joint capsule and the collateral ligaments.

Goniometer Alignment

See Figures 7–12 and 7–13.

1. Center the fulcrum of the goniometer over the dorsal aspect of the MCP joint.
2. Align the proximal arm over the dorsal midline of the metacarpal.
3. Align the distal arm over the dorsal midline of the proximal phalanx.

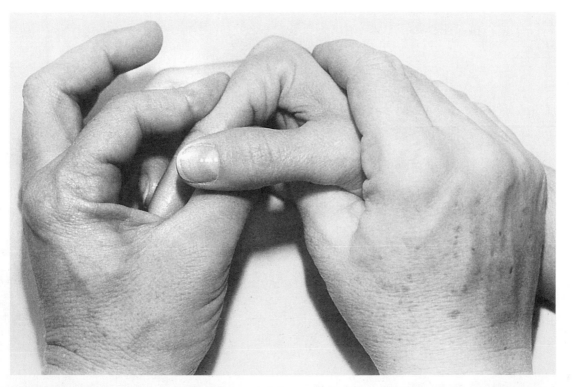

FIGURE 7–11 During flexion of the metacarpophalangeal joint, the examiner uses one hand to stabilize the subject's metacarpal and to maintain the wrist in a neutral position. The index finger and the thumb of the examiner's other hand grasp the subject's proximal phalanx to move it into flexion.

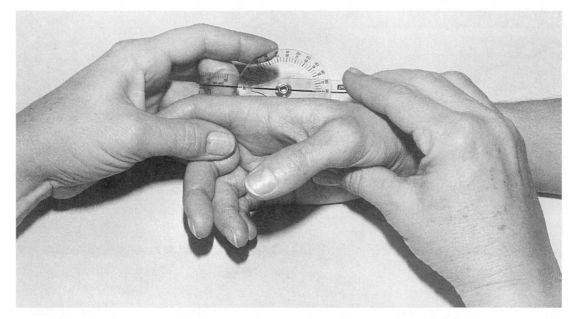

FIGURE 7–12 The alignment of the goniometer at the beginning of metacarpophalangeal flexion range of motion (ROM). In this photograph, the examiner is using a 6-inch plastic goniometer in which the arms have been trimmed to approximately 2 inches to make it easier to align over the small joints of the hand. Most examiners use goniometers with arms that are 6 inches or shorter when measuring ROM in the hand.

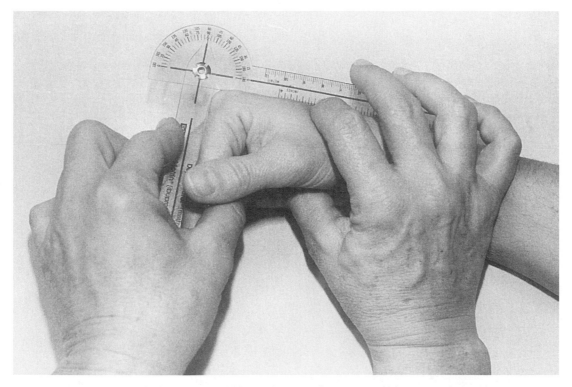

FIGURE 7–13 At the end of metacarpophalangeal (MCP) flexion range of motion, the examiner uses one hand to hold the proximal goniometer arm in alignment and to stabilize the subject's metacarpal. The examiner's other hand maintains the proximal phalanx in MCP flexion and aligns the distal goniometer arm. Note that the goniometer arms make direct contact with the dorsal surfaces of the metacarpal and proximal phalanx, causing the fulcrum of the goniometer to lie somewhat distal and dorsal to the MCP joint.

METACARPOPHALANGEAL EXTENSION

Motion occurs in the sagittal plane around a medial-lateral axis. Mean MCP finger extension ROM is 20 degrees according to the AMA[8] and 45 degrees according to the AAOS.[7] Passive MCP extension ROM is greater than active extension. Mallon, Brown, and Nunley[10] report that extension ROM at the MCP joints is similar across all fingers, whereas Skvarilova and Plevkova[11] note that the little finger has the greatest amount of MCP extension. See Tables 7–1 and 7–2 for additional information.

Testing Position

Position the subject sitting, with the forearm and hand resting on a supporting surface. Place the forearm midway between pronation and supination; the wrist in 0 degrees of flexion, extension, and radial and ulnar deviation; and the MCP joint in a neutral position relative to abduction and adduction. Avoid extension or extreme flexion of the PIP and DIP joints of the finger being tested. (If the PIP and DIP joints are positioned in extension, tension in the flexor digitorum superficialis and profundus muscles may restrict the motion. If the PIP and DIP joints are positioned in full flexion, tension in the lumbricalis and interossei muscles will restrict the motion.)

Stabilization

Stabilize the metacarpal to prevent wrist motion. Do not hold the MCP joints of the other fingers in full flexion because tension in the transverse metacarpal ligament will restrict the motion.

Testing Motion

Extend the MCP joint by pushing on the palmar surface of the proximal phalanx, moving the finger away from the palm (Fig. 7–14). Maintain the MCP joint in a neutral position relative to abduction and adduction. The end of flexion ROM occurs when resistance to further motion is felt and attempts to overcome resistance cause the wrist to extend.

Normal End-feel

The end-feel is firm because of tension in the palmar joint capsule and in the palmar plate.

Goniometer Alignment

See Figures 7–15 and 7–16 for alignment of the goniometer over the dorsal aspect of the fingers.

1. Center the fulcrum of the goniometer over the dorsal aspect of the MCP joint.
2. Align the proximal arm over the dorsal midline of the metacarpal.
3. Align the distal arm over the dorsal midline of the proximal phalanx.

Alternative Goniometer Alignment

See Figure 7–17 for alignment of the goniometer over the palmar aspect of the finger. This alignment should not be used if swelling or hypertrophy is present in the palm of the hand.

1. Center the fulcrum of the goniometer over the palmar aspect of the MCP joint.
2. Align the proximal arm over the palmar midline of the metacarpal.
3. Align the distal arm over the palmar midline of the proximal phalanx.

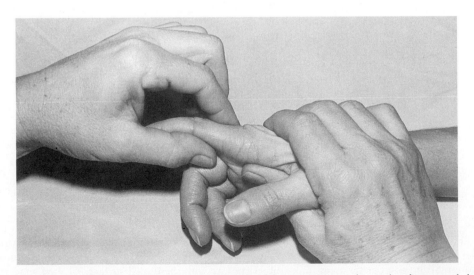

FIGURE 7–14 During metacarpophalangeal extension, the examiner uses her index finger and thumb to grasp the subject's proximal phalanx and to move the phalanx dorsally. The examiner's other hand maintains the subject's wrist in the neutral position, stabilizing the metacarpal.

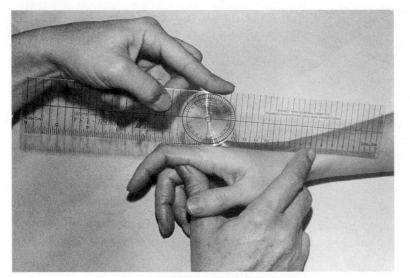

FIGURE 7–15 A full-circle, 6-inch plastic goniometer is being used to measure the beginning range of motion for metacarpophalangeal extension. The proximal arm of the goniometer is slightly longer than necessary for optimal alignment. If a goniometer of the right size is not available, the examiner can cut the arms of a plastic model to a suitable length.

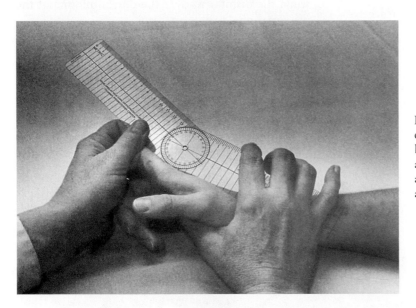

FIGURE 7–16 The alignment of the goniometer at the end of metacarpophalangeal (MCP) extension. The body of the goniometer is aligned over the dorsal aspect of the MCP joint, whereas the goniometer arms are aligned over the dorsal aspect of the metacarpal and proximal phalanx.

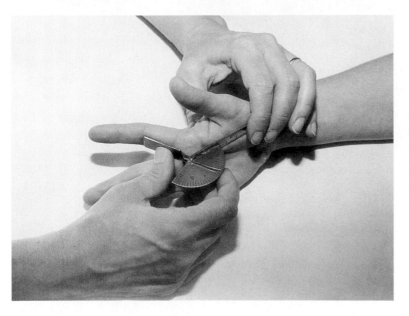

FIGURE 7–17 An alternative alignment of a finger goniometer over the palmar aspect of the proximal phalanx, the metacarpophalangeal joint, and the metacarpal. The shorter goniometer arm must be used over the palmar aspect of the proximal phalanx so that the proximal interphalangeal and distal interphalangeal joints are allowed to relax in flexion.

METACARPOPHALANGEAL ABDUCTION

Motion occurs in the frontal plane around an anterior-posterior axis. No sources were found for MCP abduction ROM values.

Testing Position

Position the subject sitting, with the forearm and hand resting on a supporting surface. Place the wrist in 0 degrees of flexion, extension, and radial and ulnar deviation; the forearm fully pronated so that the palm of the hand faces the ground; and the MCP joint in 0 degrees of flexion and extension.

Stabilization

Stabilize the metacarpal to prevent wrist motions.

Testing Motion

Abduct the MCP joint by pushing on the medial surface of the proximal phalanx, moving the finger away from the midline of the hand (Fig. 7–18). Maintain the MCP joint in a neutral position relative to flexion and extension. The end of flexion ROM occurs when resistance to further motion is felt and attempts to overcome the resistance cause the wrist to move into radial or ulnar deviation.

Normal End-feel

The end-feel is firm because of tension in the collateral ligaments of the MCP joints, the fascia of the web space between the fingers, and the palmar interossei muscles.

Goniometer Alignment

See Figures 7–19 and 7–20.

1. Center the fulcrum of the goniometer over the dorsal aspect of the MCP joint.
2. Align the proximal arm over the dorsal midline of the metacarpal.
3. Align the distal arm over the dorsal midline of the proximal phalanx.

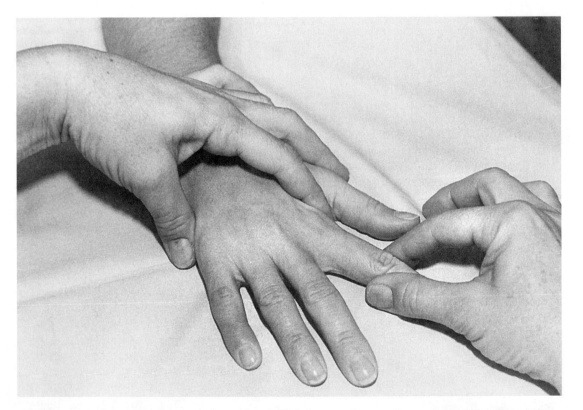

FIGURE 7–18 During metacarpophalangeal (MCP) abduction, the examiner uses the index finger of one hand to press against the subject's metacarpal and prevent radial deviation at the wrist. With the other index finger and thumb holding the distal end of the proximal phalanx, the examiner moves the subject's second MCP joint into abduction.

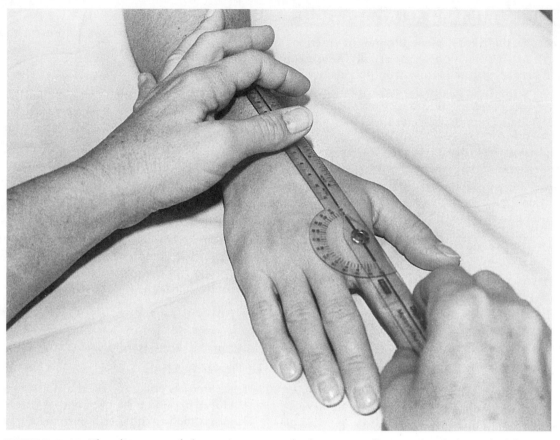

FIGURE 7–19 The alignment of the goniometer at the beginning of metacarpophalangeal abduction range of motion.

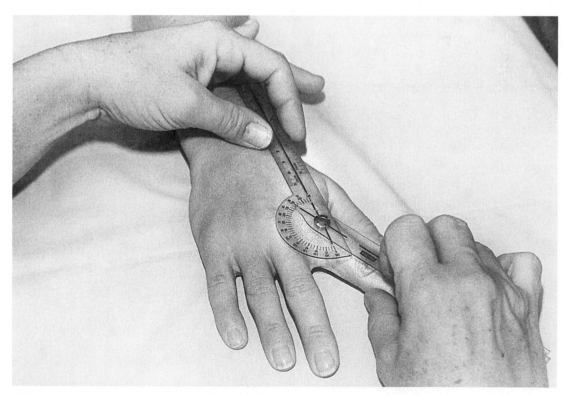

FIGURE 7–20 At the end of metacarpophalangeal abduction, the examiner aligns the arms of the goniometer with the dorsal midline of the metacarpal and proximal phalanx rather than with the contour of the hand and finger.

METACARPOPHALANGEAL ADDUCTION

Motion occurs in the frontal plane around an anterior-posterior axis. MCP adduction is not usually measured and recorded because it is the return from full abduction to the 0 starting position. There is very little adduction ROM beyond the 0 starting position. No sources were found for MCP adduction ROM values.

PROXIMAL INTERPHALANGEAL FLEXION

Motion occurs in the sagittal plane around a medial-lateral axis. Mean PIP finger flexion ROM values are 100 degrees according to the AAOS[7] and the AMA[8] and 105 degrees according to Hume and coworkers[9] and Mallon, Brown, and Nunley.[10] PIP flexion is similar between the fingers.[10] See Tables 7–1 and 7–2 for additional information.

Testing Position

Place the subject sitting, with the forearm and hand resting on a supporting surface. Position the forearm in 0 degrees of supination and pronation; the wrist in 0 degrees of flexion, extension, and radial and ulnar deviation; and the MCP joint in 0 degrees of flexion, extension, abduction, and adduction. (If the wrist and MCP joints are positioned in full flexion, tension in the extensor digitorum communis, extensor indicis, or extensor digiti minimi muscles will restrict the motion. If the MCP joint is positioned in full extension, tension in the lumbricalis and interossei muscles will restrict the motion.)

Stabilization

Stabilize the proximal phalanx to prevent motion of the wrist and the MCP joint.

Testing Motion

Flex the PIP joint by pushing on the dorsal surface of the middle phalanx, moving the finger toward the palm (Fig. 7–21). The end of flexion ROM occurs when resistance to further motion is felt and attempts to overcome the resistance cause the MCP joint to flex.

Normal End-feel

Usually, the end-feel is hard because of contact between the palmar aspect of the middle phalanx and the proximal phalanx. In some individuals, the end-feel may be soft because of compression of soft tissue between the palmar aspect of the middle and proximal phalanges. In other individuals, the end-feel may be firm because of tension in the dorsal joint capsule and the collateral ligaments.

Goniometer Alignment

See Figures 7–22 and 7–23.

1. Center the fulcrum of the goniometer over the dorsal aspect of the PIP joint.
2. Align the proximal arm over the dorsal midline of the proximal phalanx.
3. Align the distal arm over the dorsal midline of the middle phalanx.

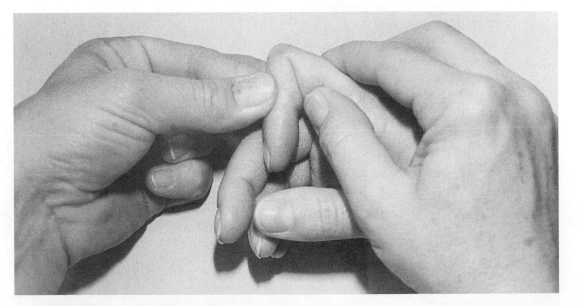

FIGURE 7–21 During proximal interphalangeal (PIP) flexion, the examiner stabilizes the subject's proximal phalanx with her thumb and index finger. The examiner uses her other thumb and index finger to move the subject's PIP joint into full flexion.

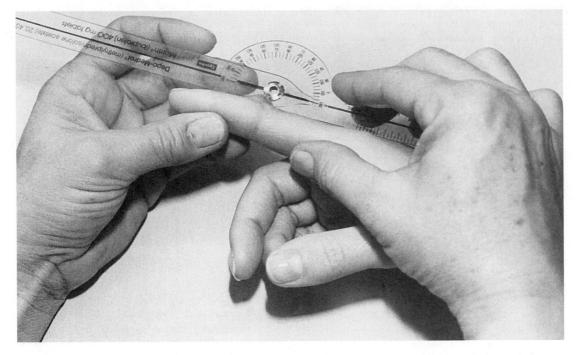

FIGURE 7–22 The alignment of the goniometer at the beginning of proximal interphalangeal flexion range of motion.

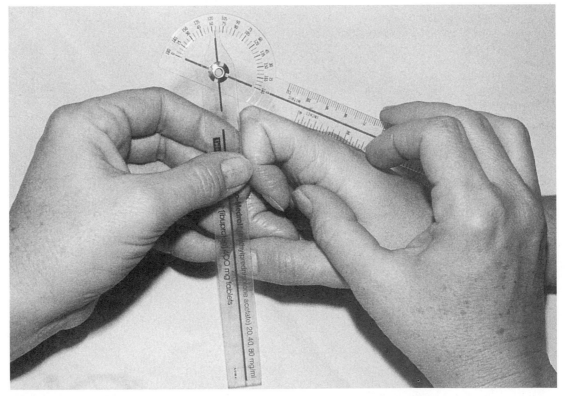

FIGURE 7–23 At the end of proximal interphalangeal (PIP) flexion, the examiner continues to stabilize and align the proximal goniometer arm over the dorsal midline of the proximal phalange with one hand. The examiner's other hand maintains the PIP joint in flexion and aligns the distal goniometer arm with the dorsal middline of the middle phalanx.

PROXIMAL INTERPHALANGEAL EXTENSION

Motion occurs in the sagittal plane around a medial-lateral axis. Mean PIP finger extension ROM values are 0 degrees according to the AAOS[7] and the AMA.[8] Data from Mallon, Brown, and Nunley[10] indicate a mean of 7 degrees of active PIP extension and 16 degrees of passive PIP extension. PIP extension is generally equal for all fingers.[10] See Tables 7–1 and 7–2 for additional information.

Testing Position

Place the subject sitting, with the forearm and hand resting on a supporting surface. Position the forearm in 0 degrees of supination and pronation, the wrist in 0 degrees of flexion, extension, and radial and ulnar deviation, and the MCP joint in 0 degrees of flexion, extension, abduction, and adduction. (If the MCP joint and wrist are extended, tension in the flexor digitorum superficialis and profundus muscles will restrict the motion.)

Stabilization

Stabilize the proximal phalanx to prevent motion of the wrist and the MCP joint.

Testing Motion

Extend the PIP joint by pushing on the palmar surface of the middle phalanx, moving the finger away from the palm. The end of extension ROM occurs when resistance to further motion is felt and attempts to overcome the resistance cause the MCP joint to extend.

Normal End-feel

The end-feel is firm because of tension in the palmar joint capsule and palmar plate (palmar ligament).

Goniometer Alignment

1. Center the fulcrum of the goniometer over the dorsal aspect of the PIP joint.
2. Align the proximal arm over the dorsal midline of the proximal phalanx.
3. Align the distal arm over the dorsal midline of the middle phalanx.

DISTAL INTERPHALANGEAL FLEXION

Motion occurs in the sagittal plane around a medial-lateral axis. DIP finger flexion ROM values are 90 degrees according to the AAOS[7] and 70 degrees according to the AMA.[8] Hume and coworkers[9] and Skvarilova and Plevkova[11] report a mean of 85 degrees of active DIP flexion. DIP flexion is generally equal for all fingers.[10] See Tables 7–1 and 7–2 for additional information.

Testing Position

Position the subject sitting, with the forearm and hand resting on a supporting surface. Place the forearm in 0 degrees of supination and pronation; the wrist in 0 degrees of flexion, extension, and radial and ulnar deviation; and the MCP joint in 0 degrees of flexion, extension, abduction, and adduction; Place the PIP joint in approximately 70 to 90 degrees of flexion. (If the wrist and the MCP and PIP joints are fully flexed, tension in the extensor digitorum communis, extensor indicis, or extensor digiti minimi muscles may restrict DIP flexion. If the PIP joint is extended, tension in the oblique retinacular ligament may restrict DIP flexion.)

Stabilization

Stabilize the middle and proximal phalanx to prevent further flexion of the wrist, MCP joints, and PIP joints.

Testing Motion

Flex the DIP joint by pushing on the dorsal surface of the distal phalanx, moving the finger toward the palm (Fig. 7–24). The end of flexion ROM occurs when resistance to further motion is felt and attempts to overcome the resistance cause the PIP joint to flex.

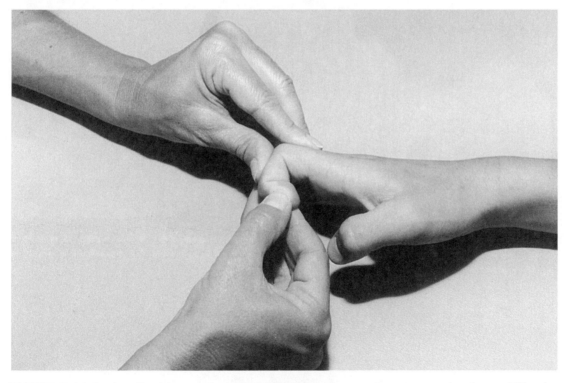

FIGURE 7–24 During distal interphalangeal (DIP) flexion, the examiner uses one hand to stabilize the middle phalanx and keep the proximal interphalangeal joint in 70 to 90 degrees of flexion. The examiner's other hand pushes on the distal phalanx to flex the DIP joint.

Normal End-feel

The end-feel is firm because of tension in the dorsal joint capsule, collateral ligaments, and oblique retinacular ligament.

Goniometer Alignment

See Figures 7–25 to 7–27.

1. Center the fulcrum of the goniometer over the dorsal aspect of the DIP joint.
2. Align the proximal arm over the dorsal midline of the middle phalanx.
3. Align the distal arm over the dorsal midline of the distal phalanx.

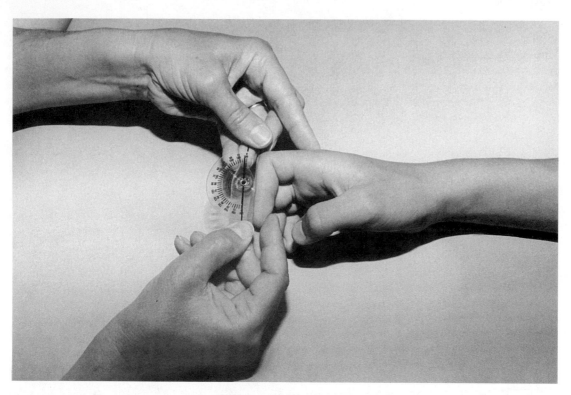

FIGURE 7–25 Measurement of the beginning of distal interphalangeal (DIP) flexion range of motion is being conducted by means of a half-circle plastic goniometer with 6-inch arms that have been trimmed to accommodate the small size of the DIP joint.

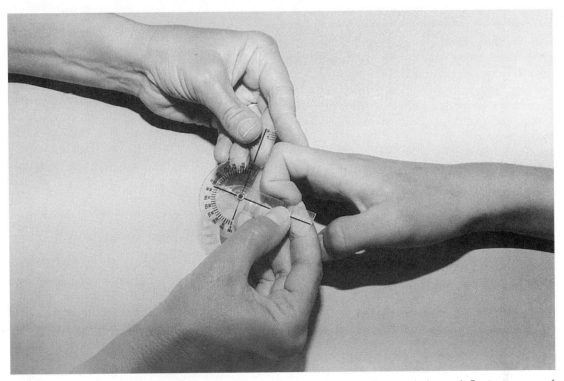

FIGURE 7–26 The alignment of the goniometer at the end of distal interphalangeal flexion range of motion. Note that the fulcrum of the goniometer lies distal and dorsal to the proximal interphalangeal joint axis so that the arms of the goniometer stay in direct contact with the dorsal surfaces of the middle and distal phalanges .

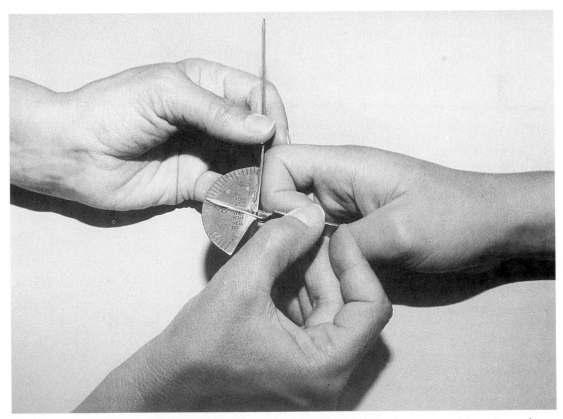

FIGURE 7–27 Distal interphalangeal flexion range of motion also can be measured by using a finger goniometer that is placed on the dorsal surface of the middle and distal phalanges. This type of goniometer is appropriate for measuring the small joints of the fingers, thumb, and toes.

DISTAL INTERPHALANGEAL EXTENSION

Motion occurs in the sagittal plane around a medial-lateral axis. Most references, such as the AAOS[7] and the AMA,[8] report DIP finger extension ROM values to be 0 degrees. However, Mallon, Brown, and Nunley[10] report a mean of 8 degrees of active DIP extension and 20 degrees of passive DIP extension. DIP extension is generally equal for all fingers.[10] See Tables 7–1 and 7–2 for additional information.

Testing Position

Position the subject sitting, with the forearm and hand resting on a supporting surface. Place the forearm in 0 degrees of supination and pronation; the wrist in 0 degrees of flexion, extension, and radial and ulnar deviation; and the MCP joint in 0 degrees of flexion, extension, abduction, and adduction. Position the PIP joint in approximately 70 to 90 degrees of flexion. (If the PIP joint, MCP joint, and wrist are fully extended, tension in the flexor digitorum profundus muscle may restrict DIP extension.)

Stabilization

Stabilize the middle and proximal phalanx to prevent extension of the wrist, MCP joints, and PIP joints.

Testing Motion

Extend the DIP joint by pushing on the palmar surface of the distal phalanx, moving the finger away from the palm. The end of extension ROM occurs when resistance to further motion is felt and attempts to overcome the resistance cause the PIP joint to extend.

Normal End-feel

The end-feel is firm because of tension in the palmar joint capsule and the palmar plate (palmar ligament).

Goniometer Alignment

1. Center the fulcrum of the goniometer over the dorsal aspect of the DIP joint.
2. Align the proximal arm over the dorsal midline of the middle phalanx.
3. Align the distal arm over the dorsal midline of the distal phalanx.

Range of Motion Testing Procedures: Thumb

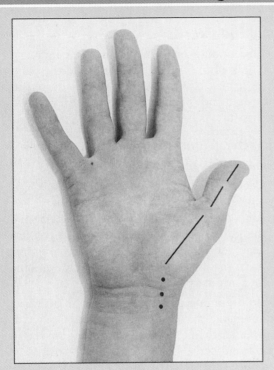

FIGURE 7–28 Anterior (palmar) view of the hand showing surface anatomy landmarks for goniometer alignment during the measurement of thumb range of motion.

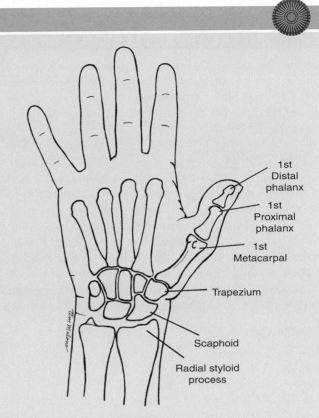

FIGURE 7–29 Anterior (palmar) view of the hand showing bony anatomical landmarks for goniometer alignment during the measurement of thumb range of motion.

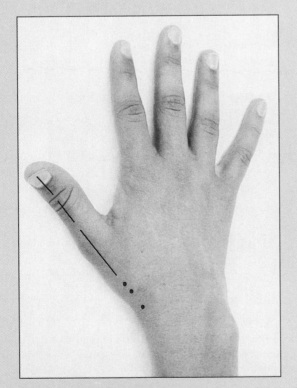

FIGURE 7–30 Posterior view of the hand showing surface anatomy landmarks for goniometer alignment during the measurement of thumb range of motion.

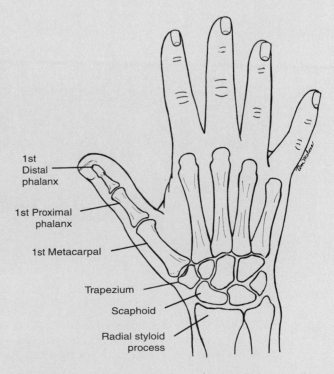

FIGURE 7–31 Posterior view of the hand showing bony anatomical landmarks for goniometer alignment during the measurement of thumb range of motion.

Range of Motion Testing Procedures: Thumb

CARPOMETACARPAL FLEXION

Motion occurs in the plane of the hand. When the subject is in the anatomical position, the motion occurs in the frontal plane around an anterior-posterior axis. Mean CMC thumb flexion ROM is 15 degrees, according to the AAOS.[7]

Testing Position

Position the subject sitting, with the forearm and hand resting on a supporting surface. Place the forearm in full supination; the wrist in 0 degrees of flexion, extension, and radial and ulnar deviation; and the CMC joint of the thumb in 0 degrees of abduction. The MCP and IP joints of the thumb are relaxed in a position of slight flexion. (If the MCP and IP joints of the thumb are positioned in full flexion, tension in the extensor pollicis longus and brevis muscles may restrict the motion.)

Stabilization

Stabilize the carpals, radius, and ulna to prevent wrist motions.

Testing Motion

Flex the CMC joint of the thumb by pushing on the dorsal surface of the metacarpal, moving the thumb toward the ulnar aspect of the hand (Fig. 7–32).

Maintain the CMC joint in 0 degrees of abduction. The end of flexion ROM occurs when resistance to further motion is felt and attempts to overcome the resistance cause the wrist to deviate ulnarly.

Normal End-feel

The end-feel may be soft because of contact between muscle bulk of the thenar eminence and the palm of the hand, or it may be firm because of tension in the dorsal joint capsule and the extensor pollicis brevis and abductor pollicis brevis muscles.

Goniometer Alignment

See Figures 7–33 and 7–34.

1. Center the fulcrum of the goniometer over the palmar aspect of the first CMC joint.
2. Align the proximal arm with the ventral midline of the radius using the ventral surface of the radial head and radial styloid process for reference.
3. Align the distal arm with the ventral midline of the first metacarpal.

In the beginning positions for flexion and extension, the goniometer may indicate approximately 30 to 50 degrees rather than 0 degrees, depending on the shape of the hand and wrist position. The end-position degrees should be subtracted from the beginning-position degrees. A measurement that begins at 35 degrees and ends at 10 degrees should be recorded as 0 to 25 degrees.

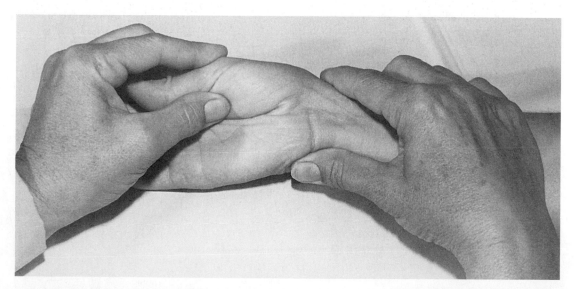

FIGURE 7–32 During carpometacarpal (CMC) flexion, the examiner uses the index finger and thumb of one hand to stabilize the carpals, radius, and ulna to prevent ulnar deviation of the wrist. The examiner's the other index finger and thumb flex the CMC joint by moving the first metacarpal medially.

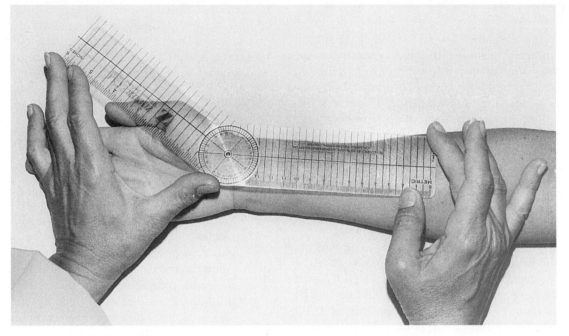

FIGURE 7–33 The alignment of the goniometer at the beginning of carpometacarpal flexion range of motion of the thumb. Note that the goniometer does not read 0 degrees.

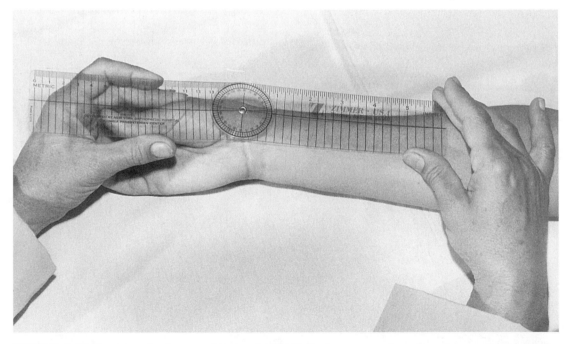

FIGURE 7–34 At the end of carpometacarpal (CMC) flexion range of motion, the examiner uses the hand that was stabilizing the wrist to align the proximal arm of the goniometer with the radius. The examiner's other hand maintains CMC flexion and aligns the distal arm of the goniometer with the first metacarpal. During the measurement, the examiner must be careful not to move the subject's wrist further into ulnar deviation or the goniometer reading will be incorrect (too high).

CARPOMETACARPAL EXTENSION

Motion occurs in the plane of the hand. When the subject is in the anatomical position, the motion occurs in the frontal plane around an anterior-posterior axis. Reported values for CMC thumb extension ROM are 50 degrees, according to the AMA,[8] and vary from 20 degrees[7] to 80 degrees,[38] according to the AAOS. However, the measurement methods used by the AAOS and the AMA appear to differ from the method suggested here. This motion is also called radial abduction.

Testing Position

Position the subject sitting, with the forearm and hand resting on a supporting surface. Place the forearm in full supination; the wrist in 0 degrees of flexion, extension, and radial and ulnar deviation; and the CMC joint of the thumb in 0 degrees of abduction. The MCP and IP joints of the thumb are relaxed in a position of slight flexion. (If the MCP and IP joints of the thumb are positioned in full extension, tension in the flexor pollicis longus muscle may restrict the motion.)

Stabilization

Stabilize the carpals, radius, and ulna to prevent wrist motions.

Testing Motion

Extend the CMC joint of the thumb by pushing on the palmar surface of the metacarpal, moving the thumb toward the radial aspect of the hand (Fig. 7–35). Maintain the CMC joint in 0 degrees of abduction. The end of extension ROM occurs when resistance to further motion is felt and attempts to overcome the resistance cause the wrist to deviate radially.

Normal End-feel

The end-feel is firm because of tension in the anterior joint capsule and the flexor pollicis brevis, adductor pollicis, opponens pollicis, and first dorsal interossei muscles.

Goniometer Alignment

See Figures 7–36 and 7–37.

1. Center the fulcrum of the goniometer over the palmar aspect of the first CMC joint.
2. Align the proximal arm with the ventral midline of the radius, using the ventral surface of the radial head and the radial styloid process for reference.
3. Align the distal arm with the ventral midline of the first metacarpal.

In the beginning positions for flexion and extension, the goniometer may indicate approximately 30 to 50 degrees rather than 0 degrees, depending on the shape of the hand and wrist position. The end-position degrees should be subtracted from the beginning-position degrees. A measurement that begins at 35 degrees and ends at 55 degrees should be recorded as 0 to 20 degrees.

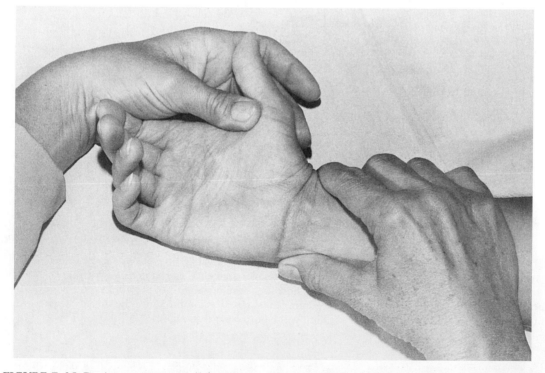

FIGURE 7–35 During carpometacarpal extension of the thumb, the examiner uses one hand to stabilize the carpals, radius, and ulnar thereby preventing radial deviation of the subject's wrist; the examiner's other hand is used to pull the first metacarpal laterally into extension.

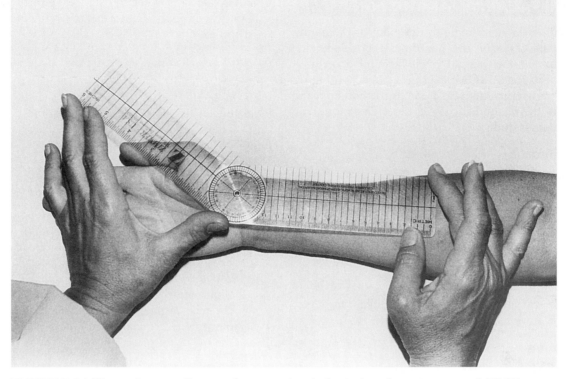

FIGURE 7–36 The goniometer alignment for measuring the beginning of carpometacarpal (CMC) extension range of motion is the same as for measuring the beginning of CMC flexion.

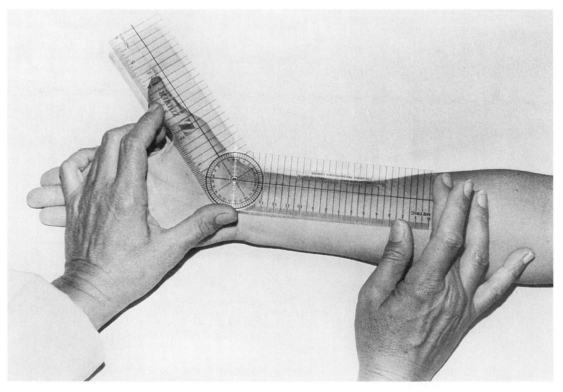

FIGURE 7–37 The alignment of the goniometer at the end of carpometacarpal (CMC) extension range of motion of the thumb. The examiner must be careful to move only the CMC joint into extension and not to change the position of the wrist during the measurement.

CARPOMETACARPAL ABDUCTION

Motion occurs at a right angle to the palm of the hand. When the subject is in the anatomical position, the motion occurs in the sagittal plane around a medial-lateral axis. Abduction ROM is 70 degrees, according to the AAOS;[10] however, the measurement method appears to differ from the method suggested here. This motion is also called palmar abduction.

Testing Position

Position the subject sitting, with the forearm and hand resting on a supporting surface. Place the forearm midway between supination and pronation; the wrist in 0 degrees of flexion, extension, and radial and ulnar deviation; and the CMC, MCP, and IP joints of the thumb in 0 degrees of flexion and extension.

Stabilization

Stabilize the carpals and the second metacarpal to prevent wrist motions.

Testing Motion

Abduct the CMC joint by moving the metacarpal away from the palm of the hand (Fig. 7–38). The end of abduc-tion ROM occurs when resistance to further motion is felt and attempts to overcome the resistance cause the wrist to flex.

Normal End-feel

The end-feel is firm because of tension in the fascia and the skin of the web space between the thumb and the index finger. Tension in the adductor pollicis and first dorsal interossei muscles also contributes to the firm end-feel.

Goniometer Alignment

See Figures 7–39 and 7–40.

1. Center the fulcrum of the goniometer over the lateral aspect of the radial styloid process.
2. Align the proximal arm with the lateral midline of the second metacarpal, using the center of the second MCP joint for reference.
3. Align the distal arm with the lateral midline of the first metacarpal, using the center of the first MCP joint for reference.

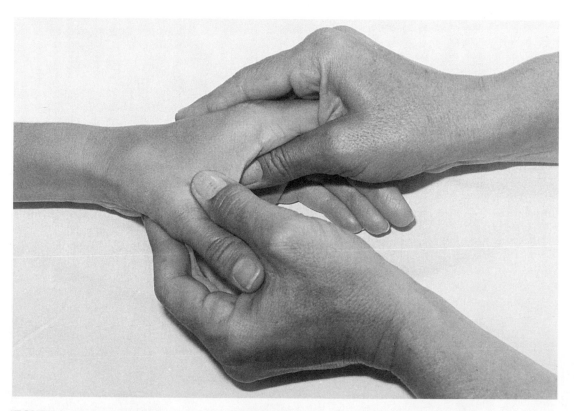

FIGURE 7–38 During carpometacarpal abduction, the examiner uses one hand to stabilize the subject's second metacarpal. Her other hand grasps the subject's first metacarpal just proximal to the metacarpophalangeal joint to move it away from the palm and into abduction.

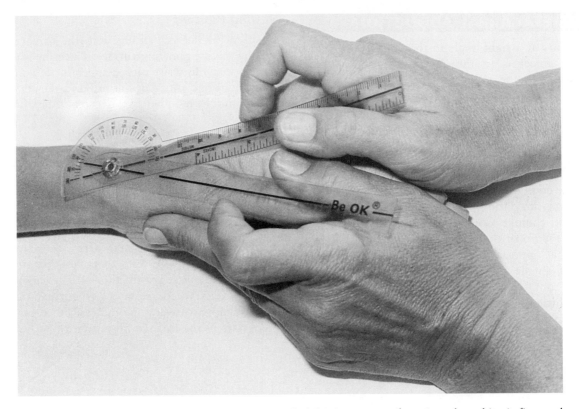

FIGURE 7–39 At the beginning of carpometacarpal abduction range of motion, the subject's first and second metacarpals are in firm contact with each other. However, when the arms of the goniometer are aligned with the first and second metacarpals, the goniometer will not be at 0 degrees.

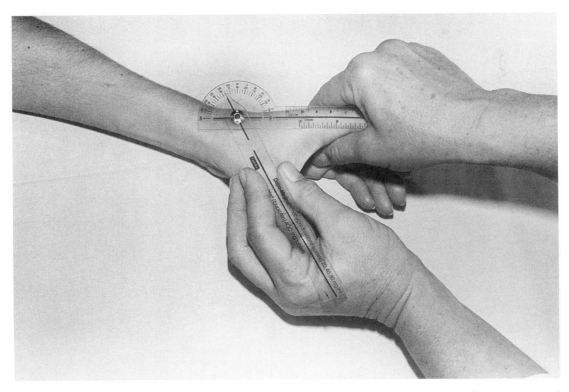

FIGURE 7–40 The alignment of the goniometer at the end of carpometacarpal abduction range of motion.

CARPOMETACARPAL ADDUCTION

Motion occurs at a right angle to the palm of the hand. When the subject is in the anatomical position, the motion occurs in the sagittal plane around a medial-lateral axis. Adduction of the CMC joint of the thumb is not usually measured and recorded because it is the return to the 0 starting position from full abduction.

CARPOMETACARPAL OPPOSITION

Motion is a combination of abduction, flexion, medial axial rotation (pronation), and adduction at the CMC joints of the thumb. Contact between the tip of the thumb and the tip of the little finger is usually possible, providing that opposition at the CMC joint of the little finger and slight flexion at the MCP joints are allowed. Alternately, contact between the tip of the thumb and the base of the little finger is usually possible, providing that slight flexion of the MCP and IP joints of the thumb is allowed.

Testing Position

Position the subject sitting with the forearm and hand resting on a supporting surface. Place the forearm in full supination; the wrist in 0 degrees of flexion, extension, and radial and ulnar deviation; and the IP joints of the thumb and little finger in 0 degrees of flexion and extension.

Stabilization

Stabilize the fifth metacarpal to prevent wrist motions.

Testing Motion

Move the first metacarpal away from the palm of the hand and then in an ulnar direction toward the little finger, allowing the first metacarpal to rotate (Figs. 7–41 and 7–42). Move the fifth metacarpal in a palmar and radial direction toward the thumb. The end of opposition ROM occurs when resistance to further motion is felt and attempts to overcome the resistance cause the wrist to deviate or the forearm to pronate.

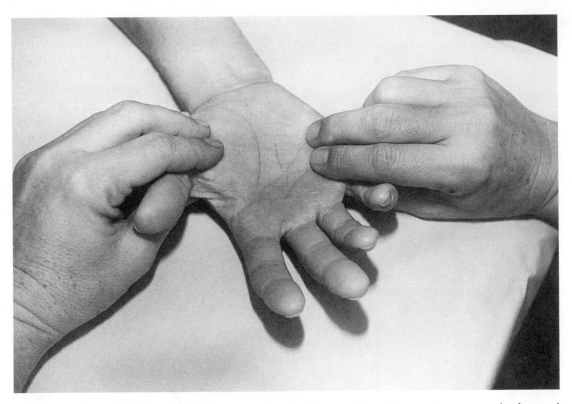

FIGURE 7–41 At the beginning of the range of motion in opposition, the examiner grasps the first and fifth metacarpals. The subject's hand is supported by the table.

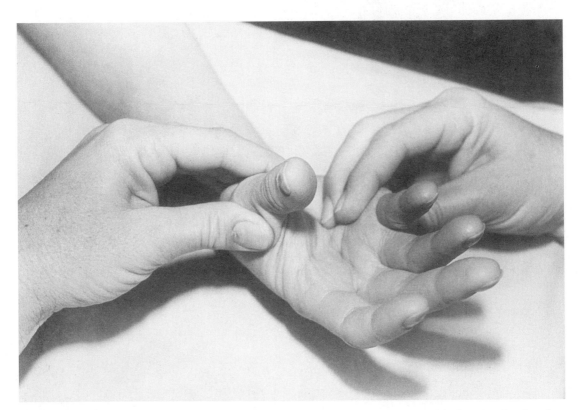

FIGURE 7–42 During opposition, the first and fifth metacarpals are moved toward each other by placing pressure on their dorsal surfaces. This subject's hand does not have full range of motion.

Normal End-feel

The end-feel may be soft because of contact between the muscle bulk of the thenar eminence and the palm; or it may be firm because of tension in the CMC joint capsule, fascia, and skin of the web space between the thumb and the index finger; and in the adductor pollicis, first dorsal interossei, extensor pollicis brevis, and extensor pollicis longus muscles; and in the transverse metacarpal ligament (which affects the little finger).

Goniometer Alignment

The goniometer is not commonly used to measure the range of opposition. Instead, a ruler is often used to measure the distance between the tip of the thumb and the tip of the little finger (Fig. 7–43). Alternatively, a ruler may be used to measure the distance between the tip of the thumb and the base of the little finger at the palmar digital crease or the distal palmar crease.[40]

The AMA *Guides to the Evaluation of Permanent Impairment*[8] recommends measuring the longest distance from the flexion crease of the thumb IP joint to the distal palmar crease directly over the third MCP joint (Fig. 7–44). However, this measurement method seems more consistent with the measurement of CMC abduction.

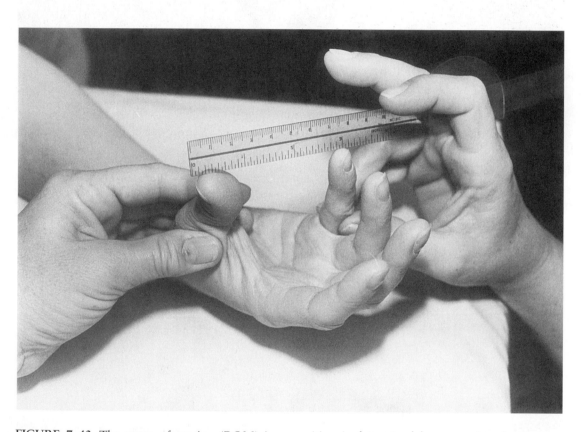

FIGURE 7–43 The range of motion (ROM) in opposition is determined by measuring the distance between the lateral tips of the subject's thumb and the little finger. The examiner is using the arm of the goniometer to measure, but any ruler would suffice. The photograph does not show the complete ROM of opposition because its purpose is to demonstrate how the ROM is measured. When full ROM in opposition is reached, the tips of the little finger and the thumb are touching.

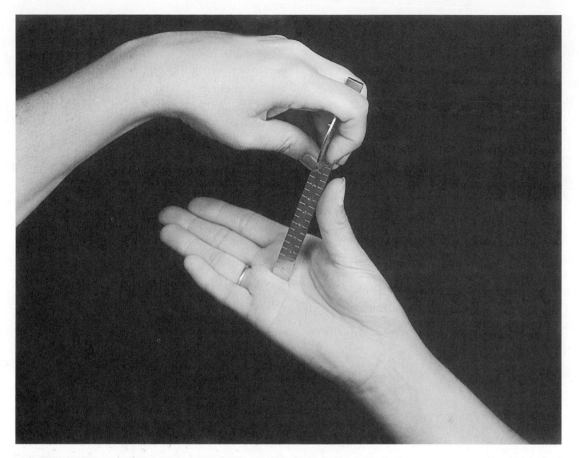

FIGURE 7–44 In an alternative method of measuring thumb opposition, the examiner uses a ruler to find the longest possible distance between the distal palmar crease directly over the metacarpophalangeal joint of the middle finger and the flexion crease of the thumb interphalangeal joint. (From Stanley, BG, and Tribuzi, SM: Concepts in Hand Rehabilitation. FA Davis, Philadelphia, 1992, p 546, with permission.)

METACARPOPHALANGEAL FLEXION

Motion occurs in the frontal plane around an anterior-posterior axis when the subject is in the anatomical position. Mean flexion ROM values are 50 degrees according to the AAOS,[7] 60 degrees according to the AMA,[8] and 55 degrees according to DeSmet and colleagues.[14] See Table 7–3 for more information.

Testing Position

Position the subject sitting, with the forearm and hand resting on a supporting surface. Place the forearm in full supination; the wrist in 0 degrees of flexion, extension, and radial and ulnar deviation; the CMC joint of the thumb in 0 degrees of flexion, extension, abduction, adduction, and opposition; and the IP joint of the thumb is in 0 degrees of flexion and extension. (If the wrist and IP joint of the thumb are positioned in full flexion, tension in the extensor pollicis longus muscle will restrict the motion.)

Stabilization

Stabilize the first metacarpal to prevent wrist motion and flexion of the CMC joint of the thumb.

Testing Motion

Flex the MCP joint by pushing on the dorsal aspect of the proximal phalanx, moving the thumb toward the ulnar aspect of the hand (Fig. 7–45). The end of flexion ROM occurs when resistance to further motion is felt and attempts to overcome the resistance cause the CMC joint to flex.

Normal End-feel

The end-feel may be hard because of contact between the palmar aspect of the proximal phalanx and the first metacarpal, or it may be firm because of tension in the dorsal joint capsule, the collateral ligaments, and the extensor pollicis brevis muscle.

Goniometer Alignment

See Figures 7–46 and 7–47.

1. Center the fulcrum of the goniometer over the dorsal aspect of the MCP joint.
2. Align the proximal arm over the dorsal midline of the metacarpal.
3. Align the distal arm with the dorsal midline of the proximal phalanx.

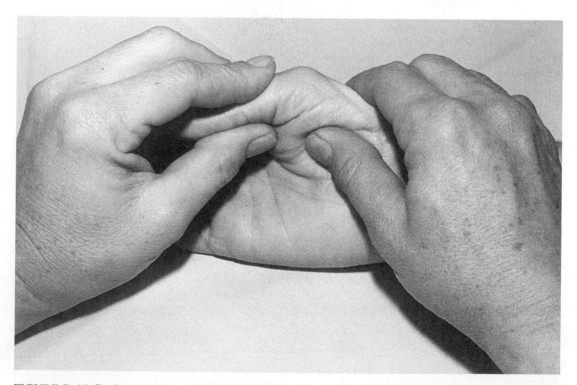

FIGURE 7–45 During metacarpophalangeal flexion of the thumb, the examiner uses the index finger and thumb of one hand to stabilize the subject's first metacarpal and maintain the wrist in a neutral position. The examiner's other index finger and thumb grasp the subject's proximal phalanx to move it into flexion.

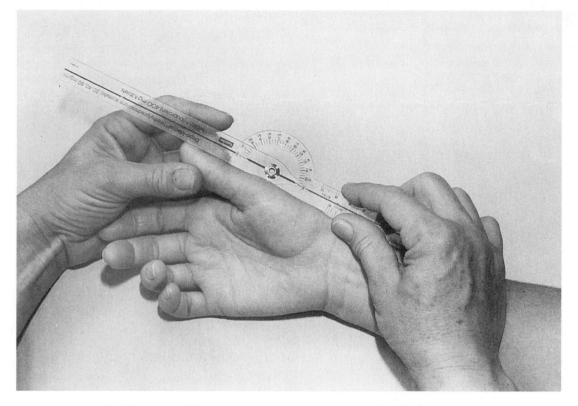

FIGURE 7–46 The alignment of the goniometer on the dorsal surfaces of the first metacarpal and proximal phalanx at the beginning of metacarpophalangeal flexion range of motion of the thumb. If a bony
deformity or swelling is present, the goniometer may be aligned with the lateral surface of these bones.

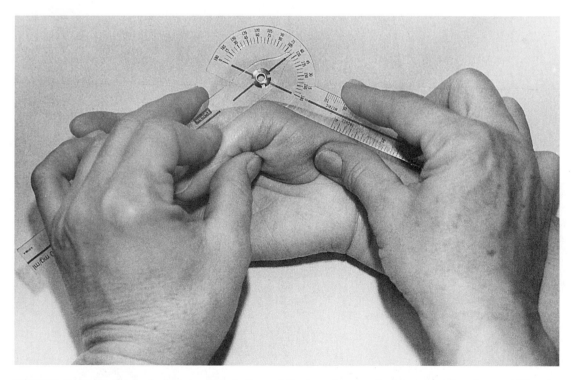

FIGURE 7–47 At the end of metacarpophalangeal flexion, the examiner uses one hand to stabilize the
subject's first metacarpal and align the proximal arm of the goniometer. The examiner uses her other
hand to maintain the proximal phalanx in flexion and align the distal arm of the goniometer.

METACARPOPHALANGEAL EXTENSION

Motion occurs in the frontal plane around an anterior-posterior axis when the subject is in the anatomical position. Mean extension ROM values are 0 degrees according to the AAOS,[7] and 14 degrees (actively) and 23 degrees (passively) according to Skvarilova and Plevkova.[11]

Testing Position

Position the subject sitting, with the forearm and hand resting on a supporting surface. Place the forearm in full supination; the wrist in 0 degrees of flexion, extension, and radial and ulnar deviation; the CMC joint of the thumb in 0 degrees of flexion, extension, abduction, and opposition; and the IP joint of the thumb in 0 degrees of flexion and extension. (If the wrist and the IP joint of the thumb are positioned in full extension, tension in the flexor pollicis longus muscle may restrict the motion.)

Stabilization

Stabilize the first metacarpal to prevent motion at the wrist and at the CMC joint of the thumb.

Testing Motion

Extend the MCP joint by pushing on the palmar surface of the proximal phalanx, moving the thumb toward the radial aspect of the hand. The end of extension ROM occurs when resistance to further motion is felt and attempts to overcome the resistance cause the CMC joint to extend.

Normal End-feel

The end-feel is firm because of tension in the palmar joint capsule, palmar plate (palmar ligament), inter-sesamoid (cruciate) ligaments, and flexor pollicis brevis muscle.

Goniometer Alignment

1. Center the fulcrum of the goniometer over the dorsal aspect of the MCP joint.
2. Align the proximal arm over the dorsal midline of the metacarpal.
3. Align the distal arm with the dorsal midline of the proximal phalanx.

INTERPHALANGEAL FLEXION

Motion occurs in the frontal plane around an anterior-posterior axis when the subject is in the anatomical position. Mean IP flexion ROM of the thumb is 67 degrees, according to Jenkins and associates,[13] and 80 degrees, according to DeSmet and colleagues,[14] and Skvarilova and Plevkova.[11] See Table 7–3 for more information.

Testing Position

Position the subject sitting, with the forearm and hand resting on a supporting surface. Place the forearm in full supination; the wrist in 0 degrees of flexion, extension, and radial and ulnar deviation; the CMC joint in 0 degrees of flexion, extension, abduction, and opposition; and the MCP joint of the thumb in 0 degrees of flexion and extension. (If the wrist and MCP joint of the thumb are flexed, tension in the extensor pollicis longus muscle may restrict the motion. If the MCP joint of the thumb is fully extended, tension in the abductor pollicis brevis and the oblique fibers of the adductor pollicis may restrict the motion through their insertion into the extensor mechanism.)

Stabilization

Stabilize the proximal phalanx to prevent flexion or extension of the MCP joint.

Testing Motion

Flex the IP joint by pushing on the distal phalanx, moving the tip of the thumb toward the ulnar aspect of the hand (Fig. 7–48). The end of flexion ROM occurs when resistance to further motion is felt and attempts to overcome the resistance cause the MCP joint to flex.

Normal End-feel

Usually, the end-feel is firm because of tension in the collateral ligaments and the dorsal joint capsule. In some individuals, the end-feel may be hard because of contact between the palmar aspect of the distal phalanx, the palmar plate, and the proximal phalanx.

Goniometer Alignment

See Figures 7–49 and 7–50.

1. Center the fulcrum of the goniometer over the dorsal surface of the IP joint.
2. Align the proximal arm with the dorsal midline of the proximal phalanx.
3. Align the distal arm with the dorsal midline of the distal phalanx.

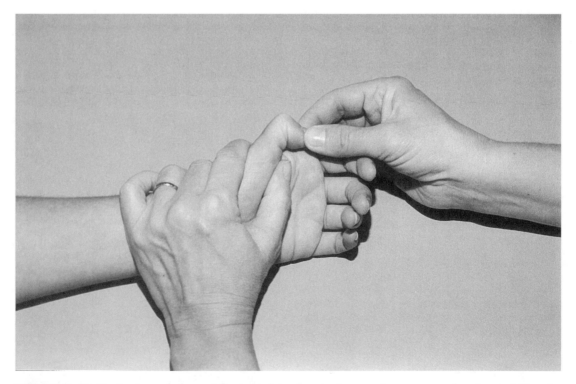

FIGURE 7–48 During interphalangeal flexion of the thumb, the examiner uses one hand to stabilize the proximal phalanx and keep the metacarpophalangeal joint in 0 degrees of flexion and the carpometacarpal joint in 0 degrees of flexion, abduction, and opposition. The examiner uses her other index finger and thumb to flex the distal phalanx.

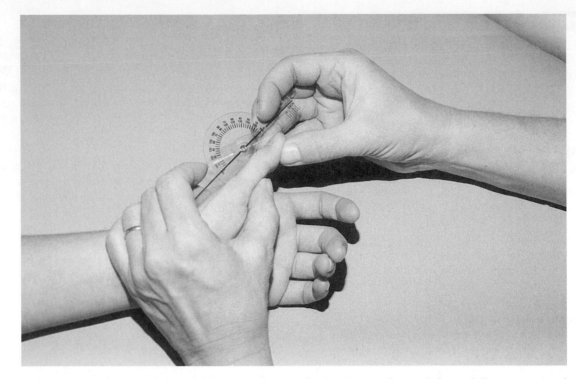

FIGURE 7–49 The alignment of the gon-iometer at the beginning of interphalangeal flexion range of motion. The arms of the goniometer are placed on the dorsal surfaces of the proximal and distal phalanges. However, the arms of the goniometer could instead be placed on the lateral surfaces of the proximal and distal phalanges if the nail protruded or if there was a bony prominence or swelling.

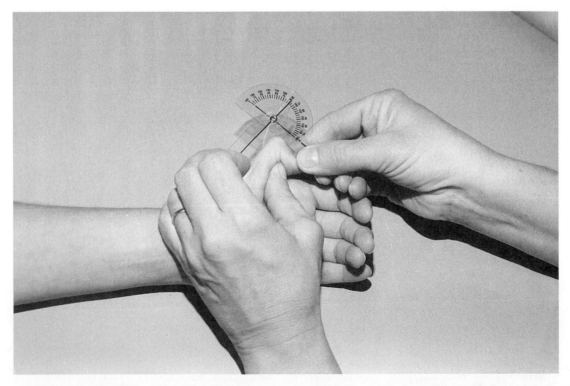

FIGURE 7–50 The alignment of the gon-iometer at the end of interphalangeal flexion range of motion. The examiner holds the arms of the goniometer so that they maintain close contact with the dorsal surfaces of the proximal and distal phalanges.

INTERPHALANGEAL EXTENSION

Motion occurs in the frontal plane around an anterior-posterior axis when the subject is in the anatomical position. Mean extension ROM at the IP joint of the thumb is 20 degrees, according to the AAOS[7], and 23 degrees (actively) and 35 degrees (passively) according to Skvarilova and Plevkova.[11]

Testing Position

Position the subject sitting, with the forearm and hand resting on a supporting surface forearm. Place the forearm in full supination; the wrist in 0 degrees of flexion, extension, and radial and ulnar deviation; the CMC joint of the thumb in 0 degrees of flexion, extension, abduction, and opposition; and the MCP joint of the thumb in 0 degrees of flexion and extension. (If the wrist and MCP joint of the thumb are extended, tension in the flexor pollicis longus muscle may restrict the motion.)

Stabilization

Stabilize the proximal phalanx to prevent extension or flexion of the MCP joint.

Testing Motion

Extend the IP joint by pushing on the palmar surface of the distal phalanx, moving the thumb toward the radial aspect of the hand. The end of extension ROM occurs when resistance to further motion is felt and attempts to overcome the resistance cause the MCP joint to extend.

Normal End-feel

The end-feel is firm because of tension in the palmar joint capsule and the palmar plate (palmar ligament).

Goniometer Alignment

1. Center the fulcrum of the goniometer over the dorsal surface of the IP joint.
2. Align the proximal arm with the dorsal midline of the proximal phalanx.
3. Align the distal arm with the dorsal midline of the distal phalanx.

Muscle Length Testing Procedures: Fingers

LUMBRICALS, PALMAR AND DORSAL INTEROSSEI

The lumbrical, palmar, and dorsal interossei muscles cross the MCP, PIP, and DIP joints. The first and second **lumbricals** originate proximally from the radial sides of the tendons of the flexor digitorum profundus of the index and middle fingers, respectively (Fig. 7–51). The third lumbrical originates on the ulnar side of the tendon of the flexor digitorum profundus of the middle finger and the radial side of the tendon of the ring finger. The fourth lumbrical originates on the ulnar side of the tendon of the flexor digitorum profundus of the ring finger, and the radial side of the tendon of the little finger. Each lumbrical passes to the radial side of the corresponding finger and inserts distally into the extensor mechanism of the extensor digitorum profundus.

The first palmar **interossei muscle** originates proximally from the ulnar side of the metacarpal of the index finger and inserts distally into the ulnar side of the proximal phalanx, and the extensor mechanism of the exten-sor digitorum profundus of the same finger (Fig. 7–52). The second and third palmar interossei muscles originate proximally from the ulnar sides of the metacarpal of the ring and little fingers, respectively, and insert distally into the ulnar side of the proximal phalanx and the extensor mechanism of the extensor digitorum profundus of the same fingers.

The four **dorsal interossei** are bipenniform muscles that originate proximally from two adjacent metacarpals (Fig. 7–53): the first dorsal interossei from the metacarpals of the thumb and index finger, the second from the metacarpals of the index and middle fingers, the third from the metacarpals of the middle and ring fingers, and the fourth from the metacarpals of the ring and little fingers. The dorsal interossei insert distally into the bases of the proximal phalanges and the extensor mechanism of the extensor digitorum profundus of the same fingers.

When these muscles contract, they flex the MCP joints and extend the PIP and DIP joints. These muscles are passively lengthened by placing the MCP joints in exten-sion and the PIP and DIP joints in full flexion. If the

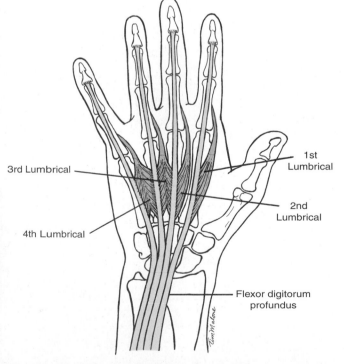

FIGURE 7–51 An anterior (palmar) view of the hand showing the proximal attachments of the lumbricals. The lumbricals insert distally into the extensor digitorum on the posterior surface of the hand.

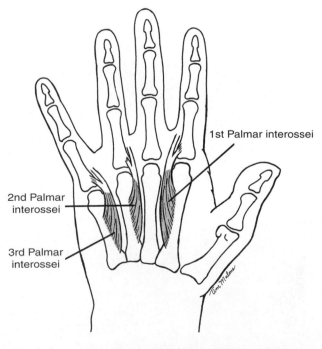

FIGURE 7–52 An anterior (palmar) view of the hand showing the proximal and distal attachments of the palmar interossei. The palmar interossei also attach distally to the extensor digi-torum on the posterior surface of the hand.

lumbricals and the palmar and dorsal interossei are short, they will limit MCP extension when the PIP and DIP joints are positioned in full flexion.

If MCP flexion is limited regardless of the position of the PIP and DIP joints, the limitation is due to abnormalities of the joint surfaces of the MCP joint or shortening of the palmar joint capsule and the palmar plate.

Starting Position

Position the subject sitting, with the forearm and hand resting on a supporting surface. Place the forearm midway between pronation and supination; and the wrist in 0 degrees of flexion, extension, and radial and ulnar deviation. Flex the MCP, PIP, and DIP joints (Fig. 7–54). The MCP joints should be in a neutral position relative to abduction and adduction.

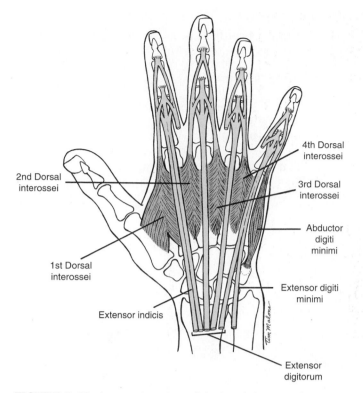

2nd Dorsal interossei

1st Dorsal interossei

Extensor indicis

4th Dorsal interossei

3rd Dorsal interossei

Abductor digiti minimi

Extensor digiti minimi

Extensor digitorum

FIGURE 7–53 A posterior view of the hand showing the proximal attachments of the dorsal interossei on the metacarpals, and the distal attachments into the extensor mechanism of the extensor digitorum, extensor indicis, and extensor digiti minimi muscles.

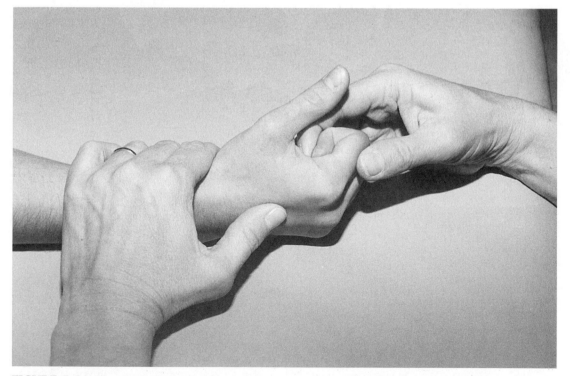

FIGURE 7–54 The starting position for testing the length of the lumbricals and the palmar and dorsal interossei. The examiner uses one hand to stabilize the subject's wrist, and the other hand to position the subject's metacarpophalangeal, proximal interphalangeal, and distal interphalangeal joints in full flexion.

Stabilization

Stabilize the metacarpals and the carpal bones to prevent wrist motion.

Testing Motion

Hold the PIP and DIP joints in full flexion while extending the MCP joint (Figs. 7–55 and 7–56). All of the fingers may be screened together, but if abnormalities are found, testing should be conducted on individual fingers. The end of flexion ROM occurs when resistance to further motion is felt and attempts to overcome the resistance cause the PIP, DIP, or wrist joints to extend.

Normal End-feel

The end-feel is firm because of tension in the lumbrical, palmar and dorsal interossei muscles.

Goniometer Alignment

See Figure 7–57.

1. Center the fulcrum of the goniometer over the dorsal aspect of the MCP joint.
2. Align the proximal arm over the dorsal midline of the metacarpal.
3. Align the distal arm over the dorsal midline of the proximal phalanx.

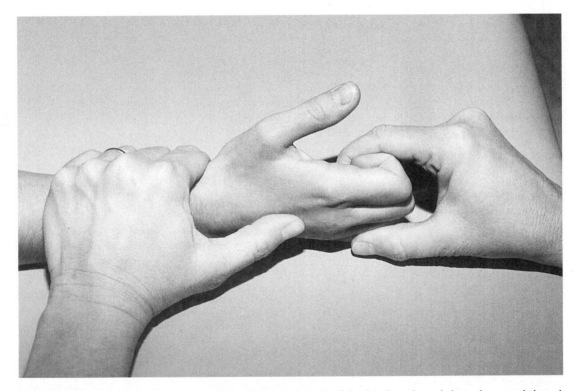

FIGURE 7–55 The end of the motion for testing the length of the lumbricals and the palmar and dorsal interossei. The examiner holds the subject's proximal interphalangeal and distal interphalangeal joints in full flexion while moving the metacarpophalangeal joint into extension.

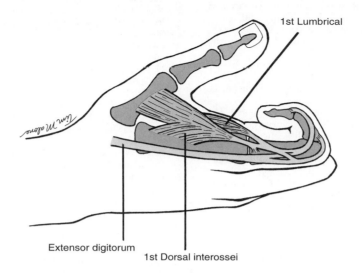

FIGURE 7–56 A lateral view of the hand showing the first lumbrical and the first dorsal interossei muscles being stretched over the metacarpophalangeal, proximal interphalangeal, and distal interphalangeal joints.

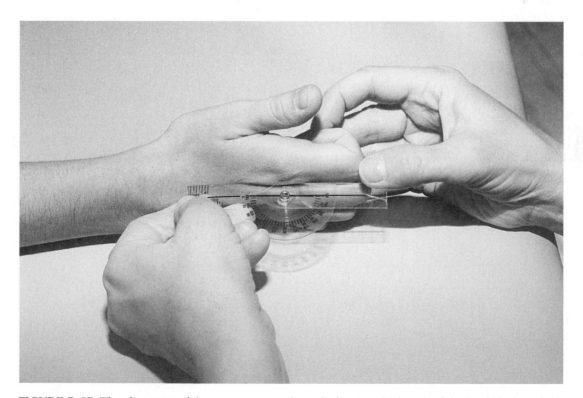

FIGURE 7–57 The alignment of the goniometer at the end of testing the length of the lumbricals and the palmar and dorsal interossei muscles. The arms of the goniometer are placed on the dorsal midline of the metacarpal and proximal phalanx of the finger being tested.

REFERENCES

1. Levangie, PL, and Norkin, CC: Joint Structure and Function: A Comprehensive Analysis, ed 3. FA Davis, Philadelphia, 2001.
2. Tubiana, R: Architecture and functions of the hand. In Tubiana, R, Thomine, JM, and Mackin, E (eds): Examination of the Hand and Upper Limb. WB Saunders, Philadelphia, 1984.
3. Krishnan, J, and Chipchase, L: Passive axial rotation of the metacarpophalangeal joint. J Hand Surg 22B:270, 2000.
4. Cyriax, JH, and Cyriax, PJ: Illustrated Manual of Orthopaedic Medicine. Butterworths, London, 1983.
5. Kaltenborn, FM: Manual Mobilization of the Joints: The Extremities, ed 5. Olaf Norlis Bokhandel, Oslo, Norway, 1999.
6. Ranney, D: The hand as a concept: Digital differences and their importance. Clin Anat 8:281, 1995.
7. American Academy of Orthopaedic Surgeons: Joint Motion: Methods of Measuring and Recording. AAOS, Chicago, 1965.
8. American Medical Association: Guides to the Evaluation of Permanent Impairment, ed 3. AMA, Chicago, 1990.
9. Hume, M, et al: Functional range of motion of the joints of the hand. J Hand Surg (Am) 15:240, 1990.
10. Mallon, WJ, Brown, HR, and Nunley, JA: Digital ranges of motion: Normal values in young adults. J Hand Surg (Am) 16:882, 1991.
11. Skvarilova, B, and Plevkova, A: Ranges of joint motion of the adult hand. Acta Chir Plast 38:67, 1996.
12. Kisner, C, and Colby, LA: Therapeutic Exercise: Foundations and Techniques, ed 4. FA Davis, Philadelphia, 2002.
13. Jenkins, M, et al: Thumb joint motion: What is normal? J Hand Surg (Br) 23:796, 1998.
14. DeSmet, L, et al: Metacarpophalangeal and interphalangeal flexion of the thumb: Influence of sex and age, relation to ligamentous injury. Acta Orthop Belg 59:357, 1993.
15. Beighton, P, Solomon, L, and Soskolne, CL: Articular mobility in an African population. Ann Rheum Dis 32:413, 1973.
16. Allander, E, et al: Normal range of joint movements in shoulder, hip, wrist and thumb with special reference to side: A comparison between two populations. Int J Epidemiol 3:253, 1974.
17. Joseph, J: Further studies of the metacarpophalangeal and interphalangeal joints of the thumb. J Anat 85:221, 1951.
18. Shaw, SJ, and Morris, MA: The range of motion of the metacarpophalangeal joint of the thumb and its relationship to injury. J Hand Surg (Br) 17:164, 1992.
19. Fairbank, JCT, Pynsett, PB, and Phillips, H: Quantitative measurements of joint mobility in adolescents. Ann Rheum Dis 43:288, 1984.
20. Nicholson, B: Clinical evaluation. In Stanley, BG, and Tribuzi, SM: Concepts in Hand Rehabilitation. FA Davis, Philadelphia, 1992.
21. Knutson, JS, et al: Intrinsic and extrinsic contributions to the passive moment at the metacarpophalangeal joint. J Biomech 33:1675, 2000.
22. Casanova, JS, and Grunert, BK: Adult prehension: Patterns and nomenclature for pinches. J Hand Ther 2:231, 1989.
23. Melvin, J: Rheumatic Disease: Occupation Therapy and Rehabilitation, ed 2. FA Davis, Philadelphia, 1982.
24. Swanson, AB: Evaluation of disabilities and record keeping. In Swanson, AB: Flexible Implant Resection Arthroplasty in the Hand and Extremities. CV Mosby, St Louis, 1973.
25. Napier, JR: Prehensile movements of the human hand. J Anat 89:564, 1955.
26. Totten, PA, and Flinn-Wagner, S: Functional evaluation of the hand. In Stanley, BG, and Tribuzi, SM (eds): Concepts in Hand Rehabilitation. FA Davis, Philadelphia, 1992.
27. Hunter, JM, et al: Rehabilitation of the Hand: Surgery and Therapy, ed 3. CV Mosby, St Louis, 1990.
28. American Society of Hand Therapists: Clinical Assessment Recommendations, ed 2. ASHT, Chicago, 1992.
29. Lee, JW, and Rim, K: Measurement of finger joint angles and maximum finger forces during cylinder grip activity. J Biomed Eng 13:152, 1991.
30. Sperling, L, and Jacobson-Sollerman, C: The grip pattern of the healthy hand during eating. Scand J Rehabil Med 9:115, 1977.
31. Bear-Lehman, J, and Abreu, BC: Evaluating the hand: Issues in reliability and validity. Phys Ther 69:1025, 1989.
32. Adams, LS, Greene, LW, and Topoozian, E: Range of motion. In American Society of Hand Therapists: Clinical Assessment Recommendations, ed 2. ASHT, Chicago, 1992.
33. Hamilton, GF, and Lachenbruch, PA: Reliability of goniometers in assessing finger joint angle. Phys Ther 49:465, 1969.
34. Groth, G, et al: Goniometry of the proximal and distal interphalangeal joints. Part II: Placement preferences, interrater reliability, and concurrent validity. J Hand Ther 14:23, 2001.
35. Weiss, PL, et al: Using the Exos Handmaster to measure digital range of motion: Reliability and validity. Med Eng Phys 16:323, 1994.
36. Ellis, B, Bruton, A, and Goddard, JR: Joint angle measurement: A comparative study of the reliability of goniometry and wire tracing for the hand. Clin Rehabil 11:314, 1997.
37. Brown, A, et al: Validity and reliability of the Dexter Hand Evaluation and Therapy System in hand-injured patients. J Hand Ther 13:37, 2000.
38. Greene, WB, and Heckman, JD (eds): The Clinical Measurement of Joint Motion. American Academy of Orthopaedic Surgeons, Rosemont, Ill., 1994.
39. MacDermid, JC, et al: Validity of pulp-to-palm distance as a measure of finger flexion. J Hand Surg 26B:432, 2001.
40. Cambridge, CA: Range-of-motion measurements of the hand. In Hunter, JM, et al (eds): Rehabilitation of the Hand: Surgery and Therapy, ed 3. CV Mosby, St Louis, 1990.

PART III

Lower-Extremity Testing

Objectives

ON COMPLETION OF PART III, THE READER WILL BE ABLE TO:

1. **Identify:**

   appropriate planes and axes for each lower-extremity joint motion

   structures that limit the end of the range of motion at each lower-extremity joint

   expected normal end-feel

2. **Describe:**

   testing positions used for each lower-extremity joint motion and muscle length test

   goniometer alignment

   capsular pattern of limitation

   range of motion necessary for selected functional activities at each major lower-extremity joint

3. **Explain:**

   how age, gender, and other variables may affect the range of motion

   how sources of error in measurement may affect testing results

4. **Perform a goniometric measurement of any lower-extremity joint, including:**

   a clear explanation of the testing procedure

   proper positioning of the subject

   adequate stabilization of the proximal joint component

   use of appropriate testing motion

   correct determination of the end of the range of motion

   correct identification of the end-feel

   palpation of the appropriate bony landmarks

   accurate alignment of the goniometer and correct reading and recording of goniometric measurements

5. **Plan goniometric measurements of the hip, knee, ankle, and foot that are organized by body position**

6. **Assess the intratester and intertester reliability of goniometric measurements of the lower-extremity joints using methods described in Chapter 3.**

7. **Perform tests of muscle length at the hip, knee, and ankle, including:**

   a clear explanation of the testing procedure

   proper placement of the subject in the starting position

   adequate stabilization

   use of appropriate testing motion

   correct identification of end-feel

   accurate alignment of the goniometer and correct reading and recording

The testing positions, stabilization techniques, testing motions, end-feels, and goniometer alignment for the joints of the lower extremities are presented in Chapters 8 through 10. The goniometric evaluation should follow the 12-step sequence that was presented in Exercise 5 in Chapter 2.

CHAPTER 8

The Hip

Structure and Function

Iliofemoral Joint

Anatomy

The hip joint, or coxa, links the lower extremity with the trunk. The proximal joint surface is the acetabulum, which is formed superiorly by the ilium, posteroinferiorly by the ischium, and anteroinferiorly by the pubis (Fig. 8–1). The concave acetabulum faces laterally, inferiorly, and anteriorly and is deepened by a fibrocartilaginous acetabular labrum. The distal joint surface is the convex head of the femur. The joint is enclosed by a strong, thick capsule, which is reinforced anteriorly by the iliofemoral and pubofemoral ligaments (Fig. 8–2) and posteriorly by the ischiofemoral ligament (Fig. 8–3).

Osteokinematics

The hip is a synovial ball-and-socket joint with 3 degrees of freedom. Motions permitted at the joint are flexion-extension in the sagittal plane around a medial-lateral axis, abduction-adduction in the frontal plane around an anterior-posterior axis, and medial and lateral rotation in the transverse plane around a vertical or longitudinal

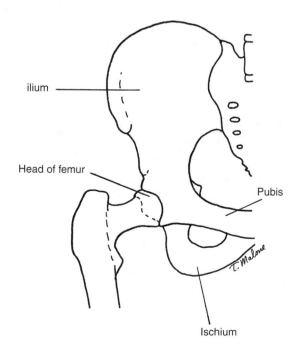

FIGURE 8–1 An anterior view of the hip joint.

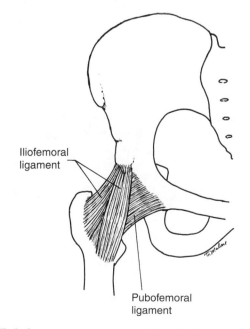

FIGURE 8–2 An anterior view of the hip joint showing the iliofemoral and pubofemoral ligaments.

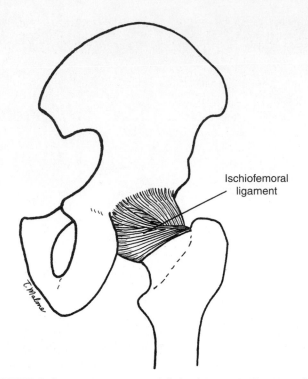

FIGURE 8–3 A posterior view of the hip joint showing the ischiofemoral ligament.

axis.[1] The axis of motion goes through the center of the femoral head.

Arthrokinematics

In an open kinematic (non–weight-bearing) chain, the convex femoral head slides on the concave acetabulum in a direction opposite to the movement of the shaft of the bone. In flexion, the femoral head slides posteriorly and inferiorly on the acetabulum, whereas in extension, the femoral head slides anteriorly and superiorly. In medial rotation, the femoral head slides posteriorly on the acetabulum. During lateral rotation, the femoral head slides anteriorly. In abduction, the femoral head slides inferiorly. In adduction, the femoral head slides superiorly.

Capsular Pattern

The capsular pattern is characterized by a marked restriction of medial rotation accompanied by limitations in flexion and abduction. A slight limitation may be present in extension, but no limitation is present in either lateral rotation or adduction.[2]

Research Findings

Effects of Age, Gender, and Other Factors

Table 8–1 shows hip range of motion (ROM) values from various sources. The age, gender, measurement instrument used, and number of subjects measured to obtain the AAOS[3] and AMA[4] values were not reported. Boone and Azen,[5] Svenningsen and associates,[6] and Roach and Miles[7] used a universal goniometer. Svenningsen and associates[6] measured passive ROM in both males and females, whereas Roach and Miles[7] measured active ROM. Boone and Azen[5] also measured active ROM but only in males.

Age

Researchers tend to agree that age affects hip ROM[8–22] and that the effects are motion specific and gender specific. Table 8–2 shows passive ROM values for neonates as reported in five studies.[8–12] All values presented in Table 8–2 were obtained by means of a universal goniometer. A comparison of the neonate's passive ROM values shown in Table 8–2 with the values of older children and adults shown in Table 8–1 reveals

TABLE 8–1	Hip Motion: Values in Degrees					
	AAOS[3]	AMA[4]	Boone and Azen[5]	Svenningsen et al[6]		Roach and Miles[7]
				Males 23 yrs	*Females 23 yrs*	
			18 mos–54 yrs n = 109	*n = 102*	*n = 104*	*25–74 yrs n = 1683*
Motion			*Mean (SD)*	*Mean*	*Mean*	*Mean (SD)*
Flexion	120	100	122.3 (6.1)	137	141	121.0 (13.0)
Extension	20	30	9.8 (6.8)	23	26	19.0 (8.0)
Abduction		40	45.9 (9.3)	40	42	42.0 (11.0)
Adduction		20	26.9 (4.1)	29	30	
Medial rotation	45	40*	47.3 (6.0)	38	52	32.0 (8.0)
Lateral rotation	45	50*	47.2 (6.3)	43	41	32.0 (9.0)

(SD) = Standard deviation.
* Measurements taken with subjects in the supine position.

TABLE 8–2   Effects of Age on Hip Motion in Neonates 6 Hours to 4 Weeks of Age: Mean Values in Degrees

Motion	Waugh et al[8] 6–65 hrs n = 40 Mean (SD)	Drews et al[11] 12 hrs–6 days n = 54 Mean (SD)	Schwarze and Denton[9] 1–3 days n = 1000 Mean	Broughton et al[10] 1–7 days n = 57 Mean (SD)	Wanatabe et al[12] 4 wks n = 62 Mean
Flexion					138.0
Extension*	46.3 (8.2)[†]	28.3 (6.0)[‡]	20.0	34.1 (6.3)	12.0
Abduction		55.5 (9.5)[†]	78.0[†]		51.0
Adduction		6.4 (3.9)[†]	15.0[†]		
Medial Rotation		79.8 (9.3)[†]	58.0		24.0
Lateral Rotation		113.7 (10.4)[†]	80.0		66.0

(SD) = Standard deviation.

* All values in this row represent the magnitude of the extension limitation.

[†] Tested with subjects in the supine position.

[‡] Tested with subjects in the side-lying position.

that the neonates studied have larger passive ROM in most hip motions except for extension, which is limited. The neonate's ROM in hip lateral and medial rotation and abduction is much larger than the ROM values of adults and older children for the same motions. Also, the relationship between hip lateral rotation and medial rotation appears to differ from that found in a majority of older children and adults. Hip lateral rotation values for the neonates are considerably greater than the values for medial rotation, whereas in children and adults the lateral rotation values are either about the same or less than the values for medial rotation.[15] Kozic and colleagues,[17] in a study of passive medial and lateral rotation in 1140 children aged 8 to 9 years, found that 90 percent of the children had less than 10 degrees difference between lateral and medial rotation. Ellison and coworkers,[18] in a study of 100 healthy adults and 50 patients with back problems found that only 27 percent of healthy subjects compared with 48 percent of patients had greater lateral rotation than medial rotation. The large number of patients who had greater lateral than medial rotation suggests a rotational imbalance that may be related to back problems.

However, as seen in Table 8–2 the most dramatic effect of age is on hip extension ROM. Newborns and infants are unable to extend the hip from full flexion to the neutral position (returning to 0 degrees from the end of the flexion ROM).[8–15] Waugh and associates[8] found that all 40 infants tested lacked complete hip extension, with limitations ranging from 21.7 degrees to 68.3 degrees. Schwarze and Denton[9] found mean limitations of 19 degrees for boys and 21 degrees for girls, and Broughton, Wright, and Menelaus[10] found a mean hip extension limitation of 34.1 degrees in 57 boys and girls. Forero, Okamura, and Larson[15] found that all 60 healthy full-term neonates studied had hip extension limitations.

Limitations in hip extension found in the very young are considered to be normal and to decrease with age as seen in Table 8–3. The term "physiological limitation of motion" has been used by Waugh and associates[8] and Walker[13] to describe the normal extension limitation of motion in infants. According to Walker,[13] movement into extension evolves without the need for intervention and should not be considered pathological in newborns and infants. Usually, a return from flexion to the neutral position is attained in children by 2 years of age. Extension ROM beginning at the neutral position usually approaches adult values by early adolescence. Broughton, Wright, and Menelaus[10] found that by 6 months of age, mean hip extension limitations in infants had decreased to 7.5 degrees, and 27 of 57 subjects had

TABLE 8–3   Hip Extension Limitations in Infants and Young Children 4 Weeks to 5 Years of Age: Mean Values in Degrees

Wanatabe et al[12] 4–8 Mos n = 54 Mean (SD)	Broughton et al[10] 3 Mos n = 57 Mean (SD)	Broughton et al[10] 6 Mos n = 57 Mean (SD)	Phelps et al[14] 9 Mos n = 25 Mean (SD)	Phelps et al[14] 18 Mos n = 18 Mean (SD)	Boone[20] 1–5 Yrs n = 19 Mean (SD)
4.0	18.9 (6.0)	7.5 (5.7)	10.0 (2.6)	4.0 (3.2)	0.8 (3.4)

(SD) = Standard deviation.

TABLE 8–4   Effects of Age on Hip Motion in Individuals 4–74 Years of Age: Mean Values in Degrees

	Svenningsen[6]		Boone[20]		Roach and Miles[7]		
	Female	Male	Males		Males and Females		
	4 yrs	4 yrs	6–12 yrs	13–19 yrs	25–39 yrs	40–59 yrs	60–74 yrs
	n = 52	n = 51	n = 17	n = 17	n = 433	n = 727	n = 523
Motion	Mean	Mean	Mean (SD)	Mean (SD)	Mean (SD)	Mean (SD)	Mean (SD)
Flexion	151	149	124.4 (5.9)	122.6 (5.2)	122.0 (12)	120.0 (14)	118.0 (13)
Extension	29	28	10.4 (7.5)	11.6 (5.0)	22.0 (8)	18.0 (7)	17.0 (8)
Abduction	55	53	48.1 (6.3)	46.8 (6.0)	44.0 (11)	42.0 (11)	39.0 (12)
Adduction	30	30	27.6 (3.8)	26.3 (2.9)			
Medial rotation	60	51	48.4 (4.8)	47.1 (5.2)	33.0 (7)	31.0 (8)	30.0 (7)
Lateral rotation	44	48	47.5 (3.2)	47.4 (5.2)	34.0 (8)	32.0 (8)	29.0 (9)

(SD) = Standard deviation.

no limitation.[9] Phelps, Smith, and Hallum[14] found that 100 percent of the 9- and 12-month-old infants tested (n = 50) had some degree of hip extension limitation. At 18 months of age, 89 percent of infants had limitations, and at 24 months, 72 percent still had limitations.

The values in Table 8–4 supplied by Svenningsen and associates[6] were obtained by means of a universal goniometer from measurements of passive ROM, whereas the values supplied by the other authors[7,20] were obtained by means of a universal goniometer from measurements of active ROM. Very little difference is evident between the ROM values for hip flexion and hip abduction across the life span of 4 to 74 years in contrast to hip medial and lateral rotation, which have the greatest decrease in ROM. Roach and Miles[7] have suggested that differences in active ROM representing less than 10 percent of the arc of motion are of little clinical significance, and that any substantial loss of mobility in individuals between 25 and 74 years of age should be viewed as abnormal and not attributable to aging. In the data from Roach and Miles[7] hip extension was the only motion in which the difference between the youngest and the oldest groups constituted a decrease of more than 20 percent of the available arc of motion.

Other authors who have investigated age or gender effects on the hip include Allander and colleagues;[21] Walker and colleagues;[22] Boone, Walker, and Perry;[23] James and Parker;[24] Mollinger and Steffan;[25] and Svenningsen and associates.[6] Allander and colleagues[21] measured the ROM of different joints (i.e., shoulder, hip, wrist, and thumb metacarpophalangeal joints) in a population of 517 females and 203 males between 33 and 70 years of age. These authors found that older groups had significantly less hip rotation ROM than younger groups. Walker and colleagues[22] measured 28 active motions (including all hip motions) in 30 women and 30 men ranging from 60 to 84 years of age. Although Walker and colleagues[22] found no differences in hip ROM between the group aged 60 to 69 years and the group aged 75 to 84 years, both age groups demon-

strated a reduced ability to attain a neutral starting position for hip flexion. The mean starting position for both groups for measurements of flexion ROM was 11 degrees instead of 0 degrees. The mean ROM values obtained for both age groups for hip rotation, abduction, and adduction were 14 to 25 degrees less than the average values published by the AAOS.[3] This finding provides strong support for the use of age-appropriate norms.

James and Parker[24] measured active and passive ROM at the hip, knee, and ankle in 80 healthy men and women ranging from 70 years to 92 years of age. Measurements of hip abduction ROM were taken with a universal goniometer. All other measurements were taken with a Leighton flexometer. Systematic decreases in both active and passive ROM were found in subjects between 70 and 92 years of age. Hip abduction decreased the most with age and was 33.4 percent less in the oldest group of men and women (those aged 85 to 92 years) compared with the youngest group (those aged 70 to 74 years). Medial and lateral rotation also decreased considerably, but the decrease was not as great as that seen in abduction. In contrast, hip flexion with the knee either extended or flexed was least affected by age, with a significant reduction occurring only in those older than 85 years of age. Passive ROM was greater than active ROM for all joint motions tested, with the largest difference (7 degrees) occurring in hip flexion with the knee flexed.

Although Svenningsen and associates[6] studied hip ROM in fairly young subjects (761 males and females aged 4 to 28 years), these authors found that even in this limited age span, the ROM for most hip motions showed a decrease with increasing age. However, the reductions in ROM varied according to the motion. Decreases in flexion, abduction, medial rotation, and total rotation were greater than decreases in extension, adduction, and lateral rotation.

Nonaka and associates,[16] in a study of 77 healthy male volunteers aged 15 to 73 years, found that passive hip ROM decreased progressively with increasing age, but no change was observed in knee ROM in the same population.

Gender

The effects of gender on ROM are usually age specific and motion specific and account for only a relatively small amount of total variance in measurement. Boone and coworkers[23] found significant differences for most hip motions when gender comparisons were made for three age groupings of males and females. Female children (1 to 9 years of age), young adult females (21 to 29 years of age) and older adult females (61 to 69 years of age) had significantly more hip flexion than their male counterparts. However, female children and young adult females had less hip adduction and lateral rotation than males in comparison groups. Both young adult females and older adult females had less hip extension ROM than males. Allander and colleagues[21] found that in five of eight age groups tested, females had a greater amount of hip rotation than males. Walker and colleagues[22] found that 30 females aged 60 to 84 years had 14 degrees more ROM in hip medial rotation than their male counterparts. Simoneau and coworkers[26] found that females (with a mean age of 21.8 years) had higher mean values in both medial and lateral rotation than age-matched male subjects. The authors used a universal metal goniometer to measure active ROM of hip rotation in 39 females and 21 males. In contrast to Walker and colleagues[22] and Simoneau and coworkers,[26] Phelps, Smith, and Hallum[14] found no gender differences in hip rotation in 86 infants and young children (aged 9 to 24 months).

Svenningsen and associates[6] measured the passive ROM of 1552 hips in 761 healthy males and females between 4 years of age and 28 years of age. Females of all age groups in this study had greater passive ROM than males for total passive ROM, total rotation, medial rotation, and abduction. Female children in the 11-year-old age group and the 15-year-old age group and female adults had greater passive ROM in hip flexion and adduction than males in the same age groups. Males had greater passive ROM in hip lateral rotation than females in the 4-year-old group and the 6-year-old group and in adults. This finding is in agreement with that of Boone.[20]

James and Parker[24] found that women were significantly more mobile than men in 7 of the 10 motions tested at the hip, knee, and ankle. At the hip, women had greater mobility than men in all hip motions except abduction. This finding is in agreement with that of Boone but opposite to the findings of Svenningsen and associates.[6] Men and women had similar mean values in hip flexion ROM, both with the knee flexed and with the knee extended in the group aged 70 to 74 years, but in the group between 70 and 85-plus years of age, men had

an approximate 25 percent decrease in ROM, whereas women had a decrease of only about 11 percent.

Body-Mass Index

Kettunen and colleagues[27] found that former elite athletes with a high body-mass index (BMI) had lower total amount of hip passive ROM compared with former elite athletes with a low BMI. Subjects in the study included 117 former elite athletes between the ages of 45 and 68 years. Measurements were taken by means of a Myrin goniometer, with the subjects in the prone position. Escalante and coworkers[28] determined that there was a loss of at least one degree of passive range of motion in hip flexion for each unit increase in BMI in a group of 687 community-dwelling elders (those who were 65 years of age to 78 years of age). Severely obese subjects had an average of 18 degrees less hip flexion than nonobese subjects as measured in the supine position with an inclinometer. BMI explained a higher proportion of the variance in hip flexion ROM than any other variable examined by the authors. Lichtenstein and associates[29] studied interrelationships among the variables in the study by Escalante and coworkers[28] and concluded that BMI could be considered a primary direct determinant of hip flexion passive ROM.

On the other hand, Bennell and associates[19] found no effect of BMI on active ROM in hip rotation in a study comparing 77 novice ballet dancers and 49 age-matched controls between the ages of 8 and 11 years. The control subjects, who had a higher BMI than the dancers, also had a significantly greater range of lateral and medial hip rotation.

Testing Position

Simoneau and coworkers[26] found that measurement position (sitting versus prone) had little effect on active hip medial rotation in 60 healthy male and female college students (aged 18 to 21 years), but that position had a significant effect on lateral rotation ROM. Lateral rotation measured with a universal goniometer on subjects in the sitting position was statistically less (mean, 36 degrees) than it was when measured on subjects in the prone position (mean, 45 degrees). Bierma-Zeinstra and associates[30] found that both lateral and medial rotation ROMs were significantly less when measured in subjects in the sitting and supine positions compared with those in the prone position. However, Schwarze and Denton[9] found no difference in hip medial and lateral rotation passive ROM measurements taken in subjects in the prone position than in measurements taken in 1000 neonates in the supine position.

Van Dillen and coworkers[31] compared the effects of knee and hip position on passive hip extension ROM in 10 patients (mean age, 33 years) with low back pain and 35 healthy subjects (mean age, 31 years). Both groups had less hip extension when the hip was in neutral abduc-

TABLE 8–5   Effects of Position on Hip ROM: Mean Values in Degrees

Author	Motion	Position		
		Seated Mean (SD)	Prone Mean (SD)	Supine Mean
Simoneau et al[26]	Lateral rotation*	36 (7)	45 (10)	
	Medial rotation*	33 (7)	36 (9)	
	Total rotation*	69 (9)	81 (12)	
Bierma-Zeinstra et al[30]	Lateral rotation*	33.9	47.0	33.1
	Medial rotation*	33.6	46.3	36.0
	Lateral rotation†	37.6	51.9	34.2
	Medial rotation†	38.8	53.2	39.9

(SD) = Standard deviation.
* Active ROM measured with a universal goniometer.
† Passive ROM measured with a universal goniometer.

tion than when the hip was fully abducted. Both groups also displayed less hip extension ROM when the knee was flexed to 80 degrees than when the knee was fully extended (Table 8–5). This finding lends support for Kendall, McCreary, and Provance,[32] who maintain that changing the knee joint angle during the Thomas test for hip flexor length can affect the passive ROM in hip extension (see Muscle Length Testing Procedures Section later in this chapter for information on the Thomas test).

Arts and Sports

A sampling of articles related to the effects of ballet, ice hockey, and running on ROM are presented in the following paragraphs. As expected, the effects of the activity on ROM vary with the activity and involve motions that are specific to the particular activity. Gilbert, Gross, and Klug[33] conducted a study of 20 female ballet dancers (aged 11 to 14 years) to determine the relationship between the dancer's ROM in hip lateral rotation and the turnout angle. An ideal turnout angle is a position in which the longitudinal axes of the feet are rotated 180 degrees from each other. The authors found that turnout angles were significantly greater (between 13 and 17 degrees) than measurements of hip lateral rotation ROM. This finding indicates that the dancers were using excessive movements at the knee and ankle to attain an acceptable degree of turnout. According to the authors, the use of compensatory motions at the knee and ankle predisposes the dancers to injury. The dancers had had 3 years of classical ballet training and still had not been able to attain the degree of hip lateral rotation that would give a 180-degree turnout angle. Consequently, the authors suggest that hip ROM may be genetically determined.

Bennell and associates[19] determined that age-matched control subjects had significantly greater active ROM in hip lateral and medial rotation than a group of 77 ballet dancers (aged 8 to 11 years), although there was no significant difference in the degree of turnout between the two groups. The amount of non-hip lateral rotation was significantly greater in the dancers than in the control

subjects. Non-hip lateral rotation as a percentage of active hip ROM was 40 percent in dancers compared with 20 percent in control subjects. The increased torsional forces on the medial aspect of the knee, ankle, and foot in the young dancers puts this group at high risk of injury. Similar to the findings of Gilbert, Gross, and Klug,[33] the authors found no relationship between number of years of training and lateral rotation ROM, which again suggests a genetic component of ROM. The authors did not offer an explanation for the fact that the control subjects had a greater ROM in lateral motion than the dancers; instead, they hypothesized that a shortening of the hip extensors (resulting from constant use) and the dancers' avoidance of full hip medial rotation might account for the fact that the dancers had less hip medial rotation than the control subjects.

Tyler and colleagues[34] found that a group of 25 professional male ice hockey players had about 10 degrees less hip extension ROM than a group of 25 matched control subjects. The authors postulated that the loss of hip extension in the hockey players was probably due to tight anterior hip capsule structures and tight iliopsoas muscles. The flexed hip and knee posture assumed by the players during skating probably contributed to the muscle shortness and loss of hip extension ROM. Van Mechelen and colleagues[35] used goniometry to measure hip ROM in 16 male runners who had sustained running injuries during the year but who were fit at the time of the study. No right-left differences in hip ROM were found either in the previously injured group or in a control group of runners who had not sustained an injury. However, hip ROM in the injured group was on average 59.4 degrees or about 10 degrees less than the average ROM of 68.1 degrees in runners without injuries.

Disability

Steultjens and associates[36] used a universal goniometer to measure bilateral active assistive ROM at the hip and knee in 198 patients with osteoarthritis (OA) of the hip or knee. These authors found that generally a decrease in hip ROM was associated with an increase in disability, but that association was motion specific. Flexion contractures of either hip or knee or both were found in 72.5 percent of the patients. Hip flexion contractures were present in 15 percent of the patients, whereas contractures at the knee were found in 31.5 percent of the patients. Hip extension and lateral rotation showed significant relationships with disability in patients with knee OA, whereas knee flexion ROM was associated with disability in hip OA patients. Twenty-five percent of the variation in disability levels was accounted for by differences in ROM.

Mollinger and Steffan,[25] in a study of 111 nursing home residents, found a mean hip extension of only 4 degrees (measured with the residents in the supine position with the leg off the side of the table and the contralateral knee flexed). Beissner, Collins, and Holmes[37] found that lower-extremity passive ROM and upper-extremity muscle force are important predictors of function for elderly individuals living in assisted living residences or skilled nursing facilities. Conversely, upper extremity ROM and age are the strongest predictors of function in elderly individuals residing in independent living situations.

Functional Range of Motion

Table 8–6 shows the hip flexion ROM necessary for selected functional activities as reported in several sources. An adequate ROM at the hip is important for meeting mobility demands such as walking, stairclimbing (Fig. 8–4), and performing many activities of daily living that require sitting and bending. According to Magee,[38] ideal functional ranges are 120 degrees of flexion, 0 degrees of abduction, and 20 degrees of lateral rotation. However, as can be seen in Table 8–6, considerably less ROM is necessary for gait on level surfaces.[39] Livingston, Stevenson, and Olney[40] studied ascent and descent on stairs of different dimensions, using 15 female subjects between 19 years of age and 26 years of age. McFayden and Winter[41] also studied stairclimbing; however, these authors used eight repeated trials of one subject.

In a study to determine the effects of age-related ROM on functional activity, Oberg, Krazinia, and Oberg[42]

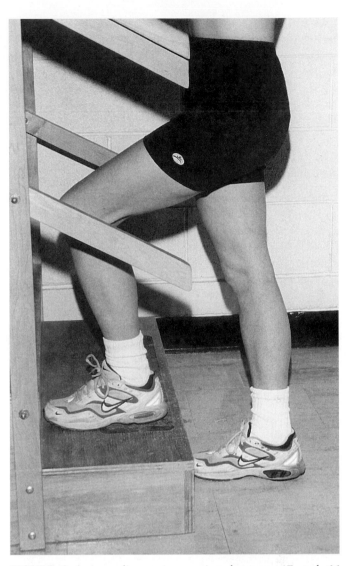

FIGURE 8–4 Ascending stairs requires between 47 and 66 degrees of hip flexion depending on stair dimensions.[40]

measured hip and knee active ROM with an electrogoniometer during gait in 240 healthy male and female individuals aged 10 to 79 years of age. Age-related changes were slightly more pronounced at slow gait speeds than at fast speeds, but the rate of changes was less than 1 degree per decade, and no distinct pattern was evident,

TABLE 8–6 Hip Flexion Range of Motion Required for Functional Activities: Values in Degrees from Selected Sources				
	Livingston et al[40]	Ranchos Los Amigos Medical Center[39]	McFayden and Winter[41]	
Activity	Range	Range	Mean	(SD)
Walking on level surfaces	0–30	0–30	44	(4.5)
Ascending stairs	1–0–66		60	
Descending stairs	1–0–45		66	(0.1)

except that hip flexion-extension appeared to be affected less than other motions.

Other functional and self-care activities require a larger ROM at the hip. For example, sitting requires at least 90 to 112 degrees of hip flexion with the knee flexed (Fig. 8–5). Additional flexion ROM (120 degrees) is necessary for putting on socks (Fig. 8–6), squatting (115 degrees), and stooping (125 degrees).[38]

Reliability and Validity

Studies of the reliability of hip measurements have included both active and passive motion and different types of measuring instruments. Therefore, comparisons among studies are difficult. Boone and associates[43] and Clapper and Wolf[44] investigated the reliability of measurements of active ROM. Ekstrand and associates,[45] Pandya and colleagues,[46] Ellison and coworkers,[18] Van Mechelen and colleagues,[35] Van Dillen and coworkers,[31] Croft and associates,[47] Cibulka and colleagues,[48] and Cadenhead and coworkers[49] studied passive motion. Bierma-Zeinstra and associates[30] studied the reliability

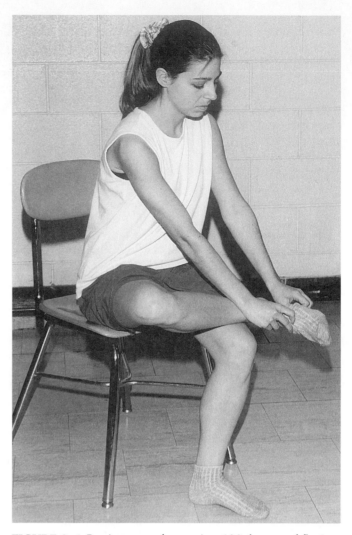

FIGURE 8–6 Putting on socks requires 120 degrees of flexion, 20 degrees of abduction and 20 degrees of lateral rotation.[38]

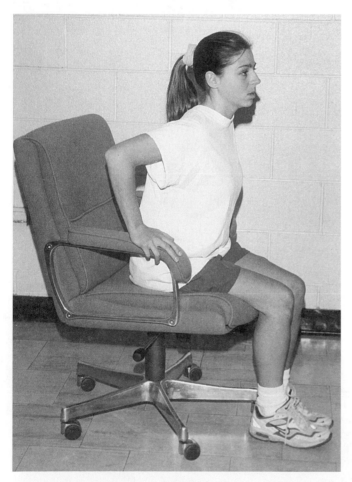

FIGURE 8–5 Sitting in a chair with an average seat height requires 112 degrees of hip flexion.[38]

of both active and passive ROM. Table 8–7 provides a sampling of intratester and intertester reliability studies.

Boone and associates[43] conducted a study in which four physical therapists used a universal goniometer to measure active ROM of three upper-extremity motions and three lower-extremity motions in 12 male volunteers aged 26 to 54 years. One of the motions tested was hip abduction. Three measurements were taken by each tester at each of four sessions scheduled on a weekly basis for 4 weeks. Intratester reliability for hip abduction was r = 0.75, with a total standard deviation between measurements of 4 degrees taken by the same testers. Intertester reliability for hip abduction was r = 0.55, with a total standard deviation of 5.2 degrees between measurements taken by different testers.

Clapper and Wolf[44] compared the reliability of the Orthoranger (Orthotronics, Daytona Beach, Fla.), an electronic computed pendulum goniometer, with that of the universal goniometer in a study of active hip motion

TABLE 8–7   Intratester Reliability

Author	n	Sample	Position	Motion	ICC
Van Dillen et al[31]	35	Healthy subjects	Supine: Hip in neutral and Knee in 80 degrees flexion.	Extension	Right hip 0.70 Left hip 0.89
			Hip in neutral and Knee in full extension.	Extension	Right hip 0.72 Left hip 0.76
			Hip in full abduction and Knee in 80 degrees flexion	Extension	Right hip 0.87 Left hip 0.76
			Hip in full abduction flexion and Knee in full extension	Extension	Right hip 0.96 Left hip 0.90
Ellison et al[18]	22	Healthy subjects	Prone: hip in neutral position and knee flexed to 90 degrees	Medial rotation Lateral rotation	Right hip 0.99 Right hip 0.96
Cadenhead et al[49]	6	Adults with cerebral palsy	Supine	Abduction	Right hip 0.99
			Prone	Extension	Right hip 0.98
			Supine	Lateral rotation	Right hip 0.79

ICC = Intraclass correlation coefficient.

involving 10 males and 10 females between the ages of 23 and 40 years. The authors found that the universal goniometer showed significantly less variation within sessions than the Orthoranger, except for measurements of hip adduction and lateral rotation. The authors concluded that the universal goniometer was a more reliable instrument than the Orthoranger. The poor correlation between the Orthoranger and the universal goniometer for measurement of hip adduction and abduction ROM values demonstrated that the two instruments could not be used interchangeably.

Ekstrand and associates[45] measured the passive ROM of hip flexion, extension, and abduction in 22 healthy men aged 20 to 30 years. They used a specially constructed goniometer to measure hip abduction and a flexometer to measure hip flexion and extension in two testing series. In the first series, the testing procedures were not controlled. In the second series, procedures were standardized and anatomical landmarks were indicated. The intratester coefficient of variation was lower than the intertester coefficient of variation for both

series. Standardization of procedures improved reliability considerably. The intertester coefficient of variation was significantly lower in the second series than in the first when the procedures were not standardized.

In a study by Pandya and colleagues,[46] five physical therapists using universal goniometers measured passive joint motions including hip extension in the upper and lower extremities of 105 children and adolescents, aged 1 to 20 years, who had Duchenne muscular dystrophy. Intratester reliability was high for all measurements; the intraclass correlation coefficient (ICC) ranged from 0.81 to 0.94. The intratester reliability for measurements of hip extension was good (ICC = 0.85). The overall ICC for intertester reliability for all measurements ranged from 0.25 to 0.91. Intertester reliability for measurements of hip extension was fair (ICC = 0.74). The results indicated the need for the same examiner to take measurements for long-term follow-up and to assess the results of therapeutic intervention.

Ellison and coworkers[18] compared passive ROM measurements of hip rotation taken with an inclinometer

TABLE 8–8   Intertester Reliability

Author	n	Sample	Position	Motion	ICC
Simoneau et al[26]	60	Healthy subjects (18–27 yrs)	Prone	Medial rotation	0.82, 0.96, 0.97
			Seated	Medial rotation	0.89, 0.85, 0.93
			Prone	Lateral rotation	0.89, 0.79, 0.98
			Seated	Lateral rotation	0.90, 0.76, 0.95
Ellison et al[18]	22	Healthy subjects (20–41 yrs)	Prone	Left medial rotation	0.98
			Prone	Left lateral rotation	0.97
			Prone	Right medial rotation	0.99
			Prone	Right lateral rotation	0.96
	15	Adults with back pain (23–61 yrs)	Prone	Left medial rotation	0.97
			Prone	Left lateral rotation	0.95
			Prone	Right medial rotation	0.96
			Prone	Right lateral rotation	0.95

ICC = Intraclass correlation coefficient.

and a universal goniometer and found no significant differences between the means. Both instruments were found to be reliable, but the authors preferred the inclinometer because it was easier to use. Croft and associates[47] used a fluid-filled inclinometer called a Plurimeter to determine the intertester reliability of passive hip flexion and rotation ROM measurements taken by six clinicians. The clinicians took ROM measurements of both hips in six patients with osteoarthritis involving only one hip joint. Flexion was measured with the patient in the supine position either to maximum flexion or to the point when further motion was restricted by pain. The results showed no difference between the measurements taken by one examiner and those taken by other examiners, but the degree of agreement was greatest for measurements of hip flexion. Cibulka and colleagues,[48] in a study of passive ROM in medial and lateral hip rotation in 100 patients with low back pain, determined that for this group of patients, measurements of rotation taken in the prone position were more reliable than those taken in the sitting position. Bierma-Zeinstra and associates[30] compared the reliability of hip ROM measurements taken by means of an electronic inclinometer with those taken by means of a universal goniometer. The two instruments showed equal intratester reliability for both active and passive hip ROM in general; however, the intratester reliability of the inclinometer was higher than that of the goniometer for passive hip rotation. The inclinometer also had higher intertester reliability for active medial rotation than the goniometer, and the authors cautioned that the instruments should not be used interchangeably.

Range of Motion Testing Procedures: Hip

Landmarks for Goniometer Alignment

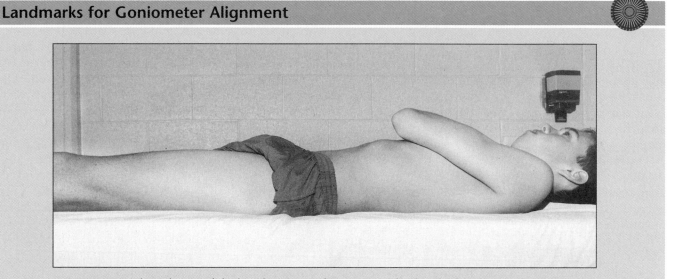

FIGURE 8–7 A lateral view of the hip showing surface anatomy landmarks for aligning the goniometer for measuring hip flexion and extension.

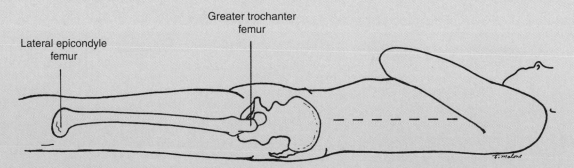

FIGURE 8–8 A lateral view of the hip showing bony anatomical landmarks for aligning the goniometer.

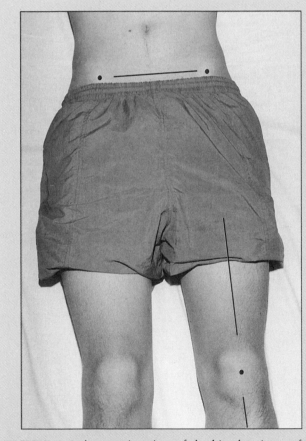

FIGURE 8–9 An anterior view of the hip showing surface anatomy landmarks for aligning the goniometer.

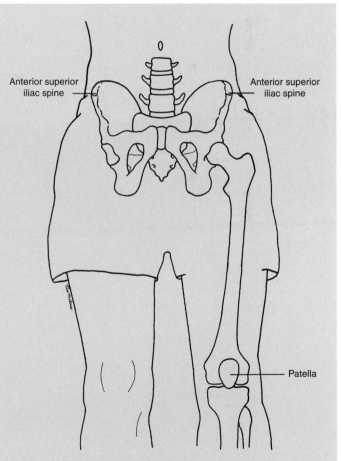

FIGURE 8–10 An anterior view of the pelvis showing the anatomical landmarks for aligning the goniometer for measuring abduction and adduction.

FLEXION

Motion occurs in the sagittal plane around a medial-lateral axis. The mean hip flexion ROM for adults is 100 degrees according to the AMA [4] and 121 degrees according to the study by Roach and Miles.[7] See Tables 8–1, 8–2, and 8–5 for additional ROM information.

Testing Position

Place the subject in the supine position, with the knees extended and both hips in 0 degrees of abduction, adduction, and rotation.

Stabilization

Stabilize the pelvis with one hand to prevent posterior tilting or rotation. Keep the contralateral lower extremity flat on the table in the neutral position to provide additional stabilization.

Testing Motion

Flex the hip by lifting the thigh off the table. Allow the knee to flex passively during the motion to lessen tension in the hamstring muscles. Maintain the extremity in neutral rotation and abduction and adduction throughout the motion (Fig. 8–11). The end of the ROM occurs when resistance to further motion is felt and attempts at overcoming the resistance cause posterior tilting of the pelvis.

Normal End-feel

The end-feel is usually soft because of contact between the muscle bulk of the anterior thigh and the lower abdomen. However, the end-feel may be firm because of tension in the posterior joint capsule and the gluteus maximus muscle.

Goniometer Alignment

See Figures 8–12 and 8–13.

1. Center the fulcrum of the goniometer over the lateral aspect of the hip joint, using the greater trochanter of the femur for reference.
2. Align the proximal arm with the lateral midline of the pelvis.
3. Align the distal arm with the lateral midline of the femur, using the lateral epicondyle as a reference.

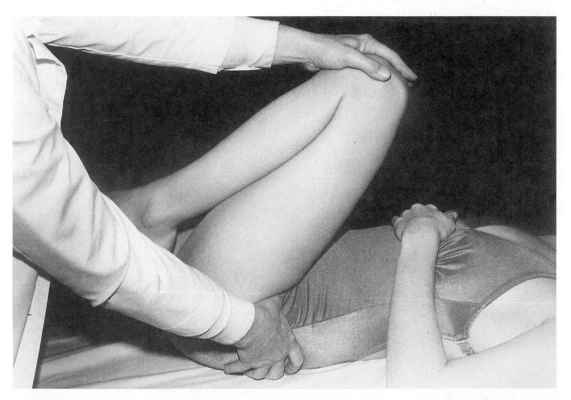

FIGURE 8–11 The end of hip flexion passive ROM. The placement of the examiner's hand on the pelvis allows the examiner to stabilize the pelvis and to detect any pelvic motion.

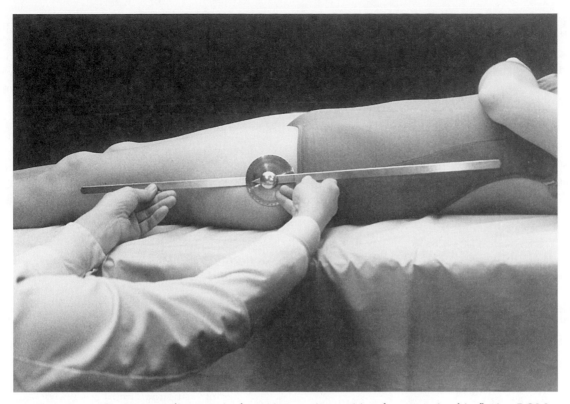

FIGURE 8–12 Goniometer alignment in the supine starting position for measuring hip flexion ROM.

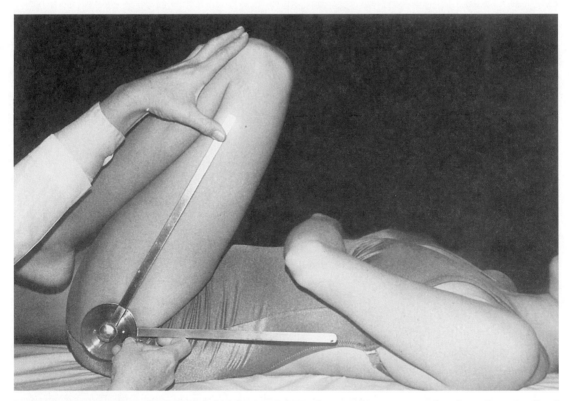

FIGURE 8–13 At the end of the left hip flexion ROM, the examiner uses one hand to align the distal goniometer arm and to maintain the hip in flexion. The examiner's other hand shifts from the pelvis to hold the proximal goniometer arm aligned with the lateral midline of the subject's pelvis.

EXTENSION

Motion occurs in a sagittal plane around a medial-lateral axis. The mean hip extension ROM for adults is 19 degrees according to Roach and Miles[7] and 30 degrees according to the AMA.[4] See Tables 8–1, 8–2, 8–4, and 8–5 for additional ROM information.

Testing Position

Place the subject in the prone position, with both knees extended and the hip to be tested in 0 degrees of abduction, adduction, and rotation. A pillow may be placed under the abdomen for comfort, but no pillow should be placed under the head.

Stabilization

Hold the pelvis with one hand to prevent an anterior tilt. Keep the contralateral extremity flat on the table to provide additional pelvic stabilization

Testing Motion

Extend the hip by raising the lower extremity from the table (Figure 8–-14). Maintain the knee in extension throughout the movement to ensure that tension in the two-joint rectus femoris muscle does not limit the hip extension ROM. The end of the ROM occurs when resistance to further motion of the femur is felt and attempts at overcoming the resistance causes anterior tilting of the pelvis and/or extension of the lumbar spine.

Normal End-feel

The end-feel is firm because of tension in the anterior joint capsule and the iliofemoral ligament, and, to a lesser extent, the ischiofemoral and pubofemoral ligaments. Tension in various muscles that flex the hip, such as the iliopsoas, sartorius, tensor fasciae latae, gracilis, and adductor longus, may contribute to the firm end-feel.

Goniometer Alignment

See Figures 8–15 and 8–16.

1. Center the fulcrum of the goniometer over the lateral aspect of the hip joint, using the greater trochanter of the femur for reference.
2. Align the proximal arm with the lateral midline of the pelvis.
3. Align the distal arm with the lateral midline of the femur, using the lateral epicondyle as a reference.

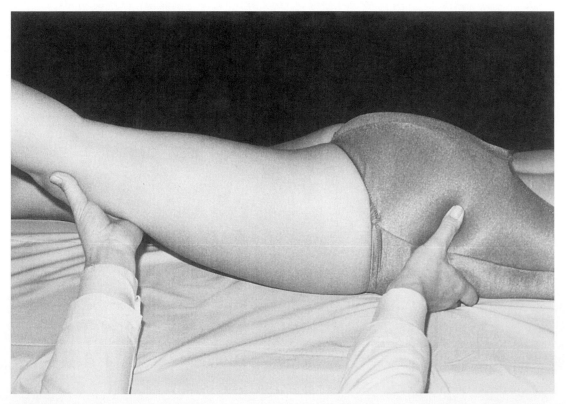

FIGURE 8–14 The subject's right lower extremity at the end of hip extension ROM. The examiner uses one hand to support the distal femur and maintain the hip in extension while her other hand grasps the pelvis at the level of the anterior superior iliac spine. Because the examiner's hand is on the subject's pelvis the examiner is able to detect pelvic tilting.

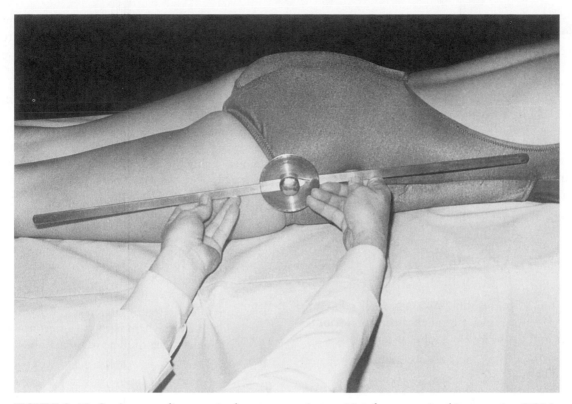

FIGURE 8–15 Goniometer alignment in the prone starting position for measuring hip extension ROM.

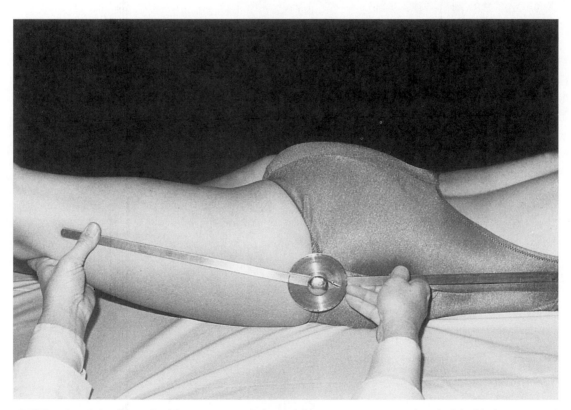

FIGURE 8–16 At the end of hip extension ROM, the examiner uses one hand to hold the proximal goniometer arm in alignment. The examiner's other hand supports the subject's femur and keeps the distal goniometer arm in alignment.

ABDUCTION

Motion occurs in the frontal plane around an anterior-posterior axis. The mean ROM in abduction is 40 degrees according to the AMA[4] and 42 degrees according to Roach and Miles.[7] (See Tables 8–1, 8–2, and 8–5 for additional ROM information.)

Testing Position

Place the subject in the supine position, with the knees extended and the hips in 0 degrees of flexion, extension, and rotation.

Stabilization

Keep a hand on the pelvis to prevent lateral tilting and rotation. Watch the trunk for lateral trunk flexion.

Testing Motion

Abduct the hip by sliding the lower extremity laterally (Fig. 8–17). Do not allow lateral rotation or flexion of the hip. The end of the ROM occurs when resistance to further motion of the femur is felt and attempts to overcome the resistance causes lateral pelvic tilting, pelvic rotation, or lateral flexion of the trunk.

Normal End-feel

The end-feel is firm because of tension in the inferior (medial) joint capsule, pubofemoral ligament, ischiofemoral ligament, and inferior band of the iliofemoral ligament. Passive tension in the adductor magnus, adductor longus, adductor brevis, pectineus, and gracilis muscles may contribute to the firm end-feel.

Goniometer Alignment

See Figures 8–18 and 8–19.

1. Center the fulcrum of the goniometer over the anterior superior iliac spine (ASIS) of the extremity being measured.
2. Align the proximal arm with an imaginary horizontal line extending from one ASIS to the other.
3. Align the distal arm with the anterior midline of the femur, using the midline of the patella for reference.

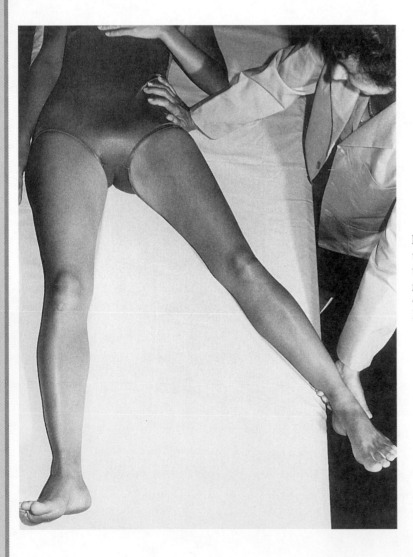

FIGURE 8–17 The left lower extremity at the end of the hip abduction ROM. The examiner uses one hand to pull the subject's leg into abduction. (The examiner's grip on the ankle is designed to prevent lateral rotation of the hip.) The examiner's other hand not only stabilizes the pelvis but also is used to detect pelvic motion.

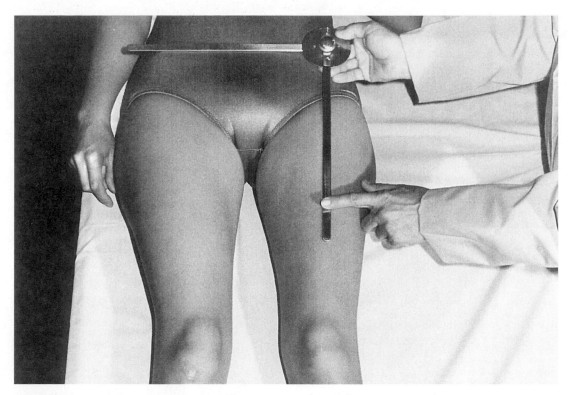

FIGURE 8-18 In the starting position for measuring hip abduction ROM, the goniometer is at 90 degrees. This position is considered to be the 0-degree starting position. Therefore, the examiner must transpose her reading from 90 degrees to 0 degrees. For example, an actual reading of 90-120 degrees on the goniometer is recorded as 0-30 degrees.

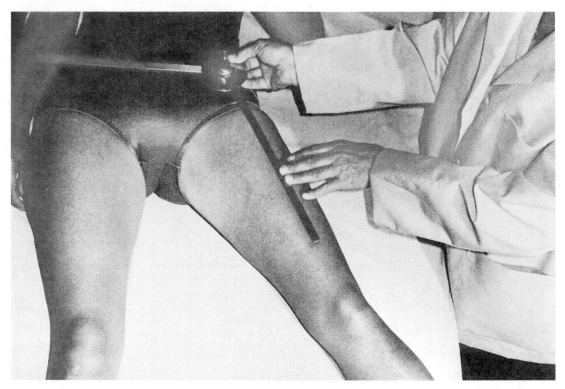

FIGURE 8-19 Goniometer alignment at the end of the abduction ROM. The examiner has determined the end-feel and has moved her right hand from stabilizing the pelvis in order to hold the goniometer in correct alignment.

ADDUCTION

Motion occurs in a frontal plane around an anterior-posterior axis. The mean ROM in adduction for adults is 20 degrees according to the AMA[4] and 30 degrees according to the AAOS.[3] See Tables 8–1, 8–2, and 8–5 for additional ROM information.

Testing Position

Place the subject in the supine position, with both knees extended and the hip being tested in 0 degrees of flexion, extension, and rotation. Abduct the contralateral extremity to provide sufficient space to complete the full ROM in adduction.

Stabilization

Stabilize the pelvis to prevent lateral tilting.

Testing Motion

Adduct the hip by sliding the lower extremity medially toward the contralateral lower extremity (Fig. 8–20). Place one hand at the knee to move the extremity into adduction and to maintain the hip in neutral flexion and rotation. The end of the ROM occurs when resistance to further adduction is felt and attempts to overcome the resistance cause lateral pelvic tilting, pelvic rotation, and/or lateral trunk flexion.

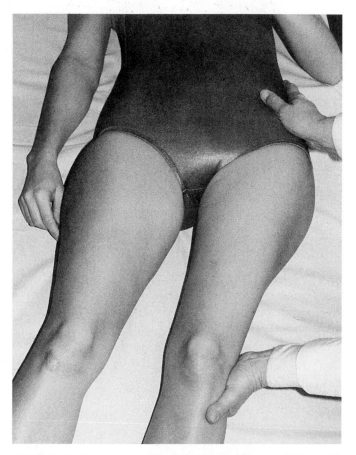

FIGURE 8–20 At the end of the hip adduction ROM, the examiner maintains the hip in adduction with one hand and stabilizes the pelvis with her other hand.

Normal End-feel

The end-feel is firm because of tension in the superior (lateral) joint capsule and the superior band of the iliofemoral ligament. Tension in the gluteus medius and minimus and the tensor fasciae latae muscles may also contribute to the firm end-feel.

Goniometer Alignment

See Figures 8–21 and 8–22.

1. Center the fulcrum of the goniometer over the ASIS of the extremity being measured.
2. Align the proximal arm with an imaginary horizontal line extending from one ASIS to the other.
3. Align the distal arm with the anterior midline of the femur, using the midline of the patella for reference.

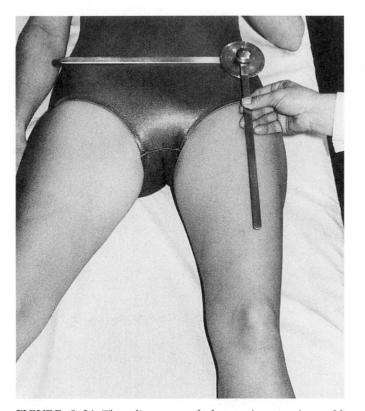

FIGURE 8–21 The alignment of the goniometer is at 90 degrees. Therefore, when the examiner records the measurement, she will have to transpose the reading so that 90 degrees is equivalent to 0 degrees. For example, an actual reading of 90 -60 degrees is recorded as 0-30 degrees.

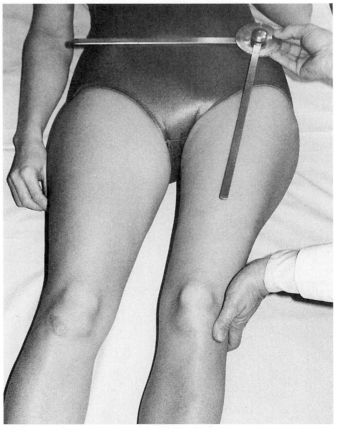

FIGURE 8–22 At the end of the hip adduction ROM, the examiner uses one hand to hold the goniometer body over the subject's anterior superior iliac spine. The examiner prevents hip rotation by maintaining a firm grasp at the subject's knee with her other hand.

MEDIAL (INTERNAL) ROTATION

Motion occurs in a transverse plane around a vertical axis when the subject is in anatomical position. The mean adult values for the ROM in medial rotation are 32 degrees according Roach and Miles[7] and 40 degrees according to the AMA.[4] See Tables 8–1, 8–2, 8–3, and 8–5 for additional ROM information.

Testing Position

Seat the subject on a supporting surface, with the knees flexed to 90 degrees over the edge of the surface. Place the hip in 0 degrees of abduction and adduction and in 90 degrees of flexion. Place a towel roll under the distal end of the femur to maintain the femur in a horizontal plane.

Stabilization

Stabilize the distal end of the femur to prevent abduction, adduction, or further flexion of the hip. Avoid rotations and lateral tilting of the pelvis.

Testing Motion

Place one hand at the distal femur to provide stabilization and use the other hand at the distal tibia to move the lower leg laterally. The hand performing the motion also holds the lower leg in a neutral position to prevent rotation at the knee joint (Fig. 8–23). The end of the ROM occurs when attempts at resistance are felt and attempts at further motion cause tilting of the pelvis or lateral flexion of the trunk.

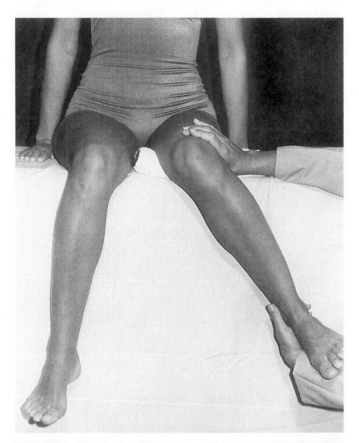

FIGURE 8–23 The left lower extremity at the end of the ROM of hip medial rotation. One of the examiner's hands is placed on the subject's distal femur to prevent hip flexion and abduction. Her other hand pulls the lower leg laterally.

Normal End-feel

The end-feel is firm because of tension in the posterior joint capsule and the ischiofemoral ligament. Tension in the following muscles may also contribute to the firm end-feel: piriformis, obturatorii (internus and externus), gemelli (superior and inferior), quadratus femoris, gluteus medius (posterior fibers), and gluteus maximus.

Goniometer Alignment

See Figures 8–24 and 8–25.

1. Center the fulcrum of the goniometer over the anterior aspect of the patella.
2. Align the proximal arm so that it is perpendicular to the floor or parallel to the supporting surface.
3. Align the distal arm with the anterior midline of the lower leg, using the crest of the tibia and a point midway between the two malleoli for reference.

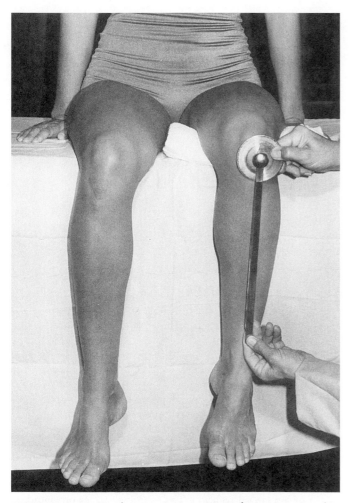

FIGURE 8–24 In the starting position for measuring hip medial rotation, the fulcrum of the goniometer is placed over the patella. Both arms of the instrument are together.

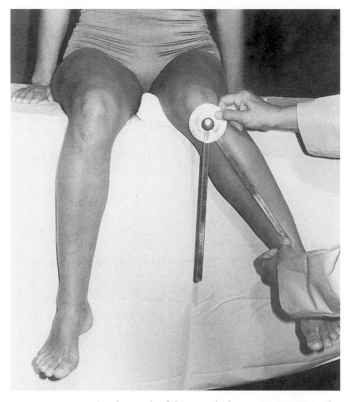

FIGURE 8–25 At the end of hip medial rotation ROM, the proximal arm of the goniometer hangs freely so that it is perpendicular to the floor.

LATERAL (EXTERNAL) ROTATION

Motion occurs in a transverse plane around a longitudinal axis when the subject is in anatomical position. The mean ROM values for lateral rotation are 32 degrees according to Roach and Miles[7] and 50 degrees according to the AMA.[4] See Tables 8–1, 8–2, 8–3, and 8–5 for additional ROM information.

Testing Position

Seat the subject on a supporting surface with knees flexed to 90 degrees over the edge of the surface. Place the hip in 0 degrees of abduction and adduction and in 90 degrees of flexion. Flex the contralateral knee beyond 90 degrees to allow the hip being measured to complete its full range of lateral rotation.

Stabilization

Stabilize the distal end of the femur to prevent abduction or further flexion of the hip. Avoid rotation and lateral tilting of the pelvis.

Testing Motion

Place one hand at the distal femur to provide stabilization and place the other hand on the distal fibula to move the lower leg medially (Fig. 8–26). The hand on the fibula also prevents rotation at the knee joint. The end of the motion occurs when resistance is felt and attempts at overcoming the resistance cause tilting of the pelvis or trunk lateral flexion.

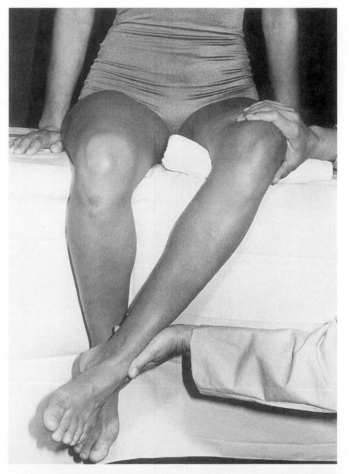

FIGURE 8–26 The left lower extremity is at the end of the ROM of hip lateral rotation. The examiner places one hand on the subject's distal femur to prevent both hip flexion and hip abduction. The subject assists with stabilization by placing her hands on the supporting surface and shifting her weight over her left hip. The subject flexes her right knee to allow the left lower extremity to complete the ROM.

Normal End-feel

The end-feel is firm because of tension in the anterior joint capsule, iliofemoral ligament, and pubofemoral ligament. Tension in the anterior portion of the gluteus medius, gluteus minimus, adductor magnus, adductor longus, pectineus, and piriformis muscles also may contribute to the firm end-feel.

Goniometer Alignment

See Figures 8–27 and 8–28.

1. Center the fulcrum of the goniometer over the anterior aspect of the patella.
2. Align the proximal arm so that it is perpendicular to the floor or parallel to the supporting surface.
3. Align the distal arm with the anterior midline of the lower leg, using the crest of the tibia and a point midway between the two malleoli for reference.

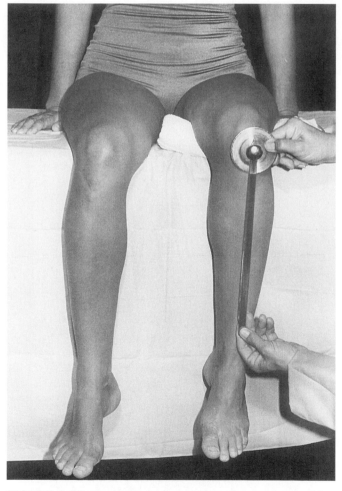

FIGURE 8–27 Goniometer alignment in the starting position for measuring hip lateral rotation.

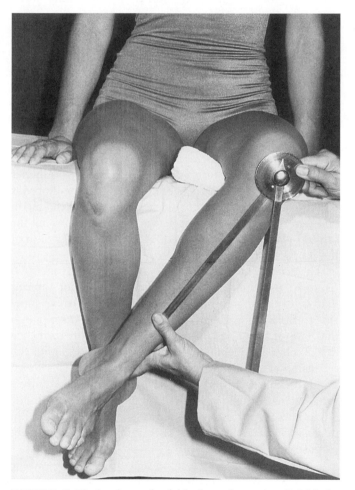

FIGURE 8–28 At the end of hip lateral rotation ROM the examiner uses one hand to support the subject's leg and to maintain alignment of the distal goniometer arm.

Muscle Length Testing Procedures: Hip

HIP FLEXORS (THOMAS TEST)

The iliacus and psoas major muscles flex the hip in the sagittal plane of motion. Other muscles, because of their attachments, create hip flexion in combination with other motions. The rectus femoris flexes the hip and extends the knee. The sartorius flexes, abducts, and laterally rotates the hip while flexing the knee. The tensor fasciae latae abducts, flexes, and medially rotates the hip and extends the knee. Several muscles that primarily adduct the hip, such as the pectineus, adductor longus, and adductor brevis, also lie anterior to the axis of the hip joint and can contribute to hip flexion. Short muscles that flex the hip limit hip extension ROM. Hip extension can also be limited by abnormalities of the joint surfaces, shortness of the anterior joint capsule, and short iliofemoral and ischiofemoral ligaments.

The anatomy of the major muscles that flex the hip is illustrated in Figure 8–29A and B. The **iliacus** originates proximally from the upper two thirds of the iliac fossa, the inner lip of the iliac crest, the lateral aspect (ala) of the sacrum, and the sacroiliac and iliolumbar ligaments. It inserts distally on the lesser trochanter of the femur. The **psoas major** originates proximally from the sides of the vertebral bodies and intervertebral discs of T12-L5, and the transverse processes of L1-L5. It inserts distally on the lesser trochanter of the femur. These two muscles are commonly referred to as the **iliopsoas**. If the iliopsoas is short, it limits hip extension without pulling the hip in another direction of motion; the thigh remains in the sagittal plane. Knee position does not affect the length of the iliopsoas muscle.

The **rectus femoris** arises proximally from two tendons: the anterior tendon from the anterior inferior iliac spine, and the posterior tendon from a groove superior to the brim of the acetabulum. It inserts distally into the base of the patella and into the tibial tuberosity via the patellar ligament. A short rectus femoris limits hip extension and knee flexion. If the rectus femoris is short, and hip extension is attempted, the knee passively moves into extension to accommodate the shortened muscle. Sometimes, when the rectus femoris is shortened and hip extension is attempted, the knee remains flexed but hip extension is limited.

The **sartorius** arises proximally from the ASIS and the upper aspect of the iliac notch. It inserts distally into the proximal aspect of the medial tibia. If the sartorius is short it limits hip extension, hip adduction, and knee extension. If the sartorius is short and hip extension is attempted, the hip passively moves into hip abduction and knee flexion to accommodate the short muscle.

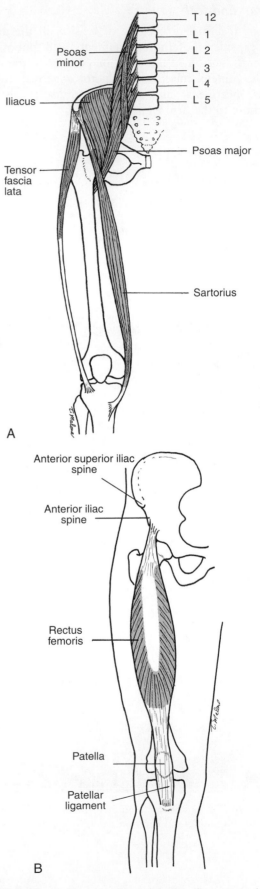

FIGURE 8–29 An anterior view of the hip flexor muscles.

The **tensor fasciae latae** arises proximally from the anterior aspect of the outer lip of the iliac crest and the lateral surface of the ASIS and iliac notch. It inserts distally into the iliotibial band of the fascia lata about one-third of the distance down the thigh. The iliotibial band inserts into the lateral anterior surface of the proximal tibia. A short tensor fascia latae can limit hip adduction, extension and lateral rotation, and knee flexion. If hip extension is attempted, the hip passively moves into abduction and medial rotation to accommodate the short muscle.

The **pectineus** originates from the pectineal line of the pubis, and inserts in a line from the lesser trochanter to the linea aspera of the femur. The **adductor longus** arises proximally from the anterior aspect of the pubis and inserts distally into the linea aspera of the femur. The **adductor brevis** originates from the inferior ramus of the pubis. It inserts into a line that extends from the lesser trochanter to the linea aspera and the proximal part of the linea aspera just posterior to the pectineus and proximal part of the adductor longus. Shortness of these muscles limits hip abduction and extension. If these muscles are short and hip extension is attempted, the hip passively moves into adduction to accommodate the shortened muscles.

Starting Position

Place the subject in the sitting position at the end of the examining table, with the lower thighs, knees, and legs off the table. Assist the subject into the supine position by supporting the subject's back and flexing the hips and knees (Fig. 8–30). This sequence is used to avoid placing a strain on the subject's lower back while the starting test position is being assumed. Once the subject is supine, flex the hips by bringing the knees toward the chest just enough to flatten the low back and pelvis against the table (Fig. 8–31). In this position, the pelvis is in about 10 degrees of posterior pelvic tilt. Avoid pulling the knees too far toward the chest because this will cause the low back to go into excessive flexion and the pelvis to go into an exaggerated posterior tilt. This low back and pelvis position gives the appearance of tightness in the hip flexors when, in fact, no tightness is present.

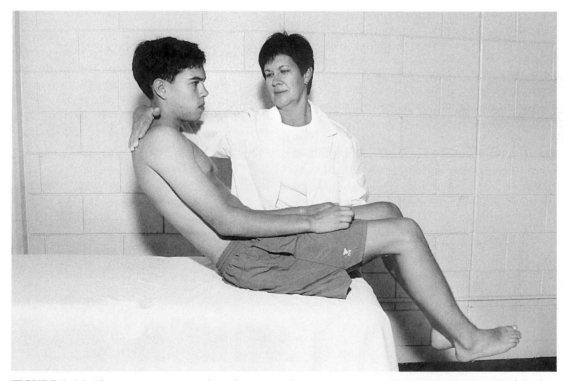

FIGURE 8–30 The examiner assists the subject into the starting position for testing the length of the hip flexors. Ordinarily the examiner stands on the same side as the hip being tested to visualize the hip region and take measurements, but the examiner is standing on the contralateral side for the photograph.

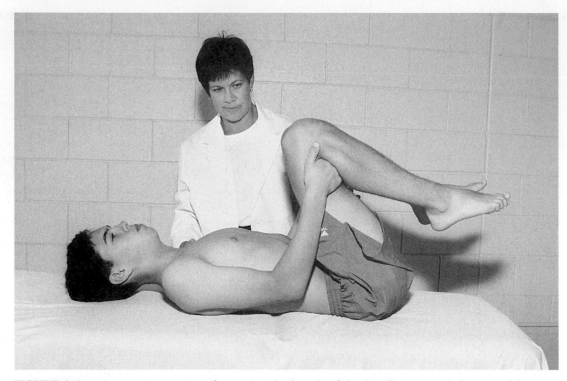

FIGURE 8–31 The starting position for testing the length of the hip flexors. Both knees and hips are flexed so that the low back and pelvis are flat on the examining table.

Stabilization

Either the examiner or the subject holds the hip not being tested in flexion (knee toward the chest) to maintain the low back and pelvis flat against the examining table.

Testing Motion

Information as to which muscles are short can be gained by varying the position of the knee and carefully observing passive motions of the hip and knee while hip extension is attempted. Extend the hip being tested by lowering the thigh toward the examining table. The knee is relaxed in approximately 80 degrees of flexion. The lower extremity should remain in the sagittal plane.

If the thigh lies flat on the examining table and the knee remains in 80 degrees of flexion, the iliopsoas and rectus femoris muscles are of normal length[32] (Figs. 8–32 and 8–33). At the end of the test, the hip is in 10 degrees of extension because the pelvis is being held in 10 degrees of posterior tilt. At this point, the test would be concluded.

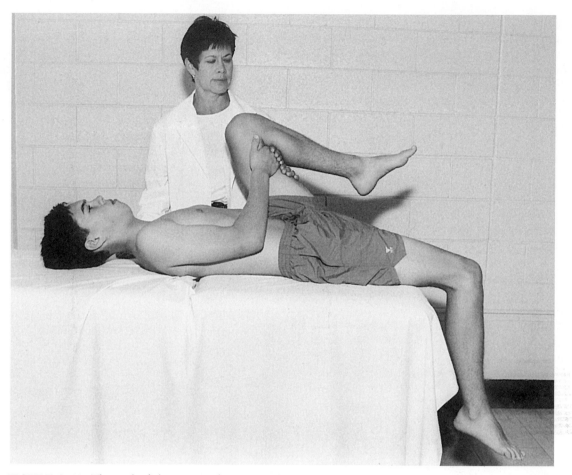

FIGURE 8–32 The end of the motion for testing the length of the hip flexors. The subject has normal length of the right hip flexors: the hip is able to extend to 10 degrees (thigh is flat on table), the knee remains in 80 degrees of flexion, and the lower extremity remains in the sagittal plane.

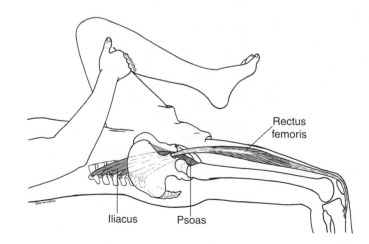

FIGURE 8–33 A lateral view of the hip showing the hip flexors at the end of the Thomas test.

If the thigh does not lie flat on the table, hip extension is limited, and further testing is needed to determine the cause (Fig. 8–34). Repeat the starting portion by flexing the hips and bringing the knee toward the chest. Extend the hip by lowering the thigh toward the examining table, but this time support the knee in extension (Fig. 8–35). When the knee is held in extension, the rectus femoris is slack over the knee joint. If the hip extends with the knee held in extension so that thigh is able to lie on the examining table, the rectus femoris can be ascertained to have been short. If the hip cannot extend with the knee held in extension and the thigh does not lie on the examining table, the iliopsoas, anterior joint capsule, iliofemoral ligament, and ischiofemoral ligament may be short.

When the hip is extending toward the examining table, observe carefully to see if the lower extremity stays in the sagittal plane. If the hip moves into lateral rotation and abduction, the sartorius muscle may be short. If the hip moves into medial rotation and abduction, the tensor fasciae latae may be short. The Ober test can be used specifically to check the length of the tensor fasciae latae. If the hip moves into adduction, the pectineus, adductor longus, and adductor brevis may be short. Hip abduction ROM can be measured to test more specifically for the length of the hip adductors.

Normal End-feel

When the knee remains flexed at the end of hip extension ROM, the end-feel is firm owing to tension in the rectus femoris. When the knee is extended at the end of hip extension ROM, the end-feel is firm owing to tension in the anterior joint capsule, iliofemoral ligament, ischiofemoral ligament, and iliopsoas muscle. If one or more of the following muscles are shortened they may also contribute to a firm end-feel: sartorius, tensor fasciae latae, pectineus, adductor longus, and adductor brevis.

Goniometer Alignment

See Figure 8–36.

1. Center the fulcrum of the goniometer over the lateral aspect of the hip joint, using the greater trochanter of the femur for reference.
2. Align the proximal arm with the lateral midline of the pelvis.
3. Align the distal arm with the lateral midline of the femur, using the lateral epicondyle for reference.

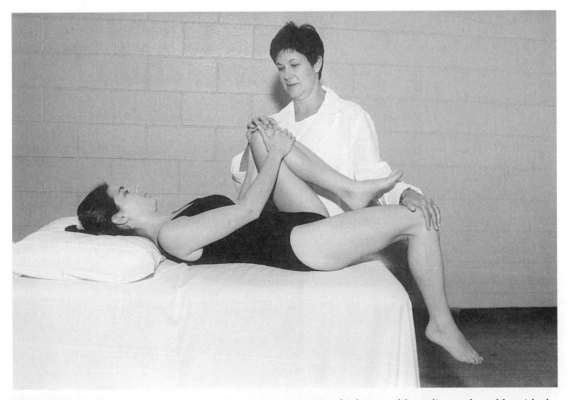

FIGURE 8–34 This subject has restricted hip extension. Her thigh is unable to lie on the table with the knee flexed to 80 degrees. Further testing is needed to determine which structures are short.

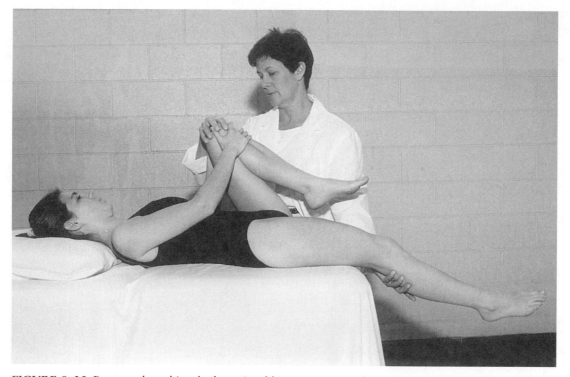

FIGURE 8–35 Because the subject had restricted hip extension at the end of the testing motion (see Fig. 8–34), the testing motion needs to be modified and repeated. This time, the knee is held in extension when the extremity is lowered toward the table. At the end of the test, the hip extends to 10 degrees, and the thigh lies flat on the table. Therefore, one may conclude that the rectus femoris is short and that the iliopsoas, anterior joint capsule, and iliofemoral and ischiofemoral ligaments are of normal length.

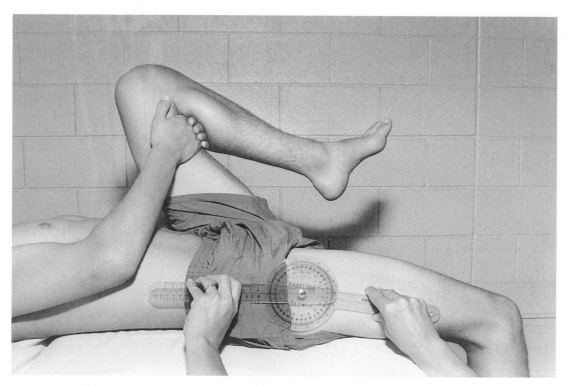

FIGURE 8–36 Goniometer alignment for measuring the length of the hip flexors.

THE HAMSTRINGS: SEMITENDINOSUS, SEMIMEMBRANOSUS, AND BICEPS FEMORIS (STRAIGHT LEG TEST)

The hamstring muscles, composed of the semitendinosus, semimembranosus, and biceps femoris, cross two joints—the hip and the knee. When they contract, they extend the hip and flex the knee. The **semitendinosus** originates proximally from the ischial tuberosity and inserts distally on the proximal aspect of the medial surface of the tibia (Fig. 8–37A). The **semimembranosus** originates from the ischial tuberosity and inserts on the posterior medial aspect of the medial condyle of the tibia (Fig. 8–37B). The long head of the **biceps femoris** originates from the ischial tuberosity and the sacrotuberous ligament, whereas the short head of the biceps femoris originates proximally from the lateral lip of the linea aspera, the lateral supracondylar line, and the lateral intermuscular septum (Fig. 8–37A). The biceps femoris inserts onto the head of the fibula with a small portion extending to the lateral condyle of the tibia and the lateral collateral ligament.

Because the hamstrings are two-joint muscles, shortness can limit hip flexion and knee extension. If hamstrings are short and the knee is held in full extension, hip flexion is limited. However, if hip flexion is limited when the knee is flexed, abnormalities of the joint surfaces, shortness of the posterior joint capsule, or a short gluteus maximus may be present.

Starting Position

Place the subject in the supine position, with both knees extended and hips in 0 degrees of flexion, extension, abduction, adduction, and rotation (Fig. 8–38). If possible remove clothing covering the ilium and low back so the pelvis and lumbar spine can be observed during the test.

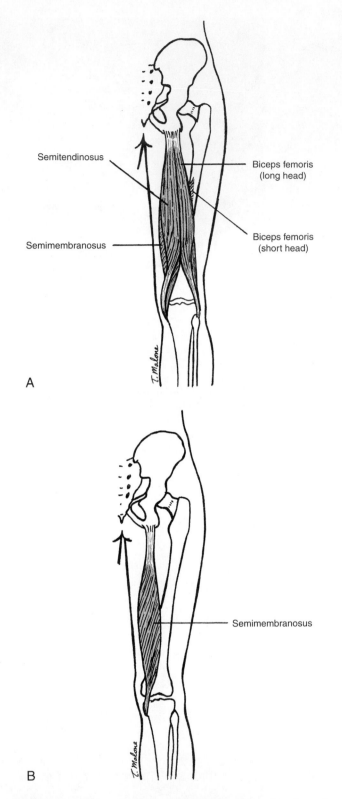

Semitendinosus

Biceps femoris (long head)

Biceps femoris (short head)

Semimembranosus

A

Semimembranosus

B

FIGURE 8–37 A posterior view of the hip showing the hamstring muscles (*A* and *B*).

Stabilization

Hold the knee of the lower extremity being tested in full extension. Keep the other lower extremity flat on the examining table to stabilize the pelvis and prevent excessive amounts of posterior pelvic tilt and lumbar flexion. Usually, the weight of the lower extremity provides adequate stabilization, but a strap securing the thigh to the examining table can be added if necessary.

Testing Motion

Flex the hip by lifting the lower extremity off the table (Figs. 8–39 and 8–40). Keep the knee in full extension by applying firm pressure to the anterior thigh. As the hip flexes, the pelvis and low back should flatten against the examining table. The end of the testing motion occurs when resistance is felt from tension in the posterior thigh and further flexion of the hip causes knee flexion, posterior pelvic tilt, or lumbar flexion. If the hip can flex to between 70 and 80 degrees with the knee extended, the test indicates normal length of the hamstring muscles.[32]

Shortness of muscles in the hip and lumbar region influences the results of the straight leg raising test. If the subject has short hip flexors on the side that is not being tested, the pelvis is held in an anterior tilt when that lower extremity is lying on the examining table. An anterior pelvic tilt decreases the distance that the leg being tested can lift off the examining table, thus giving the appearance of less hamstring length than is actually present. To remedy this situation, have the subject flex the hip not being tested by resting the foot on the table or by supporting the thigh with a pillow (Fig. 8–41). This position slackens the short hip flexors and allows the low back and pelvis to flatten against the examining table. Be careful to avoid an excessive amount of posterior pelvic tilt and lumbar flexion.

If the subject has short lumbar extensors, the low back has an excessive lordotic curve and the pelvis is in an anterior tilt. The distance that the leg can lift off the examining table is decreased if the pelvis is in an anterior tilt. This gives the appearance of less hamstring length than is actually present. In this case, the examiner needs to carefully align the proximal arm of the goniometer with the lateral midline of the pelvis when measuring hip flexion ROM, not being misled by the height of the lower extremity from the examining table.

Normal End-feel

The end-feel is firm owing to tension in the semimembranosus, semitendinosus, and biceps femoris muscles.

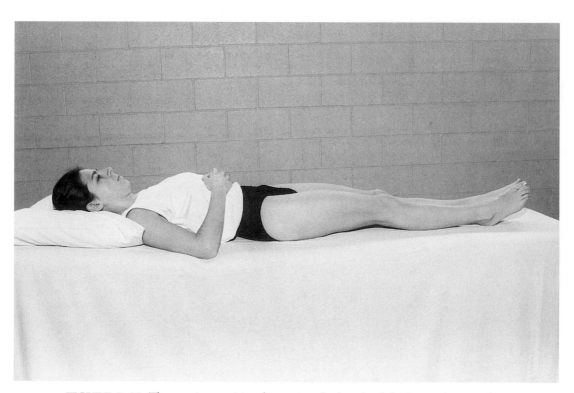

FIGURE 8–38 The starting position for testing the length of the hamstring muscles.

Goniometer Alignment

See Figure 8–42.

1. Center the fulcrum of the goniometer over the lateral aspect of the hip joint, using the greater trochanter of the femur for reference.

2. Align the proximal arm with the lateral midline of the pelvis.

3. Align the distal arm with the lateral midline of the femur, using the lateral epicondyle for reference.

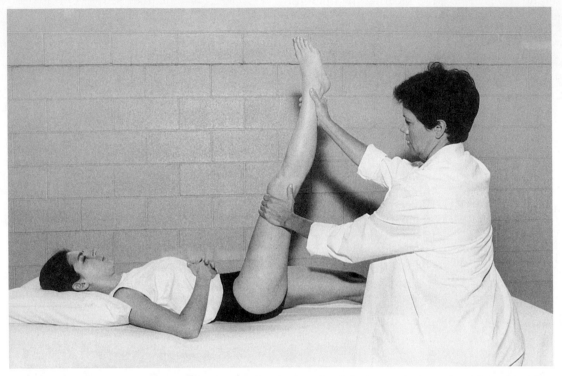

FIGURE 8–39 The end of the testing motion for the length of the hamstring muscles. The subject has normal length of the hamstrings: the hip can be passively flexed to 70 to 80 degrees with the knee held in full extension. This test is also called the straight leg raise test.

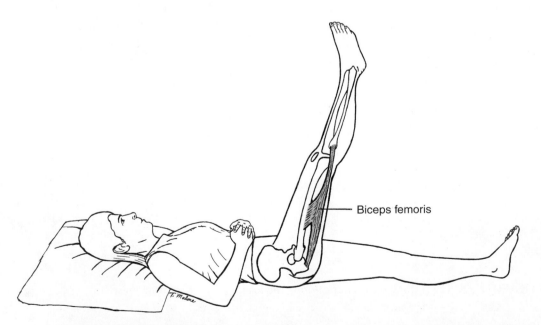

Biceps femoris

FIGURE 8–40 A lateral view of the hip showing the biceps femoris at the end of the testing motion for the length of the hamstrings.

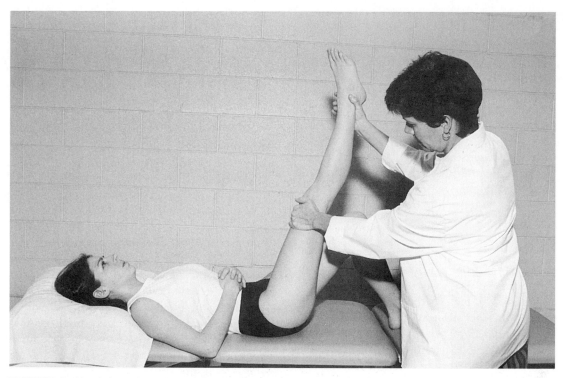

FIGURE 8–41 If the subject has shortness of the contralateral hip flexors, flex the contralateral hip to prevent an anterior pelvic tilt.

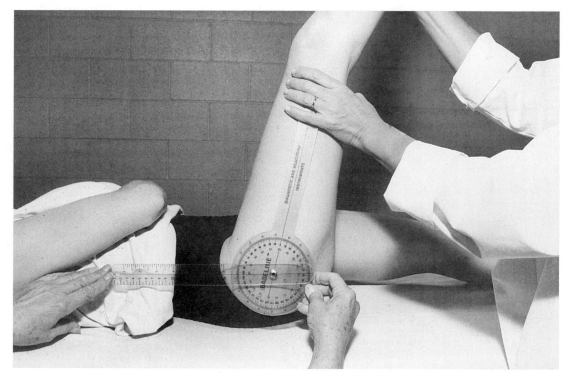

FIGURE 8–42 Goniometer alignment for measuring the length of the hamstring muscles. Another examiner will need to take the measurement while the first examiner supports the leg being tested.

TENSOR FASCIAE LATAE (OBER TEST)[50]

The **tensor fasciae latae** crosses two joints—the hip and knee. When this muscle contracts, it abducts, flexes, and medially rotates the hip and extends the knee. The tensor fascia latae arises proximally from the anterior aspect of the outer lip of the iliac crest, and the lateral surface of the ASIS and the iliac notch (Fig. 8–43). It attaches distally into the iliotibial band of the fascia latae about one third of the way down the thigh. The iliotibial band inserts into the lateral anterior surface of the proximal tibia. If the tensor fascia latae is short it limits hip adduction and, to a lesser extent, hip extension, hip lateral rotation, and knee flexion.

Starting Position

Place the subject in the sidelying position, with the hip being tested uppermost. Position the subject near the edge of the examining table, so that the examiner can stand directly behind the subject. Initially, extend the uppermost knee and place the hip in 0 degrees of flexion, extension, adduction, abduction, and rotation. The patient flexes the bottom hip and knee to stabilize the trunk, flatten the lumbar curve, and keep the pelvis in a slight posterior tilt.

Stabilization

Place one hand on the iliac crest to stabilize the pelvis. Firm pressure is usually required to prevent the pelvis from laterally tilting during the testing motion. Having the patient flex the bottom hip and knee can also help to stabilize the trunk and pelvis.

Testing Motion

Support the leg being tested by holding the medial aspect of the knee and the lower leg. Flex the hip and the knee to 90 degrees (Fig. 8–44). Keep the knee flexed and move the hip into abduction and extension to position the tensor fasciae latae over the greater trochanter of the femur (Fig. 8–45). Test the length of the tensor fasciae latae by lowering the leg into hip adduction, bringing it toward the examining table (Figs. 8–46 and 8–47). Do not allow the pelvis to tilt laterally or the hip to flex because these motions slacken the muscle. Keep the knee flexed to control medial rotation of the hip and to maintain the stretch of the muscle. If the thigh drops to slightly below horizontal (10 degrees of hip adduction), the test is negative and the tensor fasciae latae is of normal length.[32] If the thigh remains above horizontal in hip abduction, the tensor fasciae latae is tight.

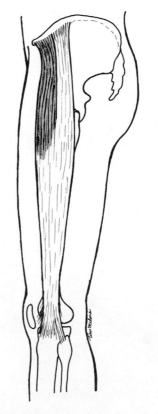

FIGURE 8–43 A lateral view of the hip showing the tensor fasciae latae and iliotibial band.

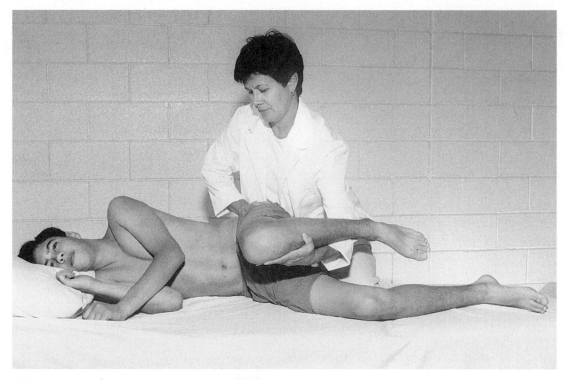

FIGURE 8–44 The first step in the testing motion for the length of the tensor fasciae latae is to flex the hip and knee.

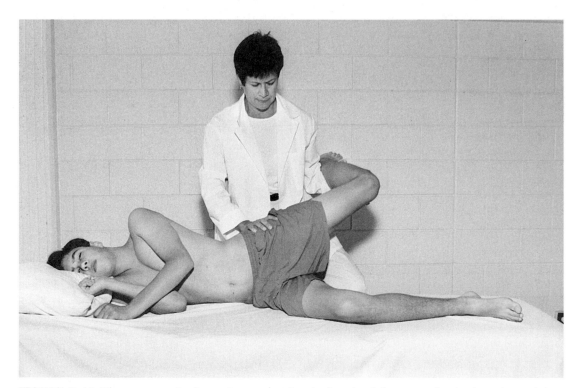

FIGURE 8–45 The next step in the testing motion for the length of the tensor fasciae latae is to abduct and extend the hip. These first two steps in the testing motion will help position the tensor fasciae latae over the greater trochanter of the femur.

Some authors have stated that the tensor fasciae latae is of normal length when the hip adducts to the examining table.[51,52] However, stabilization of the pelvis to prevent a lateral tilt and avoidance of hip flexion and medial rotation limit hip adduction to 10 degrees during the testing motion, causing the thigh to drop slightly below the horizontal position.[32] Even more conservative hip adduction values have been reported as normal by Cade and associates,[53] who found that only 7 of 50 young female subjects had normal (or not short) bent leg Ober test values when the horizontal leg position was used as the test parameter.

Note that at least 0 degrees of hip extension is needed to perform length testing of the tensor fascia lata. If the iliopsoas is tight, it prevents the proper positioning of the tensor fascia lata over the greater trochanter. If the rectus femoris is short, the knee may be extended during the test,[32] but extreme care must be taken to avoid medial rotation of the hip as the leg is lowered into adduction. This change in test position is called a modified Ober test.

Normal End-feel

The end-feel is firm owing to tension in the tensor fascia lata.

Goniometer Alignment

See Figure 8–48.

1. Center the fulcrum of the goniometer over the ASIS of the extremity being measured.
2. Align the proximal arm with an imaginary line extending from one ASIS to the other.
3. Align the distal arm with the anterior midline of the femur, using the midline of the patella for reference.

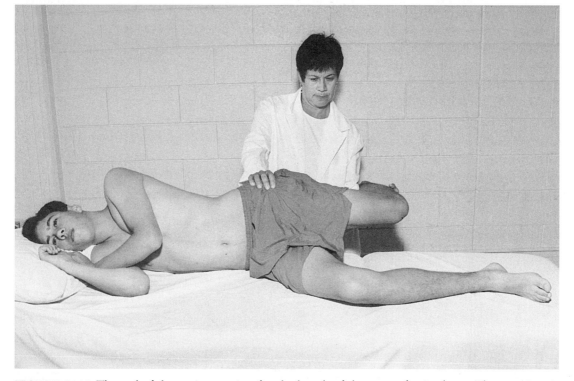

FIGURE 8–46 The end of the testing motion for the length of the tensor fasciae latae. The examiner is firmly holding the iliac crest to prevent a lateral tilt of the pelvis while the hip is lowered into adduction. No flexion or medial rotation of the hip is allowed. The subject has a normal length of the tensor fasciae latae; the thigh drops to slightly below horizontal.

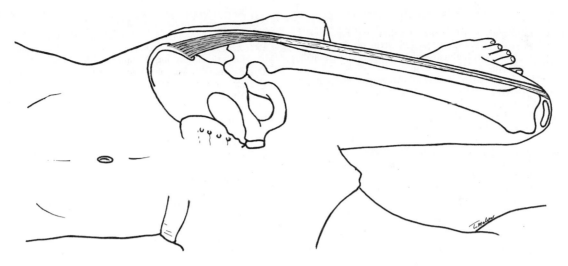

FIGURE 8–47 An anterior view of the hip showing the tensor fasciae latae at the end of the Ober test.

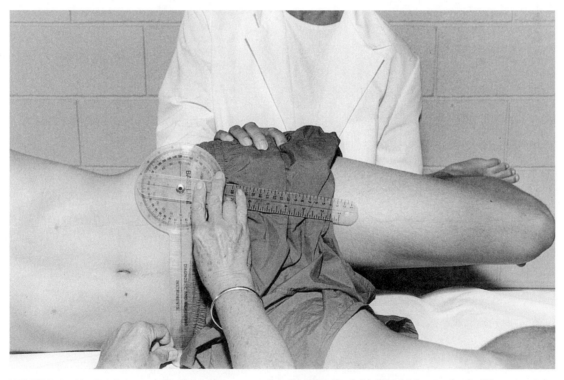

FIGURE 8–48 Goniometer alignment for measuring the length of the tensor fasciae latae. The examiner stabilizes the pelvis and positions the leg being tested while another examiner takes the measurement. If another examiner is not available, a visual estimate will have to be made.

REFERENCES

1. Levangie, PK, and Norkin, CC: Joint Structure and Function: A Comprehensive Analysis, ed 3. FA Davis, Philadelphia, 2001.
2. Cyriax, JH, and Cyriax, PJ: Illustrated Manual of Orthopaedic Medicine. Butterworths, London, 1983.
3. Greene, WB, and Heckman, JD (eds): American Academy of Orthopaedic Surgeons: The Clinical Measurement of Joint Motion: AAOS, Chicago, 1994.
4. American Medical Association: Guides to The Evaluation of Permanent Impairment, ed 3. AMA, Chicago, 1990.
5. Boone, DC, and Azen, SP: Normal range of motion of joints in male subjects. J Bone Joint Surg Am 61:756, 1979.
6. Svenningsen, S, et al: Hip motion related to age and sex. Acta Orthop Scand 60:97, 1989.
7. Roach, KE, and Miles, TP: Normal hip and knee active range of motion: The relationship to age. Phys Ther 71:656, 1991.
8. Waugh, KG, et al: Measurement of selected hip, knee and ankle joint motions in newborns. Phys Ther 63:1616, 1983.
9. Schwarze, DJ, and Denton, JR: Normal values of neonatal limbs: An evaluation of 1000 neonates. J Pediatr Orthop 13:758, 1993.
10. Broughton, NS, Wright, J, and Menelaus, MB: Range of knee motion in normal neonates. J Pediatr Orthop 13:263, 1993.
11. Drews, JE, Vraciu, JK, and Pellino, G: Range of motion of the joints of the lower extremities of newborns. Phys Occup Ther Pediatr 4:49, 1984.
12. Wanatabe, H, et al: The range of joint motions of the extremities in healthy Japanese people: The difference according to age. Cited in Walker, JM: Musculoskeletal development: A review. Phys Ther 71:878, 1991.
13. Walker, JM: Musculoskeletal development: A review. Phys Ther 71:878, 1991.
14. Phelps, E, Smith, LJ, and Hallum, A: Normal range of hip motion of infants between 9 and 24 months of age. Dev Med Child Neurol 27:785, 1985.
15. Forero, N, Okamura, LA, and Larson, MA: Normal ranges of hip motion in neonates. J Pediatr Orthop 9:391, 1989.
16. Nonaka, H, et al: Age-related changes in the interactive mobility of the hip and knee joints: A geometrical analysis. Gait Posture 15:236, 2002.
17. Kozic, S, et al: Femoral anteversion related to side differences in hip rotation. Passive rotation in 1140 children aged 8–9 years. Acta Orthop Scand 68:533, 1997.
18. Ellison, JB, Rose, SJ, and Sahrman, SA: Patterns of hip rotation: A comparison between healthy subjects and patients with low back pain. Phys Ther 70:537, 1990.
19. Bennell, K, et al: Hip and ankle range of motion and hip muscle strength in young novice female ballet dancers and controls. Br J Sports Med 33:340, 1999.
20. Boone, DC: Techniques of measurement of joint motion. (Unpublished supplement to Boone, DC, and Azen, SP: Normal range of motion in male subjects. J Bone Joint Surg Am 61:756, 1979.)
21. Allander, E, et al: Normal range of joint movements in shoulder, hip, wrist and thumb with special reference to side: A comparison between two populations. Int J Epidemiol 3:253, 1974.
22. Walker, JM, et al: Active mobility of the extremities in older subjects. Phys Ther 64:919, 1984.
23. Boone, DC, Walker, JM, and Perry, J: Age and sex differences in lower extremity joint motion. Presented at the National Conference of the American Physical Therapy Association, Washington, DC, 1981.
24. James, B, and Parker, AW: Active and passive mobility of lower limb joints in elderly men and women. Am J Phys Med Rehabil 68:162, 1989.
25. Mollinger, LA, and Steffan, TM: Knee flexion contractures in institutionalized elderly: Prevalence, severity, stability and related variables. Phys Ther 73:437, 1993.
26. Simoneau, GG, et al: Influence of hip position and gender on active hip internal and external rotation. J Orthop Sports Phys Ther 28:158, 1998.
27. Kettunen, J, et al: Factors associated with hip joint rotation in former elite athletes. Br J Sports Med 34:44, 2000.
28. Escalante, A, et al: Determinants of hip and knee flexion range: Results from the San Antonio Longitudinal Study of Aging. Arthritis Care Res 12:8, 1999.
29. Lichtenstein, MJ, et al: Modeling impairment: Using the disablement process as a framework to evaluate determinants of hip and knee flexion. Aging (Milan) 12:208, 2000.
30. Bierma-Zeinstra, SMA, et al: Comparison between two devices for measuring hip joint motions. Clin Rehabil 12:497, 1998.
31. Van Dillen, LR, et al: Effect of knee and hip position on hip extension range of motion in individuals with and without low back pain. J Orthop Sports Phys Ther 30:307, 2000.
32. Kendall, FP, McCreary, EK, and Provance, PG. Muscles Testing and Function. ed. 4. Williams & Wilkins Philadelphia, 1993.
33. Gilbert, CB, Gross, MT, and Klug, KB : Relationship between hip external rotation and turnout angle for the five classical ballet positions, J Orthop Sports Phys Ther 27:339, 1998.
34. Tyler, T, et al: A new pelvic tilt detection device: Roentgenographic validation and application to assessment of hip motion in professional hockey players. J Orthop Sports Phys Ther 24:303, 1996.
35. Van Mechelen, W, et al: Is range of motion of the hip and ankle joint related to running injuries? A case control study. Int J Sports Med 13:606, 1992.
36. Steultjens, MPM, et al: Range of motion and disability in patients with osteoarthritis of the knee or hip. Rheumatology 39:955, 2000.
37. Beissner, KL, Collins, JE, and Holmes, H: Muscle force and range of motion as predictors of function in older adults. Phys Ther 80:556, 2000
38. Magee, DJ: Orthopedic Physical Assessment, ed 4. WB Saunders, Philadelphia, 2002.
39. The Pathokinesiology Service and the Physical Therapy Department: Observational Gait Analysis Handbook. Ranchos Los Amigos Medical Center, Downey, Cal., 1989.
40. Livingston, LA, Stevenson, JM, and Olney, SJ: Stairclimbing kinematics on stairs of differing dimensions. Arch Phys Med Rehabil 72:398, 1991.
41. McFayden, BJ, and Winter, DA: An integrated biomechanical analysis of normal stair ascent and descent. J Biomech 21:733, 1988.
42. Oberg T, Krazinia, A, and Oberg, K: Joint angle parameters in gait: Reference data for normal subjects 10–79 years of age. J Rehabil Res Dev 31:199, 1994.
43. Boone, DC, et al: Reliability of goniometric measurements. Phys Ther 58:1355, 1978.
44. Clapper, MP, and Wolf, SL: Comparison of the reliability of the Orthoranger and the standard goniometer for assessing active lower extremity range of motion. Phys Ther 68:214, 1988.
45. Ekstrand, J, et al: Lower extremity goniometric measurements: A study to determine their reliability. Arch Phys Med Rehabil 63:171, 1982.
46. Pandya, S, et al: Reliability of goniometric measurements in patients with Duchenne muscular dystrophy. Phys Ther 65:1339, 1985.
47. Croft, PR, et al: Interobserver reliability in measuring flexion, internal rotation and external rotation of the hip using a pleurimeter. Ann Rheum Dis 55:320, 1996.
48. Cibulka, MT, et al: Unilateral hip rotation range of motion asymmetry in patients with sacroiliac joint regional pain. Spine 23:1009, 1998.46.
49. Cadenhead, SL, McEwen, IR, and Thompson, DM: Effect of passive range of motion exercises on lower extremity goniometric measurements of adults with cerebral palsy: A single subject study design. Phys Ther 82:658, 2002.
50. Ober, FR: The role of the iliotibial band and fascia lata as a factor in the causation of low-back disabilities and sciatica. J Bone Joint Surg 18:105, 1936.
51. Hoppenfeld, S: Physical Examination of the Spine and Extremities. Appleton-Century-Crofts, New York, 1976, p 167
52. Gose, JC, and Schweizer, P: Iliotibial band tightness. J Orthop Sports Phys Ther 10:399, 1989.
53. Cade, DL, et al: Indirectly measuring length of the iliotibial band and related hip structures: A correlational analysis of four adduction tests. Abstract Platform Presentation at APTA Mid-Winter. Tex J Orthop Sports Phys Ther 31:A22, 2001.

CHAPTER 9

The Knee

Structure and Function

Tibiofemoral and Patellofemoral Joints

Anatomy

The knee is composed of two distinct articulations enclosed within a single joint capsule: the tibiofemoral joint and the patellofemoral joint. At the tibiofemoral joint, the proximal joint surfaces are the convex medial and the lateral condyles of the distal femur (Fig. 9–1). Posteriorly and inferiorly, the longer medial condyle is separated from the lateral condyle by a deep groove called the intercondylar notch. Anteriorly, the condyles are separated by a shallow area of bone called the femoral patellar surface. The distal articulating surfaces are the two shallow concave medial and lateral condyles on the proximal end of the tibia. Two bony spines called the intercondylar tubercles separate the medial condyle from the lateral condyle. Two joint discs called menisci are attached to the articulating surfaces on the tibial condyles (Fig. 9–2). At the patellofemoral joint, the artic-

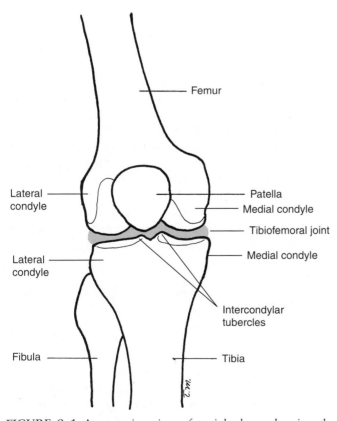

FIGURE 9–1 An anterior view of a right knee showing the tibiofemoral joint.

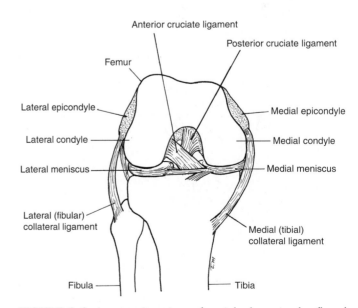

FIGURE 9–2 An anterior view of a right knee in the flexed position showing femoral and tibial condyles, medial and lateral menisci, and cruciate and collateral ligaments.

ulating surfaces are the posterior surface of the patella and the femoral patellar surface (Fig. 9–3).

The joint capsule that encloses both joints is large, loose, and reinforced by tendons and expansions from the surrounding muscles and ligaments. The quadriceps tendon, patellar ligament, and expansions from the extensor muscles provide anterior stability (see Fig. 9–3). The lateral and medial collateral ligaments, iliotibial band, and pes anserinus help to provide medial-lateral stability, and the knee flexors help to provide posterior stability. In addition, the tibiofemoral joint is reinforced by the anterior and posterior cruciate ligaments, which are located within the joint (see Fig. 9–2).

Osteokinematics

The tibiofemoral joint is a double condyloid joint with 2 degrees of freedom. Flexion-extension occurs in the sagittal plane around a medial-lateral axis; rotation occurs in the transverse plane around a vertical (longitudinal) axis.[1] The incongruence and asymmetry of the tibiofemoral joint surfaces combined with muscle activity and ligamentous restraints produce an automatic rotation. This automatic rotation is involuntary and occurs primarily at the extreme of extension when motion stops on the shorter lateral condyle but continues on the longer medial condylar surface. During the last portion of the active extension range of motion (ROM), automatic rotation produces what is referred to as either the screw-home mechanism, or "locking," of the knee. To begin flexion, the knee must be unlocked by rotation in the opposite direction. For example, during non–weight-bearing active knee extension, lateral rotation of the tibia occurs during the last 10 to 15 degrees of extension to lock the knee.[2] To unlock the knee, the tibia rotates medially. This rotation is not under voluntary control and should not be confused with the voluntary rotation movement possible at the joint.

Passive ROM in flexion is generally considered to be between 130 and 140 degrees. The range of extension beyond 0 degrees is about 5 to 10 degrees in young children, whereas 0 degrees is considered to be within normal limits for adults.[3] The greatest range of voluntary knee rotation occurs at 90 degrees of flexion; at this point, about 45 degrees of lateral rotation and 15 degrees of medial rotation are possible.

Arthokinematics

The incongruence of the tibiofemoral joint and the fact that the femoral articulating surfaces are larger than the tibial articulating surfaces, dictates that when the femoral condyles are moving on the tibial condyles (in a weight-bearing situation), the femoral condyles must roll and slide to remain on the tibia. In weight-bearing flexion, the femoral condyles roll posteriorly and slide anteriorly. The menisci follow the roll of the condyles by distorting posteriorly in flexion. In extension, the femoral condyles roll anteriorly and slide posteriorly.[1] In the last portion of extension, motion stops at the lateral femoral condyle, but sliding continues on the medial femoral condyle to produce locking of the knee.

In non–weight-bearing active motion, the concave tibial articulating surfaces slide on the convex femoral condyles in the same direction as the movement of the shaft of the tibia. The tibial condyles slide posteriorly on the femoral condyles during flexion. During extension from full flexion, the tibial condyles slide anteriorly on the femoral condyles.

The patella slides superiorly in extension and inferiorly in flexion. Some patellar rotation and tilting accompany the sliding during flexion and extension.[1]

Capsular Pattern

The capsular pattern at the knee is characterized by a smaller limitation of extension than of flexion and no restriction of rotations.[4,5] Fritz and associates[6] found that patients with a capsular pattern defined as a ratio of extension loss to flexion loss between 0.03 and 0.50, were 3.2 times more likely to have arthritis or arthroses of the knee. Hayes reported a mean ratio of extension loss to flexion loss of 0.40 in a study of 79 patients with osteoarthritis.[7,8]

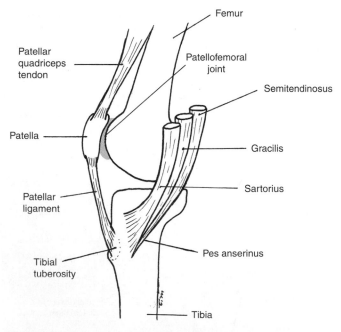

FIGURE 9–3 A view of a right knee showing the medial aspect, where the cut tendons of the three muscles that insert into the anteromedial aspect of the tibia make up the pes anserinus. Also included are the patellofemoral joint, the patellar ligament, and the patellar tendon.

TABLE 9-1	Knee Flexion Range of Motion: Values in Degrees	
AMA[9]	Boone 18 mos–54 yrs n = 109	Roach and Miles[11] 25–74 yrs n = 1683
	Mean (SD)	Mean (SD)
150	142.5 (5.4)	132.0 (10.0)

(SD) = Standard deviation.

Research Findings

Table 9–1 provides knee ROM values from selected sources. The number, age, and gender of the subjects measured to obtain the AMA[9] values are unknown. Boone and Azen[10] used a universal goniometer to measure active ROM on male subjects. Roach and Miles[11] also used a universal goniometer to measure active ROM, but their measurements were obtained from both males and females.

Effects of Age, Gender, and Other Factors

Age

Limitations of knee extension at birth are normal and similar to extension limitations found at birth at the hip joint. We have chosen to use the term "extension limitation" rather than "flexion contracture" because contracture refers to an abnormal condition caused by fixed muscle shortness, which may be permanent.[12] Knee extension limitations in the neonate gradually disappear, and extension, instead of being limited, may become excessive in the toddler. Waugh and colleagues[13] and Drews and coworkers[14] found that newborns lacked approximately 15 to 20 degrees of knee extension. Schwarze and Denton,[15] in a study of 1000 neonates (527 girls and 473 boys) in the first 3 days of life, found a mean extension limitation of 15 degrees. These findings agree with the findings of Wanatabe and associates,[16]

who found that newborns lacked 14 degrees of knee extension. The extension limitation gradually disappears as shown by comparing Tables 9–2 and 9–3. Broughton, Wright, and Menelaus[17] measured extension limitations in normal neonates at birth and again at 3 months and 6 months. At birth, 53 of the 57 (93 percent) neonates had extension limitations of 15 degrees or greater, whereas only 30 of 57 (53 percent) infants had extension limitations at 6 months of age. The mean reduction in extension limitations was 3.5 degrees per month from birth to 3 months, and 2.8 degrees between 3 and 6 months (see Table 9–3). The 2-year-olds in the study conducted by Wanatabe and associates[16] (see Table 9–3) had no evidence of a knee extension limitation.

Extension beyond 0 degrees at the knee is a normal finding in young children but is not usually observed in adults,[3] who may have slightly less than full knee extension. Wanatabe and associates[16] found that the two-year-olds had up to 5 degrees of extension. This finding is similar to the mean of 5.4 degrees of extension noted by Boone[18] for the group of children between 1 year and 5 years of age. Beighton, Solomon, and Soskolne,[19] in a study of joint laxity in 1081 males and females, found that joint laxity decreased rapidly throughout childhood in both genders and decreased at a slower rate during adulthood. The authors used a ROM of greater than 10 degrees of knee extension as one of the criteria of joint laxity. Cheng and colleagues,[20] in a study of 2360 Chinese children, found that the average of 16 degrees of knee extension ROM in children of 3 years of age

TABLE 9-2	Knee Extension Limitations in Neonates 6 Hours to 7 Days of Age: Mean Values in Degrees			
Motion	Waugh et al[13] 6–65 hrs n = 40	Drews et al[14] 12 hrs–6 days n = 54	Schwarze and Denton[10] 1–3 days n = 1000	Broughton et al[17] 1–7 days n = 57
	Mean (SD)	Mean (SD)	Mean	Mean (SD)
Extension limitation	15.3 (9.9)	20.4 (6.7)	15.0	21.4 (7.7)

(SD) = Standard deviation.
All values were obtained from passive range of motion measurements with use of a universal goniometer.

TABLE 9–3   Knee Range of Motion in Infants and Young Children 0 to 12 Years of Age: Mean Values in Degrees

| | Broughton et al[17] | | Wanatabe et al[16] | Boone[18] | |
| | 3 mos
n = 57 | 6 mos
n = 57 | 0–2 yrs
n = 109 | 1–5 yrs
n = 19 | 6–12 yrs
n = 17 |
Motion	Mean (SD)	Mean (SD)	Range of means	Mean (SD)	Mean (SD)
Flexion	145.5 (5.3)	141.7 (6.3)	148–159	141.7 (6.2)	147.1 (3.5)
Extension	10.7 (5.1)*	3.3 (4.3)*		5.4 (3.1)†	0.4 (0.9)

(SD) = Standard deviation.
* Indicates extension limitations.
† Indicates extension beyond 0 degrees.

decreased to 7 degrees by the time the children reached 9 years of age. A comparison of the knee extension mean values for the group aged 13 to 19 years in Table 9–4 with the extension values for the group aged 1 to 5 years in Table 9–3 demonstrates the decrease in extension that occurs in childhood.

In Table 9–4, the mean values obtained by Boone[18] are from male subjects, whereas the values obtained by Roach and Miles[11] are from both genders. If values presented for the oldest groups (those aged 40 to 74 years) in both studies are compared with the values for the youngest group (those aged 13 to 19 years), it can be seen that the oldest groups have smaller mean values of flexion. However, with a SD of 11 in the oldest groups, the difference between the youngest and the oldest groups is not more than 1 SD. Roach and Miles[11] concluded that, at least in individuals up to 74 years of age, any substantial loss (greater than 10 percent of the arc of motion) in joint mobility should be viewed as abnormal and not attributable to the aging process. The flexion values obtained by these authors were considerably smaller than the 150-degree average value published by the AMA[9].

Walker and colleagues[21] included the knee in a study of active ROM of the extremity joints in 30 men and 30 women ranging in age from 60 to 84 years. The men and women in the study were selected from recreational centers. No differences were found in knee ROM between the group aged 60 to 69 years and a group aged 75 to 84 years. However, average values indicated that the subjects had a limitation in extension (inability to attain a neutral 0-degree starting position). This finding was similar to the loss of extension noted at the hip, elbow, and first metatarsophalangeal (MTP) joints. The 2-degree extension limitation found at the knee was much smaller than that found at the hip joint. Using two large studies of adult males as the basis for their conclusions, the American Association of Orthopaedic Surgeons (AAOS) Handbook[3] states that extension limitations of 2 degrees (SD = 3) are considered to be normal in adults.

Extension limitations greater than 5 degrees in adults may be considered as knee flexion contractures. These contractures often occur in the elderly because of disease, sedentary lifestyles, and the effects of the aging process on connective tissues. Mollinger and Steffan[22] used a universal goniometer to assess knee ROM among 112 nursing home residents with an average age of 83 years. The authors found that only 13 percent of the subjects had full (0 degrees) passive knee extension bilaterally. Thirty-seven of the 112 subjects (33 percent) had bilateral knee extension limitations of 5 degrees or less bilaterally. Forty-seven subjects (42 percent) had greater than 10 degrees of limitations in extension (flexion contrac-

TABLE 9–4   Effects of Age on Knee Motion in Individuals 13–74 Years of Age: Mean Values in Degrees

| | Boone[18] | | | Roach and Miles[11] | |
| | 13–19 yrs
n = 17 | 20–29 yrs
n = 19 | 40–45 yrs
n = 19 | 40–59 yrs
n = 727 | 60–74 yrs
n = 523 |
Motion	Mean (SD)	Mean (SD)	Mean (SD)	Mean (SD)	Mean (SD)
Flexion	142.9 (3.7)	140.2 (5.2)	142.6 (5.6)	132.0 (11.0)	131.0 (11.0)
Extension	0.0 (0.0)	0.4 (0.9)	1.6 (2.4)		

(SD) = Standard deviation.

tures). Residents with a 30-degree loss of knee extension had an increase in resistance to passive motion and a loss of ambulation. Steultjens and coworkers[23] found knee flexion contractures in 31.5 percent of 198 patients with osteoarthritis of the knee or hip. Generally a decrease in active assistive ROM was associated with an increase in disability but was action specific. The motions that had the strongest relationship with disability were knee flexion, hip extension, and lateral rotation. A surprising finding of this study was the strong relationship between flexion ROM of the left knee with flexion ROM of the right knee.

Despite the knee flexion contractures found in the elderly by Mollinger and Steffan,[22] many elderly individuals appear to have at least a functional flexion ROM. Escalante and coworkers[24] used a universal goniometer to measure knee flexion passive ROM in 687 community-dwelling elderly subjects between the ages of 65 and 79 years. More than 90 degrees of knee flexion was found in 619 (90.1 percent) of the subjects. The authors used a cutoff value of 124 degrees of flexion as being within normal limits. Subjects who failed to reach 124 degrees of flexion were classified as having an abnormal ROM. Using this criterion, 76 (11 percent) right knees and 63 (9 percent) left knees had abnormal (limited) passive ROM in flexion.

Gender

Beighton, Solomon, and Soskolne[19] used more than 10 degrees of knee extension from 0 (hyperextension) as one of their criteria in a study of joint laxity in 1081 males and females. They determined that females had more laxity than males at any age. Loudon, Goist, and Loudon[25] operationally defined knee hyperextension (genu recurvatum) as more than 5 degrees of extension from 0. Clinically, the authors had observed that not only was hyperextension more common in females than males, but that the condition might be associated with functional deficits in muscle strength, instability, and poor proprioceptive control of terminal knee extension. The authors cautioned that the female athlete with hyperextended knees may be at risk for anterior cruciate ligament injury. Hall and colleagues[26] found that 10 female patients diagnosed with hypermobility syndrome had alterations in proprioceptive acuity at the knee compared with an age-matched and gender-matched control group.

James and Parker[27] studied knee flexion ROM in 80 men and women who were aged 70 years to older than 85 years. Women in this group had greater ROM in both active and passive knee flexion than men. Overall knee flexion values were lower than expected for both genders, possibly owing to the fact that the subjects were measured in the prone position, where the two-joint rectus femoris muscle may have limited the ROM. In contrast to the findings of James and Parker,[27] Escalante and coworkers[24] found that female subjects had reduced

passive knee flexion ROM compared with males of the same age. However, the women had on average only 2 degrees less knee flexion than the men. The women also had a higher body-mass index (BMI) than the men, which may have contributed to their reduced knee flexion. Schwarze and Denton[15] observed no differences owing to gender in a study of 527 girls and 473 boys aged 1 to 3 days.

Body-Mass Index

Lichtenstein and associates[28] found that among 647 community-dwelling elderly subjects (aged 64 to 78 years), those with high BMI had lower knee ROM than their counterparts with low BMI. Severely obese elderly subjects had an average loss of 13 degrees of knee flexion ROM compared with nonobese counterparts. The authors determined that a loss of knee ROM of at least 1 degree occurred for each unit increase in BMI. Escalante and coworkers[24] found that obesity was significantly associated with a decreased passive knee flexion ROM. Sobti and colleagues[29] found that obesity was significantly associated with the risk of pain or stiffness at the knee or hip in a survey of 5042 Post Office pensioners.

Functional Range of Motion

Table 9–5 provides knee ROM values required for various functional activities. Figures 9–4 to 9–6 show a variety of functional activities requiring different amounts of knee flexion. Among the activities measured by Jevesar and coworkers[30] (stair ascent and descent, gait, and rising from a chair), stair ascent required the greatest range of knee motion.

Livingston and associates[31] used three testing staircases with different dimensions. Shorter subjects had a greater maximum mean knee flexion range (92 to 105 degrees) for stair ascent in comparison with taller subjects (83 to 96 degrees). Laubenthal, Smidt, and Kettlekamp[33] used an electrogoniometric method to measure knee motion in three planes (sagittal, coronal, and transverse). Stair dimensions used by McFayden and Winter[34] were 22 cm for stair height and 28 cm for stair tread. The Rancho Los Amigos Medical Center's[35] values for knee motion in gait are presented in Table 9–5 because these values are used as norms by many physical therapists. However, specific information about the population from which the values were derived was not supplied by the authors.

Oberg, Karsznia, and Oberg[36] used electrogoniometers to measure knee joint motion in midstance and swing phases of gait in 233 healthy males and females aged 10 to 79 years. Only minor changes were attributable to age, and the authors determined that an increase in knee angle of about 0.5 degrees per decade occurred at midstance and a decrease of 0.5 to 0.8 degrees in knee angle in swing phase.

TABLE 9–5   Knee Flexion Range of Motion Necessary for Functional Activities: Values in Degrees

Motion	Jevsevar et al*[30] Mean	(SD)	Livingston et al†[31] Mean range	Laubenthal et al‡[33] Mean range (SD)	McFayden and Winter§[34] Mean range	Rancho Los Amigos Medical Center¶[35] Mean range
Walk on level surfaces	63.1	(7.7)				5–60.0
Ascend stairs	92.9	(9.4)	2–105.0	0–83.0 (8.4)	10–100.0	
Descend stairs	86.9	(5.7)	1–107.0	0–83.0 (8.2)	20–100.0	
Rise from chair	90.1	(9.8)				
Sit in chair				0–93.0 (10.3)		
Tie shoes				0–106.0 (9.3)		
Lift object from floor				0–117.0 (13.1)		

(SD) = Standard deviation.
* Sample consisted of a control group of 11 healthy subjects (6 males and 5 females) with a mean age of 53 years.
† Sample consisted of 15 healthy women aged 19 to 26 years.
‡ Sample consisted of 30 healthy men with a mean age of 25 years.
§ Sample consisted of 1 subject measured during eight trials.
¶ "Large Sample" data collected over a number of years.

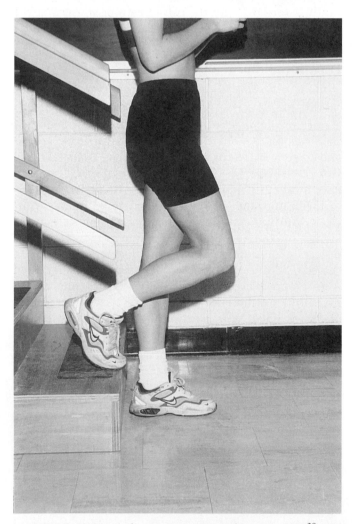

FIGURE 9–4 Descending stairs requires between 86.9[30] and 107[31] degrees of knee flexion depending on the stair dimensions.

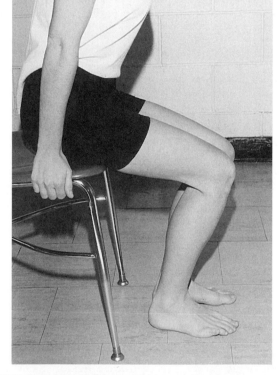

FIGURE 9–5 Rising from a chair requires a mean range of knee flexion of 90.1 degrees.[30]

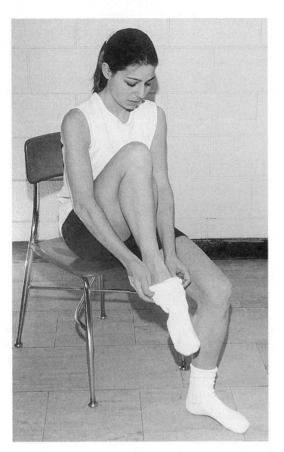

FIGURE 9–6 Putting on socks requires approximately 117 degrees of knee flexion.[32]

Reliability and Validity

Reliability studies of active and passive range of knee motion have been conducted in healthy subjects[37–41] and in patient populations.[42–45] Boone and associates,[37] in a study in which four testers using universal goniometers measured active knee flexion and extension ROM at four weekly sessions, found that intratester reliability was higher than intertester reliability. The total intratester SD for measurements at the knee was 4 degrees, whereas the intertester SD was 5.9 degrees. The authors recommended that when more than one tester measures the range of knee motion, changes in ROM should exceed 6 degrees to show that a real change has occurred.

Gogia and colleagues[38] measured knee joint angles between 0 and 120 degrees of flexion. These measurements were immediately followed by radiographs. Intertester reliability was high (Table 9–6). The intraclass correlation coefficients (ICC) for validity also was high, 0.99. The authors concluded that the knee angle measurements taken with a universal goniometer were both reliable and valid.

Rheault and coworkers[39] investigated intertester reliability and concurrent validity of a universal goniometer and a fluid-based goniometer for measurements of active knee flexion. These investigators found good intertester reliability for the universal goniometer (Table 9–6), and the fluid-based goniometer (r = 0.83). However, significant differences were found between the instruments. Therefore, the authors concluded that although the

TABLE 9–6   Intratester and Intertester Reliability: Knee Range of Motion Measured with a Universal Goniometer

Author	n	Motion	Sample	(Intra) ICC	(Inter) ICC	(Intra) r	(Inter) r
Boone et al [37]	12	AROM Flexion	Healthy adult males (25–54 yrs)	0.87	0.50		
Rheault et al [39]	20	AROM Flexion	Healthy adults (mean age (24.8 yrs)				0.87
Gogia et al [38]	30	PROM Flexion	Healthy adults (20–60 yrs)		0.99		0.98
Drews et al [14]	9	PROM	Healthy infants (12 hrs–6 days)				0.69 left 0.89 right
Rothstein et al [42]	24	PROM Flexion Extension	Patients (ages not reported)	0.97–0.99 0.91–0.97	0.91–0.99 0.64–0.71		0.88–0.91 0.63–0.70
Watkins et al [43]	43	PROM Flexion Extension	Patients (mean age 39.5 yrs)	0.99 0.98	0.90 0.86		
Pandya et al [44]	150 21	PROM Extension	Duchenne muscular dystrophy (younger than 1 yr–20 yrs)	0.93	0.73		
Mollinger and Steffan [22]	10	Extension	Nursing home residents	0.99	0.97		
Beissner et al [45]	10	PROM Flexion Extension	Nursing home and Independent living Residents (mean age 81.0 yrs)			0.70–0.93	

AROM = Active range of motion; ICC = intraclass correlation coefficient; PROM = passive range of motion; r = Pearson Product Moment Correlation Coefficient.

universal and fluid-based goniometers each appeared to have good reliability and validity, they should not be used interchangeably in the clinical setting. Bartholomy, Chandler, and Kaplan[40] had similar findings. These authors compared measurements of passive knee flexion ROM taken with a universal goniometer with measurements taken with a fluid goniometer and an Optotrak motion analysis system. Subjects for the study were 80 individuals aged 22 to 43 years. All subjects were tested in the prone position, and a hand-held dynamometer was used to apply 10 pounds of force on the distal tibia. Individually, the universal goniometer and the fluid goniometer were found to be reliable instruments for measuring knee flexion passive ROM. ICCs for the universal goniometer were 0.97 and for the fluid goniometer 0.98. However, there were significant differences among the three devices used, and the authors caution that these instruments should not be used interchangeably.

Enwemeka[41] compared the measurements of six knee joint positions (0, 15, 30, 45, 60, and 90 degrees) taken with a universal goniometer with bone angle measurements provided by radiographs. The measurements were taken on 10 healthy adult volunteers (four women and six men) between 21 and 35 years of age. The mean differences ranged from 0.52 to 3.81 degrees between goniometric and radiographic measurements taken between 30 and 90 degrees of flexion. However, mean differences were higher (4.59 degrees) between goniometric and radiographic measurements of the angles between 0 and 15 degrees.

Rothstein, Miller, and Roettger[42] investigated intratester, intertester, and interdevice reliability in a study involving 24 patients referred for physical therapy. Intratester reliability for passive ROM measurements for flexion and extension was high. Intertester reliability also was high among the 12 testers for passive ROM measurements for flexion, but was relatively poor for knee extension measurements (see Table 9–6). Intertester reliability was not improved by repeated measurements, but was improved when testers used the same patient positioning. Interdevice reliability was high for all measurements. Neither the composition of the universal goniometer (metal or plastic) nor the size (large or small) had a significant effect on the measurements.

Mollinger and Steffan[22] collected intratester reliability data on measurement of knee extension made by two testers using a universal goniometer. ICCs for knee extension repeated measurements were high (see Table 9–6), with differences between repeated measurements averaging 1 degree. Pandya and colleagues[44] studied intratester and intertester reliability of passive knee extension measurements in 150 children aged 1 to 20 years, who had a diagnosis of Duchenne muscular dystrophy. Intratester reliability with use of the universal goniometer was high, but intertester reliability was only fair (see Table 9–6).

Watkins and associates[43] compared passive ROM measurements of the knees of 43 patients made by 14 physical therapists who used a universal goniometer and visual estimates. These authors found that intratester reliability with the universal goniometer was high for both knee flexion and knee extension. Intertester reliability for goniometric measurements also was high for knee flexion but only good for knee extension (see Table 9–6). Intratester and intertester reliability were lower for visual estimation than for goniometric measurement. The authors suggested that therapists should not substitute visual estimates for goniometric measurements when assessing a patient's range of knee motion because of the additional error that is introduced with use of visual estimation. A patient's diagnosis did not appear to affect reliability, except in the case of below-knee amputees. However, the small number of amputees in the patient sample prevented the authors from making any conclusions about reliability in this type of patient.

Range of Motion Testing Procedures: Knee

Landmarks for Goniometer Alignment

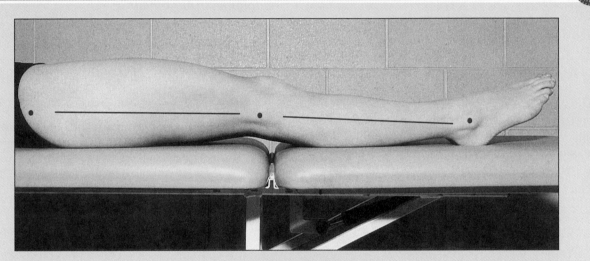

FIGURE 9–7 A lateral view of the subject's right lower extremity showing surface anatomy landmarks for goniometer alignment.

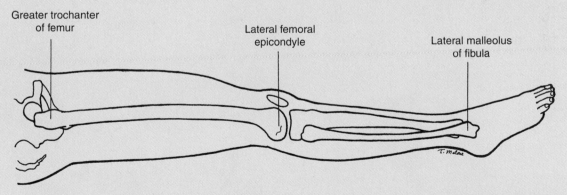

FIGURE 9–8 A lateral view of the subject's right lower extremity showing bony anatomical landmarks for goniometer alignment for measuring knee flexion ROM.

FLEXION

Motion occurs in the sagittal plane around a medial-lateral axis. The range of motion for flexion ranges from 132.0 degrees (Roach and Miles[11]) to 142.5 degrees (Boone and Azen[10]) to 150.0 degrees (AMA[9]). Please refer to Tables 9–1 through 9–4 for additional ROM information.

Testing Position

Place the subject supine, with the knee in extension. Position the hip in 0 degrees of extension, abduction, and adduction. Place a towel roll under the ankle to allow the knee to extend as much as possible.

Stabilization

Stabilize the femur to prevent rotation, abduction, and adduction of the hip.

Testing Motion

Hold the subject's ankle in one hand and move the posterior thigh with the other hand. Move the subject's thigh to approximately 90 degrees of hip flexion and move the knee into flexion (Fig. 9–9). Stabilize the thigh to prevent further motion and guide the lower leg into knee flexion. The end of the range of knee flexion occurs when resistance is felt and attempts to overcome the resistance cause additional hip flexion.

Normal End-feel

Usually, the end-feel is soft because of contact between the muscle bulk of the posterior calf and the thigh or between the heel and the buttocks. The end-feel may be firm because of tension in the vastus medialis, vastus lateralis, and vastus intermedialis muscles.

Goniometer Alignment

See Figures 9–10 and 9–11.

1. Center the fulcrum of the goniometer over the lateral epicondyle of the femur.
2. Align the proximal arm with the lateral midline of the femur, using the greater trochanter for reference.
3. Align the distal arm with the lateral midline of the fibula, using the lateral malleolus and fibular head for reference.

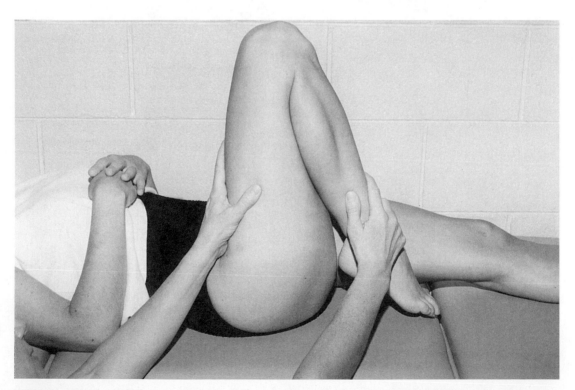

FIGURE 9–9 The right lower extremity at the end of knee flexion ROM. The examiner uses one hand to move the subject's thigh to approximately 90 degrees of hip flexion and then stabilizes the femur to prevent further flexion. The examiner's other hand guides the subject's lower leg through full knee flexion ROM.

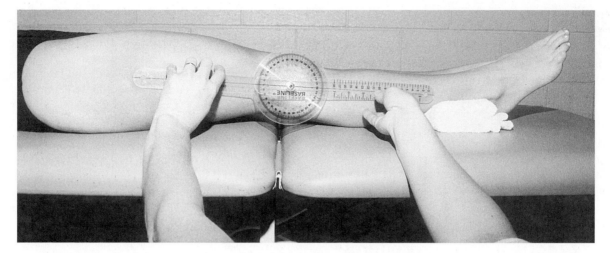

FIGURE 9–10 In the starting position for measuring knee flexion ROM, the subject is supine with the upper thigh exposed so that the greater trochanter can be visualized and palpated. The examiner either kneels or sits on a stool to align and read the goniometer at eye level.

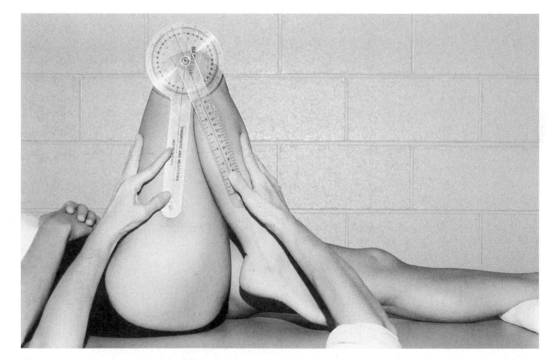

FIGURE 9–11 At the end of the knee flexion ROM, the examiner uses one hand to maintain knee flexion and also to keep the distal arm of the goniometer aligned with the lateral midline of the leg.

EXTENSION

Motion occurs in the sagittal plane around a medial-lateral axis. Extension is not usually measured and recorded because it is a return to the starting position from the end of the knee flexion ROM.

Normal End-feel

The end-feel is firm because of tension in the posterior joint capsule, the oblique and arcuate popliteal ligaments, the collateral ligaments, and the anterior and posterior cruciate ligaments.

Muscle Length Testing Procedures: Knee

RECTUS FEMORIS: ELY TEST

The rectus femoris is one of the four muscles that make up the muscle group called the quadriceps femoris. The rectus femoris is the only one of the four muscles that crosses both the hip and the knee joints. The muscle arises proximally from two tendons: an anterior tendon from the anterior inferior iliac spine, and a posterior tendon from a groove superior to the brim of the acetabulum. Distally, the muscle attaches to the base of the patella by way of the thick, flat quadriceps tendon and attaches to the tibial tuberosity by way of the patellar ligament (Fig. 9–12).

Goniometer Alignment

1. Center the fulcrum of the goniometer over the lateral epicondyle of the femur.
2. Align the proximal arm with the lateral midline of the femur, using the greater trochanter for reference.
3. Align the distal arm with the lateral midline of the fibula, using the lateral malleolus and fibular head for reference.

When the rectus femoris muscle contracts, it flexes the hip and extends the knee. If the rectus femoris is short, knee flexion is limited when the hip is maintained in a neutral position. If knee flexion is limited when the hip is in a flexed position, the limitation is not owing to a short rectus femoris muscle but to abnormalities of joint structures or short one-joint knee extensor muscles.

Starting Position

Place the subject prone, with both feet off the end of the examining table. Extend the knees and position the hips in 0 degrees of flexion, extension, abduction, adduction, and rotation (Fig. 9–13).

Stabilization

Stabilize the hip to maintain the neutral position. Do not allow the hip to flex.

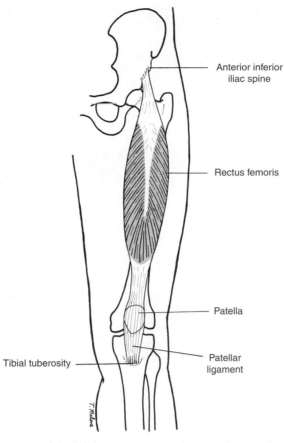

FIGURE 9–12 An anterior view of the left lower extremity showing the attachments of the rectus femoris muscle.

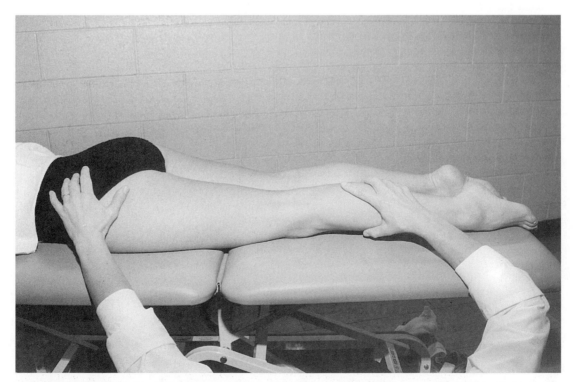

FIGURE 9–13 The subject is shown in the prone starting position for testing the length of the rectus femoris muscle. Ideally, the feet should be extended over the edge of the table.

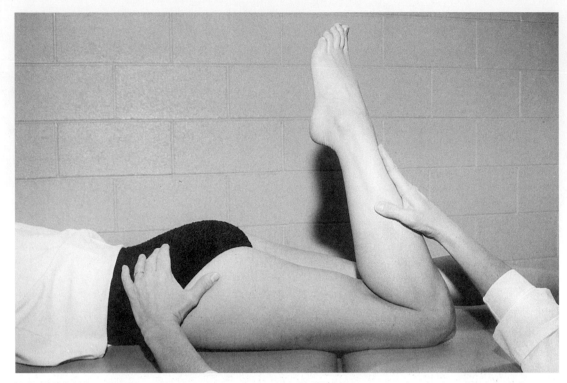

FIGURE 9–14 A lateral view of the subject at the end of the testing motion for the length of the left rectus femoris muscle.

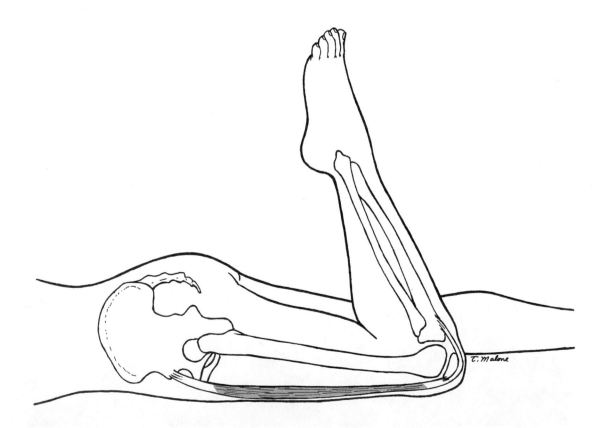

FIGURE 9–15 A lateral view of the left rectus femoris muscle being stretched over the hip and knee joints at the end of the testing motion.

Testing Motion

Flex the knee by lifting the lower leg off the table. The end of the ROM occurs when resistance is felt from tension in the anterior thigh and further knee flexion causes the hip to flex. If the knee can be flexed to at least 90 degrees with the hip in the neutral position, the length of the rectus femoris is normal (Figs. 9–14 and 9–15).

Goniometer Alignment

See Figure 9–16.

1. Center the fulcrum of the goniometer over the lateral epicondyle of the femur.
2. Align the proximal arm with the lateral midline of the femur, using the greater trochanter as a reference.
3. Align the distal arm with the lateral midline of the fibula, using the lateral malleolus and the fibular head for reference.

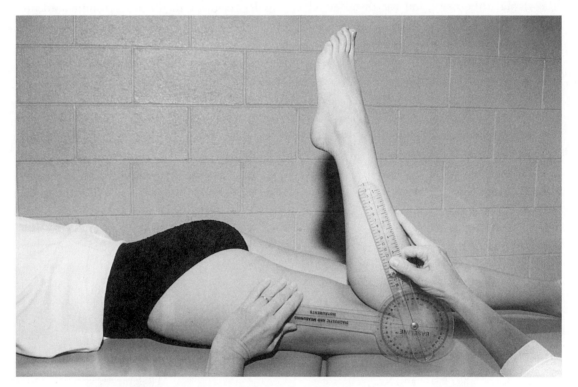

FIGURE 9–16 Goniometer alignment for measuring the position of the knee.

HAMSTRING MUSCLES: SEMITENDINOSUS, SEMIMEMBRANOSUS, AND BICEPS FEMORIS: DISTAL HAMSTRING LENGTH TEST

The hamstring muscles are composed of the semitendinosus, semimembranosus and biceps femoris. The semitendinosus and semimembranosus as well as the long head of the biceps femoris cross both the hip and the knee joints. The proximal attachment of the semitendinosus is on the ischial tuberosity and the distal attachment is on the proximal aspect of the medial surface of the tibia (Fig. 9–17A). The proximal attachment of the semimembranosus is on the ischial tuberosity and the distal attachment is on the medial aspect of the medial tibial condyle. (Fig. 9–17B) The biceps femoris muscle arises from two heads; the long head attaches to the ischial tuberosity and the sacrotuberous ligament, whereas the short head attaches along the lateral lip linear aspera, the lateral

supracondylar line, and the lateral intermuscular septum. The distal attachments of the biceps femoris are on the head of the fibula, with a small portion attaching to the lateral tibial condyle and the lateral collateral ligament (see Fig. 9–17A).

When the hamstring muscles contract, they extend the hip and flex the knee. In the following test, the hip is maintained in 90 degrees of flexion while the knee is extended to determine whether the muscles are of normal length. If the hamstrings are short, the muscles limit knee extension ROM when the hip is positioned at 90 degrees of flexion.

Gajdosik and associates,[46] in a study of 30 healthy males aged 18 to 40 years found a mean value of 31 degrees (SD = 7.5) for knee flexion during this test. Values for knee flexion ranged from 17 to 45 degrees. Examiners reported that end-feel was firm and easily identified.

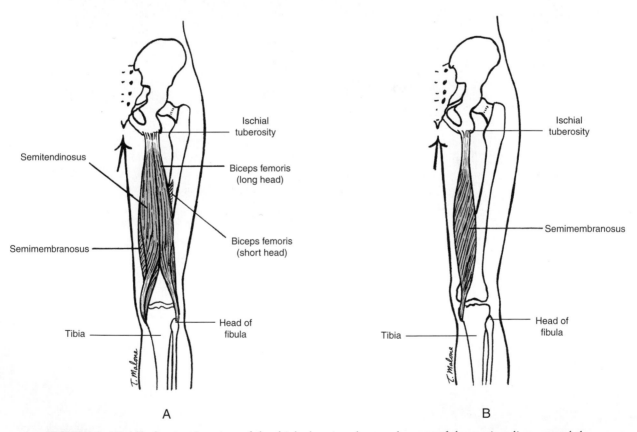

A   B

FIGURE 9–17 (*A*). A posterior view of the thigh showing the attachments of the semitendinosus and the biceps femoris muscles. (*B*). A posterior view of the thigh showing the attachments of the semimembranosus muscle which lies under the two hamstring muscles shown in Figure 9-17A.

Starting Position

Position the subject supine with the hip on the side being tested in 90 degrees of flexion and 0 degrees of abduction, adduction, and rotation (Fig. 9–18). Initially, the knee being tested is allowed to relax in flexion. The lower extremity that is not being tested rests on the examining table with the knee fully extended and the hip in 0 degrees of flexion, extension, abduction, adduction, and rotation.

Stabilization

Stabilize the femur to prevent rotation, abduction, and adduction at the hip and to maintain the hip in 90 degrees of flexion.

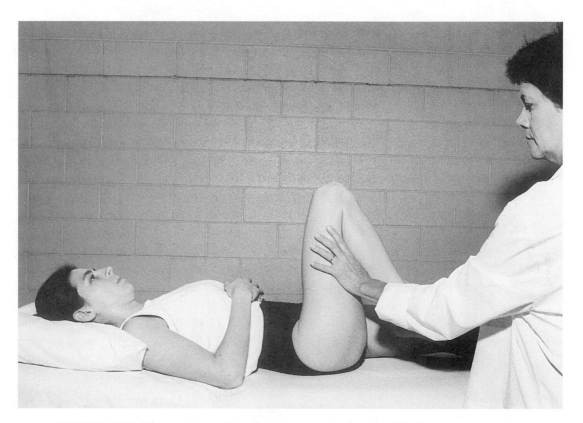

FIGURE 9–18 The starting position for measuring the length of the hamstring muscles.

Testing Motion

Extend the knee to the end of the ROM. The end of the testing motion occurs when resistance is felt from tension in the posterior thigh and further knee extension causes the hip to move toward extension (Figs. 9–19 and 9–20).

Normal End-feel

The end-feel is firm owing to tension in the semimembranosus, semitendinosus, and biceps femoris muscles.

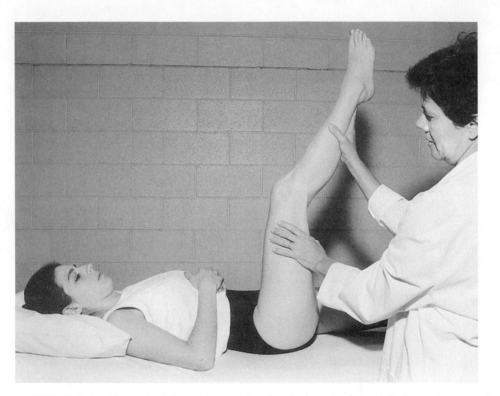

FIGURE 9–19 The end of the testing motion for the length of the right hamstring muscles.

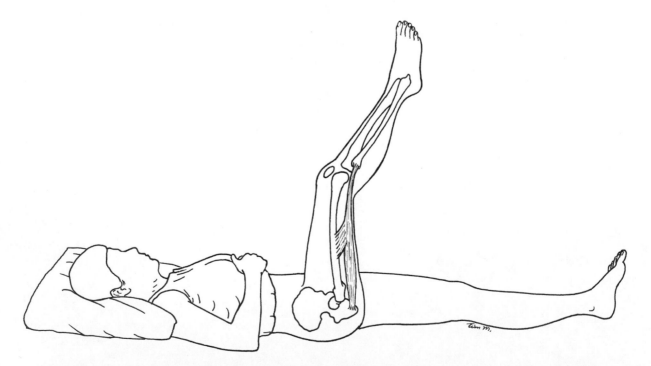

FIGURE 9–20 A lateral view of the right lower extremity shows the hamstring muscles being stretched over the hip and knee joints at the end of the testing motion.

Goniometer Alignment

See Figure 9–21.

1. Center the fulcrum of the goniometer over the lateral epicondyle of the femur.

2. Align the proximal arm with the lateral midline of the femur, using the greater trochanter for a reference.

3. Align the distal arm with the lateral midline of the fibula, using the lateral malleolus and fibular head for reference.

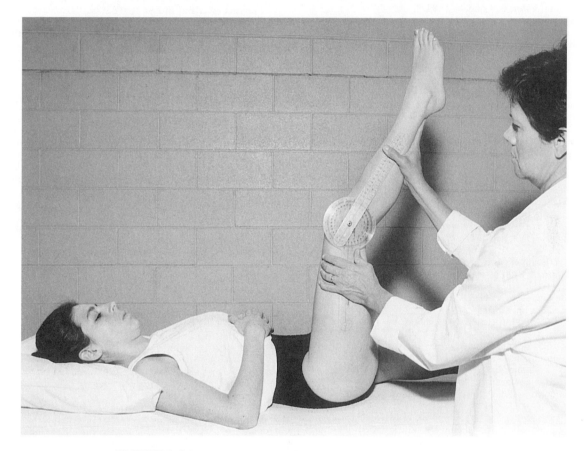

FIGURE 9–21 Goniometer alignment for measuring knee position.

REFERENCES

1. Levangie, PK, and Norkin, CC: Joint Structure and Function: A Comprehensive Analysis, ed 3. FA Davis, Philadelphia, 2001.
2. Williams, PL (ed): Gray's Anatomy, ed 38. Churchill Livingstone, New York, 1995.
3. Greene, WB, and Heckman, JD (eds): The Clinical Measurement of Joint Motion. American Academy of Orthopaedic Surgeons, Chicago, 1994.
4. Kaltenborn, FM: Mobilization of the Extremity Joints, ed 5. Olaf Norlis Bokhandel, Oslo, 1999.
5. Cyriax, JH, and Cyriax, PJ: Illustrated Manual of Orthopaedic Medicine. Butterworths, London, 1983.
6. Fritz, JM, et al: An examination of the selective tissue tension scheme, with evidence for the concept of a capsular pattern of the knee. Phys Ther 78:1046, 1998.
7. Hayes, KW: Invited commentary. Phys Ther 78:1057, 1998.
8. Hayes KW, Petersen C, and Falcone, J: An examination of Cyriax's passive motion tests with patients having osteoarthirits of the knee. Phys Ther 74:697, 1994.
9. American Medical Association: Guides to the Evaluation of Permanent Impairment, ed 3 (revised). AMA, Chicago, 1990.
10. Boone, DC, and Azen, SP: Normal range of motion of joints in male subjects. J Bone Joint Surg Am 61:756, 1979.
11. Roach, KE, and Miles, TP: Normal hip and knee active range of motion: The relationship to age. Phys Ther 71:656, 1991.
12. Rothstein, JM, Roy, SH, and Wolf, SL: The Rehabilitation Specialist's Handbook, ed 2. FA Davis, Philadelphia, 1998.
13. Waugh, KG, et al: Measurement of selected hip, knee, and ankle joint motions in newborns. Phys Ther 63:1616, 1983.
14. Drews, JE, Vraciu, JK, and Pellino, G: Range of motion of the lower extremities of newborns. Phys Occup Ther Pediatr 4:49, 1984.
15. Schwarze, DJ, and Denton, JR: Normal values of neonatal limbs: An evaluation of 1000 neonates. J Pediatr Orthop 13:758, 1993.
16. Wanatabe, H, et al: The range of joint motions of the extremities in healthy Japanese people: The difference according to age. Nippon Seikeigeka Gakkai Zasshi 53: 275, 1979 (Cited by Walker, JM: Musculoskeletal development: A review. Phys Ther 71:878, 1991.)
17. Broughton NS, Wright J, and Menelaus, MB: Range of knee motion in normal neonates. J Pediatr Orthop 13:263, 1993.
18. Boone, DC: Techniques of measurement of joint motion. (Unpublished supplement to Boone, DC, and Azen, SP: Normal range of motion in male subjects. J Bone Joint Surg Am 61:756, 1979.)
19. Beighton, P, Solomon, L, and Soskolne, CL: Articular mobility in an African population. Ann Rheum Dis 32:23, 1973.
20. Cheng, JC, Chan, PS, and Hui, PW: Joint laxity in children. J Pediatr Orthop 11: 752, 1991.
21. Walker, JM, et al: Active mobility of the extremities in older subjects. Phys Ther 64:919, 1984.
22. Mollinger, LA, and Steffan, TM: Knee flexion contractures in institutionalized elderly: Prevalence, severity, stability and related variables. Phys Ther 73:437, 1993.
23. Steultjens, MPM, et al: Range of motion and disability in patients with osteoarthritis of the knee or hip. Rheumatology 39:955, 2000.
24. Escalante, A, et al: Determinants of hip and knee flexion range: Results from the San Antonio Longitudinal Study of Aging. Arthritis Care Res 12:8, 1999.
25. Loudon, JK, Goist, HL, and Loudon, KL: Genu recurvatum syndrome. J Orthop Sports Phys Ther 27:361, 1998.
26. Hall, MG, et al: The effect of hypermobility syndrome on knee joint proprioception. Br J Rheumatol 34:121, 1995.
27. James, B, and Parker, AW: Active and passive mobility of the lower limb joints in elderly men and women. Am J Phys Med and Rehab 68:162, 1989.
28. Lichtenstein, MJ, et al: Modeling impairment: using the disablement process as a framework to evaluate determinants of hip and knee flexion. Aging (Milano) 12:208, 2000.
29. Sobti, A, et al: Occupational physical activity and long term risk of musculoskeletal symptoms: A national survey of post office pensioners. Am J Indust Med 32:76, 1997.
30. Jevsevar, DS, et al: Knee kinematics and kinetics during locomotor activities of daily living in subjects with knee arthroplasty and in healthy control subjects. Phys Ther 73:229, 1993.
31. Livingston, LA, Stevenson, JM, and Olney, SJ: Stairclimbing kinematics on stairs of differing dimensions. Arch Phys Med Rehabil 72:398, 1991.
32. Clarkson, HM: Musculoskeletal Assessment: Joint Range of Motion and Manual Muscle Strength, ed 2. Lippincott Williams & Wilkins, Philadelphia, 2000.
33. Laubenthal, KN, Smidt, GL, and Kettlekamp, DB: A quantitative analysis of knee motion during activities of daily living. Phys Ther 52:34, 1972.
34. McFayden, BJ, and Winter, DA: An integrated biomechanical analysis of normal stair ascent and descent. J Biomech 21:733, 1988.
35. The Pathokinesiology Service and Physical Therapy Department: Observational Gait Analysis, ed. 4. Los Amigos Research and Education Institute, Inc. Rancho Los Amigos National Rehabilitation Center, Downey, CA, 2001.
36. Oberg, T, Karsznia, A, and Oberg, K: Joint angle parameters in gait: Reference data for normal subjects, 10–79 years of age. J Rehabil Res Dev 31:199, 1994.
37. Boone, DC, et al: Reliability of goniometric measurements. Phys Ther 58:1355, 1978.
38. Gogia, PP, et al: Reliability and validity of goniometric measurements at the knee. Phys Ther 67:192, 1987.
39. Rheault, W, et al: Intertester reliability and concurrent validity of fluid-based and universal goniometers for active knee flexion. Phys Ther 68:1676, 1988.
40. Bartholomy, JK, Chandler, RF, and Kaplan, SE: Validity analysis of fluid goniometer measurements of knee flexion. [Abstr] Phys Ther 80:S46, 2000.
41. Enwemeka, CS: Radiographic verification of knee goniometry. Scand J Rehabil Med 18:47, 1986.
42. Rothstein, JM, Miller, PJ, and Roettger, RF: Goniometric reliability in a clinical setting. Phys Ther 63:1611, 1983.
43. Watkins, MA, et al: Reliability of goniometric measurements and visual estimates of knee range of motion obtained in a clinical setting. Phys Ther 71:90, 1991.
44. Pandya, S, et al: Reliability of goniometric measurements in patients with Duchenne muscular dystrophy. Phys Ther 65:1339, 1985.
45. Beissner K, Collins JE and Holmes H: Muscle force and range of motion as predictors of function in older adults. Phys Ther 80:556, 2000.
46. Gajdosik et al: Comparison of four clinical tests for assessing hamstring muscle length. J Orthop Sport Phys Ther 18: 614, 1993.

CHAPTER 10

The Ankle and Foot

Structure and Function

Proximal and Distal Tibiofibular Joints

Anatomy

The proximal tibiofibular joint is formed by a slightly convex tibial facet and a slightly concave fibular facet and is surrounded by a joint capsule that is reinforced by anterior and posterior ligaments. The distal tibiofibular joint is formed by a fibrous union between a concave facet on the lateral aspect of the distal tibia and a convex facet on the distal fibula. (Fig. 10–1A) Both joints are supported by the interosseous membrane, which is located between the tibia and the fibula (Fig. 10–1B) The distal joint does not have a joint capsule but is supported by anterior and posterior ligaments and the crural interosseous tibiofibular ligament. (Fig. 10–1C).

Osteokinematics

The proximal and distal tibiofibular joints are anatomically distinct from the talocrural joint but function to serve the ankle. The proximal joint is a plane synovial joint that allows a small amount of superior and inferior sliding of the fibula on the tibia and a slight amount of rotation. The distal joint is a syndesmosis, or fibrous union, but it also allows a small amount of motion.

Arthrokinematics

During dorsiflexion of the ankle, the fibula moves proximally and slightly posteriorly (lateral rotation) away from the tibia. During plantarflexion, the fibula glides distally and slightly anteriorly toward the tibia.

Capsular Pattern

The capsular pattern is not defined for the tibiofibular joints.

Talocrural Joint

Anatomy

The talocrural joint comprises the articulations between the talus and the distal tibia and fibula. Proximally, the joint is formed by the concave surfaces of the distal tibia and the tibial and fibular malleoli. Distally, the joint surface is the convex dome of the talus. The joint capsule is thin and weak anteriorly and posteriorly, and the joint is reinforced by lateral and medial ligaments. Anterior and posterior talofibular ligaments and the calcaneofibular ligament provide lateral support for the capsule and joint (Fig. 10–2A and B). The deltoid ligament provides medial support (Fig. 10–3).

Osteokinematics

The talocrural joint is a synovial hinge joint with 1 degree of freedom. The motions available are dorsiflexion and plantarflexion. These motions occur around an oblique axis and thus do not occur purely in the sagittal plane. The motions cross three planes and therefore are considered to be triplanar. Dorsiflexion of the ankle brings the foot up and slightly lateral, whereas plantarflexion brings the foot down and slightly medial. The ankle is considered to be in the 0-degree neutral position when the foot is at a right angle to the tibia.

Arthrokinematics

In dorsiflexion in the non–weight-bearing position, the talus moves posteriorly. In plantarflexion, the talus moves anteriorly. In dorsiflexion, in the weight-bearing position, the tibia moves anteriorly. In plantarflexion, the tibia moves posteriorly.

Capsular Pattern

The pattern is a greater limitation in plantarflexion than in dorsiflexion.

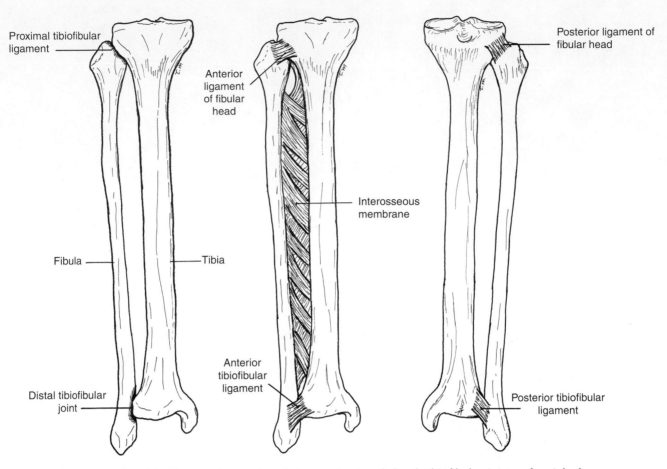

Proximal tibiofibular ligament

Anterior ligament of fibular head

Interosseous membrane

Fibula

Tibia

Anterior tibiofibular ligament

Distal tibiofibular joint

Posterior ligament of fibular head

Posterior tibiofibular ligament

FIGURE 10–1 (*A*) The anterior aspect of the proximal and distal tibiofibular joints of a right lower extremity. (*B*) The anterior tibiofibular ligaments and the interosseous membrane. (*C*) The posterior aspect of the tibiofibular joints and the posterior tibiofibular ligaments of a right lower extremity.

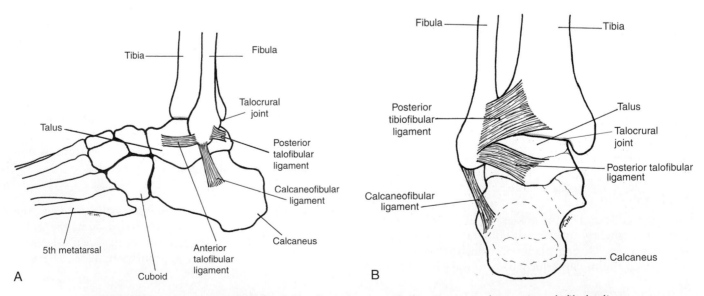

Tibia

Fibula

Talus

Talocrural joint

Posterior talofibular ligament

Calcaneofibular ligament

5th metatarsal

Anterior talofibular ligament

Cuboid

Calcaneus

A

Fibula

Tibia

Posterior tibiofibular ligament

Talus

Talocrural joint

Posterior talofibular ligament

Calcaneofibular ligament

Calcaneus

B

FIGURE 10–2 (*A*) A lateral view of a left talocrural joint with the anterior and posterior talofibular ligaments and the calcaneofibular ligament (*B*) A posterior view of a left talocrural joint shows the posterior talofibular ligament and the calcaneofibular ligament.

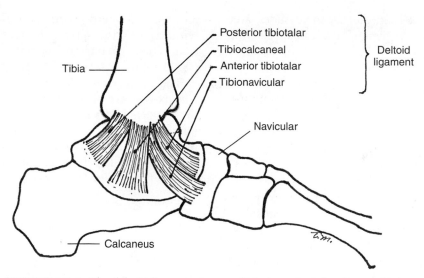

FIGURE 10-3 The deltoid ligament in a medial view of a left talocrural joint.

Subtalar Joint

Anatomy

The subtalar (talocalcaneal) joint is composed of three separate plane articulations: the posterior, anterior, and middle articulations between the talus and the calcaneus. The posterior articulation, which is the largest, includes a concave facet on the inferior surface of the talus and a convex facet on the body of the calcaneus. The anterior and middle articulations are formed by two convex facets on the talus and two concave facets on the calcaneus. The anterior and middle articulations share a joint capsule with the talonavicular joint; the posterior articulation has its own capsule. The subtalar joint is reinforced by anterior, posterior, lateral, and medial talocalcaneal ligaments and the interosseus talocalcaneal ligament. (Figs. 10-4 and 10-5).

Osteokinematics

The motions permitted at the joint are inversion and eversion, which occur around an oblique axis. These motions are composite motions consisting of abduction-adduction, flexion-extension, and supination-pronation.[1] In non--weight-bearing inversion, the calcaneus adducts around an anterior-posterior axis, supinates around a longitudinal axis, and plantar flexes around a medial-lateral axis. In eversion, the calcaneus abducts, pronates, and dorsiflexes.

Arthrokinematics

The alternating convex and concave facets limit mobility and create a twisting motion of the calcaneus on the

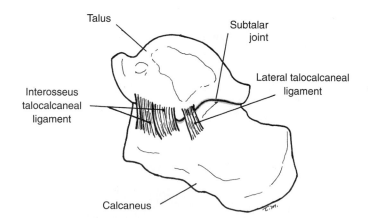
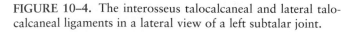

FIGURE 10-4. The interosseus talocalcaneal and lateral talocalcaneal ligaments in a lateral view of a left subtalar joint.

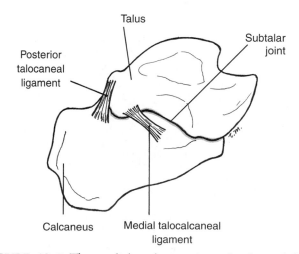

FIGURE 10-5 The medial and posterior talocalcaneal ligaments in a medial view of a left subtalar joint.

talus. In inversion of the foot, the calcaneus slides laterally on a fixed talus. In eversion, the calcaneus slides medially on the talus.

Capsular Pattern

The capsular pattern consists of a greater limitation in inversion.[3]

Transverse Tarsal (Midtarsal) Joint

Anatomy

The transverse tarsal, or midtarsal, joint is a compound joint formed by the talonavicular and calcaneocuboid joints (Fig. 10–6A). The talonavicular joint is composed of the large convex head of the talus and the concave posterior portion of the navicular bone. The concavity is enlarged by the plantar calcaneonavicular ligament (spring ligament). The joint shares a capsule with the anterior and middle portions of the subtalar joint and is reinforced by the spring, bifurcate (calcaneocuboid and calcaneonavicular), and dorsal talonavicular ligaments (Fig. 10–6B).

The calcaneocuboid joint is composed of the shallow convex-concave surfaces on the anterior calcaneus and the convex-concave surfaces on the posterior cuboid. The joint is enclosed in a capsule that is reinforced by the bifurcate (calcaneocuboid and calcaneonavicular), dorsal calcaneocuboid, plantar calcaneocuboid, and long plantar ligaments (Fig. 10–6C).

Osteokinematics

The joint is considered to have two axes, one longitudinal and one oblique. Motions around both axes are triplanar and consist of inversion and eversion. The transverse tarsal joint is the transitional link between the hindfoot and the forefoot.

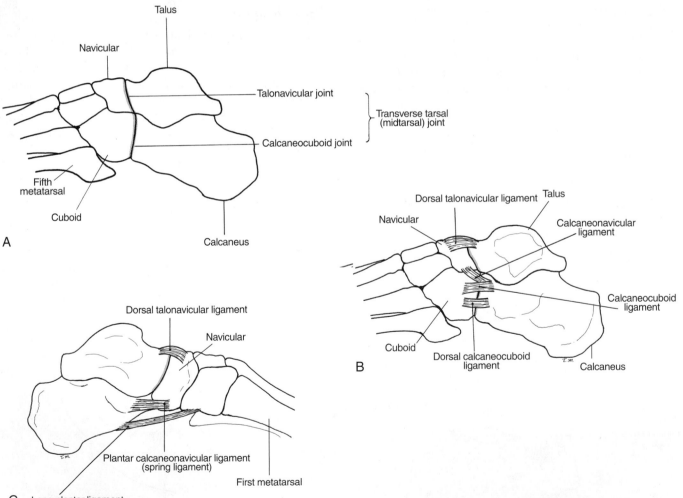

FIGURE 10–6 (A) The two joints that make up the transverse tarsal joint are shown in a lateral view of a left ankle. (B) The dorsal talonavicular ligament, the bifurcate ligament (calcaneonavicular and calcaneocuboid ligaments), and the dorsal calcaneocuboid ligament in a lateral view of a left ankle. (C) The long plantar ligament, the plantar calcaneonavicular ligament, and the dorsal talonavicular ligament in a medial view.

Arthrokinematics

In inversion, the concave navicular slides medially and dorsally on the convex talus. The calcaneus slides medially and toward the plantar surface. In eversion, the navicular slides laterally and toward the plantar surface, on the talus the calcaneus slides laterally toward the dorsal surface.

Capsular Pattern

The capsular pattern consists of a limitation in inversion (adduction and supination). Other motions are full.

Tarsometatarsal Joints

Anatomy

The five tarsometatarsal (TMT) joints link the distal tarsals with the bases of the five metatarsals (Fig. 10–7). The concave base of the first metatarsal articulates with the convex surface of the medial cuneiform. The base of the second metatarsal articulates with the mortise formed by the intermediate cuneiform and the sides of the medial and lateral cuneiforms. The base of the third metatarsal articulates with the lateral cuneiform, and the base of the fourth metatarsal articulates with the lateral cunieform

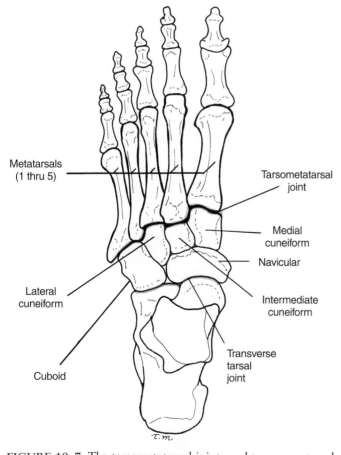

Metatarsals (1 thru 5)
Tarsometatarsal joint
Medial cuneiform
Navicular
Lateral cuneiform
Intermediate cuneiform
Transverse tarsal joint
Cuboid

FIGURE 10–7 The tarsometatarsal joints and transverse tarsal joint in a dorsal view of a left foot.

and the cuboid. The fifth metatarsal articulates with the cuboid. The first joint has its own capsule, whereas the second and third joints and the fourth and fifth joints share capsules. Each joint is reinforced by numerous dorsal, plantar, and interosseous ligaments.

Osteokinematics

The TMT joints are plane synovial joints that permit gliding motions, including flexion-extension, a minimal amount of abduction-adduction, and rotation. The type and amount of motion vary at each joint. For example, at the third TMT joint, the predominant motion is flexion-extension. The combination of motions at the various joints contributes to the hollowing and flattening of the foot, which helps the foot conform to a supporting surface.

Arthrokinematics

The distal joint surfaces glide in the same direction as the shafts of the metatarsals.

Metatarsophalangeal Joints

Anatomy

The five metatarsophalangeal (MTP) joints are formed proximally by the convex heads of the five metatarsals and distally by the concave bases of the proximal phalanges (Fig. 10–8A). The first MTP joint has two sesamoid bones that lie in two grooves on the plantar surface of the distal metatarsal. The four lesser toes are interconnected on the plantar surface by the deep transverse metatarsal ligament (Fig. 10–8B). The plantar aponeurosis helps to provide stability and limits extension.

Osteokinematics

The five MTP joints are condyloid synovial joints with 2 degrees of freedom, permitting flexion-extension and abduction-adduction. The axis for flexion-extension is oblique and is referred to as the metatarsal break. The range of motion (ROM) in extension is greater than in flexion, but the total ROM varies according to the relative lengths of the metatarsals and the weight-bearing status.

Arthrokinematics

In flexion, the bases of the phalanges slide in a plantar direction on the heads of the metatarsals. In abduction, the concave bases of the phalanges slide on the convex heads of the metatarsals in a lateral direction away from the second toe. In adduction, the bases of the phalanges slide in a medial direction toward the second toe.

Capsular Pattern

The pattern at the first MTP joint is gross limitation of extension and slight limitation of flexion. At the other

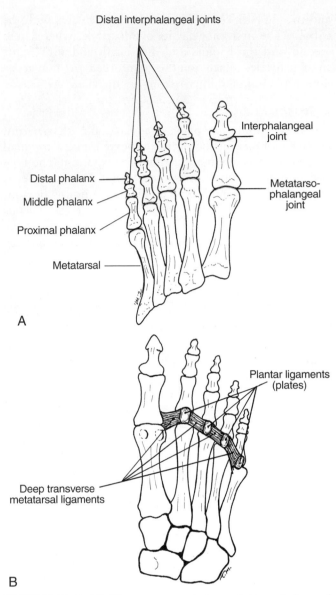

FIGURE 10–8 (A) The metatarsophalangeal, interphalangeal, and distal interphalangeal joints in a dorsal view of a left foot. (B) The deep transverse metatarsal ligaments and the plantar plates in a plantar view of a left foot.

joints (second to fifth), the limitation is more restriction of flexion than extension.[3]

Interphalangeal Joints

Anatomy

The structure of the interphalangeal (IP) joints of the feet is identical to that of the IP joints of the fingers. Each IP joint is composed of the concave base of a distal phalanx and the convex head of a proximal phalanx (see Fig. 10–8A).

Osteokinematics

The IP joints are synovial hinge joints with 1 degree of freedom. The motions permitted are flexion and extension in the sagittal plane. Each joint is enclosed in a capsule and reinforced with collateral ligaments.

Arthrokinematics

The concave base of the distal phalanx slides on the convex head of the proximal phalanx in the same direction as the shaft of the distal bone. The concave base slides toward the plantar surface of the foot during flexion and toward the dorsum of the foot during extension.

◗ Research Findings

Tables 10–1 and 10–2 provide ankle and toe ROM values from various sources. The age, gender, and number of the subjects who were measured to obtain the values reported by the American Association of Orthopaedic Surgeons (AAOS)[2] (published in 1965) and the American Medical Association (AMA)[4] are unknown. The 1994 AAOS[5] edition includes ROM values from various research studies, including the same values from Boone and Azen[6] that are included in Table 10–1 as well as a few values from the 1965 edition. Boone and Azen,[6]

TABLE 10–1   Ankle Motion: Values in Degrees from Selected Sources

	AAOS[2]	AAOS[5]	AMA[4]	Boone and Azen[†6]
Motion				Mean (SD)
Dorsiflexion	20	20	20	12.6 (4.4)
Plantarflexion	50	50	40	56.2 (6.1)
Forefoot inversion	35		30*	36.8 (4.5)
Forefoot eversion	15		20*	20.7 (5.0)
Rearfoot inversion	5			
Rearfoot eversion	5			

AMA = American Medical Association; AAOS = American Association of Orthopaedic Surgeons; (SD) = standard deviation.
* Values represent visual estimation of arc of motion.
† Subjects were 109 males 1 to 54 years of age.

TABLE 10–2   Toe Motion: Values in Degrees from Selected Sources

	Extension		Flexion	
Joint	AMA[4]	AAOS[2]	AMA[4]	AAOS[2]
MTP 1	50	70	30	45
2	40	40	30	40
3	30	40	20	40
4	20	40	10	40
5	10	40	10	40
IP 1			30	90
PIP 2–5				35
DIP 2–5				60

AMA = American Medical Association; AAOS = American Association of Orthopaedic Surgeons; DIP = distal interphalangeal; IP = interphalangeal; MTP = metatarsophalangeal; PIP = proximal interphalangeal.

TABLE 10–3   Effects of Age on Ankle Motion in Newborns and Children Aged 6 to 12 Years: Mean Values in Degrees

	Waugh et al[7]	Wanatabe et al[8]			Boone[9]	
	6–72 hrs n = 40	2–4 wks n = 57	4–8 mos n = 54	2 yrs n = 57	1–5 yrs n = 19	6–12 yrs n = 17
Motion	Mean (SD)	Mean range			Mean (SD)	Mean (SD)
Dorsiflexion	58.9 (7.9)	0–53.0	0–51.0	0–41.0	14.5 (5.0)	13.8 (4.4)
Plantarflexion	25.7 (6.3)	0–58.0	0–60.0	0–62.0	59.7 (5.4)	59.6 (4.7)

(SD) = Standard deviation.

using a universal goniometer, measured active ROM on male subjects.

Effects of Age, Gender and Other Factors

Age

A study of Table 10–3 shows that newborns, infants, and 2-year-olds have a larger dorsiflexion ROM than older children. The mean values for dorsiflexion in the youngest age groups are more than double the average adult values presented in Tables 10–1 and 10–4. However, between 1 and 5 years of age, dorsiflexion values decrease to within adult ranges (Table 10–3). Newborns also have less plantarflexion ROM than adults, but they attain adult values in the first few weeks of life. According to Walker,[10] the persistence in infants of a limited ROM in plantarflexion may indicate pathology.

Table 10–4, provides evidence that decreases in both dorsiflexion and plantarflexion ROM occur with increases in age. However, the difference between dorsiflexion values in the oldest and those in the youngest groups constitutes less than 1 standard deviation (SD). On the other hand, plantarflexion values in the oldest group are slightly more than 1 SD less than values for the youngest group.

James and Parker[12] found a consistent reduction in both active and passive ROM with increasing age in all ankle joint motions in a group of 80 active men and women ranging from 70 to 92 years of age. The most rapid reduction in ROM occurred for individuals in the ninth decade. Ankle dorsiflexion measured with the knee extended (a test of the length of the gastrocnemius muscle) showed the most marked change. The investigators suggested that shortness of the plantarflexor muscle-tendon unit was due to connective tissue changes associated with the aging process. In another study that examined the effects of aging on dorsiflexion ROM, Gajdosik, VanderLinden, and Williams[13] used an isokinetic dynamometer to passively stretch the calf muscles in 74 females (aged 20 to 84 years). The older women (aged 60 to 84 years) had a significantly smaller mean dorsiflexion angle of 15.4 degrees than the younger women (aged 20 to 39 years), who had a mean of 25.8 degrees, and the middle-aged women, who had a mean of 22.8 degrees. The decrease in dorsiflexion in the older women was associated with a decrease in plantarflexor muscle-tendon unit extensibility.

Nigg and associates[14] found that age-related changes in ankle ROM were motion specific and differed between males and females. The authors measured active ROM in 121 subjects (61 males and 60 females) between the ages of 20 and 79 years. For the whole group of subjects, decreases in active ROM with increases in age occurred in plantarflexion, inversion, abduction, and adduction but not in eversion and dorsiflexion (tested in the sitting position with the knee flexed). Plantarflexion decreased about 8 degrees from the youngest to the oldest group.

TABLE 10–4   Effects of Age on Active Ankle Motion for Individuals 13 to 69 Years of Age: Mean Values in Degrees

	Boone[9]				Boone et al[11]
	13–19 yrs n = 17	20–29 yrs n = 19	30–39 yrs n = 18	40–54 yrs n = 19	61–69 yrs n = 10
Motion	Mean (SD)	Mean (SD)	Mean (SD)	Mean (SD)	Mean (SD)
Dorsiflexion	10.6 (3.7)	12.1 (3.4)	12.2 (4.3)	12.4 (4.7)	8.2 (4.6)
Plantarflexion	55.5 (5.7)	55.4 (3.6)	54.6 (6.0)	52.9 (7.6)	46.2 (7.7)

(SD) = Standard deviation.

TABLE 10–5   Effects of Age and Gender on Dorsiflexion Range of Motion in Males and Females Aged 40 to 85 Years: Mean Values in Degrees

Nigg et al*[14]				Vandervoort et al†[15]			
Males	Females	Males	Females	Males	Females	Males	Females
40–59 yrs		70–79 yrs		55–60 yrs		81–85 yrs	
n = 15	n = 15	n = 15	n = 15	n = 20	n = 16	n = 18	n = 17
Mean (SD)	Mean (SD)	Mean (SD)	Mean (SD)	Mean (SD)	Mean (SD)	Mean (SD)	Mean (SD)
25.0 (7.0)	26.0 (6.4)	26.4 (4.7)	18.5 (4.8)	15.4 (4.3)	19.3 (3.2)	13.1 (3.5)	12.1 (5.5)

ROM = Range of motion; (SD) = standard deviation.
* A laboratory coordinate system ROM instrument was used to measure active ROM in subjects sitting with the knee flexed.
† An electric computer-controlled torque motor system was used to produce passive ROM in subjects positioned prone with the knee flexed.

Gender

Gender effects on ROM are joint specific and motion specific and are often related to age. Nigg and associates[14] found gender differences in ankle motion but determined that the differences changed with increasing age. Only in the oldest group, did women have 8 degrees more plantarflexion than men (Table 10–5). The only gender differences noted by Boone, Walker, and Perry[11] were that females in the 1-year-old to 9-year-old group and those in the 61-year-old to 69-year-old group had significantly more ROM in plantarflexion than their male counterparts. Three other studies also found that women had more plantarflexion than men. Bell and Hoshizaki[16] studied 17 joint motions in 124 females and 66 males ranging in age from 18 to 88 years. Females between 17 and 30 years of age had a greater ROM in plantarflexion as well as dorsiflexion than males in the same age groups. Walker and colleagues[17] studied active ROM in 30 men and 30 women ranging in age from 60 to 84 years. Women had 11 degrees more ankle plantarflexion than

men. James and Parker,[12] who measured both active and passive ROM, found that the only motion that showed a significant difference between the genders was ankle plantarflexion measured with the knee extended. Women and men had similar mean values in the group between 70 and 74 years of age, but the reduction in ROM over the entire age range was greater for men (25.2 percent) than for women (11.3 percent). High-heeled shoe wear has been proposed by Nigg and associates[14] as one reason why women have a greater ROM in plantarflexion than men.

In contrast to the findings that women have greater ROM than men in plantarflexion, a few investigators have found that females have less active and passive dorsiflexion ROM than males.[14,15,18] In a study by Nigg and associates,[14] males in the oldest group had a greater active range of motion in dorsiflexion (8 degrees) measured with the knee flexed than females in the same age group (Table 10–5). Females showed a significant decrease in active dorsiflexion ROM with increasing age, from 26.0 degrees in the youngest group to 18.5 degrees

TABLE 10–6   Dorsiflexion Range of Motion Measured in Non–Weight-Bearing Positions with the Knee Extended in Male and Female Subjects Aged 20 to 85 Years: Mean Values in Degrees

Gajdosik et al*[13]			Moseley et al†[19]	Jonson and Gross‡[20]	Vandervoort et al§[15]	
20–24 yrs	40–59 yrs	60–84 yrs	15–34 yrs	18–30 yrs	55–60 yrs	80–85 yrs
n = 24	n = 24	n = 33	n = 298	n = 57	n = 36	n = 35
Mean (SD)	Mean (SD)	Mean (SD)	Mean (SD)	Mean (SD)	Mean (SD)	Mean (SD)
25.83 (5.5)	22.8 (4.4)	15.4 (5.8)	18.1 (6.9)	16.2 (3.7)	20.3 (4.6)	11.8 (5.2)

ROM = Range of motion; (SD) = standard deviation.
* All measurements are of passive ROM in female subjects taken in the supine position with a universal goniometer.
† All measurements are of passive ROM in both genders taken in the prone position with use of a protractor and with the application of 12.0 Nm of torque.
‡ All measurements are of active assistive ROM in the prone position.
§ All measurements are of active ROM in the prone position with use of a footplate and a potentiometer.

TABLE 10–7   Comparison Between Dorsiflexion Range of Motion Measurements Taken with the Knee Flexed and Extended in Subjects Aged 8 to 87 Years: Mean Values in Degrees

	Bennell et al[*21]		Ekstrand et al[†22]		McPoil and Cornwall[‡23]	Mecagni et al[§24]
	8–11 yrs n = 77	8.2–11 yrs n = 49	20–25 yrs n = 10	22–30 yrs n = 12	Mean 5 26.1 yrs n = 56 feet	64–87 yrs n = 34
	Mean (SD)	Mean (SD)	Mean (SD)	Mean (SD)	Mean (SD)	Mean (SD)
Knee flexed	31.9 (6.8)	29.2 (6.4)	26.6 (2.5)	24.9 (0.8)	16.2 (3.2)	10.9 (4.2)
Knee extended	25.0 (7.6)	25.4 (8.5)	22.9 (2.5)	22.5 (0.7)	10.1 (2.2)	8.5 (3.1)

ROM = Range of motion; (SD) = standard deviation.
* All measurements were taken in weight-bearing positions with use of an inclinometer.
† All measurements were taken in weight-bearing positions with use of a Leighton Flexometer (a type of gravity inclinometer). The flexed-knee testing position was greater than 90 degrees.
‡ All measurements were taken by one tester using a masked goniometer. The testing position was not reported, but in the flexed-knee position, the knee was flexed to 90 degrees.
§ All measurements were taken in non–weight-bearing positions with use of an active assistive ROM technique

in the oldest group. Females also showed a significant decrease in eversion of 5.8 degrees with increasing age. Males, on the other hand, had little or no change in either active dorsiflexion or eversion ROM from the youngest to the oldest group. Vandervoort and coworkers[15] experienced similar findings in a study measuring passive dorsiflexion ROM with the knee flexed. The end of the ROM was defined as the maximum degree of dorsiflexion possible before muscle contraction occurred, or when the subject felt discomfort, or when the heel lifted from a floor plate. Females in the study showed a decrease in passive dorsiflexion ROM, from a high of 19.3 degrees in the youngest group (aged 55 to 60 years) to a low of 12.1 degrees in the oldest group (aged 81 to 85 years) (Table 10–5). In comparison, male subjects showed a decrease of only 2.3 degrees in dorsiflexion from the youngest group (mean = 15.4 degrees) to the oldest group (mean = 13.1 degrees). Males had greater passive elastic stiffness than females, with 10 degrees of dorsiflexion.

Grimston and associates[18] measured active ROM in 120 subjects (58 males and 62 females) ranging in age from 9 to 20 years. These authors found that females generally had a greater ROM in all ankle motions than males. Both males and females showed a consistent trend toward decreasing ROM with increasing age, but females had a larger decrease than males.

Testing Position

A variety of positions are used to measure dorsiflexion ROM, including sitting with the knee flexed, supine with the knee either flexed or extended, prone with the knee either flexed or extended, and standing with the knee either flexed or extended. Positions in which the knee is flexed are used to relax the gastrocnemius muscle so that its effect on the measurement of dorsiflexion ROM is reduced. Positions in which the knee is extended generally are used for testing the length of the gastrocnemius muscle (Table 10–6). Dorsiflexion measurements taken with the knee flexed generally are larger than measurements taken with the knee in the extended position (Table 10–7). Dorsiflexion measurements taken in the weight-bearing position are usually greater than measurements taken in the non–weight-bearing position[25] (Tables 10–6 and 10–7).

McPoil and Cornwall[23] compared dorsiflexion ROM measurements taken with the knee flexed with measurements taken with the knee extended in 27 healthy young adults. As might be expected, the mean dorsiflexion ROM (16.2 degrees) with the knee flexed was greater than the mean (10.1 degrees) with the knee extended (Table 10–7). Baggett and Young[25] compared measurements of dorsiflexion ROM taken in the non–weight-bearing supine position with those taken in the standing weight-bearing position in 10 males and 20 female patients, aged 18 to 66 years. Both supine and standing measurements were taken with the knees extended. The average dorsiflexion ROM in the supine position was 8.3 degrees, whereas the average dorsiflexion ROM in the standing position was 20.9 degrees. Little correlation was found between measurements taken in the non–weight-bearing position with those taken in the weight-bearing position. Consequently, the authors recommended that examiners not use the non–weight-bearing and weight-bearing positions interchangeably.

Lattanza, Gray, and Kanter[26] measured subtalar joint eversion in weight-bearing and non–weight-bearing postures in 15 females and 2 males . Measurements of subtalar joint eversion in a weight-bearing posture were found to be significantly greater than those in a non–weight-bearing posture. The authors advocated measurement in both positions.

Nowoczenski, Baumjauer, and Umberger[27] measured active and passive extension ROM of the MTP joint of the first toe in different positions in 14 women and 19 men between the ages of 20 and 54 years. Active and passive toe extension measurements were taken with the subject standing on a platform with toes extending over the edge. Passive measurements were taken in the non–weight-bearing seated position and during heel rise in standing. Mean values in the weight-bearing position were 37.0 degrees for passive MTP extension and 44.0 degrees for active extension compared with a mean value of 57.0 degrees obtained in the non–weight-bearing seated position and 58 degrees during heel rise in the standing position. Similar to the effects of different testing positions on ankle ROM, the results showed that the positions could not be used interchangeably, with the exception of the heel rise and seated non–weight-bearing positions.

Injury/Disease

Wilson and Gansneder[28] measured physical impairment measures (loss of passive ankle dorsiflexion, plantarflexion ROM, and swelling), functional limitations, and disability duration in 21 athletes with acute ankle sprains. Passive ROM measurements were taken with a universal goniometer, and ROM loss was obtained by subtracting the ROM total of the affected ankle from the passive ROM measurements taken on the unaffected ankle. The authors found that the combination of ROM loss and swelling predicted an acceptable estimate of disability duration, accounting for one-third of the variance. Functional limitation measures alone provided a better estimate of disability duration, accounting for 67 percent of the variance in the number of days the athletes were unable to work after the acute ankle sprain. Kaufman and associates[29] tracked 449 trainees at a Naval Special Warfare Training Center to determine whether an association existed between foot structure and the development of musculoskeletal overuse injuries of the lower extremities. Restricted dorsiflexion ROM was one of the five risk factors associated with overuse injury.

Chesworth and Vandervoort[30] measured dorsiflexion ROM after ankle fracture. They found that large differences occurred in the maximum passive dorsiflexion ROM between fractured ankles and the contralateral uninvolved ankles. Maximum passive dorsiflexion was defined as that point just prior to the initiation of muscle activity in the plantarflexor muscles. The authors hypothesized that the reflex length-tension relationship was altered in the fractured ankles and that this reflex activity acted as a protective mechanism to prevent overstretching of the plantarflexors after a period of immobilization. Reynolds and colleagues[31] found that in rats, 6 weeks of immobilization of a healthy hind limb resulted in a significant (70 percent) loss of dorsiflexion ROM when a fixed torque was applied. The authors suggested that loss of extensibility of the musculotendinous unit was probably caused by tissue remodeling that occurred during extended immobilization.

Hastings and coworkers[32] studied a single patient with diabetes mellitus who had received a tendo-achilles lengthening procedure. The operation resulted in an increase in dorsiflexion ROM with the knee extended from a preoperative level of 0 degrees to a 7 month post operative level of 18 degrees. Plantar pressure during gait was considerably reduced by 55 percent when the patient was wearing shoes and the patient's scores on the performance of a number of functional tasks was improved by 24 percent.

Salich, Mueller, and Sahrmann[33] found that patients with diabetes mellitus and peripheral neuropathy demonstrated less dorsiflexion ROM (extensibility of the musculotendinous unit) than a group of age matched control subjects. Salich, Brown, and Mueller[34] found that there was a positive relationship between body size and passive plantar flexor muscle stiffness. The lack of a correlation between stiffness (change in torque per unit change in joint angle) and a decrease in ROM led the authors to caution examiners about using the term "stiffness" to describe limited joint motion. Limitations in joint ROM may be caused by tension exerted by a fully lengthened muscle at the end of its end-range which is different than muscle stiffness. The authors suggested that older patients who complain of stiffness may actually be experiencing stretch intolerance which may halt motion early in the ROM measurement.

Functional Range of Motion

An adequate ROM at the ankle, foot, and toes is necessary for normal gait. At least 10 degrees of dorsiflexion is necessary in the stance phase of gait so that tibia can advance over the foot (Table 10–8) and at least 15 degrees of plantarflexion is necessary in preswing.[35] Five degrees of eversion is necessary at loading response to unlock the midtarsal joint for shock absorption.[35] When the midtarsal joint is unlocked the foot is able to accommodate to various surfaces by tilting medially and laterally. In normal walking the first toe extends at every step and it has been estimated that this MTP extension occurs about 900 times in walking a mile.[40] About 30 degrees of extension is required at the MTP joints in the terminal stance phase of gait. In pre-swing, extension at the MTP joints reaches a maximum of approximately 60

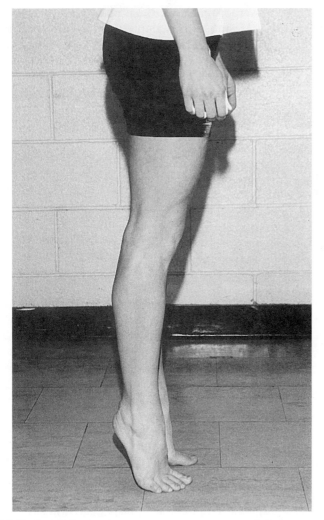

FIGURE 10–9 Standing on tiptoe requires a full range of motion in plantarflexion and 58 to 60 degrees of extension[27] at the first metatarsophalangeal joint.

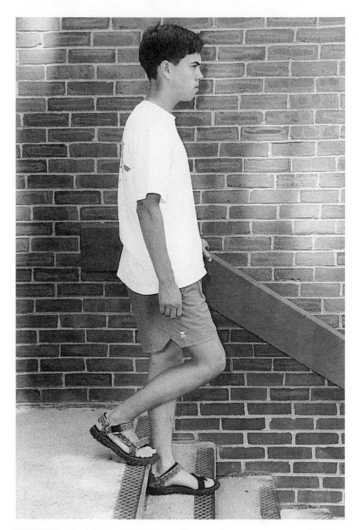

FIGURE 10–10 Descending stairs requires an average of 21 to 36 degrees of dorsiflexion.[37]

degrees when the toes maintain contact with the floor after heel rise (Fig. 10–9). If the ROM at the MTP joints is limited it will interfere with forward progression, and the step length of the contralateral leg will be decreased.[35]

Running requires 0 to 20 degrees of dorsiflexion and

0 to 30 degrees of plantarflexion,[41] these ROMs are similar to the amount of motion required for stair ascent and descent as shown in table 10–8. Descending stairs requires a maximum of between 21 and 36 degrees of dorsiflexion (Fig. 10–10). Another activity requiring maximum dorsiflexion is rising from a chair (Fig. 10–11).

TABLE 10–8   Range of Ankle Motion Necessary for Functional Locomotor Activities: Values in Degrees

	Gait Level Surfaces	Stair Ascent	Stair Descent
Dorsiflexion	0–10 (Murray) [36] 0–10 (Rancho Los Amigos) [35] 0–15 (Ostrosky et al) [39]	14–27 (Livingston et al)* [37] 15–25 (McFayden and Winter)* [38]	21–36 (Livingston et al)*
Plantarflexion	15–30 (Murray)* [36] 0–15 (Rancho Los Amigos) [35] 0–31 (Ostrosky et al) [39]	23–30 (Livingston et al)* 15–25 (McFayden and Winter)*	24–31 (Livingston et al)*

* Range of maximum mean angles observed during the activity.

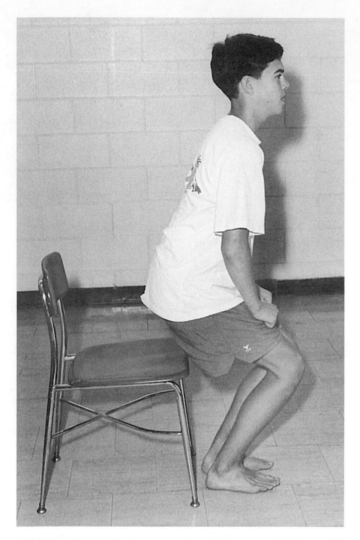

FIGURE 10–11 Getting out of a chair may require a full dorsiflexion range of motion (ROM), depending on the height of the chair seat. The lower the seat, the greater the ROM required.

Mecagni and colleagues[24] suggested that decreases in dorsiflexion ROM constituted a risk factor for decreased balance and alteration of movement patterns and Hastings and coworkers[32] identified limited dorsiflexion ROM as a risk factor for increased plantar pressures during walking and decreased functional performance.

Torburn, Perry, and Gronley[42] found that when subjects assumed a relaxed, one-legged standing position in three trials, they stood with the rearfoot in approximately the same everted position (mean of 9.8 degrees). The authors suggested that the position of the rearfoot during one-legged standing could be used as an indication of the maximum eversion ROM needed for the single support phase of gait. Garbalosa and associates[43]

measured forefoot-rearfoot frontal plane relationships in 234 feet (120 healthy males and females with a mean age of 28.1 years). Approximately 87 percent of the measured feet had forefoot varus, 8.8 percent had forefoot valgus and 4.6 percent had a neutral forefoot-rearfoot relationship.

Reliability and Validity

Reliability studies involving one or more motions at the ankle have been conducted on healthy subjects[44–49] and on patient populations.[50–51] Also, motions of the subtalar joint, the subtalar joint neutral position, and the forefoot position have been investigated. [26, 52–54]

Some joints and motions can be measured more reliably than others. Boone and associates[44] found that intratester reliability for selected motions at the ankle was better than that obtained for hip and wrist motions, but not as good as that obtained for selected motions at the shoulder, elbow, and knee.

Clapper and Wolf[45] found that both the universal goniometer and the Orthoranger (Orthotronics, Daytona Beach, FL) were reliable instruments for measuring dorsiflexion and plantarflexion but that the intraclass correlation coefficients (ICCs) were higher for the universal goniometer. The ICC for measurements of active dorsiflexion for the universal goniometer was 0.92 in comparison with 0.80 for the Orthoranger. The ICC for the goniometer for plantarflexion was 0.96, whereas the ICC for the Orthoranger was 0.93. Considering the fact that the Orthoranger, a type of pendulum goniometer, costs considerably more than the universal goniometer, the authors concluded that the additional cost involved in purchasing an Orthoranger to measure ROM could not be justified.

Bohannon, Tiberio, and Waters,[46] in a study involving 11 males and 11 females aged 21 to 43 years, investigated passive ROM for ankle dorsiflexion by means of different goniometer alignments. In one alignment, the arms of the goniometer were arranged parallel with the fibula and the heel. The second alignment used the fibula and a line parallel to the fifth metatarsal. These authors found that passive ROM measurements for dorsiflexion differed significantly according to which landmarks were used.

Bennell and colleagues[48] conducted a study to determine intertester and intratester reliability using the weight-bearing lunge method for measuring dorsiflexion. Four examiners used an inclinometer to measure the angle between the anterior border and the vertical border of the tibia and a tape measure to determine the distance of the lunging toe from the wall. Intratester and intertester reliability was extremely high (ICC = 0.97 to 0.99) for the four examiners with both methods of assessment. Refer to Tables 10–7 and 10–9.

TABLE 10–9   Intratester and Intertester Reliability: Dorsiflexion

Authors	n	Sample	Position	(Intra) ICC	(Inter) ICC	SEM
Bennell et al[48]	13	Healthy adults (mean age 18.8 yrs)	Weight bearing lunge— knee flexed	0.98	0.97	1.1° 1.4°
Clapper and Wolfe[45]	20	Healthy adults (20–36 yrs)		0.92		
McPoil and Cornwall[23]	27	Healthy adults (mean age 26.1 yrs)	Knee flexed to 90° Knee extended	0.97 0.98		
Jonson and Gross[20]	18	Healthy adults (18–30 yrs)	Knee extended—prone position	0.74	0.65	
Salsich et al[33]	34	One-half healthy/one-half with diabetes mellitus (59–63 yrs)	Knee extended—prone position	0.95		
Elveru et al[50]	43	Patients with orthopedic or neurological problems (12–81 yrs)	Passive ROM—no standard position used	0.90	0.50	
Youdas et al[51]	38	Patients with orthopedic problems (13–71 yrs)	Active ROM—no standard position used*	0.78–0.96	0.28	

ICC = Intertester or intertester correlation coefficient, as noted; ROM = range of motion; SEM = sample evaluation method.
* Knee was extended in 87.7 percent of measurement sessions.

Hopson, McPoil, and Cornwall[49] conducted four static clinical tests to measure extension of the first MTP joint in 20 healthy adult subjects between 21 and 45 years of age. All measurement techniques were found to be reliable but not interchangeable. Nowoczenski, Baumjauer, and Umberger[27] also used four clinical tests to measure the first MTP joint extension: active and passive ROM and heel rise in the weight-bearing position, and passive ROM in the non–weight-bearing position. Test values were compared with measurements of MTP extension during normal walking. Active ROM in the weight-bearing position (44 degrees) and extension measured during heel rise (58 degrees) had the strongest correlations with motion of the MTP joint (42 degrees) during normal walking (r = 0.80 and 0.87, respectively).

Elveru and associates[50] employed 12 physical therapists using universal goniometers to measure the passive ankle ROM in 43 patients with either neurological or orthopedic problems. The ICCs for intratester reliability for inversion and eversion were 0.74 and 0.75, respectively, and intertester reliability was poor (see Tables 10–9, 10–10, and 10–11). Intertester reliability also was poor for dorsiflexion, and patient diagnosis affected the reliability of dorsiflexion measurements. Sources of error were identified as variable amounts of force being exerted by the therapist, resistance to movement in neurological patients, and difficulties encountered by the

examiner in maintaining the foot and ankle in the desired position while holding the goniometer.

Youdas, Bogard, and Suman[51] used 10 examiners in a study to determine the intratester and intertester reliability for active ROM in dorsiflexion and plantarflexion. The authors compared measurements made by a universal goniometer and those obtained by visual estimation on 38 patients with orthopedic problems. A considerable measurement error was found to exist when two or more therapists made either repeated goniometric or visual estimates of the ankle ROM on the same patient (Tables 10–9 and 10–10). The authors suggested that a single therapist should use a goniometer when making repeated measurements of ankle ROM.

The subtalar joint neutral position, which has been the subject of numerous studies, is not the same as the 0 starting position for the subtalar joint as used in this book and many others, including those of the AAOS,[2] the AMA,[4] and Clarkson.[55] The subtalar joint neutral position is defined as one in which the calcaneus inverts twice as many degrees as it everts. According to Elveru and associates,[52] this position can be found when the head of the talus either cannot be palpated or is equally extended at the medial and lateral borders of the talonavicular joint. This is the position usually used in the casting of foot orthotics, but it also has been used for measurement of joint motion. However, Elveru, Rothstein, and Lamb[50]

TABLE 10–10   Intratester and Intertester Reliability: Plantarflexion

Author	n	Sample	Type of Motion	(Intra) ICC	(Inter) ICC
Clapper and Wolfe[45]	20	Healthy adults (20–36 yrs)	Active ROM	0.96	
Elveru et al[50]	43	Patients with orthopedic or neurological problems (12–81 yrs)	Passive ROM	0.86	0.72
Youdas et al[51]	38	Patients with orthopedic problems (13–71 yrs)	Active ROM	0.64–0.08	0.25

ICC = intertester or intratester coefficient; ROM = range of motion.

TABLE 10–11 Intratester and Intertester Reliability: Inversion and Eversion

Author	n	Sample	Motion	(Intra) ICC	(Inter) ICC
McPoil and Cornwall[23]	27	Healthy adults (mean age 26.1 yrs)	Inversion	0.95	
			Eversion	0.96	
Torburn et al[42]	42		Inversion		0.37
			Eversion		0.39
Elveru et al[50]	43	Patients with orthopedic and neurological problems	Inversion	0.62*	0.15*
				0.74†	0.32†
			Eversion	0.59*	0.12*
				0.75†	0.17†

ICC = Intertester and intratester correlation coefficient as noted.
* Referenced to subtalar joint neutral.
† Not referenced to subtalar joint neutral.

found that referencing passive ROM measurements for inversion and eversion to the subtalar joint neutral position consistently reduced reliability (see Table 10–11). Based on the study of Elveru, Rothstein, and Lamb[50] and information from the following studies, we have decided not to use the subtalar neutral position as defined by Elveru and associates[52] in this text.

Bailey, Perillo, and Forman[53] used tomography to study the subtalar joint neutral position in 2 female and 13 male volunteers aged 20 to 30 years. These authors found that the neutral subtalar joint position was quite variable in relation to the total ROM, and that it was not always found at one-third of the total ROM from the maximally everted position. Furthermore, the neutral position varied not only from subject to subject but also between right and left sides of each subject.

Picciano, Rowlands, and Worrell[54] conducted a study to determine the intratester and intertester reliability of measurements of open-chain and closed-chain subtalar joint neutral positions. Both ankles of 15 volunteer subjects (with a mean age of 27 years) were measured by two inexperienced physical therapy students. The students had a 2-hour training session using a universal goniometer prior to data collection. The method of taking measurements was based on the work of Elveru and associates.[52] Intratester reliability of open-chain

measurements of the subtalar joint neutral position was ICC = 0.27 for one tester and ICC = 0.06 for the other tester. Intertester reliability was 0.00. Intratester and intertester reliability also were poor for closed-kinematic-chain measurements. Picciano, Rowlands, and Worrell[54] concluded that subtalar joint neutral measurements taken by inexperienced testers were unreliable; they recommended that clinicians should practice taking measurements and performing repeated measurements to determine their own reliability for these measurements. However, Torburn, Perry, and Gronley[42] suggested that inaccuracy of measurement technique with use of a universal goniometer rather than the ability of examiners to position the subtalar joint in the neutral position might be responsible for poor reliability findings for subtalar joint neutral positioning. The ICC for intertester reliability for 3 examiners was (ICC = 0.76) for positioning the subtalar joint in the neutral position. In this study, the examiners palpated the head of the talus in 10 subjects lying in the prone position while an electrogoniometer was used to record the position.

In contrast to the low reliability found in the aforementioned studies, McPoil and Cornwall[23] found high intratester reliability for both subtalar invasion and eversion measurements taken by two testers (see Table 10–11).

Range of Motion Testing Procedures: Ankle and Foot

Landmarks for Goniometer Alignment: Talocrural Joint

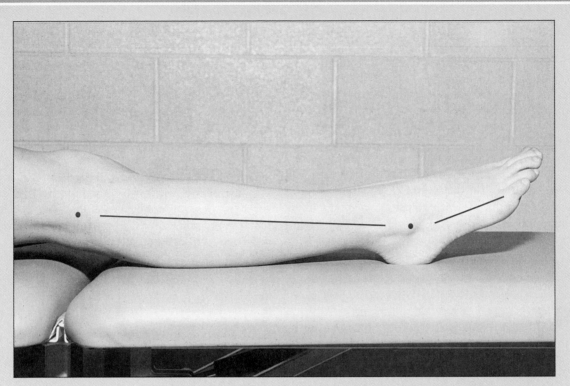

FIGURE 10–12 The subject's right lower extremity showing surface anatomy landmarks for goniometer alignment in measurement of dorsiflexion and plantarflexion range of motion.

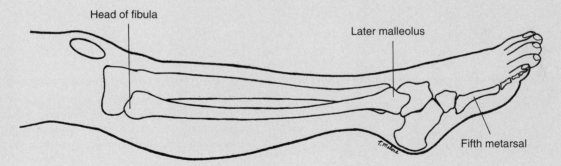

FIGURE 10–13 The subject's right lower extremity shows the bony anatomical landmarks for goniometer alignment for measurement of dorsiflexion and plantarflexion range of motion.

DORSIFLEXION: TALOCRURAL JOINT

Motion occurs in the sagittal plane around a medial-lateral axis. The mean dorsiflexion ROM according to the both the AAOS[5] and the AMA[4] is 20 degrees. The mean active dorsiflexion ROM in the non–weight-bearing position is 12.6 degrees according to Boone and Azen.[6] Refer to Tables 10–1 through 10–7 for additional information.

Dorsiflexion ROM is affected by the testing position (knee flexed or extended) and by whether the measurement is taken in the weight-bearing or non–weight-bearing position. Dorsiflexion ROM measured with the knee flexed is usually greater than that measured with the knee extended. Knee flexion slackens the gastrocnemius muscles so passive tension in the muscle does not interfere with dorsiflexion. Knee extension stretches the gastrocnemius muscle, and ROM measured in this position represents the length of the muscle. Weight-bearing dorsiflexion ROM is usually greater than non–weight-bearing measurements, and these positions should not be used interchangeably.

Testing Position

Place the subject sitting, with the knee flexed to 90 degrees position. The foot in 0 degrees of inversion and eversion.

Stabilization

Stabilize the tibia and fibula to prevent knee motion and hip rotation.

Testing Motion

Use one hand to move the foot into dorsiflexion by pushing on the bottom of the foot (Fig. 10–14). Avoid pressure on the lateral border of the foot under the fifth metatarsal and the toes. A considerable amount of force is necessary to overcome the passive tension in the soleus

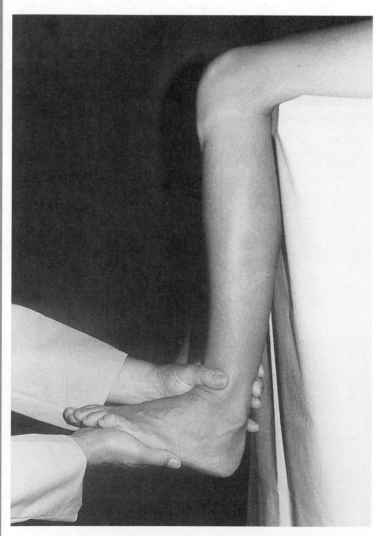

FIGURE 10–14 The subject's left ankle at the end of dorsiflexion range of motion. The examiner holds the distal portion of the lower leg with one hand to prevent knee motion and uses her other hand to push on the palmar surface of the foot to maintain dorsiflexion.

and Achilles musculotendinous unit. Often, a comparison of the active and passive ROMs for a particular individual helps to determine the amount of upward force necessary to complete the passive ROM in dorsiflexion. The end of the ROM occurs when resistance to further motion is felt and attempts to produce additional motion cause knee extension.

Normal End-feel

The end-feel is firm because of tension in the posterior joint capsule, the soleus muscle, the Achilles tendon, the posterior portion of the deltoid ligament, the posterior talofibular ligament, and the calcaneofibular ligament.

Goniometer Alignment

See Figures 10–15 and 10–16.

1. Center the fulcrum of the goniometer over the lateral aspect of the lateral malleolus.

2. Align the proximal arm with the lateral midline of the fibula, using the head of the fibula for reference.
3. Align the distal arm parallel to the lateral aspect of the fifth metatarsal. Although it is usually easier to palpate and align the distal arm parallel to the fifth metatarsal, an alternative method is to align the distal arm parallel to the inferior aspect of the calcaneus. However, if the latter landmark is used, the total ROM in the sagittal plane (dorsiflexion plus plantarflexion) may be similar to the total ROM of the preferred technique, but the separate ROM values for dorsiflexion and plantarflexion will differ considerably.

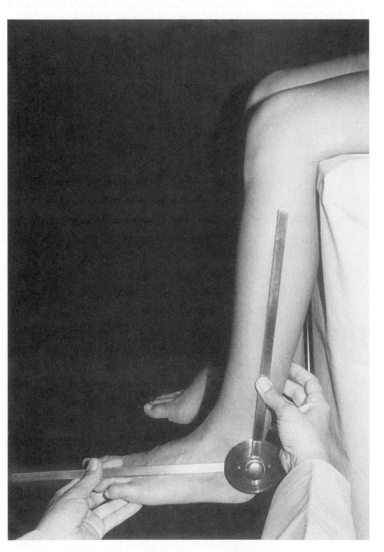

FIGURE 10–15 In the starting position for measuring dorsiflexion range of motion the ankle is positioned so that the goniometer is at 90 degrees. This goniometer reading is transposed and recorded as 0 degrees. The examiner sits on a stool or kneels in order to align the goniometer and perform the readings at eye level.

Three Alternative Positions for Measuring Dorsiflexion ROM

The supine and prone positions are two alternative non–weight-bearing positions that can be used to measure dorsiflexion ROM. Standing is an alternative weight-bearing position for this measurement. Measurements taken in different non–weight-bearing positions may not be the same; therefore, these positions should not be used interchangeably. Also, measurements taken in the weight-bearing position differ considerably from those taken in non–weight-bearing positions and therefore should not be used interchangeably. Measurements taken in the weight-bearing position compared with those taken in the non–weight-bearing position may be able to provide the examiner with information that is more relevant to the performance of functional activities such as walking. However, it may be difficult to control substitute motions of the hindfoot and forefoot in the weight-bearing position. Also, some subjects may not have the strength and balance necessary to assume the weight-bearing position.

Alternative Position for Measuring Dorsiflexion ROM: Supine

Place the subject in supine with the knee flexed to 30 degrees and supported by a pillow. Goniometer alignment is the same as that for the seated position.

Alternative Position for Measuring Dorsiflexion ROM: Prone

Position the subject prone with the knee on the side being tested flexed to 90 degrees. Position the foot in 0 degrees of inversion and eversion (Fig.10–17).

Alternative Position for Measuring Dorsiflexion ROM: Standing

Position the subject standing on the leg to be tested with the knee flexed (Fig. 10–18).

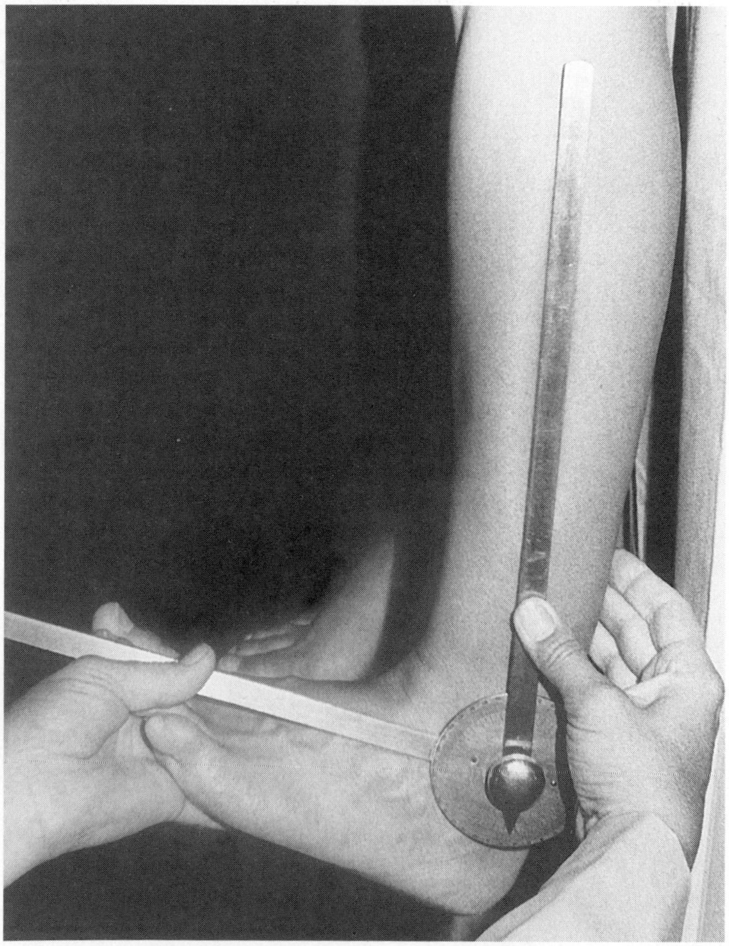

FIGURE 10–16 At the end of dorsiflexion range of motion, the examiner uses one hand to align the proximal goniometer arm while the other hand maintains dorsiflexion and alignment of the distal goniometer arm

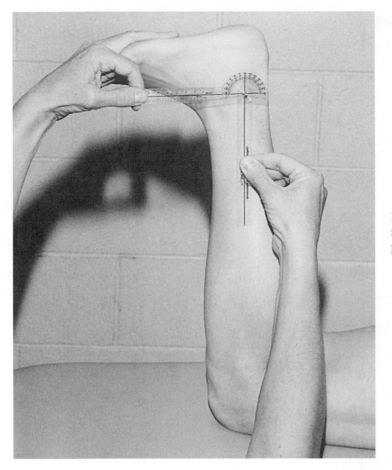

FIGURE 10–17 Goniometer alignment at the end of dorsi-flexion range of motion. The subject is in an alternative prone position with the knee flexed to 90 degrees.

FIGURE 10–18 Goniometer alignment at the end of dorsi-flexion range of motion. The subject is in an alternative weight-bearing position with the knee flexed.

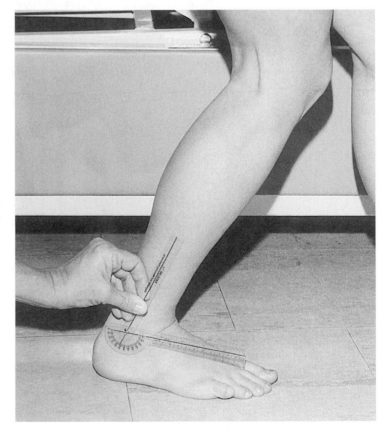

PLANTARFLEXION: TALOCRURAL JOINT

Motion occurs in the sagittal plane around a medial-lateral axis. The ROM is 50 degrees according to the AAOS,[2] 40 degrees according to the AMA,[4] and 56.1 according to Boone and Azen.[6] The ROM is affected by the testing position (knee flexed or extended) and whether or not the measurement is taken in a non–weight-bearing versus a weight-bearing position.

Please refer to Tables 10–1 through 10–4 for additional information regarding effects of age and gender.

Testing Position

Place the subject sitting with the knee flexed to 90 degrees. Position the foot in 0 degrees of inversion and eversion.

Stabilization

Stabilize the tibia and fibula to prevent knee flexion and hip rotation.

Testing Motion

Push downward with one hand on the dorsum of the subject's foot to produce plantarflexion (Fig. 10–19). Do not exert any force on the subject's toes and be careful to avoid pushing the ankle into inversion or eversion. The end of the ROM is reached when resistance is felt and attempts to produce additional plantarflexion result in knee flexion.

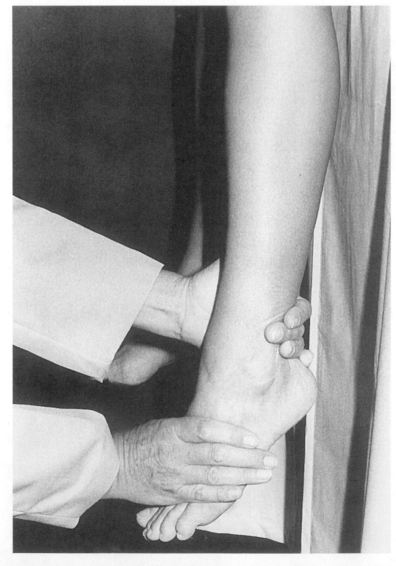

FIGURE 10–19 The subject's left ankle at the end of plantarflexion range of motion.

Normal End-feel

Usually, the end-feel is firm because of tension in the anterior joint capsule; the anterior portion of the deltoid ligament; the anterior talofibular ligament; and the tibialis anterior, extensor hallucis longus, and extensor digitorum longus muscles. The end-feel may be hard because of contact between the posterior tubercles of the talus and the posterior margin of the tibia.

Goniometer Alignment

See Figures 10–20 and 10–21.

1. Center the fulcrum of the goniometer over the lateral aspect of the lateral malleolus.
2. Align the proximal arm with the lateral midline of the fibula, using the head of the fibula for reference.

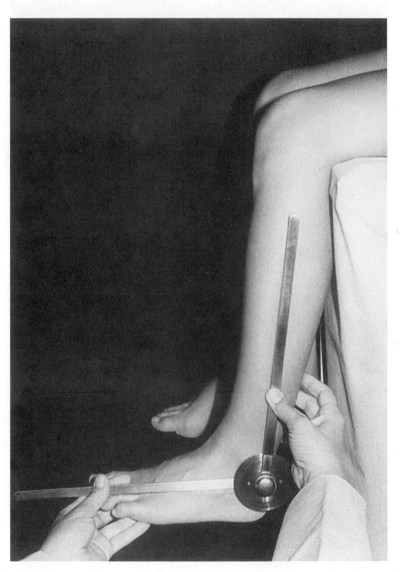

FIGURE 10–20 Goniometer alignment in the starting position for measuring plantarflexion range of motion.

3. Align the distal arm parallel to the lateral aspect of the fifth metatarsal. Although it is usually easier to palpate and align the distal arm parallel to the fifth metatarsal, as an alternative, the distal arm can be aligned parallel to the inferior aspect of the calcaneus. If the alternative landmark is used, the total ROM in the sagittal plane (dorsiflexion plus plan-

tarflexion) may be similar to the total ROM of the preferred technique, but the separate ROM values for dorsiflexion and plantarflexion will differ considerably. Measurements taken with the alternative landmark should not be used interchangeably with those taken using the fifth metatarsal landmark.

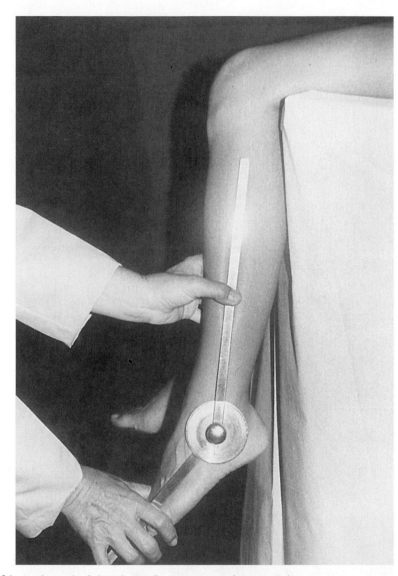

FIGURE 10–21 At the end of the plantarflexion range of motion, the examiner uses one hand to maintain plantarflexion and to align the distal goniometer arm. The examiner holds the dorsum and sides of the subject's foot to avoid exerting pressure on the toes. She uses her other hand to stabilize the tibia and align the proximal arm of the goniometer.

Landmarks for Goniometer Alignment: Tarsal Joints

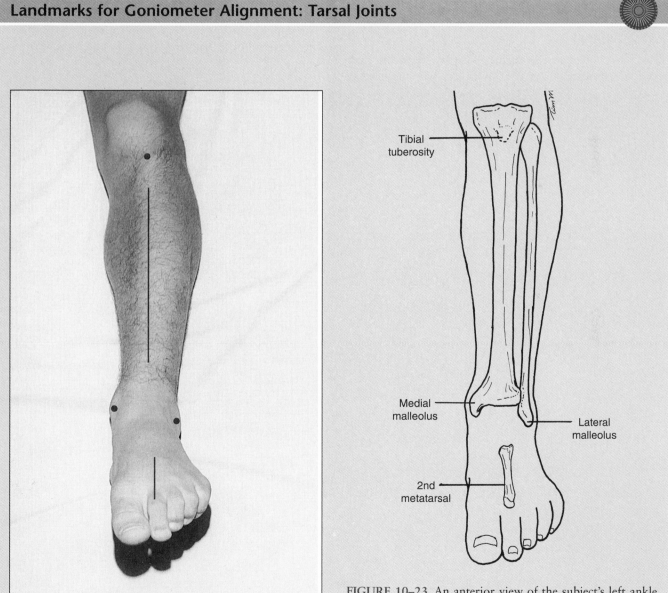

FIGURE 10–22 An anterior view of the subject's left ankle with surface anatomy landmarks to indicate goniometer alignment for measuring inversion and eversion range of motion.

FIGURE 10–23 An anterior view of the subject's left ankle with bony anatomical landmarks to indicate goniometer alignment for measuring inversion and eversion range of motion.

INVERSION: TARSAL JOINTS

This motion is a combination of supination, adduction, and plantarflexion occurring in varying degrees at the subtalar, transverse tarsal (talocalcaneonavicular and calcaneocuboid), cuboideonavicular, cuneonavicular, intercuneiform, cuneocuboid, tarsometatarsal (TMT), and intermetatarsal joints. The functional ability of the foot to adapt to the ground and to absorb contact forces depends on the combined movement of all of these joints. Because of the uniaxial limitations of the goniometer, inversion is measured in the frontal plane around an anterior-posterior axis. Methods for measuring inversion of the rearfoot and forefoot are included in the sections on the subtalar and transverse tarsal joints.

Testing Position

Place the subject in the sitting position, with the knee flexed to 90 degrees and the lower leg over the edge of the supporting surface. Position the hip in 0 degrees of rotation, adduction, and abduction. Alternatively, it is possible to place the subject in the supine position, with the foot over the edge of the supporting surface.

Stabilization

Stabilize the tibia and the fibula to prevent medial rotation and extension of the knee and lateral rotation and abduction of the hip

Testing Motion

Push the forefoot downward into plantarflexion, medially into adduction, and turn the sole of the foot medially into supination to produce inversion (Fig. 10–24). The end of the ROM occurs when resistance is felt and attempts at further motion produce medial rotation of the knee and/or lateral rotation and abduction at the hip.

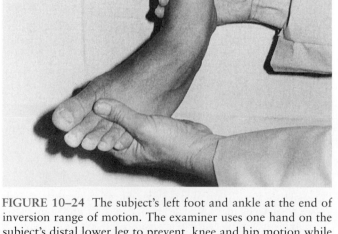

FIGURE 10–24 The subject's left foot and ankle at the end of inversion range of motion. The examiner uses one hand on the subject's distal lower leg to prevent knee and hip motion while her other hand maintains inversion.

Normal End-feel

The end-feel is firm because of tension in the joint capsules; the anterior and posterior talofibular ligament; the calcaneofibular ligament; the anterior, posterior, lateral, and interosseous talocalcaneal ligaments; the dorsal calcaneal ligaments; the dorsal calcaneocuboid ligament; the dorsal talonavicular ligament; the lateral band of the bifurcate ligament; the transverse metatarsal ligament; and various dorsal, plantar, and interosseous ligaments of the cuboideonavicular, cuneonavicular, intercuneiform, cuneocuboid, TMT, and intermetatarsal joints; and the peroneus longus and brevis muscles.

Goniometer Alignment

See Figures 10–25 and 10–26.

1. Center the fulcrum of the goniometer over the anterior aspect of the ankle midway between the malleoli. (The flexibility of a plastic goniometer makes this instrument easier to use for measuring inversion than a metal goniometer.)
2. Align the proximal arm of the goniometer with the anterior midline of the lower leg, using the tibial tuberosity for reference.
3. Align the distal arm with the anterior midline of the second metatarsal.

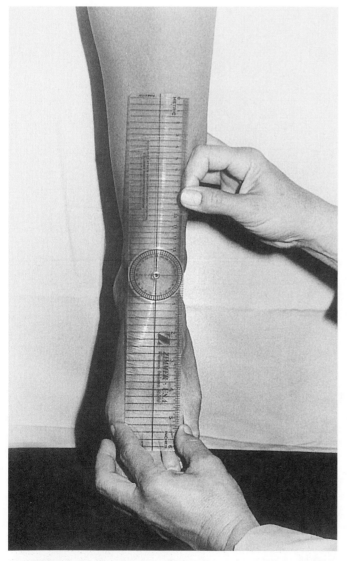

FIGURE 10–25 Goniometer alignment in the starting position for measuring inversion range of motion.

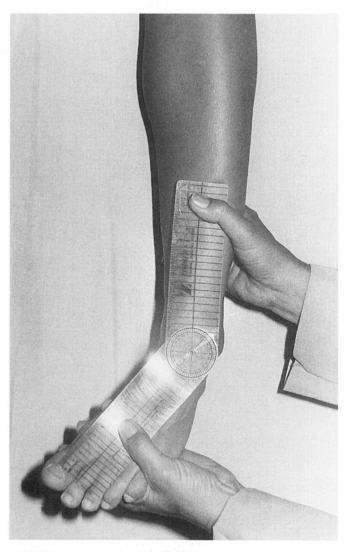

FIGURE 10–26 At the end of the range of motion, the examiner uses her one hand to maintain inversion and to align the distal goniometer arm.

EVERSION: TARSAL JOINTS

This motion is a combination of pronation, abduction, and dorsiflexion occurring in varying degrees at the subtalar, transverse tarsal (talocalcaneonavicular and calcaneocuboid), cuboideonavicular, cuneonavicular, intercuneiform, cuneocuboid, TMT, and intermetatarsal joints. The functional ability of the foot to adapt to the ground and to absorb contact forces depends on the combined movement of all of these joints. Because of the uniaxial limitations of the goniometer, this motion is measured in the frontal plane around an anterior-posterior axis. Methods for measuring eversion isolated to the rearfoot and the forefoot are included in the sections on the subtalar and transverse tarsal joints.

Testing Position

Place the subject in the sitting position, with the knee flexed to 90 degrees and the lower leg over the edge of the supporting surface. Position the hip in 0 degrees of rotation, adduction, and abduction. Alternatively, it is possible to place the subject in the supine position, with the foot over the edge of the supporting surface.

Stabilization

Stabilize the tibia and fibula to prevent lateral rotation and flexion of the knee and medial rotation and adduction of the hip.

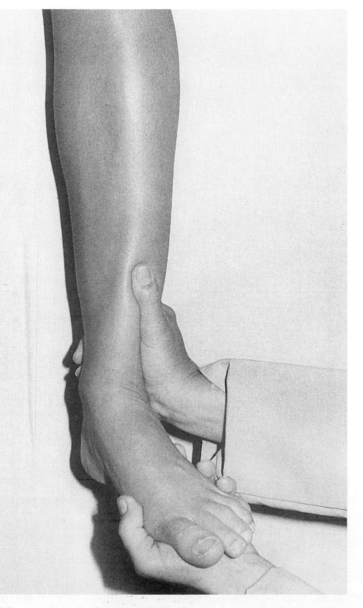

FIGURE 10–27 The left ankle and foot at the end of the range of motion in eversion. The examiner uses one hand on the subject's distal lower leg to prevent knee flexion and lateral rotation. The examiner's other hand maintains eversion.

Testing Motion

Pull the forefoot laterally into abduction and upward into dorsiflexion, turning the forefoot into pronation so that the lateral side of the foot is higher than the medial side to produce eversion (Fig. 10–27). The end of the ROM occurs when resistance is felt and attempts at further motion cause lateral rotation at the knee and/or medial rotation and adduction at the hip.

Normal End-feel

The end-feel may be hard because of contact between the calcaneus and the floor of the sinus tarsi. In some cases, the end-feel may be firm because of tension in the joint capsules; the deltoid ligament; the medial talocalcaneal ligament; the plantar calcaneonavicular and calcaneocuboid ligaments; the dorsal talonavicular ligament; the medial band of the bifurcated ligament; the transverse metatarsal ligament; various dorsal, plantar, and interosseous ligaments of the cuboideonavicular, cuneonavicular, intercuneiform, cuneocuboid, TMT, and intermetatarsal joints; and the tibialis posterior muscle.

Goniometer Alignment

See Figures 10–28 and 10–29.

1. Center the fulcrum of the goniometer over the anterior aspect of the ankle midway between the malleoli. (The flexibility of a plastic goniometer makes this instrument easier to use than a metal goniometer for measuring inversion.)
2. Align the proximal arm of the goniometer with the anterior midline of the lower leg, using the tibial tuberosity for reference.
3. Align the distal arm with the anterior midline of the second metatarsal.

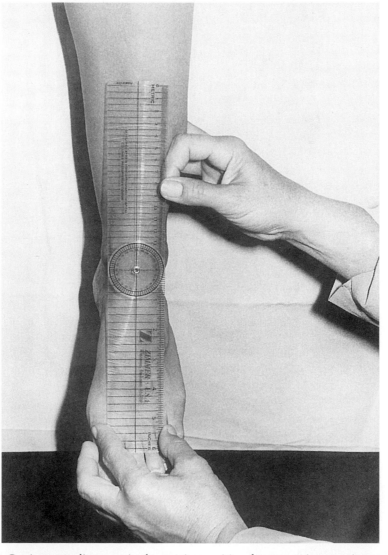

FIGURE 10–28 Goniometer alignment in the starting position for measuring eversion range of motion.

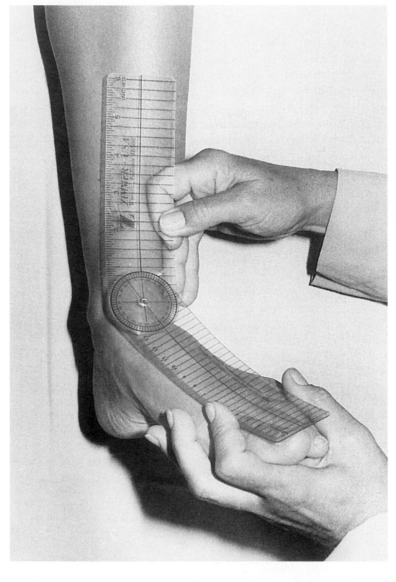

FIGURE 10–29 At the end of the eversion range of motion, the examiner's left hand maintains eversion and keeps the distal goniometer arm aligned with the subject's second metatarsal.

Landmarks for Goniometer Alignment: Subtalar Joint (Rearfoot)

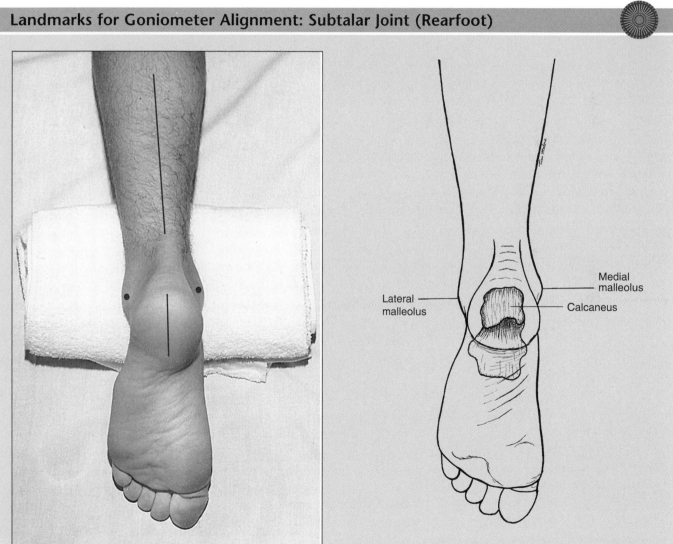

FIGURE 10–30 Surface anatomy landmarks indicate goniometer alignment for measuring rearfoot inversion and eversion range of motion in a posterior view of a subject's left lower leg and foot.

FIGURE 10–31 Bony anatomical landmarks for measuring subtalar (rearfoot) inversion and eversion range of motion in a posterior view of the subject's left lower leg and foot.

Lateral malleolus

Medial malleolus

Calcaneus

INVERSION: SUBTALAR JOINT (REARFOOT)

Motion is a combination of supination, adduction, and plantarflexion. Because of the uniaxial limitations of the goniometer, this motion is measured in the frontal plane around an anterior-posterior axis. The ROM is about 5 degrees.[2]

Testing Position

Place the subject in the prone position, with the hip in 0 degrees of flexion, extension, abduction, adduction, and rotation. Position the knee in 0 degrees of flexion and extension. Position the foot over the edge of the supporting surface.

Stablization

Stabilize the tibia and fibula to prevent lateral hip and knee rotation and hip adduction.

Testing Motion

Hold the subject's lower leg with one hand and use the other hand to pull the subject's calcaneus medially into adduction and to rotate it into supination, thereby producing rearfoot subtalar inversion (Fig. 10–32). Avoid pushing on the forefoot. The end of the ROM is reached when resistance to further motion is felt and attempts at overcoming the resistance produce lateral rotation at the hip or knee.

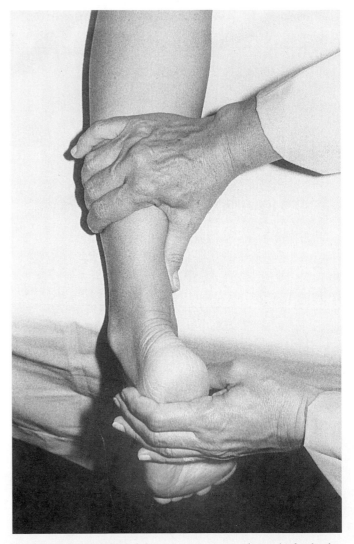

FIGURE 10–32   The left lower extremity at the end of subtalar rearfoot inversion range of motion.

Normal End-feel

The end-feel is firm because of tension in the lateral joint capsule; the anterior and posterior talofibular ligaments; the calcaneofibular ligament; and the lateral, posterior, anterior, and interosseous talocalcaneal ligaments.

Goniometer Alignment

See Figures 10–33 and 10–34.

1. Center the fulcrum of the goniometer over the posterior aspect of the ankle midway between the malleoli.
2. Align the proximal arm with the posterior midline of the lower leg.
3. Align the distal arm with the posterior midline of the calcaneus.

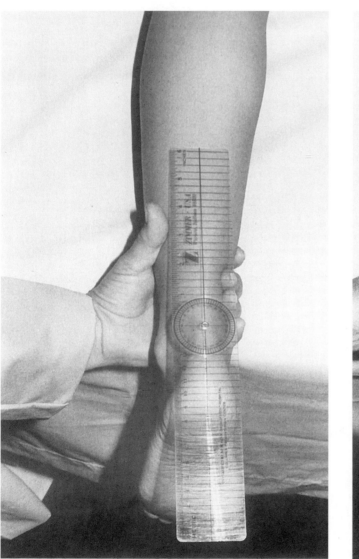

FIGURE 10–33 Goniometer alignment in the starting position for measuring subtalar rearfoot inversion range of motion. Normally, the examiner's hand would be holding the distal goniometer arm, but for the purpose of this photograph, she has removed her hand.

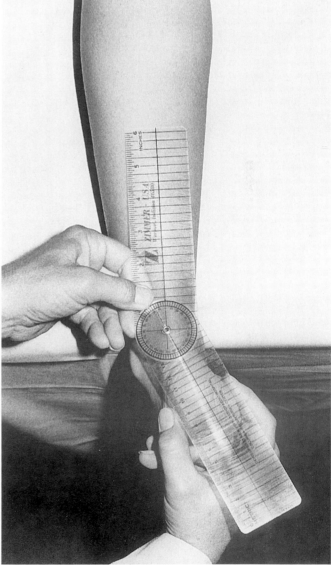

FIGURE 10–34 At the end of subtalar (rearfoot) inversion, the examiner's hand maintains inversion and keeps the distal goniometer arm in alignment.

EVERSION: SUBTALAR JOINT (REARFOOT)

Motion is a combination of pronation, abduction, and dorsiflexion. Because of the uniaxial limitations of the goniometer, this motion is measured in the frontal plane around an anterior-posterior axis. The ROM is about 5 degrees.[2]

Testing Position

Place the subject prone, with the hip in 0 degrees of flexion, extension, abduction, adduction, and rotation. Position the knee in 0 degrees of flexion and extension. Place the foot over the edge of the supporting surface.

Stabilization

Stabilize the tibia and fibula to prevent medial hip and knee rotation and hip abduction.

Testing Motion

Pull the calcaneus laterally into abduction and rotate it into pronation to produce subtalar eversion (Fig. 10–35). The end of the ROM occurs when resistance to further

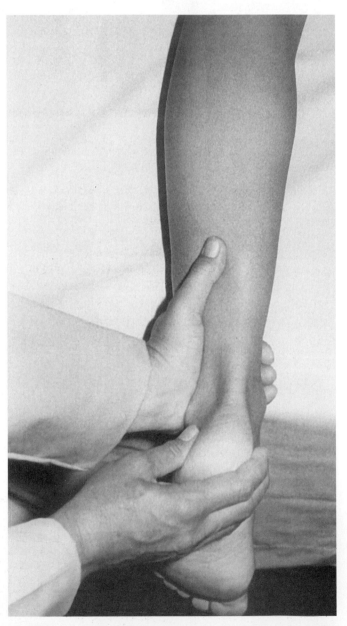

FIGURE 10–35 The left lower extremity at the end of subtalar (rearfoot) eversion range of motion. One can observe that this subject's eversion is quite limited. The examiner's hand maintains subtalar eversion by pulling the calcaneus laterally.

movement is felt and additional attempts to move the calcaneus result in medial hip or knee rotation.

Normal End-feel

The end-feel may be hard because of contact between the calcaneus and the floor of the sinus tarsi, or it may be firm because of tension in the deltoid ligament, the medial talocalcaneal ligament, and the tibialis posterior muscle.

Goniometer Alignment

See Figures 10–36 and 10–37.

1. Center the fulcrum of the goniometer over the posterior aspect of the ankle midway between the malleoli.
2. Align the proximal arm with the posterior midline of the lower leg.
3. Align the distal arm with the posterior midline of the calcaneus.

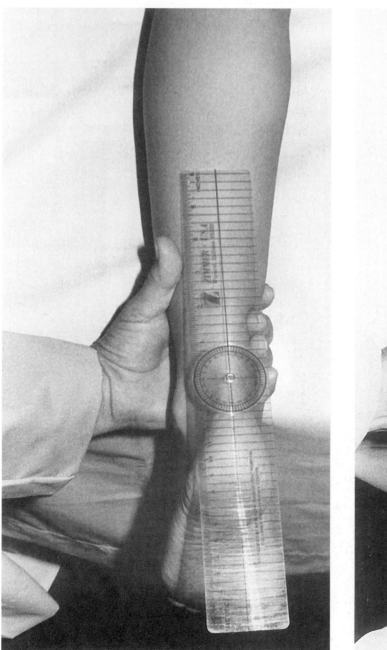

FIGURE 10–36 Goniometer alignment in the starting position for measuring subtalar (rearfoot) eversion.

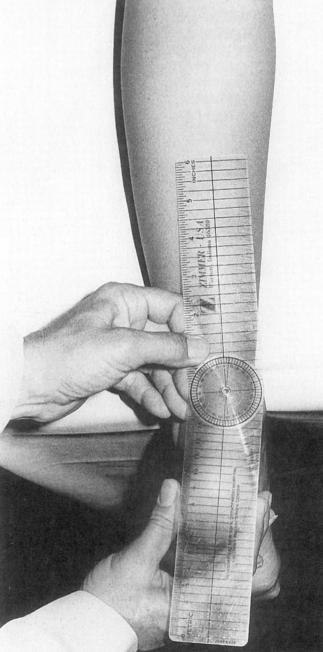

FIGURE 10–37 At the end of subtalar eversion, the examiner's hand maintains eversion and keeps the distal goniometer arm aligned.

INVERSION: TRANSVERSE TARSAL JOINT

Most of the motion in the midfoot and forefoot occurs at the talonavicular and calcaneocuboid joints. Some additional motion occurs at the cuboideonavicular, cuneonavicular, intercuneiform, cuneocuboid, and TMT joints.

Motion is a combination of supination, adduction, and plantarflexion. Because of the uniaxial limitation of the goniometer, this motion is measured in the frontal plane around an anterior-posterior axis. The normal ROM ranges from 30 to 37 degrees for the forefoot.[4,6]

Testing Position

Place the subject sitting, with the knee flexed to 90 degrees and the lower leg over the edge of the supporting surface. The hip is in 0 degrees of rotation, adduction, and abduction, and the subtalar joint is placed in the 0 starting position. Alternatively, it is possible to place the subject in the supine position, with the foot over the edge of the supporting surface.

Stabilization

Stabilize the calcaneus to prevent dorsiflexion of the ankle and inversion of the subtalar joint.

Testing Motion

Grasp the metatarsals rather than the toes and push the forefoot slightly into plantarflexion and medially into adduction. Turn the sole of foot medially into supination, being careful not to dorsiflex the ankle (Fig. 10–38). The end of the ROM occurs when resistance is felt and attempts at further motion cause dorsiflexion and/or subtalar enversion.

Normal End-feel

The end-feel is firm because of tension in the joint capsules; the dorsal calcaneocuboid ligament; the dorsal talonavicular ligament; the lateral band of the bifurcated ligament; the transverse metatarsal ligament; various dorsal, plantar, and interosseous ligaments of the cuboideonavicular, cuneonavicular, intercuneiform, cuneocuboid, TMT, and intermetatarsal joints; and the peroneus longus and brevis muscles.

Goniometer Alignment

See Figures 10–39 and 10–40.

1. Center the fulcrum of the goniometer over the anterior aspect of the ankle slightly distal to a point midway between the malleoli.
2. Align the proximal arm with the anterior midline of the lower leg, using the tibial tuberosity for reference.
3. Align the distal arm with the anterior midline of the second metatarsal.

Alternative Goniometer Alignment

See Figures 10–41 and 10–42.

1. Place the fulcrum of the goniometer at the lateral aspect of the fifth metatarsal head.
2. Align the proximal arm parallel to the anterior midline of the lower leg.
3. Align the distal arm with the plantar aspect of the first through the fifth metatarsal heads.

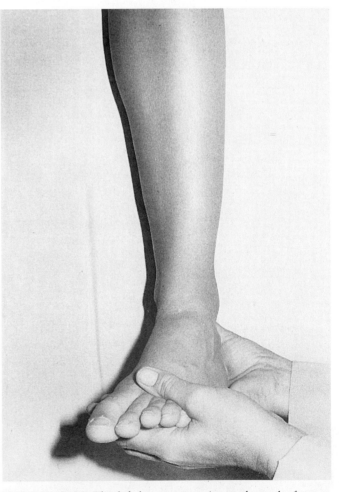

FIGURE 10–38 The left lower extremity at the end of transverse tarsal inversion range of motion (ROM). The examiner's hand stabilizes the calcaneus to prevent subtalar inversion. Notice that the ROM for the transverse tarsal joint is less than that of all of the tarsal joints combined.

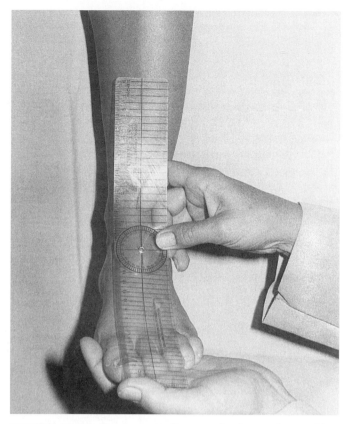

FIGURE 10–39 Goniometer alignment in the starting position for measuring transverse tarsal inversion.

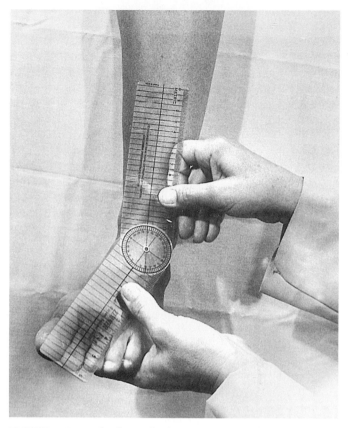

FIGURE 10–40 At the end of transverse tarsal inversion, one of the examiner's hands releases the calcaneus and aligns the proximal goniometer arm with the lower leg. The examiner's other hand maintains inversion and holds the distal goniometer arm aligned with the second metatarsal.

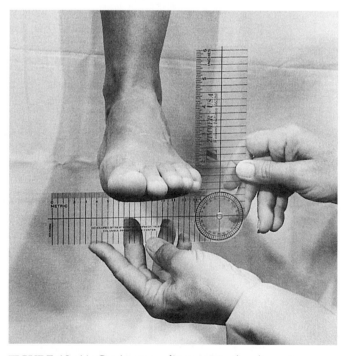

FIGURE 10–41 Goniometer alignment in the alternative starting position for measuring transverse tarsal inversion range of motion places the goniometer at 90 degrees, which is the 0 starting position. Therefore, the goniometer reading should be transposed and recorded as starting at 0 degrees.

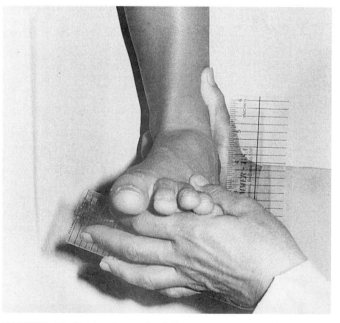

FIGURE 10–42 At the end of the transverse tarsal inversion range of motion, the examiner uses her hand to maintain inversion and to keep the distal goniometer arm aligned.

EVERSION: TRANSVERSE TARSAL JOINT

Motion is a combination of pronation, abduction, and dorsiflexion. Because of the uniaxial limitations of the goniometer, this motion is measured in the frontal plane around an anterior-posterior axis. The normal ROM for forefoot eversion ranges from 15 to 21 degrees.[4, 6]

Testing Position

Place the subject sitting, with the knee flexed to 90 degrees and the lower leg over the edge of the supporting surface. Position the hip in 0 degrees of rotation, adduction, and abduction, and the subtalar joint in the 0 starting position. Alternatively, it is possible to place the subject in the supine position, with the foot over the edge of the supporting surface.

Stabilization

Stabilize the calcaneus and talus to prevent plantarflexion of the ankle and eversion of the subtalar joint.

Testing Motion

Pull the forefoot laterally into abduction and upward into dorsiflexion. Turn the forefoot into pronation so that the lateral side of the foot is higher than the medial side (Fig. 10–43). The end of the ROM occurs when resistance is felt and attempts to produce additional motion cause plantarflexion and/or subtalar eversion.

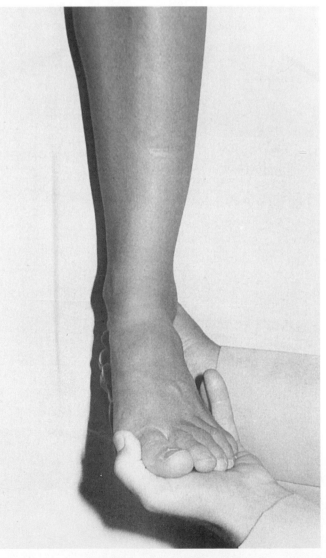

FIGURE 10–43 The end of transverse tarsal eversion range of motion. The examiner's hand stabilizes the calcaneus to prevent subtalar eversion. As can be seen in the photograph, only a small amount of motion is available at the transverse tarsal joint in this subject.

Normal End-feel

The end-feel is firm because of tension in the joint capsules; the deltoid ligament; the plantar calcaneonavicular and calcaneocuboid ligaments; the dorsal talonavicular ligament; the medial band of the bifurcated ligament; the transverse metatarsal ligament; various dorsal, plantar, and interosseous ligaments of the cuboideonavicular, cuneonavicular, intercuneiform, cuneocuboid, TMT, and intermetatarsal joints; and the tibialis posterior muscle.

Goniometer Alignment

See Figures 10–44 and 10–45.

1. Center the fulcrum of the goniometer over the anterior aspect of the ankle slightly distal to a point midway between the malleoli.
2. Align the proximal arm with the anterior midline of the lower leg, using the tibial tuberosity for reference.
3. Align the distal arm with the anterior midline of the second metatarsal.

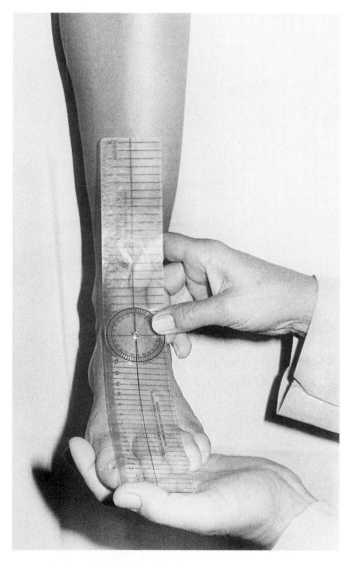

FIGURE 10–44 Goniometer alignment in the starting position for measuring transverse tarsal eversion range of motion.

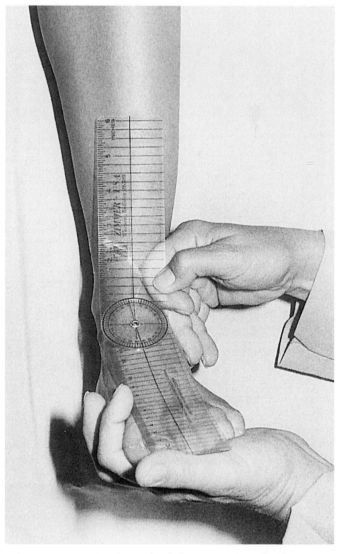

FIGURE 10–45 At the end of the transverse tarsal eversion range of motion, one of the examiner's hands releases the calcaneus and aligns the proximal goniometer arm with the lower leg. The examiner's other hand maintains eversion and alignment of the distal goniometer arm.

Alternative Goniometer Alignment

See Figures 10–46 and 10–47.

1. Place the fulcrum of the goniometer at the medial aspect of the first metatarsal head.

2. Align the proximal arm parallel to the anterior midline of the lower leg.
3. Align the distal arm with the plantar aspect from the first to the fifth metatarsal heads.

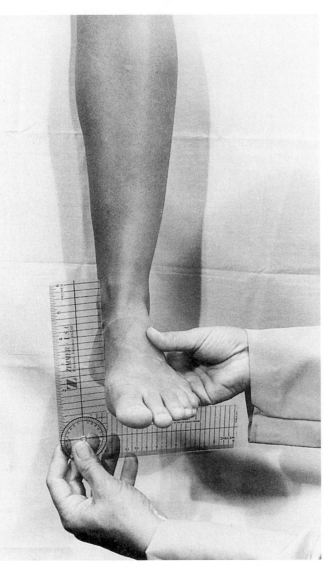

FIGURE 10–46 Goniometer alignment in the alternative starting position for measuring transverse tarsal eversion range of motion.

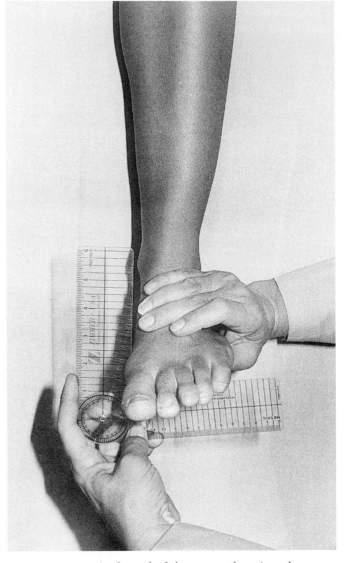

FIGURE 10–47 At the end of the range of motion, the examiner uses one hand to maintain eversion while her other hand aligns the goniometer. Because the subject is sitting on a table, the examiner sits on a low stool to align the goniometer and to read the measurements at eye level.

Landmarks for Goniometer Alignment: Metatarsophalangeal Joint

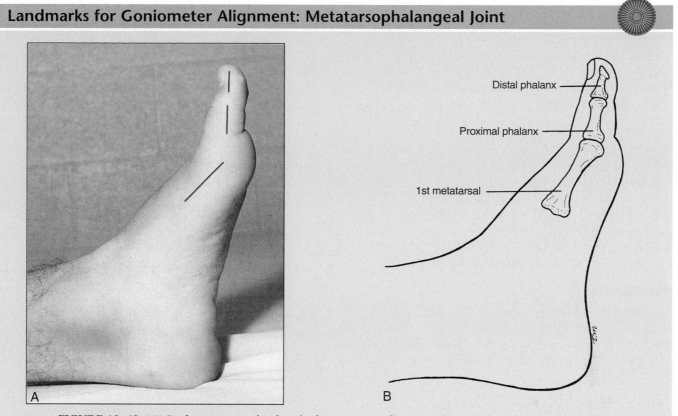

Distal phalanx

Proximal phalanx

1st metatarsal

FIGURE 10–48 (*A*) Surface anatomy landmarks for measuring flexion and extension at the first metatarsophalangeal (MTP) joint and first interphalangeal (IP) joint in a medial view of the subject's left foot. (*B*) Bony anatomical landmarks for measuring flexion and extension at the first MTP and IP joints.

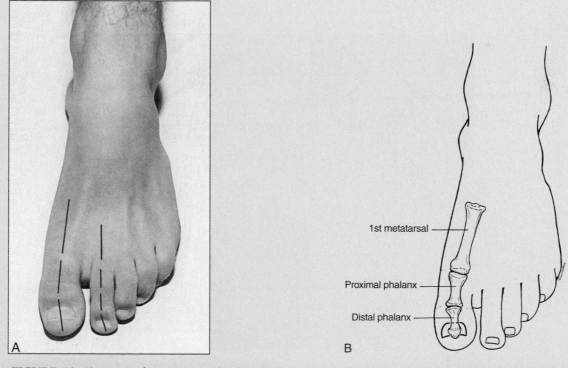

1st metatarsal

Proximal phalanx

Distal phalanx

FIGURE 10–49 (*A*) Surface anatomy landmarks for goniometer alignment for measuring flexion and extension range of motion at the first and second MTP and IP joints and abduction and adduction at the first MTP joint. (*B*) Bony anatomical landmarks for flexion and extension at the first and second MTP and IP joints and abduction and adduction at the first MTP joint.

RANGE OF MOTION TESTING PROCEDURES: ANKLE AND FOOT

FLEXION: METATARSOPHALANGEAL JOINT

Motion occurs in the sagittal plane around a medial-lateral axis. Flexion ROM at the fist MTP joint ranges between 30 degrees[4] and 45 degrees.[2] See Table 10–2 for additional information.

Testing Position

Place the subject in the supine or sitting position, with the ankle and foot in 0 degrees of dorsiflexion, plantarflexion, inversion, and eversion. Position the MTP joint in 0 degrees of abduction and adduction and the IP joints in 0 degrees of flexion and extension. (If the ankle is plantarflexed and the IP joints of the toe being tested are flexed, tension in the extensor hallucis longus or extensor digitorum longus muscle will restrict the motion.)

Stabilization

Stabilize the metatarsal to prevent plantarflexion of the ankle and inversion or eversion of the foot. Do not hold the MTP joints of the other toes in extension, because tension in the transverse metatarsal ligament will restrict the motion.

Testing Motion

Pull the great toe downward toward the plantar surface into flexion (Fig. 10–50). Avoid pushing on the distal phalanx and causing interphalangeal flexion. The end of the ROM is reached when resistance is felt and attempts at further motion cause plantarflexion at the ankle.

Normal End-feel

The end-feel is firm because of tension in the dorsal joint capsule and the collateral ligaments. Tension in the extensor digitorum brevis muscle may contribute to the firm end-feel.

Goniometer Alignment

See Figures 10–51 and 10–52.

1. Center the fulcrum of the goniometer over the dorsal aspect of the MTP joint.
2. Align the proximal arm over the dorsal midline of the metatarsal.
3. Align the distal arm over the dorsal midline of the proximal phalanx.

Alternative Goniometer Alignment for First Metatarsophalangeal Joint

1. Center the fulcrum of the goniometer over the medial aspect of the first MTP joint.
2. Align the proximal arm with the medial midline of the first metatarsal.
3. Align the distal arm with the medial midline of the proximal phalanx of the first toe.

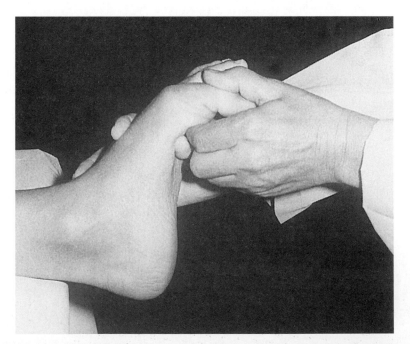

FIGURE 10–50 The left first metatarsophalangeal (MTP) joint at the end of the flexion range of motion. The subject is supine, with her foot and ankle placed over the edge of the supporting surface. However, the subject's foot could rest on the supporting surface. The examiner uses her thumb across the metatarsals to prevent ankle plantarflexion. The examiner's other hand maintains the first MTP joint in flexion.

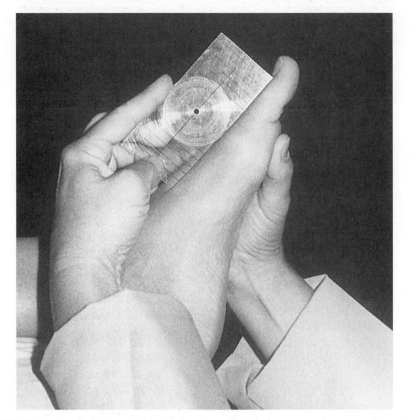

FIGURE 10–51 Goniometer alignment in the starting position for measuring metatarsophalangeal flexion range of motion. The arms of this goniometer have been cut short to accommodate the relative shortness of the proximal and distal joint segments

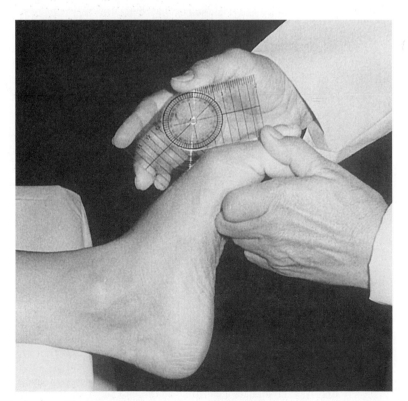

FIGURE 10–52 At the end of the range of motion, the examiner uses one hand to align the goniometer while her other hand maintains metatarsophalangeal flexion.

EXTENSION: METATARSOPHALANGEAL JOINT

Motion occurs in the sagittal plane around a medial-lateral axis. The ROM ranges between 50 degrees[4] and 70 degrees.[2] See Table 10–2 for additional information.

Testing Position

The testing position is the same as that for measuring flexion of the MTP joint. (If the ankle is dorsiflexed and the IP joints of the toe being tested are extended, tension in the flexor hallucis longus or flexor digitorum longus muscle will restrict the motion. If the IP joints of the toe being tested are in extreme flexion, tension in the lumbricalis and interosseus muscles may restrict the motion.)

Stabilization

Stabilize the metatarsal to prevent dorsiflexion of the ankle and inversion or eversion of the foot. Do not hold the MTP joints of the other toes in extreme flexion, because tension in the transverse metatarsal ligament will restrict the motion.

Testing Motion

Push the proximal phalanx toward the dorsum of the foot, moving the MTP joint into extension (Fig. 10–53). Avoid pushing on the distal phalanx, which causes IP extension. The end of the motion occurs when resistance is felt and attempts at further motion cause dorsiflexion at the ankle.

Normal End-feel

The end-feel is firm because of tension in the plantar joint capsule, the plantar pad (plantar fibrocartilaginous plate), and the flexor hallucis brevis, flexor digitorum brevis, and flexor digiti minimi muscles.

Goniometer Alignment

See Figures 10–54 and 10–55.

1. Center the fulcrum of the goniometer over the dorsal aspect of the MTP joint.
2. Align the proximal arm over the dorsal midline of the metatarsal.
3. Align the distal arm over the dorsal midline of the proximal phalanx.

Alternative Goniometer Alignment for Extension at the First Metatarsophalangeal Joint

1. Center the fulcrum of the goniometer over the medial aspect of the first MTP joint.
2. Align the proximal arm with the medial midline of the first metatarsal.
3. Align the distal arm with the medial midline of the proximal phalanx of the first toe.

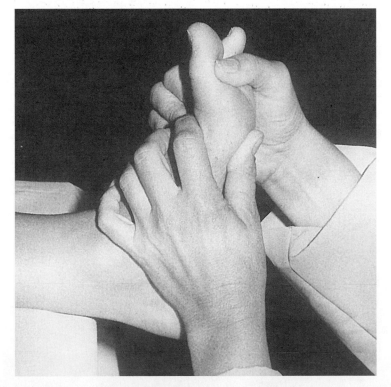

FIGURE 10–53 The left first metatarsophalangeal joint at the end of extension range of motion. The examiner places her digits on the dorsum of the subject's foot to prevent dorsiflexion and uses the thumb on her other hand to push the proximal phalanx into extension.

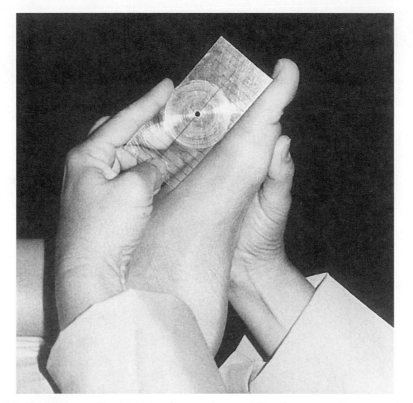

FIGURE 10–54 Goniometer alignment in the starting position for measuring extension at the first metatarsophalangeal joint.

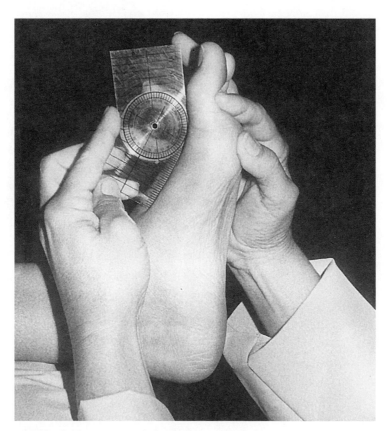

FIGURE 10–55 At the end of metatarsophalangeal extension, the examiner maintains goniometer alignment with one hand while using her the index finger of her other hand to maintain extension.

ABDUCTION: METATARSOPHALANGEAL JOINT

Motion occurs in the transverse plane around a vertical axis when the subject is in anatomical position.

Testing Position

Place the subject supine or sitting, with the foot in 0 degrees of inversion and eversion. Position the MTP and IP joints in 0 degrees of flexion and extension.

Stabilization

Stabilize the metatarsal to prevent inversion or eversion of the foot.

Testing Motion

Pull the proximal phalanx of the toe laterally away from the midline of the foot into abduction (Fig. 10–56). Avoid pushing on the distal phalanx, which places a strain on the IP joint. The end of the ROM occurs when resistance is felt and attempts at further motion cause either inversion or eversion of the foot.

Normal End-feel

The end-feel is firm because of tension in the joint capsule, the collateral ligaments, the fascia of the web space between the toes, and the adductor hallucis and plantar interosseus muscles.

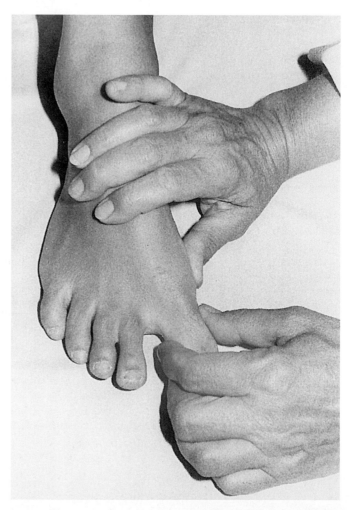

FIGURE 10–56 The subject's right first toe at the end of abduction range of motion. The examiner uses one thumb to prevent transverse tarsal inversion. She uses the index finger and thumb of her other hand to pull the proximal phalanx into abduction.

Goniometer Alignment

See Figures 10–57 and 10–58.

1. Center the fulcrum of the goniometer over the dorsal aspect of the MTP joint.

2. Align the proximal arm with the dorsal midline of the metatarsal.

3. Align the distal arm with the dorsal midline of the proximal phalanx.

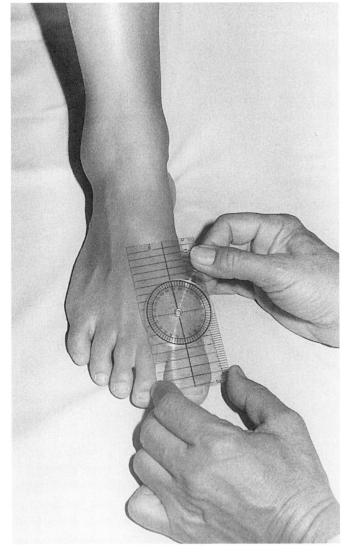

FIGURE 10–57 Goniometer alignment in the starting position for measuring metatarsophalangeal abduction range of motion.

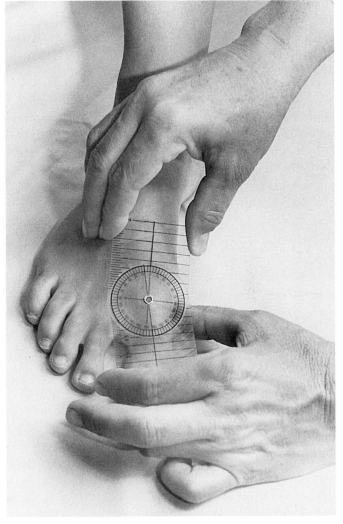

FIGURE 10–58 At the end of metatarsophalangeal (MTP) abduction, the examiner's hand maintains alignment of the distal goniometer arm while keeping the MTP in abduction.

ADDUCTION: METATARSOPHALANGEAL JOINT

Motion occurs in the transverse plane around a vertical axis when the subject is in anatomical position. Adduction is the return from abduction to the 0 starting position and is not usually measured.

FLEXION: INTERPHALANGEAL JOINT OF THE FIRST TOE AND PROXIMAL INTERPHALANGEAL JOINTS OF THE FOUR LESSER TOES

Motion occurs in the sagittal plane around a medial-lateral axis. The ROM is between 30 degrees[4] and 90 degrees for the first toe[2] and 35 degrees and 65 degrees for the four lesser toes.[2]

Testing Position

Place the subject supine or sitting, with the ankle and foot in 0 degrees of dorsiflexion, plantarflexion, inversion, and eversion. Position the MTP joint in 0 degrees of flexion, extension, abduction, and adduction. (If the ankle is positioned in plantarflexion and the MTP joint is flexed, tension in the extensor hallucis longus or extensor digitorum longus muscles will restrict the motion. If the MTP joint is positioned in full extension, tension in the lumbricalis and interosseus muscles may restrict the motion.)

Stabilization

Stabilize the metatarsal and proximal phalanx to prevent dorsiflexion or plantarflexion of the ankle and inversion or eversion of the foot. Avoid flexion and extension of the MTP joint.

Testing Motion

Pull the distal phalanx of the first toe or the middle phalanx of the lesser toes down toward the plantar surface of the foot. The end of the ROM occurs when resistance is felt and attempts at further flexion cause plantarflexion of the ankle or flexion at the MTP joint.

Normal End-feel

The end-feel for flexion of the IP joint of the big toe and the proximal interphalangeal (PIP) joints of the smaller toes may be soft because of compression of soft tissues between the plantar surfaces of the phalanges. Sometimes, the end-feel is firm because of tension in the dorsal joint capsule and the collateral ligaments.

Goniometer Alignment

1. Center the fulcrum of the goniometer over the dorsal aspect of the interphalangeal joint being tested.
2. Align the proximal arm over the dorsal midline of the proximal phalanx.
3. Align the distal arm over the dorsal midline of the phalanx distal to the joint being tested.

EXTENSION: INTERPHALANGEAL JOINT OF THE FIRST TOE AND PROXIMAL INTERPHALANGEAL JOINTS OF THE FOUR LESSER TOES

Motion occurs in the sagittal plane around a medial lateral axis. Usually this motion is not measured because it is a return from flexion to the zero starting position.

FLEXION: DISTAL INTERPHALANGEAL JOINTS OF THE FOUR LESSER TOES

Motion occurs in the sagittal plane around a medial-lateral axis. Flexion ROM is 0 to 30 degrees.[5]

Testing Position

Place the subject supine or sitting, with the ankle and foot in 0 degrees of dorsiflexion, plantarflexion, inversion, and eversion. Position the MTP and PIP joints in 0 degrees of flexion, extension, abduction, and adduction.

Stabilization

Stabilize the metatarsal, proximal, and middle phalanx to prevent dorsiflexion or plantarflexion of the ankle and inversion or eversion of the foot. Avoid flexion and extension of the MTP and PIP joints of the toe being tested.

Testing Motion

Push the distal phalanx toward the plantar surface of the foot. The end of the motion occurs when resistance is felt and attempts to produce further flexion cause flexion at the MTP and PIP joints and/or plantarflexion of the ankle.

Normal End-feel

The end-feel is firm because of tension in the dorsal joint capsule, the collateral ligaments, and the oblique retinacular ligament.

Goniometer Alignment

1. Center the fulcrum of the goniometer over the dorsal aspect of the distal interphalangeal (DIP) joint.
2. Align the proximal arm over the dorsal midline of the middle phalanx.
3. Align the distal arm over the dorsal midline of the distal phalanx.

EXTENSION: DISTAL INTERPHALANGEAL JOINTS OF THE FOUR LESSER TOES

Motion occurs in the sagittal plane around a medial-lateral axis. Usually this motion not measured becuase it is returned from flexion to the zero starting position.

Muscle Length Testing Procedures: The Ankle and Foot

GASTROCNEMIUS

The gastrocnemius muscle is a two-joint muscle that crosses the ankle and knee. The medial head of the gastrocnemius originates proximally from the posterior aspect of the medial condyle of the femur, whereas the lateral head of the gastrocnemius originates from the posterior lateral aspect of the lateral condyle (Fig. 10–59). Both heads join with the tendon of the soleus muscle to form the tendocalcaneus (Achilles) tendon which inserts distally into the posterior surface of the calcaneus. When the gastrocnemius contracts, it plantarflexes the ankle and flexes the knee.

A short gastrocnemius can limit ankle dorsiflexion and knee extension. During the test for the length of the gastrocnemius the knee is held in full extension. A short gastrocnemius results in a decrease in ankle dorsiflexion ROM when the knee is extended. If, however, ankle dorsiflexion ROM is decreased with the knee in a flexed position, the dorsiflexion limitation is due to shortness of the one-joint soleus muscle or other joint structures.

Normal values for dorsiflexion of the ankle with the knee in extension vary (see Tables 10–6 and 10–7).

Starting Position

Place the subject supine, with the knee extended and the foot in 0 degrees of inversion and eversion.

Stabilization

Hold the knee in full extension. Usually, the weight of the limb and hand pressure on the anterior leg can maintain an extended knee position.

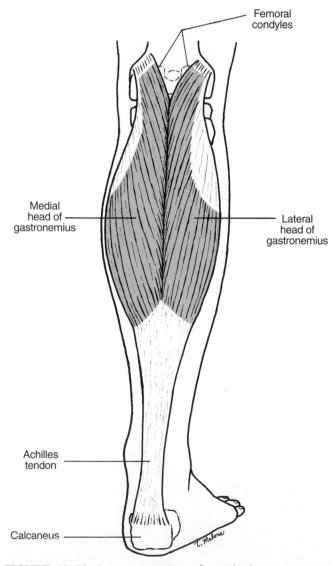

FIGURE 10–59 A posterior view of a right lower extremity shows the attachments of the gastrocnemius muscle.

Testing Motion

Dorsiflex the ankle to the end of the ROM by pushing upward across the plantar surface of the metatarsal heads (Fig. 10–60 and Fig. 10–61). Do not allow the foot to rotate and move into inversion or eversion. The end of the testing motion occurs when considerable resistance is felt from tension in the posterior calf and knee and further ankle dorsiflexion causes the knee to flex.

Normal End-feel

The end-feel is firm owing to tension in the gastrocnemius muscle.

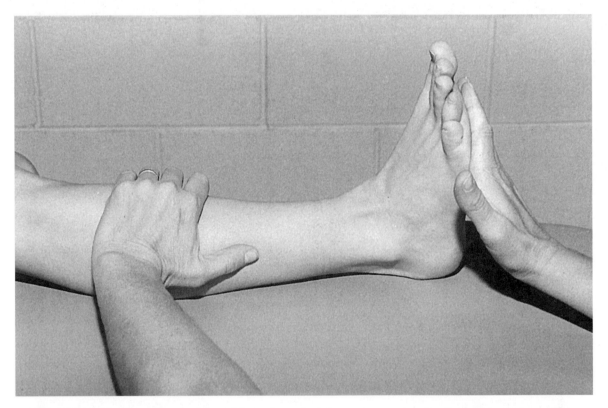

FIGURE 10–60 The subject's right ankle at the end of the testing motion for the length of the gastrocnemius muscle.

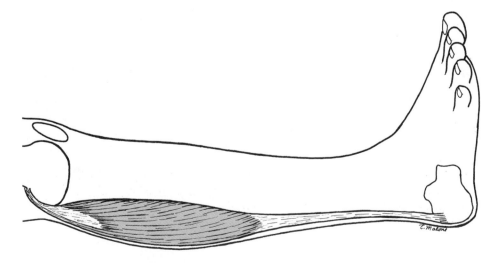

FIGURE 10–61 The gastrocnemius muscle is stretched over the extended knee and dorsiflexed ankle.

Goniometer Alignment

See Figure 10–62.

1. Center the fulcrum of the goniometer over the lateral aspect of the lateral malleolus.
2. Align the proximal arm with the lateral midline of the fibula, using the head of the fibula for reference.
3. Align the distal arm parallel to the lateral aspect of the fifth metatarsal.

Alternative Testing Position: Standing

Place the subject in the standing position, with the knee extended and the foot in 0 degrees of inversion and eversion. The foot is in line (sagittal plane) with the lower leg and knee. The subject stands facing a wall or examining table, which can be used for balance and support.

Stabilization

Maintain the knee in full extension, and the heel remains in total contact with the floor. The examiner may hold the heel in contact with the floor.

Testing Motion

The patient dorsiflexes the ankle by leaning the body forward (Fig. 10–63). The end of the testing motion occurs when the patient feels tension in the posterior calf and knee and further ankle dorsiflexion causes the knee to flex.

Goniometer Alignment

See Figure 10–64.

1. Center the fulcrum of the goniometer over the lateral aspect of the lateral malleolus.
2. Align the proximal arm with the lateral midline of the fibula, using the head of the fibula for reference.
3. Align the distal arm parallel to the lateral aspect of the fifth metatarsal.

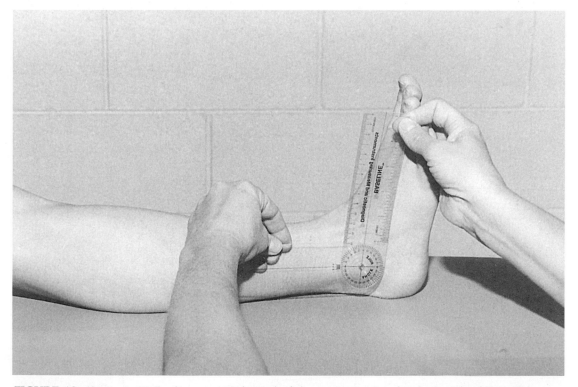

FIGURE 10–62 Goniometer alignment at the end of the testing motion for the length of the gastrocnemius muscle.

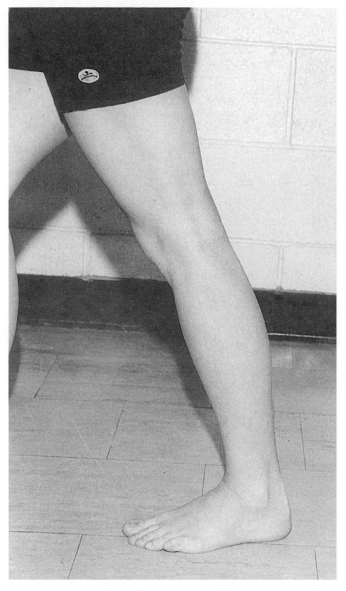

FIGURE 10–63 The subject's right ankle at the end of the weight-bearing testing motion for the length of the gastrocnemius muscle.

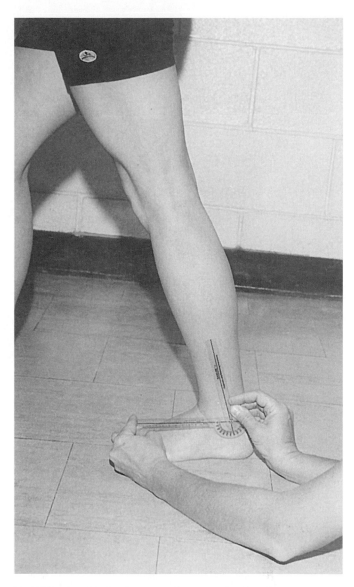

FIGURE 10–64 Goniometer alignment in the alternative testing position.

REFERENCES

1. Levangie, PK, and Norkin, CC: Joint Structure and Function: A Comprehensive Analysis, ed 3. FA Davis, Philadelphia, 2001.
2. American Academy of Orthopaedic Surgeons: Joint Motion: Method of Measuring and Recording. AAOS, Chicago, 1965
3. Cyriax, JM, and Cyriax, PJ: Illustrated Manual of Orthopaedic Medicine. Butterworths, London, 1983.
4. American Medical Association: Guides to the Evaluation of Permanent Impairment, ed 3 (revised). AMA, Chicago, 1988.
5. Greene, WB, and Heckman, JD (Eds): The Clinical Measurement of Joint Motion: American Academy of Orthopaedic Surgeons, Chicago, 1994.
6. Boone, DC, and Azen, SP: Normal range of motion of joints in male subjects. J Bone Joint Surg Am 61:756, 1979.
7. Waugh, KG, et al: Measurement of selected hip, knee and ankle joint motions in newborns. Phys Ther 63:1616, 1983.
8. Wanatabe, H, et al: The range of joint motion of the extremities in healthy Japanese people: The differences according to age. Nippon Seikeigeka Gakkai Zasshi 53:275, 1979. (Cited in Walker, JM: Musculoskeletal development: A review Phys Ther 71:878, 1991.)
9. Boone, DC: Techniques of measurement of joint motion. (Unpublished supplement to Boone, DC, and Azen, SP: Normal range of motion in male subjects. J Bone Joint Surg Am 61:756, 1979.)
10. Walker, JM: Musculoskeletal development: A review. Phys Ther 71:878, 1991.
11. Boone, DC, Walker, JM, and Perry, J: Age and sex differences in lower extremity joint motion. Presented at the National

Conference, American Physical Therapy Association, Washington, DC, 1981.

12. James, B, and Parker, AW: Active and passive mobility of lower limb joints in elderly men and women. Am J Phys Med Rehabil 68:162, 1989.

13. Gajdosik RL, VanderLinden, DW, and Williams, AK: Influence of age on length and passive elastic stiffness: Characteristics of the calf muscle-tendon unit of women. Phys Ther 79:827, 1999.

14. Nigg, BM, et al: Range of motion of the foot as a function of age. Foot Ankle 613:336, 1992.

15. Vandervoort, AA, et al: Age and sex effects on the mobility of the human ankle. J Gerontol 476:M17, 1992.

16. Bell, RD, and Hoshizaki, TB: Relationships of age and sex with range of motion of seventeen joint actions in humans. Can J Appl Sport Sci, 6:202, 1981.

17. Walker, JM, et al: Active mobility of the extremities of older subjects. Phys Ther 64:919, 1984.

18. Grimston, SK, et al: Differences in ankle joint complex range of motion as a function of age. Foot Ankle 14:215, 1993.

19. Moseley, AN, Crosbie, J, and Adams, R: Normative data for passive plantarflexion-dorsiflexion flexibility. Clin Biomech (Bristol, Avon) 16: 514, 2001.

20. Jonson, SR, and Gross, MT: Intraexaminer reliability, interexaminer reliability and mean values for nine lower extremity skeletal measures in healthy midshipmen. J Orthop Sports Phys Ther 25:253, 1997.

21. Bennell, K, et al: Hip and ankle range of motion and hip muscle strength in young female ballet dancers and controls. Br J Sports Med 33:340, 1999.

22. Ekstrand, MD, et al: Lower extremity goniometric measurements: A study to determine their reliability. Arch Phys Med Rehabil 63:171, 1982.

23. McPoil, TG, and Cornwall, MW: The relationship between static lower extremity measurements and rearfoot motion during walking. J Orthop Sports Phys Ther 24: 309, 1996.

24. Mecagni, C, et al : Balance and ankle range of motion in community-dwelling women aged 64–87 years: A correlational study. Phys Ther 80:1004, 2000.

25. Baggett, BD, and Young, G: Ankle joint dorsiflexion. Establishment of a normal range. J Am Podiatr Med Assoc 83:251, 1993.

26. Lattanza, L, Gray, GW, and Kanter, RM: Closed versus open kinematic chain measurements of subtalar joint eversion: Implications for clinical practice. J Orthop Sports Phys Ther 9:310, 1988.

27. Nawoczenski, DA, Baumhauer, JF, and Umberger, BR: Relationship between clinical measurements and motion of the first metatarsophalangeal joint during gait. J Bone Joint Surg 81:370, 1999.

28. Wilson, RW, and Gansneder, BM: Measures of functional limitation as predictors of disablement in athletes with acute ankle sprains. J Orthop Sports Phys Ther 30:528, 2000.

29. Kaufman, KR, et al: The effect of foot structure and range of motion on musculoskeletal overuse injuries. Am J Sports Med 27: 585, 1999.

30. Chesworth, BM, and Vandervoort, AA: Comparison of passive stiffness variables and range of motion in uninvolved and involved ankle joints of patients following ankle fractures. Phys Ther 75:253, 1995.

31. Reynolds, CA, et al: The effect of nontraumatic immobilization on ankle dorsiflexion stiffness in rats. J Orthop Sports Phys Ther 23: 27, 1996.

32. Hastings, MK, et al: Effects of a tendo-achilles lengthening procedure on muscle function and gait characteristics in a patient with diabetes mellitus. J Orthop Sports Phys Ther 30:85, 2000.

33. Salsich, GB, Mueller, MJ, and Sahrmann, SA: Passive ankle stiffness in subjects with diabetes and peripheral neuropathy versus an age matched comparison group. Phys Ther 80:352, 2000.

34. Salsich, GB, Brown, M, and Mueller, MJ: Relationship between plantarflexor muscle stiffness, strength and range of motion in subjects with diabetes; peripheral neuropathy compared to age-matched controls. J Orthop Sports Phys Ther 30: 473, 2000.

35. Pathokinesiology Service and Physical Therapy Dept: Observational Gait Analysis, ed 4. LAREI, Ranchos Los Amigos National Rehabilitation Center, Downey, CA, 2001.

36. Murray, MP: Gait as a total pattern of movement. Am J Phys Med Rehabil 46:290, 1967.

37. Livingston, LA, Stevenson, JM, and Olney, SJ: Stairclimbing kinematics on stairs of differing dimensions. Arch Phys Med Rehabil 72:398, 1991.

38. McFayden, BJ, and Winter, DA: An integrated biomechanical analysis of normal stair ascent and descent. J Biomech 21:733, 1988.

39. Ostrosky, KM: A comparison of gait characteristics in young and old subjects. Phys Ther 74:637, 1994.

40. Cailliet, R: Foot and Ankle, ed 3. FA Davis, Philadelphia, 1997.

41. McPoil, TG, and Cornwall, MW: Applied sports biomechanics in rehabilitation running. In Zachazeweski, JE, Magee, DJ, and Quillen, WS (Eds): Athletic Injuries and Rehabilitation.. WB Saunders, Philadelphia, 1996.

42. Torburn, L, Perry, J, and Gronley, J-AK: Assessment of rearfoot motion: Passive positioning, one-legged standing, gait. Foot Ankle Int 19:688, 1998.

43. Garbalosa, JC, et al: The frontal plane relationship of the forefoot to the rearfoot in an asymptomatic population. J Orthop Sports Phys Ther 20:200, 1994.

44. Boone, DC, et al: Reliability of goniometric measurements. Phys Ther 68:1355, 1978.

45. Clapper, MP, and Wolf, SL: Comparison of the reliability of the Orthoranger and the standard goniometer for assessing active lower extremity range of motion. Phys Ther 68:214, 1988.

46. Bohannon, RW, Tiberio, D, and Waters, G: Motion measured from forefoot and hindfoot landmarks during passive ankle dorsiflexion range of motion. J Orthop Sports Phys Ther 13:20, 1991.

47. Rome, K, and Cowieson, F: A reliability study of the universal goniometer, fluid goniometer, and electrogoniometer for the measurement of ankle dorsiflexion. Foot Ankle Int 17:28, 1996.

48. Bennell, K, et al: Interrater and intrarater reliability of a weight-bearing lunge measure of ankle dorsiflexion. Aust Physiother 44:175, 1998.

49. Hopson, MM, McPoil, TG, and Cornwall, MW: Motion of the first metatarsophalangeal joint. Reliability and validity of four measurement techniques. J Am Podiatr Med Assoc 85:198, 1995.

50. Elveru, RA, Rothstein, J, and Lamb, RL: Goniometric reliability in a clinical setting: Subtalar and ankle joint measurements. Phys Ther 68:672, 1988.

51. Youdas, JW, Bogard, CL, and Suman, VJ: Reliability of goniometric measurements and visual estimates of ankle joint range of motion obtained in a clinical setting (abstract). Phys Ther 72(Suppl):S113, 1992.

52. Elveru, RA, et al: Methods for taking subtalar joint measurements: A clinical report. Phys Ther 68:678, 1988.

53. Bailey, DS, Perillo, JT, and Forman, M: Subtalar joint neutral: A study using tomography. J Am Podiatr Assoc 74:59, 1984.

54. Picciano, AM, Rowlands, MS, and Worrell, T: Reliability of open and closed kinetic chain subtalar joint neutral positions and navicular drop test. J Orthop Sports Phys Ther 18:553, 1993.

55. Clarkson, HM: Musculoskeletal Assessment: Joint Range of Motion and Manual Muscle Strength, ed. 2. Lippincott Williams & Wilkins, Philadelphia, 2000.

PART IV

Testing of the Spine and Temporomandibular Joint

Objectives

ON COMPLETION OF PART III, THE READER WILL BE ABLE TO:

1. Identify:

   appropriate planes and axes for each spinal and jaw motion

   expected normal end-feels

   structures that limit the end of the range of motion

2. Describe:

   testing positions for motions of the spine and jaw

   goniometer alignments

   capsular patterns of restrictions

   range of motion necessary for functional tasks

3. Explain:

   how age and gender may affect the range of motion

   how sources of error in measurement may affect testing results

4. Perform an assessment of the cervical, thoracic, and lumbar spine, using a universal goniometer including:

   a clear explanation of the testing procedure

   placement of the subject in the appropriate testing position

   adequate stabilization of the proximal joint component

   correct determination of the end of the range of motion

   correct identification of the end-feel

   palpation of the correct bony landmarks

   accurate alignment of the goniometer

   correct reading and recording

5. Perform an assessment of the range of motion of the cervical spine, using each of the following methods: a tape measure, dual inclinometers, and the cervical range of motion (CROM) device.

6. Perform an assessment of the range of motion of the thoracic and lumbar spine, using a tape measure and dual inclinometers

7. Perform an evaluation of the temporomandibular joint using a ruler

8. Assess the intratester and intertester reliability of measurements of the spine and temporomandibular joint

Chapters 11 through 13 present common clinical techniques for measuring gross motions of the cervical, thoracic, and lumbar spine and the temporomandibular joint. Evaluation of the range of motion and end-feels of individual facet joints of the spine are not included.

293

CHAPTER 11

The Cervical Spine

Structure and Function

Atlanto-occipital and Atlantoaxial Joints

Anatomy

The atlanto-occipital joint is composed of the right and left slightly concave superior facets of the atlas (C1) that articulate with the right and left convex occipital condyles of the skull (Fig. 11–1).

The atlantoaxial joint is composed of three separate articulations: the median atlantoaxial and two lateral joints. The median atlantoaxial joint consists of an anterior facet on the dens (the odontoid process of C2) that articulates with a facet on the internal surface of the atlas (C1). The two lateral joints are composed of the right and left superior facets of the axis (C2) that articulate with the right and left slightly convex inferior facets on the atlas (C1) (Fig. 11–2).

The atlanto-occipital and atlantoaxial joints are reinforced by the posterior and anterior atlantoaxial ligaments, the transverse band of the cruciate ligament, the alar ligaments, and the tectorial membrane.

Osteokinematics

The atlanto-occipital joint is a plane synovial joint that permits flexion-extension, some axial rotation, and lateral flexion. Flexion-extension takes place in the sagittal plane around a medial-lateral axis. Axial rotation takes place in the transverse plane around a vertical axis

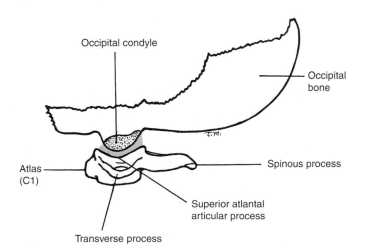

FIGURE 11–1 A lateral view of a portion of the atlanto-occipital joint shows the superior atlantal articular process of the atlas (C1) and the corresponding occipital condyle. The joint space has been widened to show the articular processes.

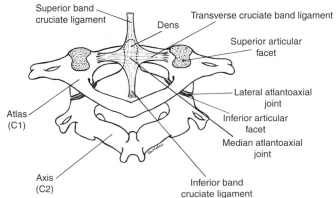

FIGURE 11–2 A posterior view of the atlantoaxial joint and the superior, inferior, and transverse bands of the cruciate ligament.

295

and lateral flexion takes place in the frontal plane around an anterior-posterior axis. Flexion is limited by osseous contact of the anterior ring of the foramen magnum with the dens and by tension in the tectorial membrane. Extension is limited by the anterior atlantoaxial ligament. Combined flexion-extension is reported to be between 20 degrees[1] and 30 degrees[2] and is usually described as the amount of motion that occurs during nodding of the head. However, according to Cailliet,[3] the range of motion (ROM) in flexion is 10 degrees and the range in extension is 30 degrees. Maximum rotation at the atlanto-occipital joint is between approximately 2.5 percent and 5 percent of the total cervical spine rotation.[4,5] Lateral flexion is approximately 10 degrees.[1]

The two lateral atlantoaxial joints are plane synovial joints that allow flexion-extension, lateral flexion, and rotation. The median atlantoaxial joint is a synovial trochoid (pivot) joint that permits rotation. Approximately 55 percent of the total cervical range of rotation occurs at the atlantoaxial joint. Rotation at the median atlantoaxial joint is limited by the two alar ligaments. About 45 degrees of rotation to the right and left sides are available. The motions permitted at the three atlantoaxial articulations are flexion-extension, lateral flexion, and rotation.

Arthokinematics

At the atlanto-occipital joint, the inferior convex condyles of the occiput articulate with the two superior concave zygapophyseal articular facets of the lateral bodies of the atlas. When the head moves on the atlas

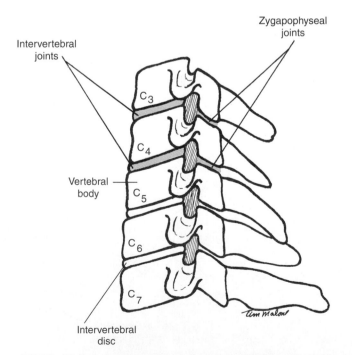

FIGURE 11–3 A lateral view of the cervical spine shows the intervertebral and zygapophyseal joints from C3 to C7.

(convex surfaces moving on concave surfaces), the occipital condyles glide in the direction opposite to the movement of the top of the head. In flexion, the condyles glide posteriorly on the atlas articular surfaces. In extension, the occipital condyles glide anteriorly on the atlas, whereas the back of the head moves posteriorly.

At the lateral atlantoaxial joints the inferior zygapophyseal articular facets of the atlas are convex and articulate with the superior concave articular facets of the axis. At the median joint the atlas forms a ring with the transverse ligament (band) of the cruciate ligament, and this ring rotates around the dens (odontoid process), which serves as a pivot for rotation. The dens articulates with a small facet in the central area of the anterior arch of the atlas.

Capsular Pattern

The capsular pattern for the atlanto-occipital joint is an equal restriction of extension and lateral flexion. Rotation and flexion are not affected.[1]

Intervertebral and Zygapophyseal Joints

Anatomy

The intervertebral joints are composed of the superior and inferior surfaces of the vertebral bodies and the adjacent intervertebral discs (Fig. 11–3). The joints are reinforced anteriorly by the anterior longitudinal ligament, which limits extension, and posteriorly by the posterior longitudinal ligament, ligamentum nuchae, and ligamentum flavum, which help to limit flexion.

The zygapophyseal joints are formed by the right and left superior articular facets (processes) of one vertebra and the right and left inferior articular facets of an adjacent superior vertebra (Fig. 11–4). Each joint has its own capsule and capsular ligaments, which are lax and permit a relatively large ROM. The ligamentum flavum helps to reinforce the joint capsules.

Osteokinematics

According to White and Punjabi,[6] one vertebra can move in relation to an adjacent vertebra in six different directions (three translations and three rotations) along and around three axes. The compound effects of sliding and tilting at a series of vertebrae produce a large ROM for the column as a whole, including flexion-extension, lateral flexion, and rotation. Some motions in the vertebral column are coupled with other motions; this coupling varies from region to region. A coupled motion is one in which one motion around one axis is consistently associated with another motion or motions around a different axis or axes. For example, left lateral flexion from C2 to C5 is accompanied by rotation to the left (spinous processes move to the right) and forward flexion. In the cervical region from C2 to C7, flexion and extension are the only motions that are not coupled.[6]

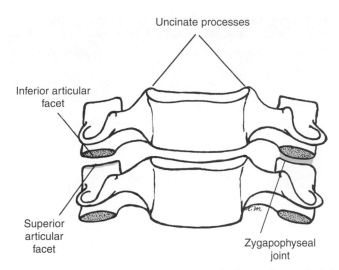

Uncinate processes

Inferior articular facet

Superior articular facet

Zygapophyseal joint

FIGURE 11–4 An anterior view of the right and left zygapophyseal joints between two cervical vertebrae. The vertebrae have been separated to provide a clear view of the inferior articular facets of the superior vertebra and the superior articular facets of the adjacent inferior vertebra.

The intervertebral joints are cartilaginous joints of the symphysis type. The zygapophyseal joints are synovial plane joints. In the cervical region, the facets are oriented at 45 degrees to the transverse plane. The inferior facets of the superior vertebrae face anteriorly and inferiorly. The superior facets of the inferior vertebrae face posteriorly and superiorly. The orientation of the articular facets, which varies from region to region, determines the direction of the tilting and sliding of the vertebra, whereas the size of the disc determines the amount of motion. In addition, passive tension in a number of soft tissues and bony contacts controls and limits motions of the vertebral column. In general, although regional variations exist, the soft tissues that control and limit extremes of motion in forward flexion include the supraspinous and interspinous ligaments, zygapophyseal joint capsules, ligamentum flavum, posterior longitudinal ligament, posterior fibers of the annulus fibrosus of the intervertebral disc, and back extensors.

Extension is limited by bony contact of the spinous processes and by passive tension in the zygapophyseal joint capsules, anterior fibers of the annulus fibrosus, anterior longitudinal ligament, and anterior trunk muscles. Lateral flexion is limited by the intertransverse ligaments, by passive tension in the annulus fibrosus on the side opposite the motion on the convexity of the curve, and by the uncinate processes. Rotation is limited by fibers of the annulus fibrosus.

Arthrokinematics

The intervertebral joints permit a small amount of sliding and tilting of one vertebra on another. In all of the motions at the intervertebral joints, the nucleus pulposus of the intervertebral disc acts as a pivot for the tilting and sliding motions of the vertebrae. Flexion is a result of anterior sliding and tilting of a superior vertebra on the interposed disc of an adjacent inferior vertebra. Extension is the result of posterior sliding and tilting.

The zygapophyseal joints permit small amounts of sliding of the right and left inferior facets on the right and left superior facets of an adjacent inferior vertebra. In flexion, the inferior facets of the superior vertebrae slide anteriorly and superiorly on the superior facets of the inferior vertebrae. In extension, the inferior facets of the superior vertebrae slide posteriorly and inferiorly on the superior facets of the inferior vertebrae. In lateral flexion and rotation, one inferior facet of the superior vertebra slides inferiorly and posteriorly on the superior facet of the inferior vertebra on the side to which the spine is laterally flexed. The opposite inferior facet of the superior vertebra slides superiorly and anteriorly on the superior facet of the adjacent inferior vertebra.

Capsular Pattern

The capsular pattern for C2 to C7 is recognizable by pain and equal limitation of all motions except flexion, which is usually minimally restricted. The capsular pattern for unilateral facet involvement is a greater restriction of movement in lateral flexion to the opposite side and in rotation to the same side. For example, if the right articular facet joint capsule is involved, lateral flexion to the left and rotation to the right are the motions most restricted.[7]

Research Findings

Effects of Age, Gender, and Other Factors

Measurement of the cervical spine ROM is complicated by the region's multiple joint structure, lack of well defined landmarks, lack of an accurate and workable definition of the neutral position, and the lack of a standardized method of stabilization to isolate cervical motion from thoracic spine motion. The search for instruments and methods that are capable of providing accurate and affordable measurements of the cervical spine ROM is ongoing, and the following sections provide a sampling of studies that have investigated cervical ROM. Tables 11–1 and 11–2 provide cervical spine ROM values from various sources and with use of a variety of methods.

Age

A large number of researchers have investigated the effects of age on cervical ROM,[14–25] but differences between the populations tested and the wide variety of instruments and procedures employed in these studies make it difficult to compare results. Generally, researchers agree that a tendency exists for cervical ROM

TABLE 11–1   Cervical Spine Range of Motion: Mean Values in Degrees

	Lantz, Chen, and Buch*[8]		AMA†[9]	Capuano-Pucci et al‡[10]	Youdas et al§[11]
	Mean age = 20–39 yrs n = 63			Mean age = 23.5 yrs n = 20	Mean age = 59.1 yrs n = 20
Motion	Mean	(SD)		Mean (SD)	Mean (SD)
Flexion	60	(8)	50	51 (9)	40 (12)
Extension	56	(11)	60	70 (9)	50 (14)
Right lateral flexion	43	(8)	45		22 (8)
Left lateral flexion	41	(7)	45	44 (8)	22 (7)
Right rotation	72	(7)	80		51 (11)
Left rotation	73	(6)	80	71 (5)	49 (9)

CROM = Cervical Range of Motion device; ROM = range of motion; (SD) = standard deviation.

* Values for active ROM were obtained with use of the CA-6000 spine motion analyzer.

† Values obtained using an inclinometer.

‡ Values obtained using the CROM device.

§ Values for active ROM obtained using a universal goniometer.

to decrease with increasing age. The only exception is axial rotation (occurring primarily at the atlantoaxial joint), which has been shown either to stay the same or to increase with age to compensate for an age-related decrease in rotation in the lower cervical spine.[17,25] Age may not account for a large amount of the variance in ROM, but age appears to have a stronger effect than gender. O'Driscoll and Tomenson[14] studied cervical ROM across age groups. These investigators used a spirit inclinometer (a hydrogoniometer that works on a pendulum principle) for their measurements. They measured 79 females and 80 males ranging in age from 0 to 79 years. ROM decreased with increasing age, and differences existed between males and females. A multiple regression analysis showed that age alone explained a significant amount of the variation, but regression lines for males and females were significantly different.

Table 11–3 shows the effects of age on cervical spine ROM. Values presented in Table 11–3 were obtained from 337 healthy volunteers (171 females and 166 males). The subjects were measured using the cervical range of motion (CROM) device; therefore, the values presented in these tables should be used for reference *only* if examiners are using a CROM device for their measuring instrument. However, the tables are useful in that they show the effects of age on cervical ROM. Ideally, the examiner should use norms that are appropriate to the method of measurement and the age and gender of the individuals being examined. In Table 11–3, the mean values for active neck flexion in the two oldest groups of males and females are less than the mean values obtained in the youngest group. Eighty- to ninety-year-old subjects show about 20 degrees less motion than 11 to 19 year-old subjects.

Pellachia and Bohannon[22] found that the mean values for lateral flexion in subjects younger than 30 years of age exceeded 42 degrees, whereas mean values for lateral flexion in subjects older than 79 years of age were less than 25 degrees. Nilsson, Hartvigsen, and Christensen,[18] in a study of 90 healthy men and women aged 20 to 60 years, concluded that the decrease in cervical passive ROM with increasing age could be explained by using a simple linear regression of ROM as a function of age. Chen and colleagues,[23] in a detailed review of the literature regarding the effects of aging on cervical spine ROM, concluded that active ROM decreased by 4 degrees per decade. This finding is very close to the 5-degree decrease found by Youdas and associates.[16]

Other investigators have found some evidence that the

TABLE 11–2   Cervical Spine Range of Motion Measured with a Tape Measure: Mean Values in Centimeters

	Hsieh and Yeung*[12]		Balogun et al†[13]
	14–31 yrs		18–26 yrs
	n = 17 Tester 1	n = 17 Tester 2	n = 21
Motion	Mean (SD)	Mean (SD)	Mean (SD)
Flexion	1.0 (1.68)	1.8 (1.60)	4.3 (2.0)
Extension	22.4 (1.56)	20.8 (2.36)	18.5 (2.0)
Right lateral flexion	11.0 (1.92)	11.5 (2.10)	12.9 (2.4)
Left lateral flexion	10.7 (1.87)	11.1 (2.07)	12.8 (2.5)
Right Rotation	11.6 (1.73)	12.6 (2.52)	11.0 (2.5)
Left Rotation	11.2 (1.88)	13.2 (2.37)	11.0 (2.5)

CI = Confidence interval; r = Pearson product moment correlation coefficient; (SD) = standard deviation.

* 99 percent confidence interval of measurement error ranged from 1.4 cm to 2.55 cm for tester 1 (experienced). CI ranged from 1.91 cm to 3.30 cm for tester 2 (inexperienced).

† r values ranged from 0.26 to 0.88 for intratester reliability and from 0.30 to 0.92 for intertester reliability.

TABLE 11–3   Effects of Age on Active Cervical Flexion Range of Motion in Males and Females Aged 11 to 89 Years: Mean Values in Degrees*

11–19 yrs n = 40	20–29 yrs n = 42	30–39 yrs n = 41	40–49 yrs n = 42	50–59 yrs n = 40	60–69 yrs n = 40	70–79 yrs n = 40	80–89 yrs n = 38
Mean (SD)	Mean (SD)	Mean (SD)	Mean (SD)	Mean (SD)	Mean (SD)	Mean (SD)	Mean (SD)
64 (9)	54 (9)	47 (10)	50 (11)	46 (9)	41 (8)	39 (9)	40 (9)

(SD) = Standard deviation.
Adapted from Youdas, JW, et al[16]: Reprinted from Physical Therapy with the permission of the American Physical Therapy Association.
* Measurements were obtained with use of a Cervical Range of Motion (CROM) device.

effects of age on ROM may be motion specific and age specific; however, the evidence appears to be somewhat controversial. Trott and colleagues[21] found a significant decrease in the means of all motions (flexion-extension, lateral flexion, and axial rotation) with increasing age, but they determined that most coupled motions were not affected by age. Pearson and Walmsley[18] and Walmsley, Kimber, and Culham[20] were the only authors to include the cervical spine motions of retraction and protraction in their studies. Pearson and Walmsley[18] found that the older age groups had less ROM in retraction, but that they showed no age difference in the neutral resting position. In contrast to Pearson and Walmsley's[18] findings, Walmsley, Kimber, and Culham[20] found age-related decreases in both protraction and retraction. Lantz, Chen, and Buch,[8] in a study of 52 matched males and females, found a significant age effect, with subjects in the third decade having greater ROM in rotation and flexion-extension than subjects in the fourth decade. Dvorak and associates[17] determined that the most dramatic decrease in ROM in 150 healthy men and women (aged 20 to 60 years and older) occurred between the 30-year-old group and the 40-year-old group. In contrast to the findings of Dvorak and associates,[17] Trott

and colleagues[21] found that the greatest decrease in flexion-extension ROM in 60 healthy men and women (aged 20 to 59 years) occurred between the 20-year-old group and the 30-year-old group.

Gender

Many of the same researchers who looked at the effects of age on cervical ROM also studied the effects of gender, but the results of these studies appear to be more inconsistent than the results of the age studies. In some studies, the trend for women to have a greater ROM than men was apparent, although differences were small and generally not significant. Also, in some instances, the effects of gender appeared to be motion specific and age specific in that some motions at some ages were affected more than others.

Castro[25] was one of the authors who found significant gender differences in cervical ROM, but these authors noted that the differences occurred primarily in the motions of lateral flexion and flexion-extension in subjects between the ages of 70 and 79 years (Tables 11–4, 11–5, and 11–6). Women older than 70 years of age were on the average more mobile in flexion-extension than men of the same age. Nilsson, Hartvigsen,

TABLE 11–4   Effects of Age and Gender on Cervical Lateral Flexion Range of Motion in Males and Females Aged 20 to 80 Years and Older: Mean Values in Degrees*

Age Groups	Nilsson et al[19] Males n = 31	Dvorak et al[17] Males n = 86	Castro et al[25] Males n = 71	Nilsson et al[19] Females n = 59	Dvorak et al[17] Females n = 64	Castro et al[25] Females n = 86
	Mean (SD)	Mean (SD)	Mean (SD)	Mean (SD)	Mean (SD)	Mean (SD)
20–29 yr	122 (4)	101 (13)	92 (14)	116 (18)	100 (9)	90 (13)
30–39 yr	111 (12)	95 (10)	89 (23)	108 (14)	106 (18)	86 (18)
40–49 yr	102 (15)	84 (14)	74 (15)	99 (11)	88 (16)	77 (12)
50–59 yr	104 (12)	88 (29)	70 (12)	97 (7)	76 (10)	69 (15)
60–69 yr		74 (14)	65 (14)		80 (18)	68 (12)
70–79 yr			47 (12)			70 (14)
80+ yr						50 (18)

(SD) = Standard deviation.
* The values in this table represent the combined total of right and left lateral flexion range of motion.
† Nilsson et al. used the Cervical Range of Motion (CROM) device to measure passive range of motion.
‡ Dvorak et al. used the CA 6000 spinal motion analyzer to measure passive range of motion.
§ Castro et al. used an ultasound-based coordinate measuring system, the CMS 50, to measure active range of motion.

TABLE 11–5   Effects of Age and Gender on Cervical Flexion/Extension Range of Motion in Males and Females Aged 20 to 80 Years and Older: Mean Values in Degrees*

Age Groups	Nilsson et al[†19] Males n = 31 Mean (SD)	Dvorak et al[‡17] Males n = 86 Mean (SD)	Castro et al[§25] Males n = 71 Mean (SD)	Nilsson et al[19] Females n = 59 Mean (SD)	Dvorak et al[17] Females n = 64 Mean (SD)	Castro et al[25] Females n = 86 Mean (SD)
20–29 yrs	129 (6)	153 (20)	149 (18)	128 (12)	149 (12)	152 (15)
30–39 yrs	120 (8)	141 (11)	135 (26)	120 (12)	156 (23)	141 (132)
40–49 yrs	110 (6)	131 (19)	129 (21)	114 (10)	140 (13)	125 (13)
50–59 yrs	111 (8)	136 (16)	116 (14)	117 (19)	127 (15)	124 (24)
60–69 yrs		116 (19)	110 (16)		133 (8)	117 (15)
70–79 yrs			102 (13)			121 (21)
80+ yrs						98 (11)

(SD) = Standard deviation.
* The values in this table represent the combined total of flexion and extension range of motion.
† Nilsson et al. used the Cervical Range of Motion device (CROM) to measure passive range of motion.
‡ Dvorak et al. used the CA-6000 spinal motion analyzer to measure passive ROM.
§ Castro et al. used an ultasound-based coordinate measuring system, the CMS 50, to measure active range of motion.

and Christensen[19] found a difference between genders in lateral flexion ROM. The differences were significant, but, in this study, males were more mobile than females (Table 11–4). Lantz, Chen, and Buch[8] studied a total of 56 healthy men and women aged 20 to 39 years. The authors found no difference between genders in total combined left and right lateral flexion, but women had greater ranges of active and passive axial rotation and flexion-extension than men of the same age. Women had an average of 12.7 degrees more active flexion-extension and an average of 6.50 degrees more active axial rotation than men of the same age. Women also had greater passive ROM in all cervical motions. Dvorak and associates[17] found that women between 40 and 49 years of age had greater ROM in all motions than men in the same

age group. However, within each of the other age groups 20 to 29 years, 60 to 69 years, 70 to 79 years, and 80 to 89 years, no differences in cervical ROM were found between genders.

Tables 11–7 and 11–8 contain information from a study by Youdas and associates[16] showing that females in almost all age groups appear to have greater mean values for active cervical motion than males. Youdas and associates[16] found a significant gender effect in all motions except flexion and determined that males and females lose about 5 degrees of active extension and 3 degrees of active lateral flexion and rotation with each 10-year increase in age. If the measurements using the CROM device are valid, one can expect to find approximately 15 degrees to 20 degrees less active neck extension in a

TABLE 11–6   Effects of Age and Gender on Cervical Rotation Range of Motion in Males and Females Aged 20 to 80 Years and Older: Mean Values in Degrees*

Age Groups	Nilsson et al[†19] Males n = 31 Mean (SD)	Dvorak et al[‡17] Males n = 86 Mean (SD)	Castro et al[§25] Males n = 71 Mean (SD)	Nilsson et al[19] Females n = 59 Mean (SD)	Dvorak et al[17] Females n = 64 Mean (SD)	Castro et al[25] Females n = 86 Mean (SD)
20–29 yrs	174 (13)	184 (12)	161 (16)	174 (13)	182 (10)	160 (14)
30–39 yrs	166 (12)	175 (10)	156 (32)	167 (13)	186 (10)	150 (15)
40–49 yrs	161 (21)	157 (20)	141 (15)	170 (10)	169 (14)	142 (15)
50–59 yrs	158 (10)	166 (14)	145 (11)	163 (12)	152 (16)	139 (19)
60–69 yrs		146 (13)	136 (18)		154 (15)	126 (14)
70–79 yrs			121 (14)			135 (16)
80+ yrs						113 (21)

(SD) = Standard deviation.
* The values in this table represent the combined total of right and left rotation range of motion.
† Nilsson et al used the Cervical Range of Motion device (CROM) to measure passive range of motion.
‡ Dvorak et al used the CA 6000 spinal motion analyzer to measure passive ROM.
§ Castro et al used an ultasound-based coordinate measuring system, the CMS 50, to measure active range of motion.

TABLE 11–7   Effects of Age and Gender on Active Cervical Spine Motion in Males and Females Aged 11 to 49 Years: Mean Values in Degrees*

	Males	Females	Males	Females	Males	Females	Males	Females
	11–19 yrs		20–29 yrs		30–39 yrs		40–49 yrs	
	n = 20	n = 20	n = 20	n = 20	n = 20	n = 21	n = 20	n = 22
Motions	Mean (SD)	Mean (SD)	Mean (SD)	Mean (SD)	Mean (SD)	Mean (SD)	Mean (SD)	Mean (SD)
Extension	86 (12)	84 (15)	77 (13)	86 (11)	68 (13)	78 (14)	63 (12)	78 (13)
Right lateral flexion	45 (8)	49 (7)	45 (7)	46 (7)	43 (9)	47 (8)	38 (11)	42 (9)
Left lateral flexion	46 (7)	47 (7)	41 (7)	43 (5)	41 (10)	44 (8)	36 (8)	41 (9)
Right rotation	74 (8)	75 (10)	70 (6)	75 (6)	67 (7)	72 (6)	65 (10)	70 (7)
Left rotation	72 (7)	71 (10)	69 (7)	72 (6)	65 (9)	66 (8)	62 (8)	64 (8)

(SD) = Standard deviation.
Adapted from Youdas, JW, et al[16]: Reprinted from Physical Therapy with the permission of the American Physical Therapy Association.
*Measurements were obtained using the Cervical Range of Motion device (CROM).

healthy 60-year-old individual compared with a healthy 20-year-old individual of the same gender.

In contrast to the preceding studies, the following investigators concluded that gender had no effect on cervical ROM. Feipel and coworkers,[24] in a study involving 250 subjects between the ages of 17 and 70 years, concluded that gender had no effect on cervical ROM. Walmsley, Kimber, and Culham[20] found no differences in axial rotation that were attributable to gender. Trott and colleagues,[21] in a study of 120 men and women between 20 and 59 years of age, also found that gender did not have a significant effect either on coupled motions or on ROM. However, age-related effects were different between males and females. Ordway and associates[26] found a nonsignificant gender effect, and Pellachia and Bohannon,[22] in a study of 135 subjects aged 15 to 95 years with a history of neck pain, concluded that neither neck pain nor gender had any effect on ROM.

Testing Position

The lack of a well-defined neutral cervical spine position is thought to be responsible for the lower reliability of cervical spine motions starting in the neutral position (half-cycle motions) compared with those starting at the end of one ROM and continuing to the end of another ROM (full-cycle motions). Studies that have attempted to better define the neutral position have used either radiographs[26,27] or motion analysis systems.[28,29] In the radiographic study conducted by Ordway and associates,[26] the authors determined that when the cervical spine is in the neutral position, the upper segments are in flexion and the lower segments have progressively less flexion; therefore, at C6 to C7, the spine is in a considerable amount of extension. Miller, Polissar, and Haas,[27] in the other radiographic study, found that the cervical spine is in the neutral position when the hard palate is in the horizontal plane. Although these findings are of considerable interest, they provide little help to the average clinician, who does not have access to radiographs for patient positioning.

Two studies that are more clinically relevant used the CA-6000 Spine Analyzer.[28,29] This motion analysis system is capable of giving the location of neutral 0 position as coordinates in three dimensions corresponding to the three planes of motion. Christensen and Nilsson[28] found that the ability of 38 healthy subjects to reproduce

TABLE 11–8   Effects of Age and Gender on Active Cervical Spine Motion in Males and Females Aged 50 to 89 Years: Mean Values in Degrees*

	Males	Females	Males	Females	Males	Females	Males	Females
	50–59 yrs		60–69 yrs		70–79 yrs		80–89 yrs	
	n = 20	n = 20	n = 20	n = 20	n = 20	n = 20	n = 20	n = 18
Motion	Mean (SD)	Mean (SD)	Mean (SD)	Mean (SD)	Mean (SD)	Mean (SD)	Mean (SD)	Mean (SD)
Extension	60 (10)	65 (16)	57 (11)	65 (13)	54 (14)	55 (10)	49 (11)	50 (15)
Right lateral flexion	36 (5)	37 (7)	30 (5)	33 (10)	26 (7)	28 (7)	24 (6)	26 (6)
Left lateral flexion	35 (7)	35 (6)	30 (5)	34 (8)	25 (8)	27 (7)	24 (7)	23 (7)
Right rotation	61 (8)	61 (9)	54 (7)	65 (10)	50 (10)	53 (9)	46 (8)	53 (11)
Left rotation	58 (9)	63 (8)	57 (7)	60 (9)	50 (9)	53 (9)	47 (9)	51 (11)

(SD) = Standard deviation.
Adapted from Youdas, JW, et al[16]: Reprinted from Physical Therapy with the permission of the American Physical Therapy Association.
*Measurements were obtained using the Cervical Range of Motion device (CROM).

the neutral spine position with eyes and mouth closed was very good. The mean difference from neutral 0 in three motion planes was 2.7 degrees in the sagittal plane, 1.0 degree in the horizontal plane, and 0.65 degrees in the frontal plane. Possibly, patients may be able to find the neutral position on their own, but the subjects in this study were healthy individuals, and the ability of patients to reproduce the neutral position is unknown. Solinger, Chen, and Lantz[29] attempted to standardize a neutral head position when measuring cervical motion in 20 subjects. For flexion and extension, the authors described a neutral position as one in which the corner of the eye was aligned with the upper angle of the ear, at the point where it meets the scalp. For lateral flexion, neutral was defined as the point at which the axis of the head was perceived to be vertically aligned. Compared with data collected using a less stringent head positioning, Solinger, Chen, and Lantz[29] demonstrated that by standardizing head position they obtained increases in reliability of 3 percent to 15 percent for rotation and lateral flexion but showed a decrease in reliability of up to 14 percent for flexion-extension. In a study using (the 3-Space Isotrak System) Pearson and Walmsley[18] found a significant difference in the neutral resting position (it became more retracted) after repeated neck retractions performed by 30 healthy subjects.

Another potential positional problem that testers need to be aware of has been identified by Lantz, Chen, and Buch.[8] These authors found that ROM measurements of the cervical spine taken in the seated position were consistently about 2.6 degrees greater than measurements taken in the standing position in all planes of motion. Greater differences occurred between seated and standing positions when flexion and extension were measured as half-cycle motions starting in the neutral 0 position as opposed to measurement of full-cycle motions.

Body Size

Castro[25] found that obese patients were not as mobile as nonobese patients. Mean values for motions in all planes decreased with increasing body weight. Chibnall, Duckro, and Baumer,[30] in a study of 42 male and female subjects, found that body size reflected by distances between specific anatomic landmarks (e.g., between the chin and the acromial process) influenced ROM measurements taken with a tape measure. Any variation in body size among subjects resulted in an underestimation of ROM for subjects with large distances between landmarks and an overestimation of ROM for subjects with small distances between landmarks. The authors concluded that the use of proportion of distance (POD) should be used when comparing testing results among subjects. The use of POD (calculated by dividing the distance between the at-rest value and the end-of-range value by the at-rest value) helps to eliminate the effect of body size on ROM values obtained with a tape measure.

Obviously, calculation of POD is not necessary if the progress of only one subject is measured.

Functional Range of Motion

Motion of the cervical spine is necessary for most activities of daily living as well as most recreational and occupational activities. Relatively small amounts of flexion, extension, and rotation are required for eating, reading, writing, and using a computer. Drinking requires more cervical extension ROM than eating, and star-gazing or simply looking up at the ceiling requires a full ROM in extension (Fig. 11–5). Using a telephone requires lateral flexion as well as rotation. Considerably more motion is required for bathing and grooming. Sports activities such as serving a tennis ball, catching or batting a baseball, canoeing, and kayaking may require a full ROM in all

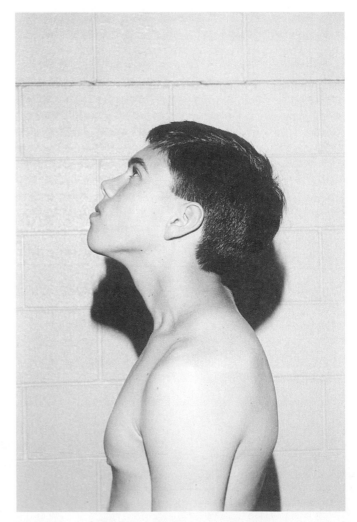

FIGURE 11–5 One needs at least 40 to 50 degrees of cervical extension range of motion (ROM) to look up at the ceiling.[1] If cervical extension ROM is limited, the person must extend the entire spine in an effort to place the head in a position whereby the eyes can look up at the ceiling.

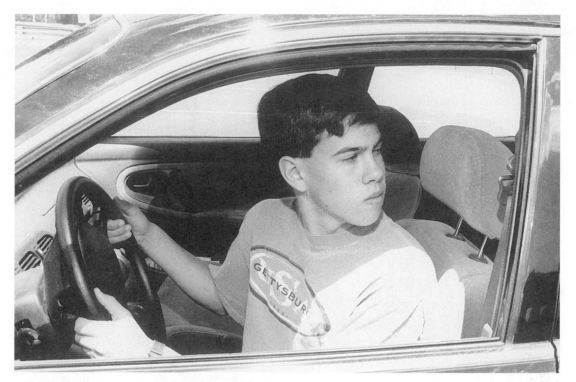

FIGURE 11–6 One needs a minimum of 60 to 70 degrees of cervical rotation to look over the shoulder.[1] If cervical rotation range of motion is limited, the person has to rotate the entire trunk to position the head to check for oncoming traffic.

planes. Guth[31] compared cervical rotation ROM in a group of 40 swimmers with that in 40 nonathletic volunteers. The swimmers aged 14 to 17 years had a mean total rotation ROM that was 9 degrees greater than the ROM of those aged 14 to 17 years in the control group. Occupational activities such as house painting or wallpapering require a full range of cervical extension and, possibly, a full range of flexion. A full ROM in cervical rotation is essential for safe driving of cars or trucks (Fig. 11–6).

Reliability and Validity

Many different methods and instruments have been employed to assess motion of the head and neck. Similar to other areas of the body, intratester reliability generally is better than intertester reliability, no matter what instrument is used. Also, some motions seems to be more reliably measured than others. For example, the total (combined) ranges of flexion-extension and right-left lateral flexion appear to be more reliably measured than single motions such as flexion or extension measured from the neutral position. This finding may be owed to the variability of the neutral position and the lack of a standardized method that an examiner can use for placing a subject in the neutral position.

According to Chen and colleagues,[23] it is not possible to obtain a true validation of cervical ROM measurements because radiographic measurement has not been subjected to reliability and validity studies. Therefore, no valid gold standard exists. The only options available for investigators at the present time are to conduct concurrent validity studies to obtain agreement between instruments and procedures. Some of the studies that have been conducted to assess reliability or validity (or both) of the various instruments and methods are reviewed in the following section.

Universal Goniometer and Gravity Goniometer

Tucci and coworkers[32] compared the intratester and intertester reliability of cervical spine motions measured with both a universal goniometer and a gravity goniometer. Intraclass correlation coefficients (ICCs) for intertester reliability ranged from -0.08 for flexion to 0.82 for extension, for measurements taken with the universal goniometer by two experienced testers on 10 volunteer subjects. ICCs for intertester reliability ranged from 0.80 for right rotation to 0.91 for left rotation, for measurements taken with the gravity goniometer by one experienced and one novice tester on 11 different volunteers. The authors concluded that the gravity goniometer that they had developed had good intertester reliability and was an accurate and reliable instrument.

TABLE 11-9 Cervical Range of Motion (CROM) Device Intratester and Intertester Reliability

Author	Tester n	Subject n	Mean age	Sample	Motions	(Intra) ICC	(Inter) ICC	(Intra) r	(Inter) r	SEM
Cupuano-Pucci et al[10]	2	20 (4 males, 16 females)	23.5 yrs	Healthy	Flexion					
					Tester 1			0.63		
					Tester 2			0.91		
					Extension					
					Tester 1			0.90		
					Tester 2			0.82		
					Right lateral flexion					
					Tester 1			0.79	0.84	
					Tester 2			0.89		
					Right rotation					
					Tester 1			0.85	0.84	
					Tester 2			0.62		
Youdas et al[16]	5	6 (Intratester)	27.2 yrs	Healthy	Flexion	0.88	0.83			
		20 (Intertester)	33.0 yrs		Extension	0.94	0.90			
					Right lateral flexion	0.88	0.87			
					Right rotation	0.82	0.82			
Garrett et al[33]	7	40	59.1 yrs		Forward head posture	0.93	0.83			
Nilsson*[34]	2 (1 experienced; 1 no experience)	14	20–45 yrs	Healthy	Flexion			0.76	0.71	6°†
					Extension			0.85	0.47	5°
					Right lateral flexion			0.61	0.58	5°
					Right rotation			0.75	0.66	6°
Nilsson et al*[35]	2	35	20–28 yrs	Healthy	Flexion		0.65		0.70	
					Extension		0.54		0.55	
					Right lateral flexion		0.64		0.70	
					Right rotation		0.41		0.41	
					Flexion–extension		0.60		0.61	
					Right–left lateral flexion		0.69		0.71	
					Right–left rotation		0.88		0.88	
Rheault et al[36]		22	37.4 yrs	Hx of cervical spine pathology	Flexion		0.76			
					Extension		0.98			
					Right lateral flexion		0.87			
					Right rotation		0.81			
Olson et al[37]	4	12	34 yrs	Neck pain	Flexion	0.88	0.58			4°‡
					Extension	0.99	0.97			3°
					Right lateral flexion	0.98	0.96			2°
					Right rotation	0.99	0.96			3°
Youdas et al[11]	11	20	55.9 yrs	Orthopedic disorders	Flexion	0.95	0.86			
					Extension	0.90	0.86			
		20	60.7 yrs		Right lateral flexion	0.92	0.88			
		20	60.8 yrs		Left lateral flexion	0.93	0.92			

ICC = Intraclass correlation coefficient, r = Pearson product moment correlation coefficient; SEM = standard error of measurement.
* Nilsson measured passive ROM.
† 95 percent CI for single subject measurement (mean of 5 measurements).
‡ Represents intersubject SEM.

Universal Goniometer, Visual Estimation, and the CROM Device

Youdas, Carey, and Garrett [11] used the following three methods to determine active cervical ROM: visual estimation, a universal goniometer, and the cervical ROM device. Prior to testing, the therapists had 1 hour of instruction and practice using standardized measurement procedures for each instrument. Intratester and intertester reliability varied among the motions tested, but, generally, intratester reliability using either the universal goniometer or the CROM device were good (ICCs greater than 0.80). ICCs for intertester reliability of both the universal goniometer and visual estimates were less than 0.80. Intertester ICCs for visual estimation were lower than those of the universal goniometer for all motions except rotation. Intertester reliability for the CROM device was good. ICCs were poor to fair for interdevice comparisons among the three methods (visual estimation, universal goniometer, and CROM device) for all cervical motions. The authors concluded that, because of poor interdevice reliability, the three methods should not be used interchangeably. The fact that intertester reliability was higher with the CROM device than with the universal goniometer suggests that use of the CROM device for measuring cervical ROM is preferable to use of either the universal goniometer or visual estimation when different therapists take measurements on a particular patient.

CROM Device

Capuano-Pucci and coworkers[10] studied intratester and intertester reliability using the CROM device and concluded that the instrument had acceptable reliability. Intertester reliability was slightly higher than intratester reliability, a finding attributed to the fact that the time interval between testers was only minutes, whereas the time interval between the first and the second trials by one tester was 2 days. See Table 11–9 for more detailed information about this study and other studies in this section.

Youdas and associates[16] determined the intratester reliability of cervical ROM measurements during repeated testing on six healthy subjects. The testers followed a written protocol and were given a 30-minute training session using the CROM device prior to testing. Intertester reliability was determined based on measurements of 20 healthy volunteers (11 females and 9 males) between 22 and 50 years of age. Each subject's active ROM in six cervical motions was measured independently by three testers within moments of each other.

Nilsson[34] found that intratester reliability for passive ROM with use of the CROM device was moderately reliable, but intertester reliability was less than acceptable. In a follow-up study, Nilsson, Christensen, and Hartvigsen[35] found that both intratester and intertester reliability was unacceptable if motions were started in the neutral position. Measurement of total ROM (combining the motions of flexion and extension by measuring from a position of full flexion to a position of full extension) improved intratester reliability to an acceptable level. Rheault and colleagues[36] found small mean differences ranging from 0.5 degrees to 3.6 degrees between two testers who measured extension with the CROM device. See Table 11–9.

CROM Device, 3-D-Space System and Radiographs

Ordway and associates[38] compared measurements of 20 volunteers' combined flexion-extension taken with a CROM device with those taken with the 3-D-Space System (an internally referenced computed tracking system with 6 degrees of freedom) and with radiographic measurements. The authors determined that flexion-extension could be measured reliably by all three methods but that there was no measurement consistency between the methods. However, the CROM device's advantages over the 3-D Space System were lower cost and ease of use.

Tousignant,[39] using radiographs to determine criterion validity of the CROM device, found that the measurements of flexion and extension in 31 healthy participants aged 18 to 25 years were highly correlated. One drawback of this study was the fact that the neutral position was not defined.

CA-6000 Spine Motion Analyzer

The CA-6000 Spine Motion Analyzer, which consists of 6 potentiometers linked by a series of hinged rods, is a very expensive piece of equipment used primarily for research purposes. Christensen and Nilsson[40] found good intratester and intertester reliability for measurements of active cervical ROM in 40 individuals tested by 2 examiners. Intratester reliability was also good for passive ROM, but intertester reliability was good only for passive ROM of combined motions. Lantz, Chen, and Buch[8] determined the validity of the CA-6000 Spine Motion Analyzer concurrent with the dual inclinometer by demonstrating almost identical mean values for flexion/extension and lateral flexion. Full-cycle ROM had less variability than ROM measured from neutral and axial rotation, and lateral flexion measurements had greater reliability than flexion-extension measurements. Intertester and intratester reliability was high for total active motion, and reliability values were consistently higher for active motion than for passive motion. Solinger, Chen, and Lantz,[29] in a study of cervical ROM in 20 healthy men and women volunteers aged 20 to 40 years, also found that reliability values were consistently lower for measurements beginning in the neutral position compared with those taken at full-cycle ROM. The range of intertester and intratester reliability values (ICCs) for full-cycle motions of left and right rotation and left and right lateral flexion were 0.93 to 0.97 compared with the single motions starting in the neutral position whose range was 0.83 to 0.95. Flexion from the neutral position was the least reliable measurement, even when taken by a single examiner.

Pendulum Goniometer

Defibaugh[41] used a pendulum goniometer with an attached mouthpiece to measure cervical motion. The 30 male subjects in this study ranged in age from 20 to 40 years. The author found coefficients of 0.90 to 0.71 for intratester reliability and coefficients of correlations of 0.94 to 0.66 for intertester reliability. Unlike the majority of other researchers, the author found that intertester reliability was higher than intratester reliability for some motions. However, 1 to 7 days elapsed between the first and the second measurements taken by the same tester, whereas only 2 hours elapsed between one tester's measurements and those taken by another tester. The higher intertester reliability was attributed to the short lapse of time between measurements.

Herrmann[42] took radiographic measurements of passive ROM of neck flexion-extension in 16 individuals aged 2 to 68 years. The radiographic measurements were compared with those obtained by means of a pendulum goniometer. ICCs of 0.98 indicated a good agreement between the two methods.

Gravity Goniometer and Tape Measure

Balogun and coworkers,[13] in a study that employed three testers and 21 healthy subjects, compared the reliability of measurements obtained with a Myrin Gravity-Reference Goniometer (Inclinometer) (OB Rehab AB, Soina, Sweden) with measurements taken by a tape measure. Intratester reliability coefficients for both the inclinometer and the tape measure were moderately high for all motions except flexion. Intertester reliability was slightly higher for the tape measure method than for the Myrin goniometric method. However, intertester reliability of flexion measurements was poor for both methods. See Table 11–2 for additional information.

In a reliability study of the tape measure method, by Hsieh and Yeung,[12] an experienced tester (tester 1) and an inexperienced tester (tester 2) measured active cervical motion. Tester 1 measured 17 subjects and tester 2 measured a different group of 17 subjects. Intratester reliability coefficients (Pearson's r) ranged from 0.80 to 0.95 for tester 1 and 0.78 to 0.91 for tester 2. See Table 11–2 for measurement error.

Visual Estimation

The reliability of visual estimates has been studied by Viikari-Juntura[43] in a neurological patient population and by Youdas, Carey, and Garrett[11] in an orthopedic patient population. In the study by Viikari-Juntura,[43] the subjects were 52 male and female neurological patients ranging in age from 13 to 66 years, who had been referred for cervical myelography. Intertester reliability between two testers of visual estimates of cervical ROM was determined by the authors to be fair. The weighted kappa reliability coefficient for intratester agreement in categories of normal limited, or markedly limited ROM, ranged from 0.50 to 0.56.

In the study by Youdas, Carey, and Garrett,[11] the subjects were 60 orthopedic patients ranging in age from 21 to 84 years. Intertester reliability for visual estimates of both active flexion and extension was poor (ICC = 0.42). Intertester reliability for visual estimates of active neck lateral flexion ROM was fair. The ICC for left lateral flexion was 0.63; for right lateral flexion it was 0.70. The intertester reliability for visual estimates of rotation was poor for left rotation (ICC = 0.69) and good for right rotation (ICC = 0.82).

Flexible Ruler

Rheault and colleagues[36] found that intertester reliability with a flexible ruler was good (r = 0.80) for obtaining measurements of the neutral cervical spine position and high (r = 0.90) for obtaining measurements of cervical spine flexion,. Measurements were taken on 20 healthy subjects (14 women and 6 men).

Summary

Each of the techniques for measuring cervical ROM discussed in this chapter has certain advantages and disadvantages. The universal goniometer, tape measure, and flexible ruler are the least inexpensive and easiest to obtain, transport, and use. Reliability tends to be motion specific, and, generally, intratester reliability is better than intertester reliability. Therefore, if these methods are used to determine a patient's progress, measurements should be taken by a single therapist.

In consideration of the cost and availability of the various instruments for measuring cervical ROM, and because of the fact that the intratester reliability of the universal goniometer and tape measure appears comparable with that of measurements taken with other instruments, we decided to retain the universal goniometer and tape measure methods in this edition, but we added the double inclinometer and the CROM device. If the tape measure is being used to compare ROM among subjects, calculation of POD should help to eliminate the effects of different body sizes on measurements.[30]

Range of Motion Testing Procedures: Cervical Spine

Landmarks for Goniometer Alignment

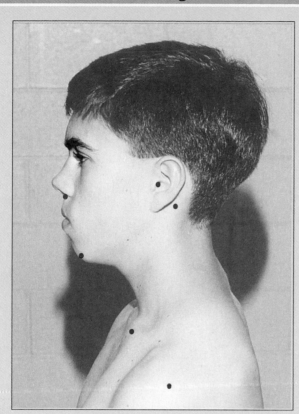

FIGURE 11–7 Surface anatomy landmarks for goniometer alignment and tape measure alignment for measuring cervical motions.

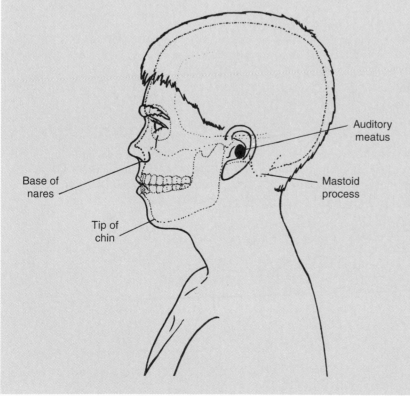

FIGURE 11–8 Bony anatomical landmarks for goniometer alignment for measuring cervical flexion and extension.

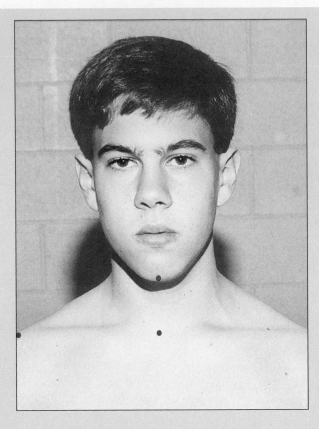

FIGURE 11–9 Surface anatomy landmarks used to measure cervical motion with a tape measure: tip of the chin, sternal notch, and acromion process. The mastoid process, which is used to measure lateral flexion, is included in Figure 11–8.

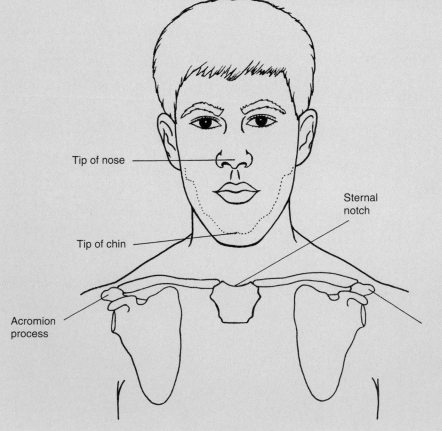

Tip of nose

Tip of chin

Sternal notch

Acromion process

FIGURE 11–10 Bony anatomical landmarks for measuring cervical spine range of motion with a tape measure.

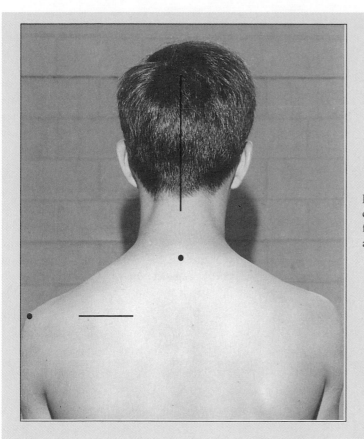

FIGURE 11-11 A posterior view of the subject's head and cervical spine shows the surface anatomy landmarks used for measuring lateral flexion with a goniometer and flexion and extension with dual inclinometers.

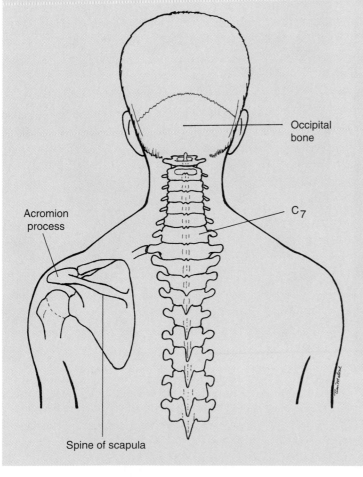

Occipital bone

C₇

Acromion process

Spine of scapula

FIGURE 11-12 Bony anatomical landmarks used to align the goniometer, inclinometers, and cervical range of motion device. All of these instruments use the spinous process of the seventh cervical vertebra as a landmark for the measurement of at least one cervical motion.

FLEXION

Motion occurs in the sagittal plane around a medial-lateral axis. The mean cervical flexion ROM measured with a universal goniometer is 40 degrees (SD = 12) degrees.[11] See Table 11–1.

Testing Position

Place the subject in the sitting position, with the thoracic and lumbar spine well supported by the back of a chair. Position the cervical spine in 0 degrees of rotation and lateral flexion. A tongue depressor can be held between the teeth for reference.

Stabilization

Stabilize the shoulder girdle either by a strap or by the examiner's arm to prevent flexion of the thoracic and lumbar spine.

Testing Motion

Put one hand on the back of the subject's head and, with the other hand, hold the subject's chin. Push gently but firmly on the back of the subject's head to move the head anteriorly. Pull the subject's chin in toward the chest to move the subject through flexion ROM (Fig. 11–13). The end of the ROM occurs when resistance to further motion is felt and further attempts at flexion cause forward flexion of the trunk.

Normal End-feel

The normal end-feel is firm owing to stretching of the posterior ligaments (supraspinous, infraspinous, ligamentum flavum, and ligamentum nuchae), posterior fibers of the annulus fibrosus in the intervertebral disks, and the zygapophyseal joint capsules; and because of impaction of the submandibular tissues against the throat and passive tension in the following muscles: iliocostalis

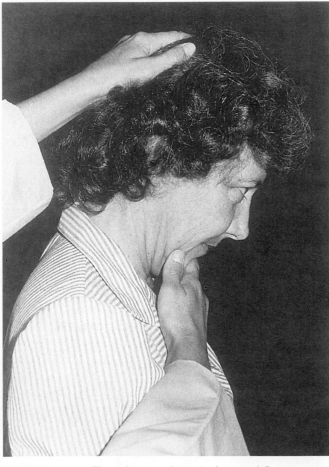

FIGURE 11–13 The subject at the end of cervical flexion range of motion.

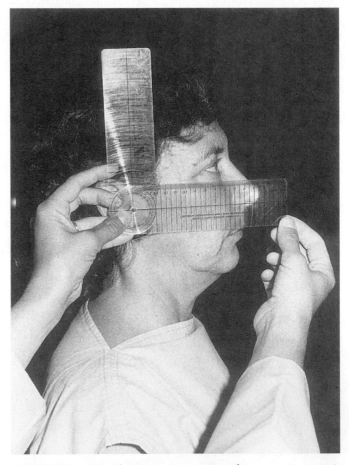

FIGURE 11–14 In the 0 starting position for measuring cervical flexion range of motion, the goniometer reads 90 degrees. This reading should be transposed and recorded as 0 degrees.

cervicis, longissimus capitis, longissimus cervicis, obliquus capitis superior, rectus capitis posterior major, rectus capitis posterior minor, semispinalis capitis, semispinalis cervicis, splenius cervicis, splenius capitis, spinalis capitis, spinalis cervicis, and upper trapezius.

Goniometer Alignment

See Figures 11–14 and 11–15.

1. Center the fulcrum of the goniometer over the external auditory meatus.
2. Align the proximal arm so that it is either perpendicular or parallel to the ground.
3. Align the distal arm with the base of the nares. If a tongue depressor is used, align the arm of the goniometer parallel to the longitudinal axis of the tongue depressor.

Alternative Measurement Method for Flexion: Tape Measure

The mean cervical flexion ROM obtained with a tape measure ranges from 1.0 to 4.3 cm [12,13] (see Table 11–2). Measure the distance between the tip of the chin and the lower edge of the sternal notch at the end of the ROM. Make sure that the subject's mouth remains closed (Fig. 11–16).

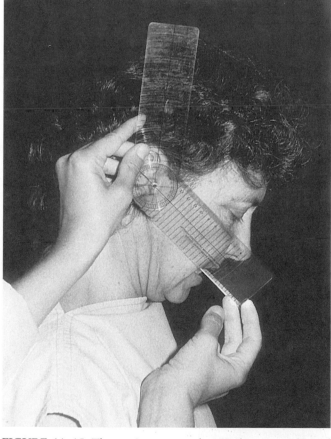

FIGURE 11–15 The goniometer reads 130 degrees at the end of the range of motion (ROM), but the ROM should be recorded as 0 to 40 degrees because the goniometer reads 90 degrees in the 0 starting position. The tongue depressor that the subject is holding between her teeth may be used as an alternative landmark for the alignment of the distal goniometer arm.

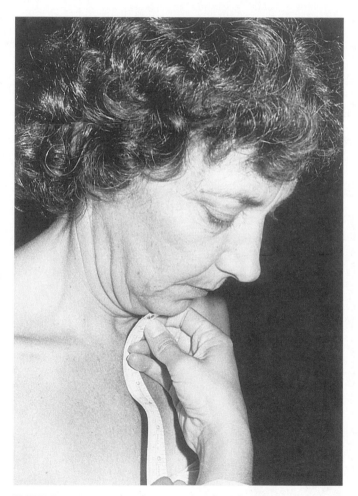

FIGURE 11–16 In the alternative method for measuring cervical flexion, the examiner uses a tape measure to determine the distance from the tip of the chin to the sternal notch.

Alternative Measurement Method for Flexion: Double Inclinometers

Both inclinometers must be zeroed after they are positioned on the subject and prior to the beginning of the measurement. To zero the inclinometer, adjust the rotating dial so the bubble or pointer is at 0 on the scale.

Inclinometer Alignment

1. Place one inclinometer directly over the spinous process of the C-7 vertebra, making sure that the inclinometer is adjusted to 0.
2. Place the second inclinometer firmly on the posterior aspect of the head, making sure that the inclinometer is adjusted to 0 (Fig. 11–17).

Testing Motion

Instruct the subject to bring the head forward into flexion while keeping the trunk straight. (Fig. 11–18). (Note that active ROM is being measured.

At the end of the motion, read and record the information on the dials of each inclinometer. The ROM is the difference between the readings of the two instruments.

Alternative Measurement Method for Flexion: CROM Device

The mean flexion ROM for the CROM device ranges from 64 degrees in subjects aged 11 to 19 years to 40 degrees in subjects aged 80 to 89 years.[16] Refer to Tables 11–1 and 11–3 for additional information.

Familiarize yourself with the CROM device prior to beginning the measurement The CROM device consists of a headpiece that supports two gravity inclinometers and a compass inclinometer. The gravity inclinometers are used to measure flexion, extension, and lateral flexion. The compass goniometer is used to measure rotation. A neckpiece containing two strong magnets is worn to ensure the accuracy of the compass inclinometer.

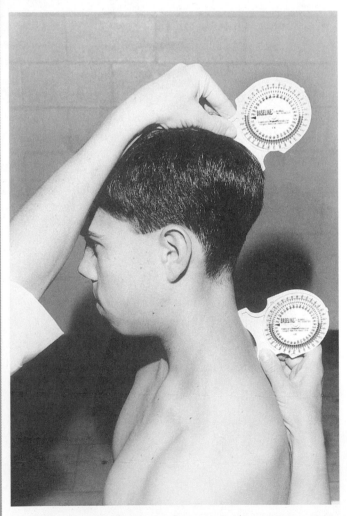

FIGURE 11–17 Inclinometer alignment in the starting position for measuring cervical flexion range of motion.

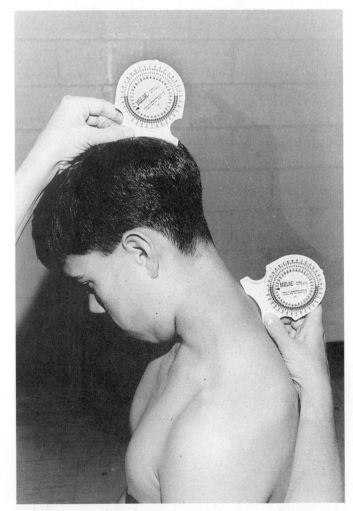

FIGURE 11–18 Inclinometer alignment at the end of cervical flexion range of motion.

The CROM device should fit comfortably over the bridge of the subject's nose. A Velcro strap that goes around the back of the head can be adjusted to make a snug fit. One size instrument fits all, and it is relatively easy for an examiner to fit the device to a subject

CROM Device Alignment[44]

1. Place the CROM device carefully on the subject's head so that the nosepiece is on the bridge of the nose and the band fits snugly across the back of the subject's head (Fig. 11–19).
2. Position the subject's head so that the inclinometer on the side of the head reads 0.

Testing Motion

Push gently but firmly on the back of the subject's head to move it anteriorly and inferiorly through flexion ROM (Fig. 11–20). At the end of the motion, read the dial on the inclinometer on the side of the head.

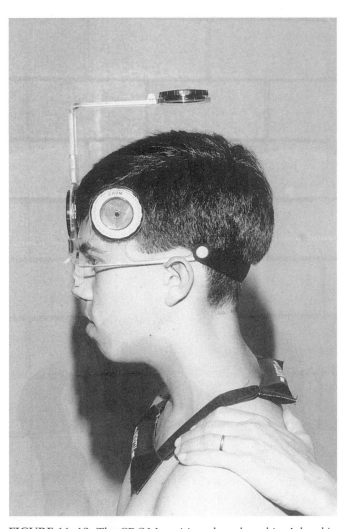

FIGURE 11–19 The CROM positioned on the subject's head in the starting position for measuring cervical flexion range of motion. The dial on the gravity inclinometer located on the side of the subjects head is at 0 degrees.

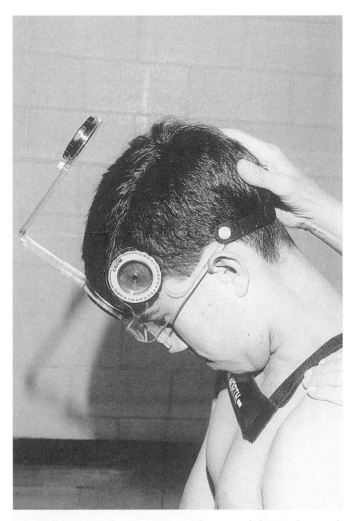

FIGURE 11–20 The examiner is shown stabilizing the trunk with one hand and maintaining the end of the flexion range of motion with her other hand.

EXTENSION

Motion occurs in the sagittal plane around a medial-lateral axis. Mean cervical extension ROM measured with a universal goniometer is 50 degrees (SD = 14 degrees).[11] Refer to Table 11–1 for additional information.

Testing Position

Place the subject in the sitting position, with the thoracic and lumbar spine well supported by the back of a chair. Position the cervical spine in 0 degrees of rotation and lateral flexion. A tongue depressor can be held between the teeth for reference.

Stabilization

Stabilize the shoulder girdle to prevent extension of the thoracic and lumbar spine. Usually, the stabilization is achieved through the cooperation of the patient and support from the back of the chair. A strap placed around the chest and the back of the chair also may be used.

Testing Motion

Put one hand on the back of the subject's head and, with the other hand, hold the subject's chin. Push gently but firmly upward and posteriorly on the chin to move the head through the ROM in extension (Fig. 11–21). The end of the ROM occurs when resistance to further motion is felt and further attempts at extension cause extension of the trunk.

Normal End-feel

The normal end-feel is firm owing to the passive tension developed by stretching of the anterior longitudinal ligament, anterior fibers of the annulus fibrosus, zygapophyseal joint capsules, and the following muscles: sternocleidomastoid, longus capitis, longus colli, rectus capitis anterior, and scalenus anterior. Extremes of exten-

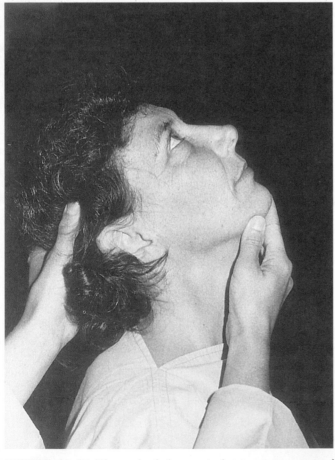

FIGURE 11–21 The end of the cervical extension range of motion. The examiner prevents both cervical rotation and lateral flexion by holding the subject's chin with one hand and the back of the subject's head with her other hand. The back of the chair (not visible) helps to prevent thoracic and lumbar extension.

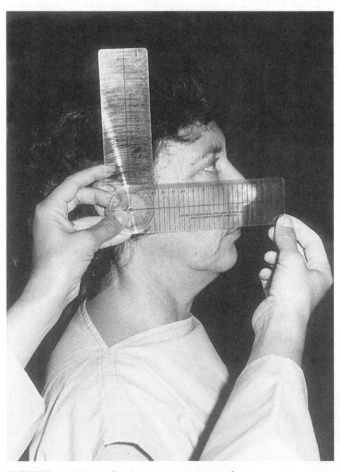

FIGURE 11–22 In the 0 starting position for measuring cervical extension range of motion the goniometer reads 90 degrees. This reading should be transposed and recorded as 0 degrees.

sion may be limited by contact between the spinous processes.

Goniometer Alignment

See Figures 11–22 and 11–23.

1. Center the fulcrum of the goniometer over the external auditory meatus.
2. Align the proximal arm so that it is either perpendicular or parallel to the ground.
3. Align the distal arm with the base of the nares. If a tongue depressor is used, align the arm of the goniometer parallel to the longitudinal axis of the tongue depressor.

Alternative Measurement Method for Extension: Tape Measure

The mean cervical extension ROM measured with a tape measure ranges from 18.5 to 22.4 cm.[12,13] See Table 11–2 for additional information.

A tape measure can be used to measure the distance between the tip of the chin and the sternal notch (Fig. 11–24). The distance between the two points of reference is recorded in centimeters at the end of the ROM. Be sure that the subject's mouth remains closed during the measurement.

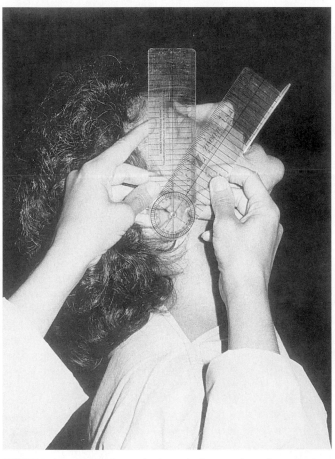

FIGURE 11–23 At the end of cervical extension, the examiner maintains the perpendicular alignment of the proximal goniometer arm with one hand. With her other hand, she aligns the distal arm with the base of the nares. The tongue depressor between the subject's teeth also can be used to align the distal arm.

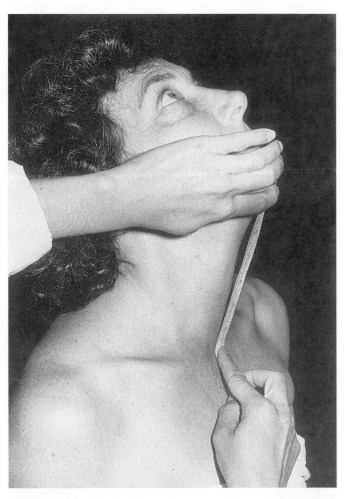

FIGURE 11–24 In the alternative method for measuring cervical extension, one end of the tape measure is placed on the tip of the subject's chin; the other end is placed at the subject's sternal notch.

Alternative Measurement Method for Extension: Double Inclinometers

Inclinometer Alignment

1. Place one inclinometer directly over the spine of the scapula. Adjust the dial of the inclinometer so that it reads 0. (If the inclinometer is placed over the seventh cervical vertebra it may impact the other inclinometer in full extension.)
2. Place the second inclinometer firmly on the posterior aspect of the head, making sure that the inclinometer reads 0 (Fig. 11–25).

Testing Motion

Instruct the subject to move the head into extension while keeping the trunk straight (Fig. 11–26). (Note that active ROM is being measured). At the end of the motion, read and record the information on the dials of each inclinometer. The ROM is the difference between the readings of the two instruments.

Alternative Measurement Method for Extension: CROM Device

The mean cervical ROM in extension measured with the CROM ranges from 86 degrees in males aged 11 to 19

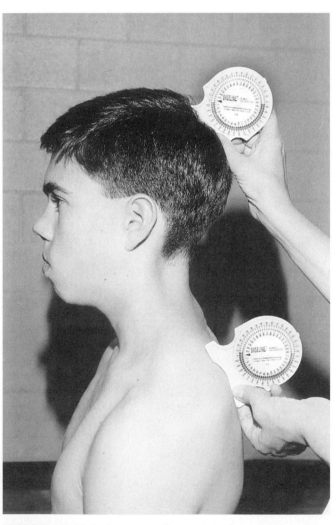

FIGURE 11–25 Inclinometer alignment in the starting position for measuring cervical extension ROM. The examiner has zeroed both inclinometers prior to beginning the motion.

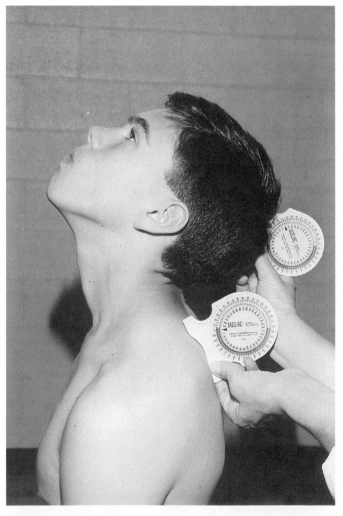

FIGURE 11–26 Inclinometer alignment at the end of cervical extension range of motion.

years and to 49 degrees in males aged 80 to 89 years.[16] Refer to Tables 11–1, 11–7, and 11–8 for additional information.

CROM Device Alignment[44]

1. Place the CROM device carefully on the subject's head so that the nosepiece is on the bridge of the nose and the band fits snugly across the back of the subject's head (Fig. 11–27).

2. Position the subject's head so that the gravity inclinometer on the side of the head reads 0.

Testing Motion

Guide the subject's head posteriorly and interiorly through extension ROM (Fig. 11–28). At the end of the motion read the dial on the inclinometer on the side of the head.

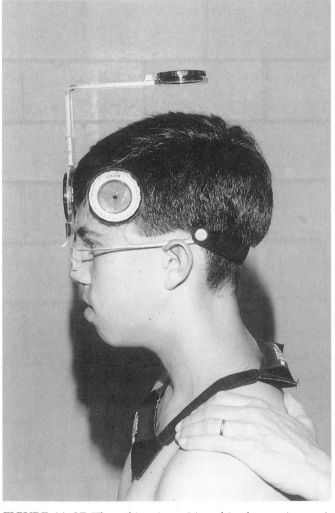

FIGURE 11–27 The subject is positioned in the starting position with the CROM device in place. The gravity inclinometer located at the side of the subject's head is at 0 prior to beginning the motion.

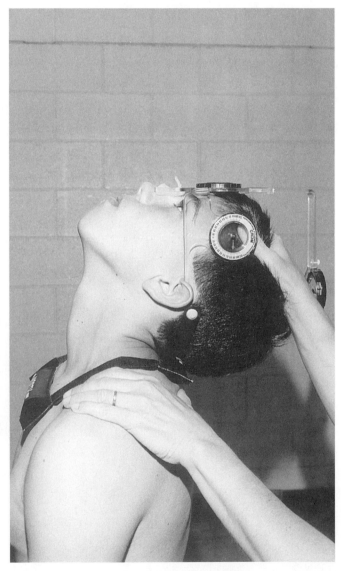

FIGURE 11–28 At the end of cervical extension range of motion (ROM), the examiner is stabilizing the trunk with one hand and maintaining the end of the ROM with her other hand on top of the subject's head. Note that this subject's passive ROM in extension is much greater than his active ROM in extension as shown in Fig. 11–26.

LATERAL FLEXION

Motion occurs in the frontal plane around an anterior-posterior axis. The mean cervical lateral flexion ROM to one side, measured with a universal goniometer, is 22 degrees (SD = 7 to 8 degrees). Refer to Table 11–1 for additional information.

Testing Position

Place the subject sitting, with the thoracic and lumbar spine well supported by the back of a chair. Position the cervical spine in 0 degrees of flexion, extension, and rotation.

Stabilization

Stabilize the shoulder girdle to prevent lateral flexion of the thoracic and lumbar spine.

Testing Motion

Grasp the subject's head at the top and side (opposite to the direction of the motion). Pull the head toward the shoulder. Do not allow the head to rotate, forward flex, or extend during the motion (Fig. 11–29). The end of the motion occurs when resistance to motion is felt and attempts to produce additional motion cause lateral trunk flexion.

Normal End-feel

The normal end-feel is firm owing to the passive tension developed in the intertransverse ligaments, the lateral annulus fibrosus fibers, and the following contralateral muscles: longus capitis, longus colli, scalenus anterior, and sternocleidomastoid.

Goniometer Alignment

See Figures 11–30 and 11–31.

1. Center the fulcrum of the goniometer over the spinous process of the C7 vertebra.
2. Align the proximal arm with the spinous processes of the thoracic vertebrae so that the arm is perpendicular to the ground.
3. Align the distal arm with the dorsal midline of the head, using the occipital protuberance for reference.

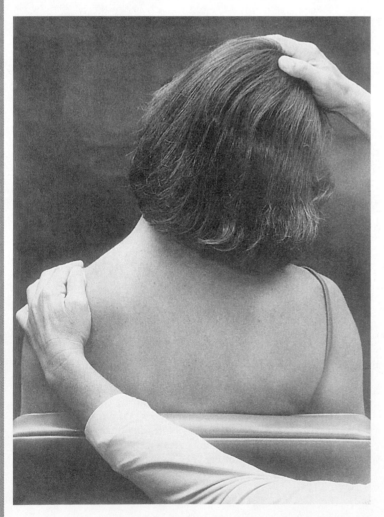

FIGURE 11–29 The end of the cervical lateral flexion range of motion. The examiner's hand holds the subject's left shoulder to prevent lateral flexion of the thoracic and lumbar spine. The examiner's other hand maintains cervical lateral flexion by pulling the subject's head laterally.

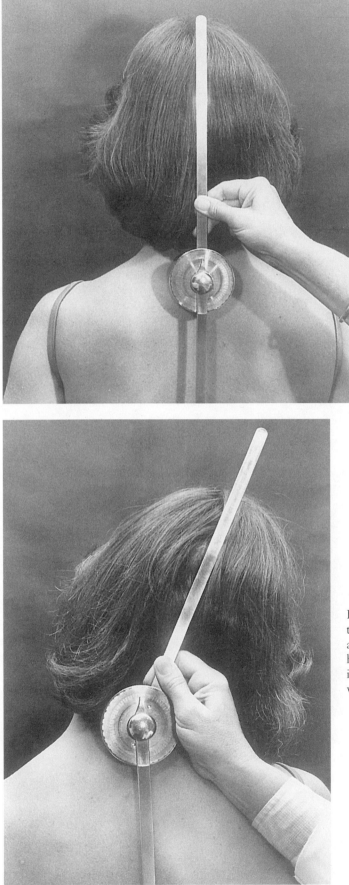

FIGURE 11–30 In the starting position for measuring cervical lateral flexion range of motion, the proximal goniometer arm is perpendicular to the floor.

FIGURE 11–31 At the end of the lateral flexion range of motion, the examiner maintains alignment of the proximal goniometer arm with one hand. In practice, the examiner would have one hand on the subject's head to maintain lateral flexion; the examiner is using only one hand so that the goniometer alignment is visible.

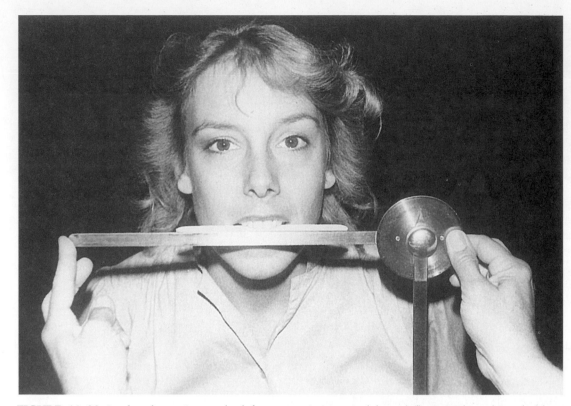

FIGURE 11–32 In the alternative method for measuring cervical lateral flexion, the subject holds a tongue depressor between her teeth (in this photograph the tongue depressor is almost completely hidden by the goniometer arm). The proximal arm is perpendicular to the floor.

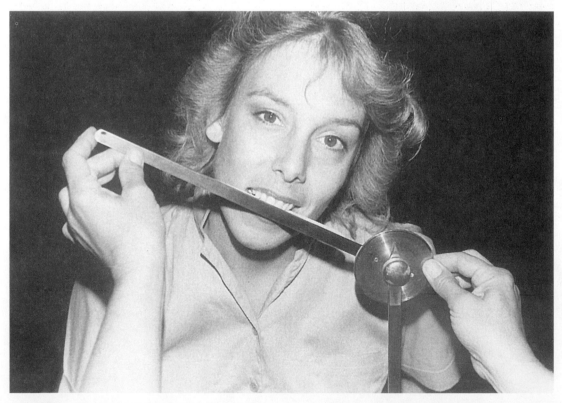

FIGURE 11–33 At the end of lateral flexion, the examiner maintains alignment of the distal goniometer arm with one hand while holding the fulcrum of the instrument with her other hand.

Alternative Goniometer Alignment

Place a tongue depressor between the upper and the lower teeth of both sides of the subject's mouth.

1. Center the fulcrum of the goniometer near one end of the tongue depressor (Fig. 11–32).
2. Align the proximal arm so that it is either perpendicular or parallel to the ground.
3. Align the distal arm with the longitudinal axis of the tongue depressor (Fig. 11-33).

Alternative Measurement Method for Lateral Flexion: Tape Measure

The mean cervical lateral flexion ROM measured with a tape measure ranges from 10.7 to 12.9 cm. Refer to Table 11–2 for additional information.

A tape measure can be used to measure the distance between the mastoid process and the lateral tip of the acromial process (Fig. 11–34). The examiner measures the distance between the subject's mastoid process and the acromial process, at the end of the ROM.

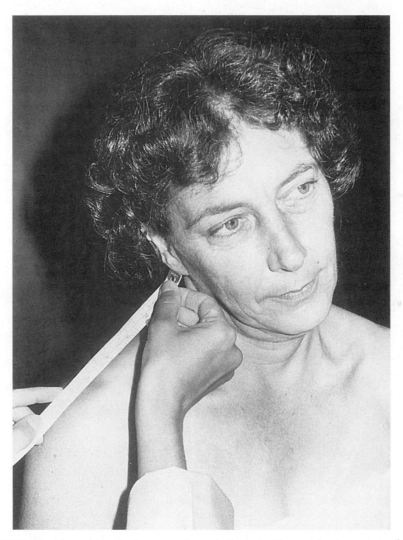

FIGURE 11–34 The subject is shown at the end of cervical lateral flexion range of motion.

Alternative Measurement Method for Lateral Flexion: Double Inclinometers

Inclinometer Alignment

1. Position one inclinometer directly over the spinous process of the seventh cervical vertebra. Adjust the rotating dial so that the bubble is at 0 on the scale.
2. Place the second inclinometer firmly on the top of the subject's head and adjust the dial so that it reads 0 (Fig. 11–35).

Testing Motion

Instruct the subject to move the head into lateral flexion while keeping the trunk straight (Fig. 11–36). (Note that active ROM is being measured.) The ROM is the difference between the two instruments.

Alternative Measurement Method for Lateral Flexion: CROM Device

The mean ROM lateral flexion using the cervical ROM device ranges from a mean of 45 degrees in subjects aged

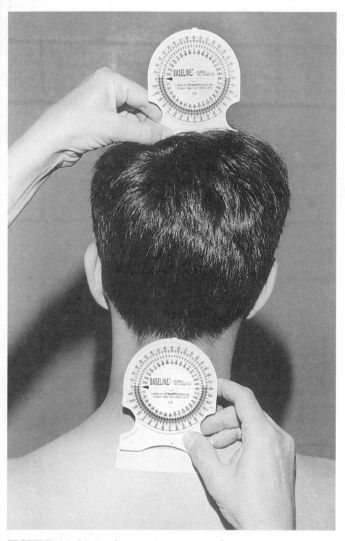

FIGURE 11–35 In the starting position for measuring cervical lateral flexion range of motion, one inclinometer is positioned at the level of the spinous process of the seventh cervical vertebra. A piece of tape has been placed at that level to help align the inclinometer. The examiner has zeroed both inclinometers prior to beginning the motion.

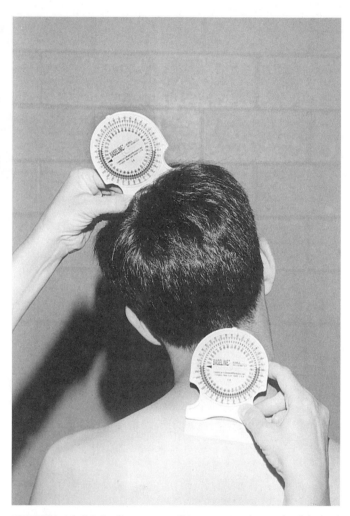

FIGURE 11–36 Inclinometer alignment at the end of lateral flexion range of motion. At the end of the motion, the examiner reads and records the information on the dials of each inclinometer. The range of motion is the difference between the readings of the two instruments.

11 to 19 years to 23 degrees in subjects aged 80 to 89 years.[16] See Tables 11–1, 11–7, and 11–8 for additional information.

CROM Device Alignment[44]

1. Place the CROM device on the subject's head so that the nosepiece is on the bridge of the nose and the band fits snugly across the back of the subject's head.

2. Position the subject in the testing position so that the gravity inclinometer on the front of the CROM device reads 0 degree (Fig. 11–37).

Testing Motion

Guide the subject's head lateral. At the end of the motion, read the dial located in front of the forehead.

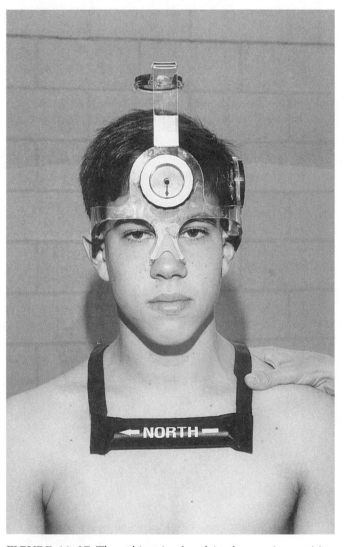

FIGURE 11–37 The subject is placed in the starting position for measuring cervical lateral flexion range of motion so that the inclinometer located in front of the subject's forehead is zeroed before starting the motion.

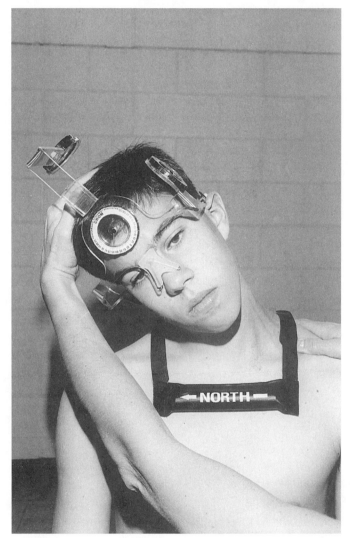

FIGURE 11–38 At the end of lateral flexion range of motion (ROM), the examiner is stabilizing the subject's shoulder with one hand and maintaining the end of the ROM with her other hand on the subject's head.

ROTATION

Motion occurs in the transverse plane around a vertical axis. The mean cervical ROM in rotation with use of a universal goniometer is 49 degrees to the left (SD = 9 degrees) and 51 degrees to the right (SD = 11 degrees).[11] See Table 11–1. Magee [1] reports that the range of motion in rotation is between 70 and 90 degrees but cautions that cervical rotation past 50 degrees may lead to kinking of the contralateral vertebral artery. The ipsilateral artery may kink at 45 degrees of rotation.[1]

Testing Position

Place the subject sitting, with the thoracic and lumbar spine well supported by the back of the chair. Position the cervical spine in 0 degrees of flexion, extension, and lateral flexion. The subject may hold a tongue depressor between the front teeth for reference.

Stabilization

Stabilize the shoulder girdle to prevent rotation of the thoracic and lumbar spine.

Testing Motion

Grasp the subject's chin and rotate the head by moving the head toward the shoulder as shown in Figure 11–39. The end of the ROM occurs when resistance to movement is felt and further movement causes rotation of the trunk.

Normal End-feel

The normal end-feel is firm owing to stretching of the alar ligament, the fibers of the zygapophyseal joint capsules, and the following contralateral muscles: longus capitis, longus colli, and scalenus anterior. Passive tension in the ipsilateral sternocleidomastoid may limit extremes of rotation.

Goniometer Alignment

See Figures 11–40 and 11–41.

1. Center the fulcrum of the goniometer over the center of the cranial aspect of the head.
2. Align the proximal arm parallel to an imaginary line between the two acromial processes.
3. Align the distal arm with the tip of the nose. If a tongue depressor is used, align the arm of the goniometer parallel to the longitudinal axis of the tongue depressor.

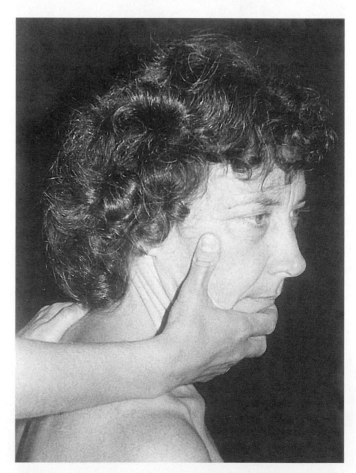

FIGURE 11–39 The end of the cervical rotation range of motion. One of the examiner's hands maintains rotation and prevents cervical flexion and extension. The examiner's other hand is placed on the subject's left shoulder to prevent rotation of the thoracic and lumbar spine.

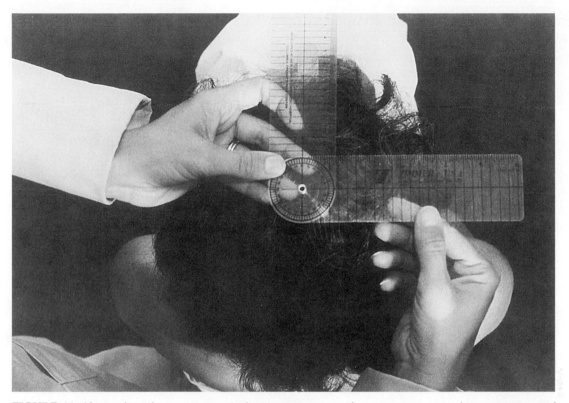

FIGURE 11–40 To align the goniometer at the starting position for measuring cervical rotation range of motion, the examiner stands in back of the subject, who is seated in a low chair.

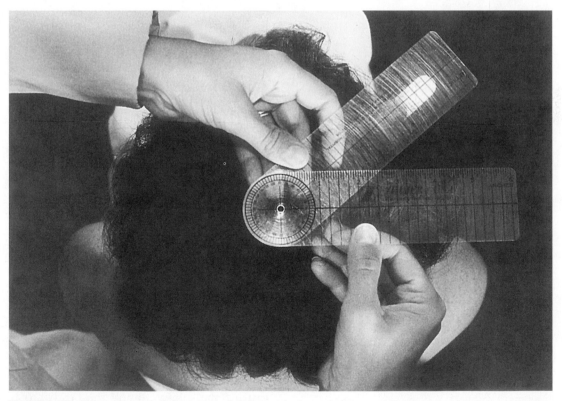

FIGURE 11–41 At the end of the range of right cervical rotation, one of the the examiner's hands maintains alignment of the distal goniometer arm with the tip of the subject's nose and with the tip of the tongue depressor. The examiner's other hand keeps the proximal arm aligned parallel to the imaginary line between the acromial processes.

Alternative Measurement Method for Rotation: Tape Measure

The mean cervical rotation ROM to the left measured with a tape measure ranges from 11.0 to 13.2 centimeters[12,13]. Measure the distance between the tip of the chin and the acromial process at the end of the motion (Fig. 11–42).

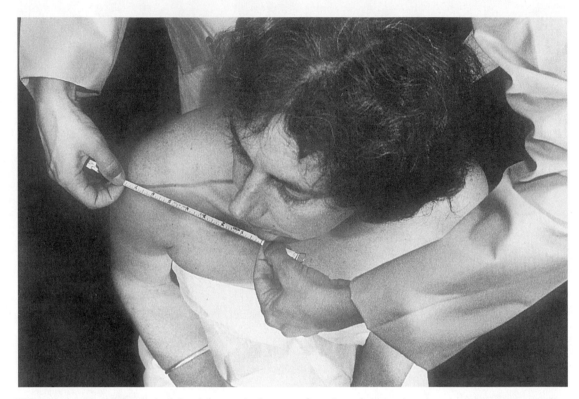

FIGURE 11–42   At the end of the right cervical range of motion, the examiner is using a tape measure to determine the distance between the tip of the subject's chin and her right acromial process.

Alternative Measurement Method for Rotation: Inclinometer

Testing Position

Place the subject supine with the head in neutral rotation, lateral flexion, flexion, and extension.

Inclinometer Alignment

1. Place the inclinometer in the middle of the subject's forehead, and zero the inclinometer (Fig. 11–43).
2. Hold the inclinometer firmly while the subject's head moves through rotation ROM (Fig. 11–44).

Testing Motion

Instruct the subject to roll the head into rotation. The ROM can be read on the inclinometer at the end of the ROM.

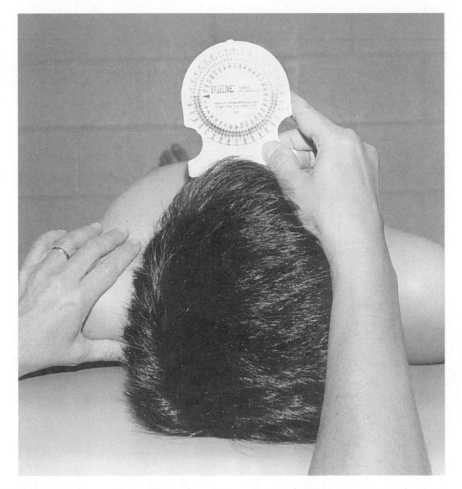

FIGURE 11–43 Inclinometer alignment in the starting position for measuring cervical rotation range of motion. Only one inclinometer is used for this measurement.

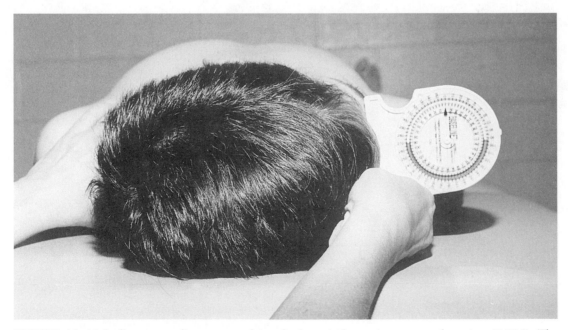

FIGURE 11–44 Inclinometer alignment at the end of cervical rotation range of motion (ROM). The number of degrees on the dial of the inclinometer equals the ROM in rotation.

Alternative Measurement Method for Rotation: CROM Device

The mean cervical ROM in rotation with use of the CROM varies from 75 degrees in subjects aged 11 to 19 years to 46 degrees in subjects aged 80 years.[16] Refer to Tables 11–1 and 11–7 and 11–8 for additional information regarding rotation ROM using the CROM device.

CROM Device Alignment[44]

1. Place the CROM device on the subject's head so that the nosepiece is on the bridge of the nose and the band fits snugly across the back of the subject's head. The arrow on the magnetic yoke should be pointing north (Fig. 11–45).
2. To ensure that the compass inclinometer is level, adjust the position of the subject's head so that both gravity inclinometers read 0 (Fig. 11–46).
3. After leveling the compass inclinometer, turn the rotation meter on the compass inclinometer until the pointer is at 0.

Testing Motion

Guide the subjects head into rotation and read the inclinometer at the end of the ROM.

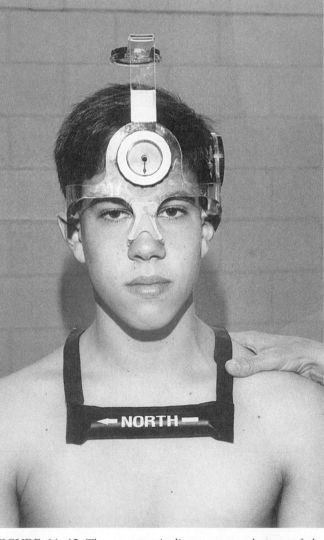

FIGURE 11–45 The compass inclinometer on the top of the CROM device has been leveled so that the examiner is able to zero it prior to the beginning of the motion.

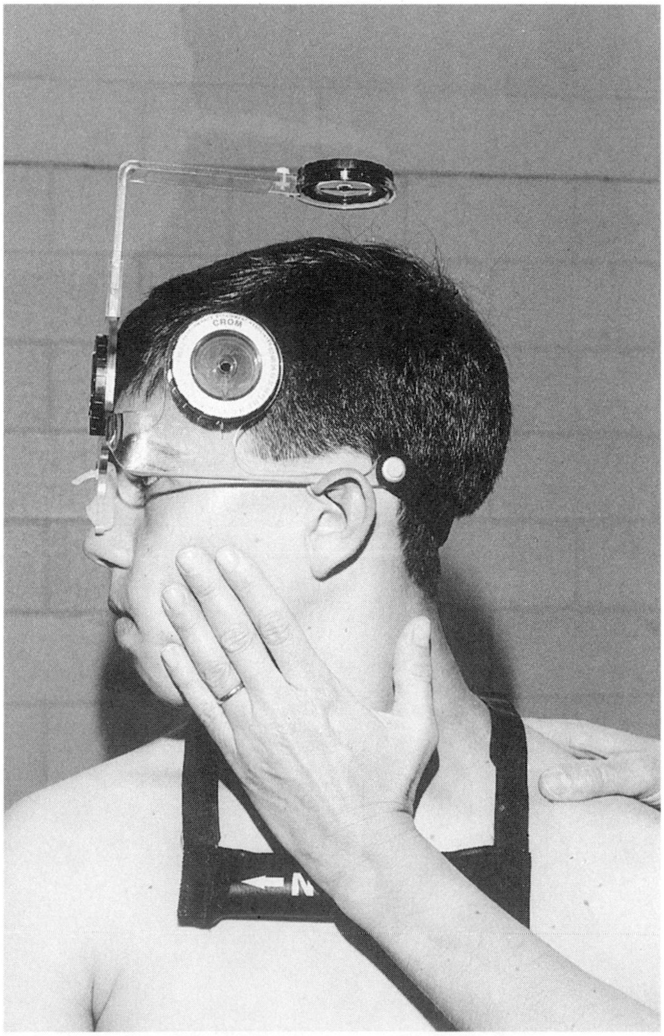

FIGURE 11–46 At the end of right rotation range of motion (ROM), the examiner is stabilizing the subject's shoulder with one hand and maintaining the end of rotation ROM with the other hand. The examiner will read the dial of the inclinometer on the top of the CROM device. Rotation ROM will be the number of degrees on the dial at the end of the ROM.

REFERENCES

1. Magee, DJ: Orthopedic Physical Assessment, ed 4. WB Saunders, Philadelphia, Elsevier Science USA, 2002.
2. Goel, VK: Moment-rotation relationships of the ligamentous occipito-atlanto-axial complex. J Biomech 8:673, 1988.
3. Caillie, R: Soft Tissue Pain and Disability,. ed 3. FA Davis, Philadelphia, 1991.
4. Crisco, JJ, Panjabi, MM, and Dvorak, J: A model of the alar ligaments of the upper cervical spine in axial rotation. J Biomech 24:607, 1991.
5. Dumas, JL, et al: Rotation of the cervical spinal column. A computed tomography in vivo study. Surg Radiol Anat 15:33, 1993.
6. White, AA, and Punjabi, MM: Clinical Biomechanics of the Spine, ed 2. JB Lippincott, Philadelphia, 1990.
7. Hertling, D, and Kessler, RM: Management of Common Musculoskeletal Disorders, ed 3. JB Lippincott, Philadelphia, 1996
8. Lantz, CA, Chen, J, and Buch, D: Clinical validity and stability of active and passive cervical range of motion with regard to total and unilateral uniplanar motion. Spine 11:1082, 1999.
9. American Medical Association: Guides to the Evaluation of Permanent Impairment, ed 3. AMA, Chicago, 1988.
10. Capuano-Pucci, D, et al: Intratester and intertester reliability of the cervical range of motion device. Arch Phys Med Rehabil 72:338, 1991.
11. Youdas, JW, Carey, JR, and Garrett, TR: Reliability of measurements of cervical spine range of motion: Comparison of three methods. Phys Ther 71:2, 1991.
12. Hsieh, C-Y, and Yeung, BW: Active neck motion measurements with a tape measure. J Orthop Sports Phys Ther 8:88, 1986.
13. Balogun, JA, et al: Inter- and intratester reliability of measuring neck motions with tape measure and Myrin gravity-reference goniometer. J Orthop Sports Phys Ther Jan:248, 1989.
14. O'Driscoll, SL, and Tomenson, J: The cervical spine. Clin Rheum Dis 8:617, 1982.
15. Keske, J, Johnson, G, and Ellingham, C: A reliability study of cervical range of motion of young and elderly subjects using an electromagnetic range of motion system (ENROM) (abstract). Phys Ther 71:S94, 1991.
16. Youdas, JW, et al: Normal range of motion of the cervical spine: An initial goniometric study. Phys Ther 72:770, 1992.
17. Dvorak, J, et al: Age and gender related normal motion of the cervical spine. Spine 17:S-393, 1992.
18. Pearson, ND, and Walmsley, RP: Trial into the effects of repeated neck retractions in normal subjects. Spine 20:1245, 1995.
19. Nilsson, N, Hartvigsen, J, and Christensen, HW: Normal ranges of passive cervical motion for women and men 20-60 years old. J Manipulative Physiol Ther 19:306, 1996.
20. Walmsley, RP, Kimber, P, and Culham, E: The effect of initial head position on active cervical axial rotation range of motion in two age populations. Spine 21:24335, 1996
21. Trott, PH, et al: Three dimensional analysis of active cervical motion: The effect of age and gender. Clin Biomech 11:201, 1996.
22. Pellachia, GL, and Bohannon, RW: Active lateral neck flexion range of motion measurements obtained with a modified goniometer: Reliability and estimates of normal. J Manipulative Physiol Ther 21:443, 1998.
23. Chen, J, et al: Meta-analysis of normative cervical motion. Spine 24:1571, 1999.
24. Feipel, V, et al: Normal global motion of the cervical spine: An electrogoniometric study. Clin Biomech (Bristol, Avon) 14:462, 1999.
25. Castro, WHM: Noninvasive three-dimensional analysis of cervical spine motion in normal subjects in relation to age and sex. Spine 25:445, 2000.
26. Ordway, NR, et al: Cervical flexion, extension, protrusion and retraction. A radiographic segmental analysis. Spine 24:240, 1999.
27. Miller, JS, Polissar, NL, and Haas, M: A radiographic comparison of neutral cervical posture with cervical flexion and extension ranges of motion. J Manipulative Physiol Ther 19:296, 1996.
28. Christiansen, HW, and Nilsson, N: The ability to reproduce the neutral zero position of the head. J Manipulative Physiol Ther 22:26, 1999.
29. Solinger, AB, Chen, J, and Lantz, CA: Standardized initial head position in cervical range-of-motion assessment: Reliability and error analysis. J Manipulative Physiol 23:20, 2000.
30. Chibnall, JT, Duckro, PN, and Baumer, K. The influence of body size on linear measurements used to reflect cervical range of motion. Phys Ther 74:1134, 1994.
31. Guth, EH: A comparison of cervical rotation in age-matched adolescent competitive swimmers and healthy males. J Orthop Sports Phys Ther 21:21, 1995.
32. Tucci, SM, et al: Cervical motion assessment: A new, simple and accurate method. Arch Phys Med Rehabil 67:225, 1986.
33. Garrett, TR, Youdas, JW, and Madson, TJ: Reliability of measuring the forward head posture in patients (abstract). Phys Ther 71:S54, 1991.
34. Nilsson N: Measuring passive cervical motion: A study of reliability. J Manipulative Physiol Ther 18:293, 1995
35. Nilsson N, Christensen, HW, and Hartvigsen, J: The interexaminer reliability of measuring passive cervical range of motion. J Manipulative Physiol Ther 19:302, 1996.
36. Rheault, W, et al: Intertester reliability of the flexible ruler for the cervical spine. J Orthop Sports Phys Ther Jan:254, 1989.
37. Olson, SL, et al: Tender point sensitivity, range of motion, and perceived disability in subjects with neck pain. J Orthop Sports Phys Ther 30:13, 2000.
38. Ordway, NR, et al: Cervical sagittal range of motion. Analysis using three methods: Cervical range-of-motion device. 3. Space and radiography. Spine 22:501, 1997.
39. Tousignant, MA: Criterion validity of the cervical range of motion (CROM) goniometer for cervical flexion and extension. Spine 25:324, 2000.
40. Christensen, HW, and Nilsson, N: The reliability of measuring active and passive cervical range of motion: An observer blinded and randomized repeated measures design. J Manipulative Physiol Ther 21:341, 1998.
41. Defibaugh, JJ: Measurement of head motion. Part II: An experimental study of head motion in adult males. Phys Ther 44:163, 1964.
42. Herrmann, DB: Validity study of head and neck flexion-extension motion comparing measurements of a pendulum goniometer and roentgenograms. J Orthop Sports Phys Ther 11:414, 1990.
43. Viikari-Juntura, E: Interexaminer reliability of observations in physical examination of the neck. Phys Ther 67:1526, 1987.
44. CROM Procedure Manual: Procedure for Measuring Neck Motion with the CROM. Performance Attainment Assoc., St Paul.

CHAPTER 12

The Thoracic and Lumbar Spine

⬤ Structure and Function

Thoracic Spine

Anatomy

The 12 vertebrae of the thoracic spine form a curve that is convex posteriorly (Fig. 12–1*A*). These vertebrae have a number of unique features. Spinous processes slope inferiorly from T1 to T10 and overlap from T5 to T8. The spinous processes of T11 and T12 take on the horizontal orientation of the spinous processes in lumbar vertebrae. The transverse processes from the T1 to the T10 area are large, with thickened ends that support paired costal facets for articulation with the ribs. The vertebral bodies from T2 to T9 have paired demifacets (superior and inferior costovertebral facets) on the posterolateral corners. The intervertebral and zygapophyseal joints in the thoracic region have essentially the same structure as described for the cervical region, except that the superior articular zygapophyseal facets face posteriorly, slightly laterally, and cranially. The superior articular facet surfaces are slightly convex, whereas the inferior articular facet surfaces are slightly concave. The inferior articular facets face anteriorly and slightly medially and caudally. In addition, the joint capsules are tighter than those in the cervical region.

The costovertebral joints are formed by slightly convex costal superior and inferior demifacets (costovertebral facets) on the head of a rib and corresponding demifacets on the vertebral bodies of a superior and an inferior vertebra (Fig. 12–1*B*). From T2 to T8, the costovertebral facets articulate with concave demifacets located on the inferior body of one vertebra and on the

superior aspect of the adjacent inferior vertebral body. Some of the costovertebral facets also articulate with the interposed intervertebral disc, whereas the 1st, 11th, and 12th ribs articulate with only one vertebra. A thin, fibrous capsule, which is strengthened by radiate ligaments and the posterior longitudinal ligament, surrounds the costovertebral joints. An intra-articular ligament lies within the capsule and holds the head of the rib to the annulus pulposus.

The costotransverse joints are the articulations between the costal tubercles of the 1st to the 10th ribs and the costal facets on the transverse processes of the 1st to the 10th thoracic vertebrae. The costal tubercles of the 1st to the 7th ribs are slightly convex, and the costal facets on the corresponding transverse processes are slightly concave (see Fig. 12–1*B*). The articular surfaces of the costal and vertebral facets are quite flat from about T7 to T10. The costotransverse joint capsules are strengthened by the medial, lateral, and superior costotransverse ligaments.

Osteokinematics

The zygapophyseal articular facets lie in the frontal plane from T1 to T6 and therefore limit flexion and extension in this region. The articular facets in the lower thoracic region are oriented more in the sagittal plane and thus permit somewhat more flexion and extension. The ribs and costal joints restrict lateral flexion in the upper and middle thoracic region, but in the lower thoracic segments, lateral flexion and rotation are relatively free because these segments are not limited by the ribs. In general, the thoracic region is less flexible than the cervi-

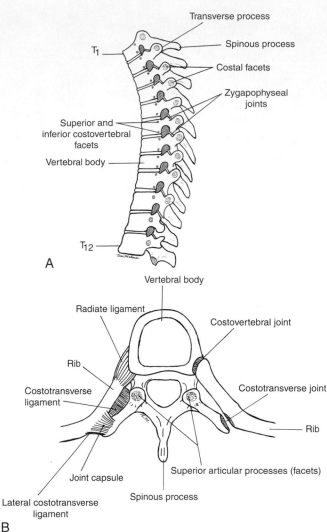

FIGURE 12–1 (*A*) A lateral view of the thoracic spine shows the costal facets on the enlarged ends of the transverse processes from T1 to T10 and the costovertebral facets on the lateral edges of the superior and inferior aspects of the vertebral bodies. The zygapophyseal joints are shown between the inferior articular facets of the superior vertebrae and the superior articular facets of the adjacent inferior vertebra. (*B*) A superior view of a thoracic vertebra shows the articulations between the vertebra and the ribs: the left and right costovertebral joints, the costotransverse joints between the costal facets on the left and right transverse processes, and the costal tubercles on the corresponding ribs.

cal spine because of the limitations on movement imposed by the overlapping spinous processes, the tighter joint capsules, and the rib cage.

Arthrokinematics

In flexion, the body of the superior vertebra tilts anteriorly, translates anteriorly and rotates slightly on the adjacent inferior vertebra. At the zygapophyseal joints, the inferior articular facets of the superior vertebra slide upwards on the superior articular facets of the adjacent inferior vertebra. In extension, the opposite motions occur: the superior vertebra tilts and translates posteriorly and the inferior articular facets glide downward on the superior articular facets of the adjacent inferior vertebra.

In lateral flexion to the right, the right inferior articular facets of the superior vertebra glide downward on the right superior articular facets of the inferior vertebra. On the contralateral side, the left inferior articular facets of the superior vertebra glide upward on the left superior articular facets of the adjacent inferior vertebra.

In axial rotation, the superior vertebra rotates on the inferior vertebra, and the inferior articular surfaces of the superior vertebra impact on the superior articular surfaces of the adjacent inferior vertebra. For example, in rotation to the left, the right inferior articular facet impacts on the right superior articular facet of the adjacent inferior vertebra. Rotation and gliding motions occur between the ribs and the vertebral bodies at the costovertebral joints. A slight amount of rotation is possible between the joint surfaces of the ribs and the transverse processes at the upper costotransverse joints, and more rotation is allowed in the gliding that occurs at the lower joints (T7 to T10). The movements at the costal joints are primarily for ventilation of the lungs but also allow some flexibility of the thoracic region.

Capsular Pattern

The capsular pattern for the thoracic spine is a greater limitation of extension, lateral flexion, and rotation than of forward flexion.

Lumbar Spine

Anatomy

The bodies of the five lumbar vertebrae are more massive than those in the other regions of the spine. Spinous processes are broad and thick and extend horizontally (Fig. 12–2A). Surfaces of the superior articular facets at the zygapophyseal joints are concave and face medially and posteriorly. Inferior articular facet surfaces are convex and face laterally and anteriorly. The fifth lumbar vertebra differs from the other four vertebrae in having a wedge-shaped body, with the anterior height greater than the posterior height. The inferior articular facets of the fifth vertebra are widely spaced for articulation with the sacrum.

Joint capsules are strong and ligaments of the region are essentially the same as those for the thoracic region, except for the addition of the iliolumbar and thoracolumbar fascia. The supraspinous ligament is well developed only in the upper lumbar spine. The interspinous ligaments connect one spinous process to another. The iliolumbar ligament helps to stabilize the lumbosacral joint and prevent anterior displacement. The intertrans-

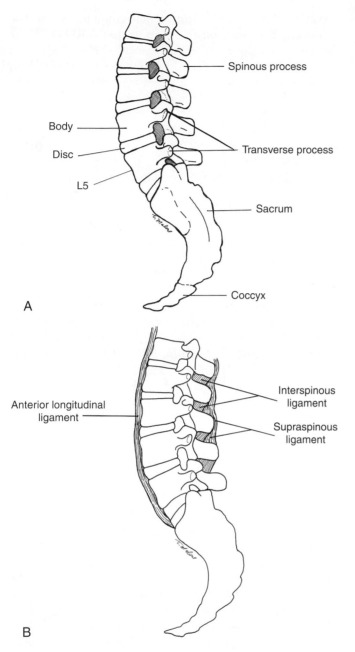

FIGURE 12–2 (*A*) A lateral view of the lumbar spine shows the broad, thick, horizontally oriented spinous processes and large vertebral bodies. (*B*) A lateral view of the lumbar spine shows the anterior longitudinal, supraspinous, and interspinous ligaments.

verse ligament is well developed in the lumbar area, and the anterior longitudinal ligament is strongest in this area (see Fig. 12–2*B*). The posterior longitudinal ligament is not well developed in the lumbar area.

Osteokinematics

The zygapophyseal articular facets of L1 to L4 lie primarily in the sagittal plane, which favors flexion and extension and limits lateral flexion and rotation. Flexion of the lumbar spine is more limited than extension. During combined flexion and extension, the greatest mobility takes place between L4 and L5. The greatest amount of flexion takes place at the lumbosacral joint, L5-S1. Lateral flexion and rotation are greatest in the upper lumbar region, and little or no lateral flexion is present at the lumbosacral joint because of the orientation of the facets.

Arthrokinematics

According to Bogduk,[1] flexion at the intervertebral joints consistently involves a combination of 8 to 13 degrees of anterior rotation (tilting), 1 to 3 mm of anterior translation (sliding), and some axial rotation. The superior vertebral body rotates, tilts, and translates (slides) anteriorly on the adjacent inferior vertebral body. During flexion at the zygapophyseal joints, the inferior articular facets of the superior vertebra slide upward on the superior articular facets of the adjacent inferior vertebra. In extension, the opposite motions occur: The vertebral body of the superior vertebra tilts and slides posteriorly on the adjacent inferior vertebra, and the inferior articular facets of the superior vertebra slide downward on the superior articular facets of the adjacent inferior vertebra. In lateral flexion, the superior vertebra tilts and translates laterally on the adjacent vertebra below.

In lateral flexion to the right, the right inferior articular facets of the superior vertebra slide downward on the right superior facets of the adjacent inferior vertebra. The left inferior articular facets of the superior vertebra slide upward on the left superior facets of the adjacent inferior vertebra. In axial rotation, the superior vertebra rotates on the inferior vertebra, and the inferior articular surfaces of the superior vertebra impact on the superior articular facet surfaces of the adjacent inferior vertebra. In rotation to the left, the right inferior articular facet impacts on the right superior facet of the adjacent inferior vertebra.

Capsular Pattern

The capsular pattern for the lumbar spine is a marked and equal restriction of lateral flexion followed by restriction of flexion and extension.[2]

◗ Research Findings

Table 12–1 shows thoracolumbar spine range of motion (ROM) values from the American Academy of Orthopaedic Surgeons (AAOS)[3] and lumbar spine ROM values from the American Medical Association (AMA).[4]

Effects of Age, Gender, and Other Factors

Age

A wide range of instruments and methods have been used to determine the range of thoracic, thoracolumbar, and

TABLE 12–1 Thoracic and Lumbar Spine Motion: Values in Inches and Degrees from Selected Sources

Motion	AAOS* [3]	AMA† [4]
Flexion	4	60
Extension	20–30	25
Right lateral flexion	35	25
Left lateral flexion	35	25
Right rotation	45	30

AAOS = American Association of Orthopaedic Surgeons; AMA = American Medical Association.

* Values represent thoracolumbar motion. Flexion measurement in inches was obtained with a tape measure with use of the spinous processes of C7 and S1 as reference points. The remaining motions were measured with a universal goniometer and are in degrees.

† Lumbosacral motion was measured from midsacrum to T12 with use of a two-inclinometer method (values in degrees).

lumbar motion. Therefore, comparisons between studies are difficult. As is true for other regions of the body, conflicting evidence exists regarding the effects of age on ROM. However, most studies indicate that age-related changes in the ROM occur and that these changes may affect certain motions more than others at the same joint or region.[5–11]

In one of the earlier studies, Loebl[5] used an inclinometer to measure active ROM of the thoracic and lumbar spine of 126 males and females between 15 and 84 years of age. He found age-related effects for both males and females and concluded that both genders should expect a loss of about 8 degrees of spinal ROM per decade with increases in age. In a more recent study, Sullivan, Dickinson and Troup[6] used double inclinometers to measure sagittal plane lumbar motion in 1126 healthy male and female subjects. These authors found that when gender was controlled, flexion, extension, and total ROM decreased with increasing age. The authors suggested that the ROM thresholds that determine impairment ratings should take age into consideration.

Different measurement methods were used in each of the following three studies to assess the effects of age on lumbar sagittal plane ROM. In each instance, the investigators found decreases in ROM with increases in age. Macrae and Wright,[7] using a modification of the Schober technique to measure forward flexion in 195 women and 147 men (18 to 71 years of age), found that active flexion ROM decreased with age. Moll and Wright[8] used skin markings and a plumb line to measure the range of lumbar extension in a study involving 237 subjects (119 men and 118 women) aged 20 to 90 years. These authors found a wide variation in normal values but detected a gradual decrease in lumbar extension in subjects between 35 and 90 years of age. Anderson and

Sweetman[9] employed a device that combined a flexible rule and a hydrogoniometer to measure the ROM of 432 working men aged 20 to 59 years. Increasing age was associated with a lower total lumbar spine ROM (flexion and extension). From a total of 74 men who had less than 50 degrees combined flexion-extension, 32 were in the category of 50-year-old to 59-year-old subjects, compared with 9 in the group of 20-year-old to 29-year-old subjects. Of the 162 men who had more than 60 degrees total ROM, 22 were in the 50-year-old to 59-year-old group and 60 were in the 20-year-old to 29-year-old category.

One of the following two studies investigated segmental mobility, whereas the other investigated lumbar spine motion in all planes. Segmental and motion-specific changes were found with increasing age. Gracovetsky and associates[10] found a significant difference between young and old in a group of 40 subjects aged 19 to 64 years. Older subjects had decreased segmental mobility in the lower lumbar spine compared with younger subjects. To compensate for the decrease in mobility, the older subjects increased the contribution of the pelvis to flexion and extension. McGregor, McCarthy, and Hughes[11] found that although age had a significant effect on all planes of motion, the effect varied for each motion, and age accounted for only a small portion of the variability seen in the 203 normal subjects studied. Maximum extension was the most affected motion, with significant decreases between each decade. Lateral flexion decreased after age 40 and each decade thereafter. Flexion decreased initially after age 30 years but stayed the same until an additional decrease after age 50 years. No similar decreases or trends were found in axial rotation.

The results of a study by Fitzgerald and associates.[12] are presented in Table 12–2. The authors investigated effects of age on thoracolumbar ROM. A review of the values in Table 12–2 shows that the oldest group had considerably less motion than the youngest group in all motions except for flexion. The coefficients of variation indicated that a greater amount of variability existed in the ROM in the oldest groups.

Gender

Investigations of the effects of gender on lumbar spine ROM indicate that they may be motion specific and possibly age specific, but controversy still exists about which motions are affected, and some authors report that gender has no effects. The fact that investigators used different instruments and methods makes comparisons between studies difficult. For example, the research cited in the following paragraph was carried out by means of tape measures, inclinometers, and plumb lines.

Macrae and Wright[7] found that females had significantly less forward flexion than males across all age groups. Sullivan, Dickinson, and Troup[6] found that when age was controlled, mean flexion ROM was greater in

TABLE 12–2   Effects of Age on Lumbar and Thoracolumbar Spine Motion: Mean Values in Degrees

Motion	20–29 yrs n = 31 Mean (SD)	30–39 yrs n = 42 Mean (SD)	40–49 yrs n = 16 Mean (SD)	50–59 yrs n = 43 Mean (SD)	60–69 yrs n = 26 Mean (SD)	70–79 yrs n = 9 Mean (SD)
Flexion*	3.7 (0.7)	3.9 (1.0)	3.1 (0.8)	3.0 (1.1)	2.4 (0.7)	2.2 (0.6)
Extension	41.2 (9.6)	40.0 (8.8)	31.1 (8.9)	27.4 (8.0)	17.4 (7.5)	16.6 (8.8)
Right lateral flexion	37.6 (5.8)	35.3 (6.5)	27.1 (6.5)	25.3 (6.2)	20.2 (4.8)	18.0 (4.7)
Left lateral flexion	38.7 (5.7)	36.5 (6.0)	28.5 (5.2)	26.8 (6.4)	20.3 (5.3)	18.9 (6.0)

(SD) = Standard deviation.
Adapted from Fitzgerald, GK, et al: Objective assessment with establishment of normal values for lumbar spine range of motion. Phys Ther 63:1776, 1983. With the permission of the American Physical Therapy Association.
* Flexion measurements were obtained with use of the Schober method and are reported in centimeters. All other measurements were obtained with use of a universal goniometer and are reported in degrees. Subjects were 172 volunteer patients without current back pain.

males, but mean extension ROM and total ROM were significantly greater in females. Subjects in the study were 1126 healthy male and female volunteers aged 15 to 65 years. The authors noted that although female total ROM was significantly greater than male total ROM, the difference of 1.5 degrees was not clinically relevant. Age and gender combined accounted for only 14 percent of the variance in flexion, 25 percent in extension and 20 percent of the variance in total ROM. Measurements of lumbar spine motion were taken with an inclinometer. Flexion was measured in the sitting position and extension in the prone position (Table 12–3). Moll and Wright's[8] findings regarding lumbar spine extension are directly opposite to the findings of Sullivan, Dickinson, and Troup[6] in that Moll and Wright[8] determined that male mobility in extension significantly exceeded female mobility by 7 percent. Differences in findings between studies may have resulted from the fact that Moll and Wright did not control for age. These authors used skin markings and a plumb line to measure the range of lumbar extension in a study involving 237 subjects (119 males and 118 females) aged 15 to 90 years, who were clinically and radiologically normal relatives of patients with psoriatic arthritis (Tables 12–4 and 12–5).

In contrast to the preceding authors, the following two studies reported no significant effects for gender on lumbar spine ROM. Loebl[5] found no significant gender differences between the 126 males and females aged 15 to 84 years of age for measurements of lumbar flexion and extension. Bookstein and associates[13] used a tape measure to measure the lumbar extension ROM in 75 elementary school children aged 6 to 11 years. The authors found no differences for age or gender, but they found a significant difference for age-gender interaction in the 6-year-old group. Girls aged 6 years had a mean range of extension of 4.1 cm in contrast to the 6-year-old boys, who had a mean range of extension of 2.1 cm.

Occupation and Lifestyle

Researchers have investigated the following factors among others in relation to their effects on lumbar ROM: occupation, lifestyle,[11,14–16] time of day,[17] and disability.[6,18–22] Similar to the findings related to age and gender, the results have been controversial.

Sughara and colleagues,[14] using a device called a spinometer, studied age-related and occupation-related changes in thoracolumbar active ROM in 1071 men and 1243 women aged 20 to 60 years. The subjects were selected from three occupational groups: fishermen, farmers, and industrial workers. Although both flexion

TABLE 12–3   Effects of Age and Gender on Lumbar Motion in Individuals 15–65 years: Mean Values in Degrees *

Motion	Male 16–24 yrs n =122 Mean (SD)	Female 15–24 yrs n =161 Mean (SD)	Male 25–34 yrs n =295 Mean (SD)	Female 25–34 yrs n =143 Mean (SD)	Male 35–65 yrs n =269 Mean (SD)	Female 35–65 yrs n =136 Mean (SD)
Flexion	33 (9)	26 (9)	31 (8)	24 (8)	27 (8)	22 (8)
Extension	54 (10)	63 (9)	52 (9)	60 (10)	47 (9)	53 (9)

(SD) = Standard deviation.
Adapted from Sullivan, MS, Dickinson, CE, and Troup, JDG: The influence of age and gender on lumbar spine sagittal plane range of motion: A study of 1126 healthy subjects. Spine 19:682, 1994.
* ROM values obtained with a fluid filled inclinometer.

TABLE 12–4 Effects of Age and Gender on Lumbar and Thoracolumbar Motion in Individuals Age 15–44 years: Mean Values in Centimeters

	Male	Female	Male	Female	Male	Female
	15–24 yrs		25–34 yrs		35–44 yrs	
	n = 21	n = 10	n = 13	n = 16	n = 14	n = 18
Motion	Mean (SD)	Mean (SD)	Mean (SD)	Mean (SD)	Mean (SD)	Mean (SD)
Flexion*	7.23 (0.92)	6.66 (1.03)	7.48 (0.82)	6.69 (1.09)	6.88 (0.88)	6.29 (1.04)
Extension*	4.21 (1.64)	4.34 (1.52)	5.05 (1.41)	4.76 (1.53)	3.73 (1.47)	3.09 (1.31)
Right lateral flexion†	5.43 (1.30)	6.85 (1.46)	5.34 (1.06)	6.32 (1.93)	4.83 (1.34)	5.30 (1.61)
Left lateral flexion†	5.06 (1.40)	7.20 (1.66)	5.93 (1.07)	6.13 (1.42)	4.83 (0.99)	5.48 (1.30)

Adapted from Moll, JMH, and Wright, V: Normal range of spinal mobility: An objective clinical study. Ann Rheum Dis 30:381, 1971. The authors used skin markings and a plumb line on the thorax for lateral flexion.
(SD) = Standard deviation.
*Lumbar motion
†Thoracolumbar motion

and extension were found to decrease with increasing age, decreases in the extension ROM were greater than decreases in flexion. Decreases in active extension ROM were less in the group of fishermen and their wives than in the farmers and industrial worker groups and their wives. The authors concluded that because the fishermen's wives, like the fishermen, had more extension than other groups, variables other than the physical demands of fishing were affecting the maintenance of extension ROM in the fisherman group.

Sjolie[16] compared low-back strength and low-back and hip mobility between a group of 38 adolescents living in a community without access to pedestrian roads and a group of 50 adolescents with excellent access to pedestrian roads. Low-back mobility was measured by means of the modified Schober technique. The results showed that adolescents living in rural areas without easy access to pedestrian roads had less low-back extension and hamstring flexibility than their counterparts in urban areas. The hypothesis that negative associations would exist between school bus use and physical performance was confirmed. The distance traveled by the school bus was inversely associated with hamstring flexibility and other hip motions but not with low-back flexion. Walking or bicycling to leisure activities was positively associated with low-back strength, low-back extension ROM and hip flexion and extension.

Freidrich and colleagues[15] conducted a comprehensive examination of spinal posture during stooped walking in 22 male sewer workers aged 24 to 49 years. Working in a stooped posture has been identified as one of the risk factors associated with spinal disorders. Five posture levels corresponding to standardized sewer heights ranging from 150 to 105 cm were taped by a video-based motion analysis system. The results showed that the lumbar spine abruptly changed from the usual lordotic position in normal upright walking to a kyphotic position in mild, 150-cm headroom restriction. As ceiling height decreased, the neck progressively assumed a more extended lordotic position, the thoracic spine extended

TABLE 12–5 Effects of Age and Gender on Lumbar and Thoracolumbar Motion in Individuals Aged 45–74 years: Mean Values in Centimeters

	Male	Female	Male	Female	Male	Female
	45–54 yrs		55–64 yrs		65–74 yrs	
	n = 19	n = 23	n = 34	n = 30	n = 14	n = 14
Motion	Mean (SD)	Mean (SD)	Mean (SD)	Mean (SD)	Mean (SD)	Mean (SD)
Flexion*	7.17 (1.20)	6.02 (1.32)	6.87 (0.89)	6.08 (1.32)	5.67 (1.31)	4.93 (0.90)
Extension*	3.88 (1.19)	3.12 (1.36)	3.56 (1.28)	3.57 (1.32)	3.41 (1.56)	2.72 (0.95)
Right lateral flexion†	4.71 (1.35)	5.37 (1.54)	5.05 (1.30)	5.10 (1.85)	4.44 (1.03)	5.56 (2.04)
Left lateral flexion†	4.55 (0.94)	5.14 (1.54)	4.94 (1.22)	4.88 (1.61)	4.38 (0.98)	5.55 (2.16)

Adapted from Moll, JMH, and Wright, V: Normal range of spinal mobility: An objective clinical study. Ann Rheum Dis 30:381, 1971. The authors used skin markings and a plumb line on the thorax for lateral flexion.
(SD) = Standard deviation.
*Lumbar Motion
†Thoracolumbar Motion

and flattened, becoming less kyphotic, and the lumbar spine became more kyphotic. As expected, the older workers showed decreased segmental mobility in the lumbar spine and an increase in cervical lordosis with decreasing ceiling height.

Disability

Sullivan, Dickinson, and Troup[6] used dual inclinometers to measure lumbar spine sagittal motion in 1126 healthy individuals. The authors found a large variation in measurements and suggested that detection of ROM impairments might be difficult because 95 percent confidence intervals yielded up to a 36-degree spread in normal ROM values. Sullivan, Shoaf, and Riddle[18] examined the relationship between impairment of active lumbar flexion ROM and disability. The authors used normative data to determine when an impairment in flexion ROM was present, and used the judgement of physical therapists to determine whether flexion ROM impairment was relevant to the patient's disability. Low correlations between lumbar ROM and disability were found, and the authors concluded that active lumbar ROM measurements should not be used as treatment goals.

Lundberg and Gerdle[19] investigated spinal and peripheral joint mobility and spinal posture in 607 female employees (mean age = 40.5 years) working at least 50 percent part time as homecare personnel. Lumbar sagittal hypomobility alone was associated with higher disability, and a combination of positive pain provocation tests and lumbar sagittal hypomobility was associated with particularly high disability levels. Peripheral joint mobility, spinal sagittal posture, and thoracic sagittal mobility showed low correlations with disability.

Kujala and coworkers[20] conducted a 3-year longitudinal study of lumbar mobility and occurrence of low-back pain in 98 adolescents. The subjects included 33 nonathletes (16 males and 17 females), 34 male athletes, and 31 female athletes. Participation in sports and low maximal lumbar flexion predicted low-back pain during the follow-up in males but accounted for only 16 percent of the variance between groups with and without low-back pain. A decreased ROM in the lower lumbar segments, low maximal ROM in extension and high body weight were predictive of low-back pain in females and accounted for 31 percent of the variability between groups.

Natrass and associates[21] used a long-arm goniometer and dual inclinometers to measure low-back ROM in 34 patients with chronic low-back pain. ROM for all subjects was compared with their ratings on commonly used impairment and disability indexes. The investigators found no relationship between the ROM measurements and the impairment ratings as determined by the tests. The authors concluded that the instruments and methods of measurement had poor validity.

Shirley and colleagues[22] compared lumbar ROM values obtained with three different instruments in 44 patients with chronic low-back pain whose mean age was 38 years. Measurements obtained with the SPINETRAK (Motion Analysis Corp., Santa Rosa, Cal.) were significantly correlated (r = .62) with ROM determined by liquid inclinometers, but only mildly correlated with the MedX (lumbar extension testing and exercise machine) ROM measurements. T-test results showed that measurements taken with the SPINETRAK were significantly lower than those taken with either the liquid inclinometer or the MedX. The SPINETRAK measurements also were about 12 to 16 degrees lower than the values set by the AMA guide for determining disability.

Functional Range of Motion

Hsieh and Pringle[23] used a CA-6000 Spinal Motion Analyzer (Orthopedic Systems, Inc., Hayward, Cal.) to measure the amount of lumbar motion required for selected activities of daily living performed by 48 healthy subjects with a mean age of 26.5 years. Activities included stand to sit, sit to stand, putting on socks, and picking up an object from the floor. The individual's peak flexion angles for the activities were normalized to the subject's own peak flexion angle in erect standing. Stand to sit and sit to stand (Fig. 12-3) required approximately 56 percent to 66 percent of lumbar flexion. The mean

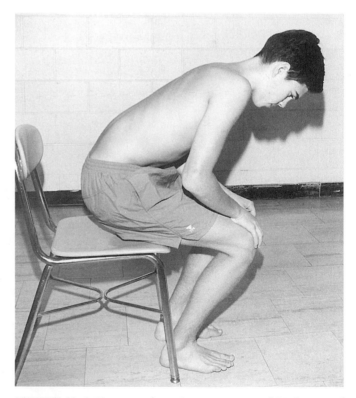

FIGURE 12–3 Sit to stand requires an average of 35 degrees of lumbar flexion.[23]

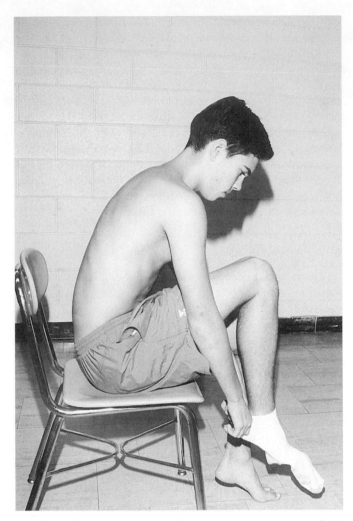

FIGURE 12–4 Putting on socks requires an average of 56 degrees of lumbar flexion.[23]

was 34.6 degrees (SD = 14 degrees) for sit to stand. The mean was 41.8 degrees (SD = 14.2 degrees) for stand to sit. Putting on socks (Fig. 12–4) required 90 percent of lumbar flexion (mean = 56.4 degrees and the SD = 15), and picking up an object from the floor (Fig. 12–5) required 95 percent of lumbar flexion (mean = 60.4 degrees). In view of these findings, one can understand how limitations in lumbar ROM may affect an individual's ability to independently carry out dressing and other activities of daily living.

Reliability and Validity

The following section on reliability and validity has been divided according to the instruments and methods used to obtain the measurements. Some overlap occurs between the sections because several investigators have compared different methods and instruments within one study.

Inclinometer

Loebl[5] has stated that the only reliable technique for measuring lumbar spine motion is radiography. However, radiography is expensive and poses a health risk to the subject; moreover, the validity of radiographic assessment of ROM is unreported. Therefore, researchers have used many different instruments and methods in a search for reliable and valid measures of lumbar spine motion. Loebl[5] used an inclinometer to measure flexion and extension in nine subjects. He found that in five repeated active measurements, the ROM varied by 5 degrees in the most consistent subject and by 23 degrees in the most inconsistent subject. Variability decreased when measurements were taken on an hourly basis rather than on a daily basis. Patel,[24] who used the double-inclinometer method to measure lumbar flexion on 25 subjects aged 21 to 37 years, found intratester reliability to be high (r = 0.91) but intertester reliability to be only moderate (r = 0.68).

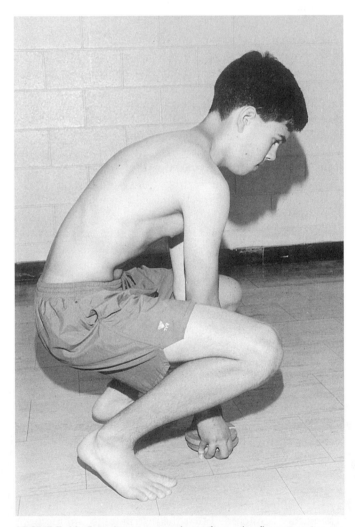

FIGURE 12–5 Picking up an object from the floor requires an average of 60 degrees of lumbar flexion.[23]

The AMA *Guides to the Evaluation of Permanent Impairment*[4] states that "measurement techniques using inclinometers are necessary to obtain reliable spinal mobility measurements." However, in a study by Williams and coworkers[25] that compared the measurements of the inclinometer with those of the tape measure, the authors found that the double-inclinometer technique had questionable reliability (Table 12–6).

Mayer and associates[26] compared repeated measurements of lumbar ROM of 18 healthy subjects taken by 14 different examiners using three different instruments: a fluid-filled inclinometer, the kyphometer, and the electrical inclinometer. The three instruments were found to be equally reliable, but significant differences were found between examiners. Poor intertester reliability was the most significant source of variance. The authors identified sources of error as being caused by differences in instrument placement among examiners and inability to locate the necessary landmarks.

Saur and colleagues[27] used Pleurimeter V inclinometers to measure lumbar ROM in 54 patients with chronic low-back pain who were between 18 and 60 years of age. Measurements were taken with and without radiographic verification of the T12 and S1 landmarks used for positioning the inclinometers. Also, correlation of radiographic ROM measurements with inclinometer ROM measurements demonstrated an almost linear correlation for flexion ($r = 0.98$) and total lumbar flexion/extension ROM ($r = 0.97$, but extension did not correlate as well ($r = 0.75$). Intertester reliability of the inclinometry technique for total ROM in a subgroup of 48 patients was high ($r = 0.94$), and flexion was good ($r = 0.88$), but extension was poor ($r = 0.42$). The authors concluded that the Pleurimeter V was a reliable and valid method for measuring lumbar ROM and that with use of this instrument it was possible to differentiate lumbar spine movements from hip movements.

In contrast to the findings of Saur and colleagues,[27] a number of authors[28-31] have reported poor criterion validity and poor intertester and intratester reliability with use of inclinometers. Samo and coworkers[28] compared radiographic measurements of lumbar ROM in 30 subjects with measurements taken with the following three instruments: a Pleurimeter V (double inclinometer), a carpenter's double inclinometer, and a computed single-sensor inclinometer. All ICCs between radiographs and for each method were below 0.90 and therefore judged by the authors to have poor criterion validity. Chen and associates[29] investigated intertester and intratester reliability using three health professionals

TABLE 12–6   Intratester and Intertester Reliability for Thoracolumbar and Lumbar ROM

Author	Subject n	Sample	Instrument	Motions	Intra ICC	Inter ICC	Intra r	Inter r
Fitzgerald[12]	17	Healthy	Tape Measure* (Schober)	Flexion				1.0
			Universal Goniometer+	Extension				.88
				R. lat. Flex.				.76
				L. lat.Flex.				.91
Breum et al [32]	47	Healthy (18–38 yrs)	BROM II*	Flexion	.91	.77		
				Extension	.63	.35		
				R. lat.Flex.	.89	.89		
				R. Rotation	.57	.35		
Madson et al[33]	40	Healthy (20–40 yrs)	BROM*	Flexion	.67			
				Extension	.78			
				R. lat. Flex.	.95			
				R. Rotation	.93			
Petersen et al[47]	21	Healthy (10–79 yrs)	OSI-CA 6000 +	Flexion	.90	.85		
				Extension	.96	.96		
				R. lat Flex.	.89	.85		
				R. Rotation	.95	.90		
Williams et al[25]	25	Back pain (25–53 yrs)	Tape Measure (MMS)*	Flexion		.72	.78–.89	
				Extension		.76	.69–.91	
			Dual Inclinometers*	Flexion		.60	.13–.87	
				Extension		.48	.28–.66	
Nitschke et al [31]	34	Back pain (20–65yrs)	Universal Goniometer +	Flexion	.92	.84		
				Extension	.81	.63		
				R. lat.Flex	.76	.62		
			Dual Inclinometers *	Flexion	.90	.52		
				Extension	.70	.35		
				R. lat Flex.	.90	.18		

BROM II= Back Range of Motion Device; OSI CA 6000 = Spine Motion Analyzer; MMS= Modified Modified Schober
* Lumbar ROM
+ Thoracolumbar ROM

to measure lumbar ROM with the same instruments used in the study by Samo and coworkers[28] Intertester reliability was poor, with all ICCs below 0.75, and with a single exception, intratester reliability was below 0.90. The authors determined that the largest source of measurement error was attributable to the examiners and associated factors and concluded that these three surface methods had only limited clinical usefulness.

Mayer and colleagues[30] used a Cybex EDI-320 (Lumex, Ron Konkoma, NY), a computed inclinometer with a single sensor, to measure lumbar ROM in 38 healthy individuals. Total sagittal ROM was the most accurate measurement and extension was the least accurate. Errors in locating T12 and S1, improper instruction of patients, lack of firm placement of the inclinometer, device error, and human variability contributed to a lack of measurement accuracy. Clinical utility of lumbar sagittal plane ROM measurement appeared to be highly sensitive to the training of the test administrator in aspects of the process such as locating bony landmarks and maintaining inclinometer placement without rocking on the sacrum. The authors determined that device error was negligible relative to the error associated with the test process itself and that practice was the most significant factor in eliminating the largest source of error when inexperienced examiners were used.

Nitschke and colleagues[31] compared the following measurement methods in a study involving 34 male and female subjects with chronic low-back pain and two examiners: dual inclinometers for lumbar spine ROM (flexion, extension, and lateral flexion) and a plastic long arm goniometer for thoracolumbar ROM (flexion, extension, lateral flexion, and rotation).

Intertester reliability was poor for all measurements except for flexion taken with the long arm goniometer (Table 12–6). The dual inclinometer method had no systematic error, but there was a large random error for all measurements. The authors concluded that the standard error of measurement might be a better indicator of reliability than the ICC.

Back Range of Motion Device

The back range of motion (BROM) II device (Performance Attainment Associates, Roseville, Minn.) has been used to measure lumbar spine motion. It is relatively expensive (see Appendix B), and we are not convinced that its measurements are better than less expensive measurement methods. Two groups of researchers investigating the reliability of the BROM II device agreed that the instrument had high reliability for measuring lumbar lateral flexion and low reliability for measuring extension. However, the two groups differed regarding the reliability of the BROM II device for measuring flexion and rotation. Breum, Wiberg, and Bolton[32] concluded that the BROM II device could measure flexion and rotation reliably, whereas Madson, Youdas, and

Suman[33] determined that rotation but not flexion could be reliably measured (see Table 12–6). Potential sources of error identified by Madson, Youdas, and Suman[33] included slippage of the device over the sacrum during flexion and extension and variations in the identification of landmarks from one measurement to another.

Tape Measure Methods

Macrae and Wright,[7] tested the validity of both the original two-mark Schober technique and a three-mark modification of the Schober technique (modified Schober). The authors found a linear relationship between measurements of lumbar flexion obtained by these methods and measurements taken radiographically. The correlation coefficient was 0.90 between the Schober technique and radiographs (x-rays) with a standard error of 6.2 degrees. The correlation coefficient was 0.97 between the modified Schober measurement and the radiographic measurements, with a standard error of 3.25 degrees. Clinical identification of the lumbosacral junction was not easy, and faulty placement of skin marks seriously impaired the accuracy of the unmodified Schober technique. Placement of marks 2 cm too low led to an overestimate of 14 degrees. Marks placed 2 cm too high led to an underestimate of 15 degrees. In the modified Schober technique, the same errors in placement led to overestimates and underestimates of 5 and 3 degrees, respectively.

Reynolds[34] compared intratester and intertester reliability with use of a spondylometer, a plumb line and skin distraction, and an inclinometer. Subjects were 30 volunteers with a mean age of 38.1 years. Intertester error was calculated by comparing the results of two testers taking 10 repeated measurements of lumbar flexion, extension, and lateral flexion on 30 volunteers with a mean age of 38.1 years. Highly significant positive correlations were found between flexion-extension ROM measured with the inclinometer and that measured with the spondylometer. Lumbar flexion measurements correlated well with skin distraction and the inclinometer. The inclinometer had acceptable intertester reliability, but the skin distraction method had acceptable intertester reliability only for extension. The highest intratester reliability was found for inclinometer measurement of lateral flexion to the right.

Miller and colleagues[35] compared the following four methods for measuring thoracolumbar mobility: the fingertip-to-floor method, the modified Schober technique, the OB Myrin gravity goniometer (LIC Rehab, Sweden), and a skin contraction 10-cm-segment method with a tape measure. Four testers using all four methods measured four subjects (one healthy subject and three patients with ankylosing spondylitis). Intertester error was not found to be a significant source of variation. The 10-cm-segment method was found to be the most sensitive in detecting a loss of spinal mobility in the upper and middle 10-cm segments. The fingertip-to-floor method was the next sensitive, followed by the 10-cm-segment technique for the lower 10-cm segment, and the modified Schober technique. The least sensitive was the OB Myrin goniometric measurement. The testers rated the fingertip-to-floor method as the most convenient, followed by the modified Schober technique, the 10-cm-segment method, and the OB Myrin goniometric technique.

Portek and colleagues[36] compared the modified Schober method and two other clinical methods with each other and with radiographs. These authors found little correlation either among the measurements obtained by two testers using three clinical techniques to measure lumbar flexion in 11 subjects or among the three clinical techniques and radiographs. A Pearson's reliability coefficient of 0.43 was found between the modified Schober technique and the radiographic measurement. The intertester error for the modified Schober method for lumbar flexion showed significant differences between testers according to paired t-tests. However, intertester error was calculated between 10 measurements on 10 different days, and the authors attributed the error to difficulties in reestablishing a neutral starting position and the mobility of the skin over the landmarks.

Gill and coworkers[37] compared the reliability of four methods of measurement including fingertip-to-floor distance, the modified Schober technique, the two-inclinometer method, and a photometric technique. The subjects of the study were 10 volunteers (five men and five women), aged 24 to 34 years. Repeatability of the fingertip-to-floor method was poor (CV = 14.1 percent). Repeatability of the inclinometer for the measurement of full flexion was also poor (CV = 33.9 percent). However, the modified Schober technique yielded a CV of 0.9 percent for full flexion and a CV of 2.8 percent for extension.

Fitzgerald and associates[12] used the Schober technique to measure forward lumbar flexion and the universal goniometer to measure thoracolumbar lateral flexion and extension. Intertester reliability was calculated from measurements taken by two testers on 17 physical therapy student volunteers. Pearson reliability coefficients were calculated on paired results of the two testers (see Table 12–6).

Williams and coworkers[25] measured flexion and extension on 15 patient volunteers (eight females and seven males) with a mean age of 35.7 years who had chronic low-back pain. The authors compared the modified–modified Schober technique (MMS),[38] which is also referred to as the simplified skin distraction method,[39] with the double-inclinometer method. Intratester Pearson correlation coefficients for the MMS were 0.89 for tester 1, 0.78 for tester 2, and 0.83 for tester 3. Intertester Pearson correlation coefficients between the three physical therapist testers were 0.72 for flexion and 0.77 for extension with use of the MMS. The therapists under-

went training in the use of standardized procedures for each method prior to testing. According to the testers, the MMS was easier and quicker to use than the double-inclinometer method. The only disadvantage to using the MMS method is that norms have not been established for all age groups.

Flexible Ruler

The flexible ruler has been investigated as a possible instrument for measuring lumbar spine ROM as well as fixed postures.[40–44] Measurements taken with the ruler must be calculated, and Youdas, Suman, and Garrett[41] determined that two commonly used methods for calculating measurements can be used interchangeably. ICCs for each motion and calculation method in this study were in the good (0.80 to 0.90) to high (0.90 to 0.99) range. Lindahl[40] described the flexible ruler as providing a "fairly accurate" method of measuring flexion and extension compared with the fingertip-to-floor method. Lovell, Rothstein, and Personius,[44] in a study involving 80 subjects, found that the intratester reliability for measuring lumbar lordosis ranged from 0.73 to 0.94. However, intertester reliability was poor. Bryan and colleagues[43] measured lumbar lordosis in 45 subjects and found a poor correlation between measurements taken with the flexible ruler and radiographs. Based upon a lack of norms and the fact that the flexible ruler has been used only for measuring flexion and extension, we decided not to include this instrument in the procedures section of the book.

Functional Axial Rotation Device

Schenkman and coworkers[45] developed a device and a measurement technique for quantifying axial rotation of the spine. The functional axial rotation (FAR) device consists of a 1-m-diameter circular hoop that is suspended by tripods at the eye level of a seated subject . It is designed to measure functional movements of the neck and trunk such as those that occur when one rotates the body to look at children in the back seat of a car. Axial motion is quantified by the distance that the head is moved in relation to the pelvis. In a study of 17 subjects aged 20 to 74 years, test retest reliability was high (ICC greater than 0.90) and intertester reliability was also high (ICC = 0.97). In a subsequent study by Schenkman and associates[46] involving 15 patients with Parkinson's disease, ranging from 64 to 84 years of age, the ICC for test retest reliability was 0.89.

Motion Analysis Systems

A number of researchers have investigated the reliability of motion analysis systems including, among others, the CA-6000 Spine Motion Analyzer,[11,12,47] the SPINE-TRAK,[48] and the FASTRAK (Polhemus, Colchester, Vt.).[49] Two research groups found that intratester reliability for measuring lumbar flexion was very high with use of the CA-6000.[11,23] In one of the studies, both intratester and intertester reliability ranged from good to high for lumbar forward flexion and extension, but intratester and intertester reliability were poor for rotation.[11] In a study using the SPINETRAK,[48] ICCs were 0.89 or greater for intratester reliability. ICCs for intertester reliability ranged from 0.77 for thoracolumbar flexion to 0.95 for thoracolumbopelvic flexion. Steffan and colleagues[49] used the FASTRAK system to measure segmental motion in forward lumbar flexion by tracking sensors attached to Kirschner wires that had been inserted into the spinous processes of L3 and L4 in 16 healthy men. Segmental forward flexion showed large intersubject variation.

Summary

The sampling of studies reviewed in this chapter reflects the amount of effort that has been directed toward finding a reliable and valid method for measuring spinal motion. Each method reviewed has advantages and disadvantages, and clinicians should first select a method that appears to be appropriate for their particular clinical situation and then determine its reliability.

Range of Motion Testing Procedures

The testing procedures that are presented in the next section include the universal goniometer, the tape measure method, the modified Schober technique as described by Macrae and Wright,[7] the MMS technique or simplified skin distraction method, and the double-inclinometer method. The first four methods were selected because they were inexpensive, were relatively easy to use, and had reliability and validity comparable with other methods. The inclinometer method has been included in this edition because examiners may find these instruments being used in the clinical setting. We hope that by the time the next edition of this textbook is being prepared, more norms will have been published for the simplified skin distraction method and that additional evidence regarding the reliability and validity of methods of measuring spinal ROM will be available.

Anatomical Landmarks: For Tape Measure Alignment

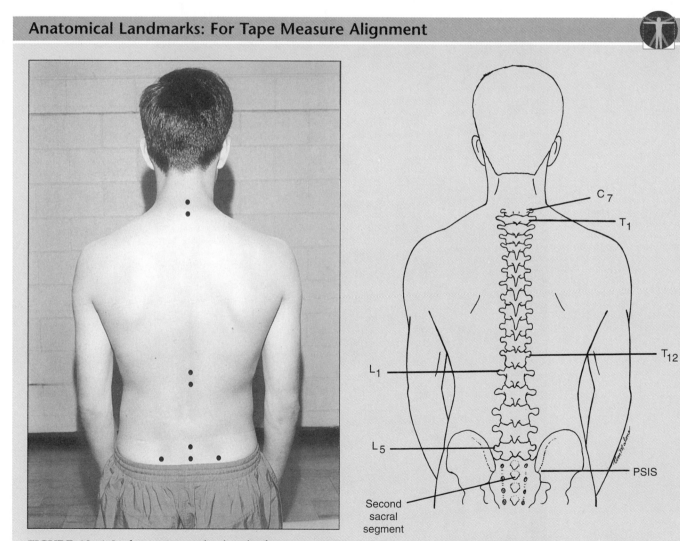

FIGURE 12–6 Surface anatomy landmarks for tape measure and inclinometer alignment for measuring the thoracic and lumbar spine motion. The dots are located over spinous processes of C7, T1, T12, L1, L5, and S2 as well as over the right and left posterior superior iliac spines (PSIS).

FIGURE 12–7 Bony anatomical landmarks for tape measure and inclinometer alignment for measuring thoracic and lumbar spine motion.

THORACIC AND LUMBAR FLEXION

Motion occurs in the sagittal plane around a medial-lateral axis.

Testing Position

Place the subject standing, with the cervical, thoracic, and lumbar spine in 0 degrees of lateral flexion and rotation.

Stabilization

Stabilize the pelvis to prevent anterior tilting.

Testing Motion

Direct the subject to bend forward gradually while keeping the arms relaxed (Fig. 12–8). The end of the motion occurs when resistance to additional flexion is experienced by the subject and the examiner feels the pelvis start to tip anteriorly.

Normal End-feel

The normal end-feel is firm owing to the stretching of the posterior longitudinal ligament (in the thoracic region), the ligamentum flavum, the supraspinous and interspinous ligaments, and the posterior fibers of the annulus pulposus of the intervertebral discs and the zygapophyseal joint capsules. Passive tension in the thoracolumbar fascia and the following muscles may contribute to the end-feel: spinalis thoracis, semispinalis thoracis, iliocostalis lumborum and iliocostalis thoracis, interspinales, intertransversarii, longissimus thoracis, and multifidus. The orientation of the zygapophyseal facets from T1 to T6 restrict flexion in the upper thoracic spine.

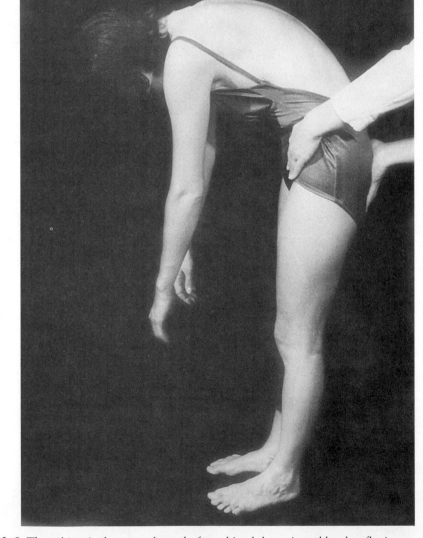

FIGURE 12–8 The subject is shown at the end of combined thoracic and lumbar flexion range of motion. The examiner is shown stabilizing the subject's pelvis to prevent anterior pelvic tilting.

Measurement Method for Thoracic and Lumbar Flexion: Tape Measure

Four inches is considered to be an average measurement for healthy adults.[3]

1. Use a skin-marking pencil to mark the spinous processes of C7 and S1.
2. Align the tape measure between the two processes and note the distance (Fig. 12–9).
3. Hold the tape measure in place as the subject performs flexion ROM. (Allow the tape measure to unwind and accommodate the motion.)
4. Record the distance at the end of the ROM (Fig. 12–10). The difference between the first and the second measurements indicates the amount of thoracic and lumbar flexion that is present.

Alternative Measurement Method for Thoracic and Lumbar Flexion: Fingertip-to-Floor

In this method the subject is asked to bend forward as far as possible in an attempt to touch the floor with the fingers while keeping knees extended. No stabilization is provided by the examiner.

At the end of flexion ROM, measure the distance between the tip of the subject's middle finger and the floor. This test combines spinal flexion and hip flexion, making it impossible to isolate and measure either motion. Therefore, this test is not recommended for measuring thoracic and lumbar flexion, but it can be used to assess general body flexibility.[50–52]

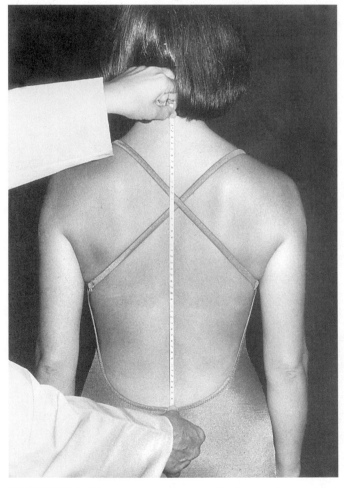

FIGURE 12–9   Tape measure alignment in the starting position for measuring thoracic and lumbar flexion range of motion.

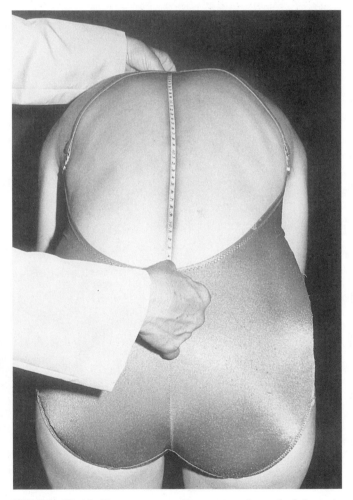

FIGURE 12–10   Tape measure alignment at the end of thoracic and lumbar flexion range of motion. The metal tape measure case (not visible in the photo) is in the examiner's right hand.

Alternative Measurement Method for Thoracic and Lumbar Flexion: Double Inclinometer

1. Use a skin-marking pencil to mark the midline of the midsacrum and the spinous process of the seventh cervical vertebra with the subject in the upright 0 starting position.
2. Position one inclinometer over the midsacrum. Position the other inclinometer over the spinous process of the seventh cervical vertebra, and zero both instruments prior to beginning the motion (Fig. 12–11).
3. At the end of the motion, read and note the information on both inclinometers (Fig. 12–12). The difference between the two inclinometers indicates the amount of thoracic and lumbar flexion ROM.

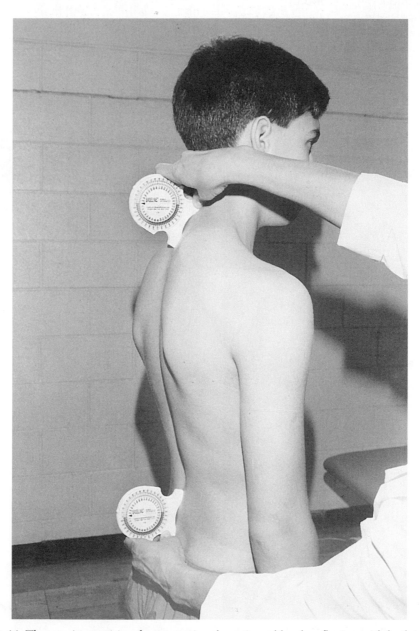

FIGURE 12–11 The starting position for measuring thoracic and lumbar flexion with both inclinometers aligned and zeroed.

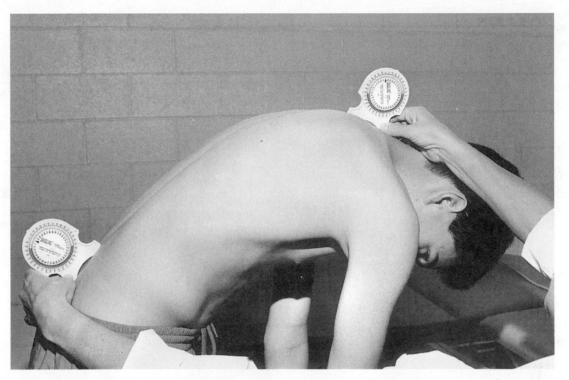

FIGURE 12–12 Inclinometer alignment at the end of thoracic and lumbar flexion range of motion.

LUMBAR FLEXION

Testing Position

Place the subject standing, with the cervical, thoracic, and lumbar spine in 0 degrees of lateral flexion and rotation.

Stabilization

Stabilize the pelvis to prevent anterior tilting

Testing Motion

Ask the subject to bend forward as far as possible while keeping the knees straight.

Normal End-feel

The end feel is firm owing to stretching of the ligamentum flavum, posterior fibers of the annulus fibrosus and zygapophyseal joint capsules, thoracolumbar fascia, iliolumbar ligaments and the multifidus, quadratus lumborum, iliocostalis lumborum, and longissimus thoracis muscles. The location of the following muscles suggests that they may limit flexion, but the actual actions of the interspinales and the intertransversarii mediales and laterales are unknown.[1]

Measurement Method for Lumbar Flexion: Modified–Modified Schober Test[25,38] or Simplified Skin Distraction Method[39]

In the original Schober method, the examiner made only two marks on the subject's back. The first mark was made at the lumbosacral junction and the second 10 cm above the first mark on the spine. Macrae and Wright[7] decided to modify the Schober method because they believed skin movement was a problem in the original method and that the skin was more firmly attached in the

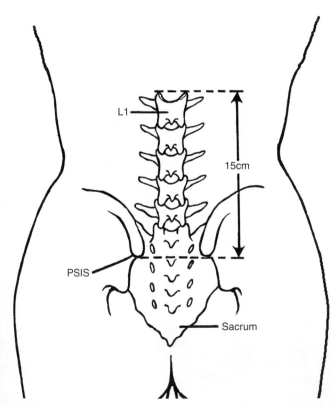

FIGURE12–13 A line is drawn between the two posterior superior iliac spines and the point at which the lower end of the tape measure should be positioned. The location of the 15-cm mark shows that all five of the lumbar vertebrae in this subject are included.

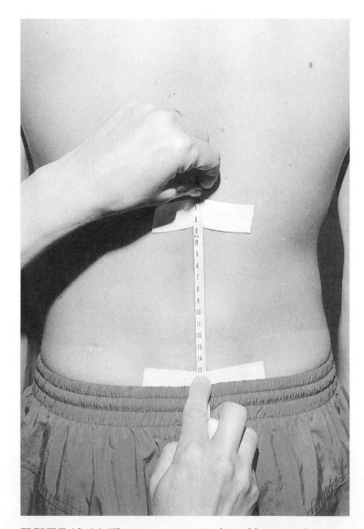

FIGURE 12–14 The tape measure is aligned between the upper and the lower landmarks at the beginning of lumbar flexion range of motion. Paper tape was placed over the skin marking pencil dots to improve visibility of landmarks for the photograph.

region below the lumbosacral junction. However, beginning the measurement 5 cm below the lumbosacral junction places the most superior mark at L2 or L3; therefore, the measurement in Macrae and Wright's[7] modified method does not include the entire lumbar spine. Furthermore, examiners experienced difficulties in accurately locating the lumbosacral junction. Macrae and Wright's method is presented in this text as an alternative measurement method following the Modified-Modified Schober Test (MMST)[38] or the simplified skin distraction method,[39] which is presented in the next paragraph.

The MMST uses two marks, one over the spine on a line connecting the two posterior-superior iliac spines (PSIS) and the other over the spine 15 cm superior to the first mark. This technique was proposed by van Adrichem and van der Korst[38] to eliminate errors in identification of the lumbosacral junction and to make sure that the entire lumbar spine was included.

Van Adrichem and van der Korst,[38] using the MMST, found a mean of 6.7 cm (SD = 1.0 cm) in male subjects between 15 and 18 years of age and a mean of 5.8 cm (SD = 0.9 cm) in female subjects in the same age group.

Tape measure alignment: MMST

1. Use a skin-marking pencil to mark the subject's two posterior superior iliac spines. Use a ruler to locate and mark a midline point on the sacrum that is on a level with the iliac spines. Make a mark on the lumbar spine that is 15 cm above the midline sacral mark (Fig. 12–13).
2. Align the tape measure between the superior and the inferior marks. (Fig. 12–14) Ask the subject to bend forward as far as possible while keeping the knees straight.
3. Maintain the tape measure against the subject's back during the movement but the allow the tape measure to unwind to accomodate the motion. At the end of the flexion ROM, note the distance between the two marks (Fig. 12–15). The ROM is the difference between 15 cm and the length measured at the end of the motion.

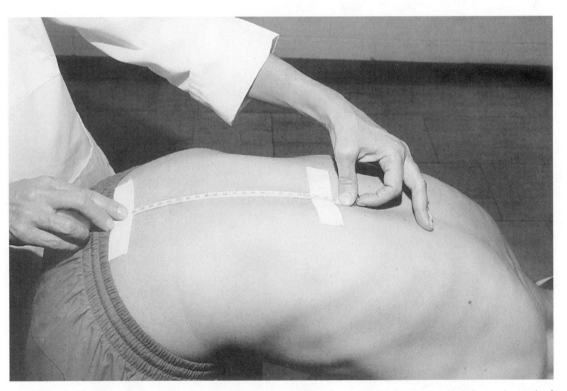

FIGURE 12–15 The tape measure is stretched between the upper and the lower landmarks at the end of lumbar flexion range of motion.

Alternative Measurement Method for Lumbar Flexion: Modified Schober Technique[7]

Macrae and Wright found an average of 6.3 cm[7] of flexion in healthy adults, and Battie and coworkers[53] found an average of 6.9 cm in a similar group of subjects.

1. Use a skin-marking pencil to place a mark at the lumbosacral junction. Place a second mark 10 centimeters above the first (measure to the nearest millimeter). Place a third mark 5 centimeters below the first (lumbosacral junction).

2. Align the tape measure between the most superior and the most inferior marks. Ask the subject to bend forward as far as possible while keeping the knees straight.

3. Maintain the tape measure against the subject's back during the movement and note the distance between the most superior and the most inferior marks at the end of the ROM. The ROM is the difference between 15 cm and the length measured at the end of the motion.

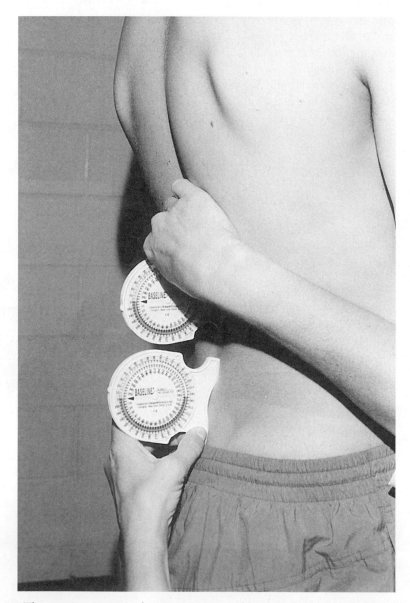

FIGURE 12–16 The starting position for measurement of lumbar flexion range of motion, with inclinometers aligned and zeroed.

Alternative Measurement Method for Lumbar Flexion: Double Inclinometer

The ROM in flexion is 60 degrees according to the AMA[4] and 0 to 66 degrees (for males 15 to 30 years of age) according to Loebl.[5]

1. Use a skin-marking pencil to place a mark in the midline of the midsacrum and a second mark over the spinous process of T12.
2. Place one inclinometer over the spinous process of T12 and the other over the midsacrum. (Fig. 12–16).

3. Zero both inclinometers, and ask the subject to bend forward as far as possible while keeping the knees straight.
4. Note the information on the inclinometers at the end of the flexion ROM (Fig. 12–17). Calculate lumbar flexion ROM by subtracting the degrees from the dial of the sacral inclinometer from those on the dial on the T12 inclinometer. The degrees on the sacral inclinometer are supposed to represent hip flexion ROM.[39]

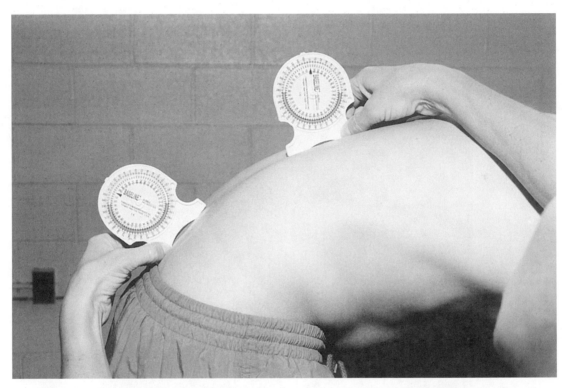

FIGURE 12–17 The end of lumbar flexion range of motion, with inclinometers aligned over the spinous processes of T12 and S1.

THORACIC AND LUMBAR EXTENSION

Motion occurs in the sagittal plane around a medial-lateral axis.

Testing Position

Place the subject standing, with the cervical, thoracic, and lumbar spine in 0 degrees of lateral flexion and rotation.

Stabilization

Stabilize the pelvis to prevent posterior tilting.

Testing Motion

Ask the subject to extend the spine as far as possible (Fig. 12–18). The end of the extension ROM occurs when the pelvis begins to tilt posteriorly.

Normal End-feel

The end feel is firm owing to stretching of the zygapophyseal joint capsules, anterior fibers of the annulus fibrosus, anterior longitudinal ligament, rectus abdominis, and external and internal oblique abdominals. The end-feel also may be hard owing to contact by the spinous processes and the zygapophyseal facets.

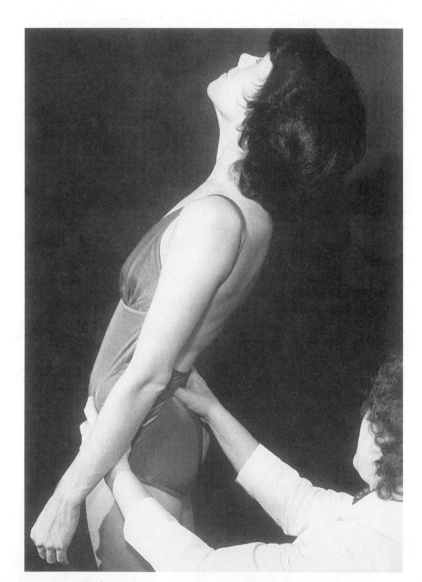

FIGURE 12–18 At the end of thoracic and lumbar extension range of motion, the examiner uses one hand on the subject's anterior pelvis and her other hand on the posterior pelvis to prevent posterior pelvic tilting. If the subject has balance problems or muscle weakness in the lower extremities, the measurement can be taken in either the prone or side-lying position.

Measurement Method for Thoracic and Lumbar Extension: Tape Measure

1. Use a skin-marking pencil to mark the spinous processes of C7 and S1.
2. Align the tape measure between the two marks and record the measurement (Fig. 12–19).

3. Keep the tape measure aligned during the motion and record the measurement at the end of the ROM (Fig. 12–20). The difference between the measurement taken at the beginning of the motion and that taken at the end indicates the amount of thoracic and lumbar extension that is present.

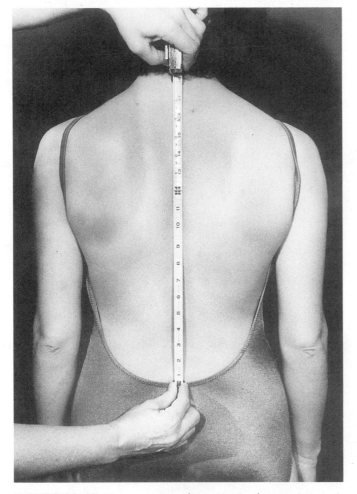

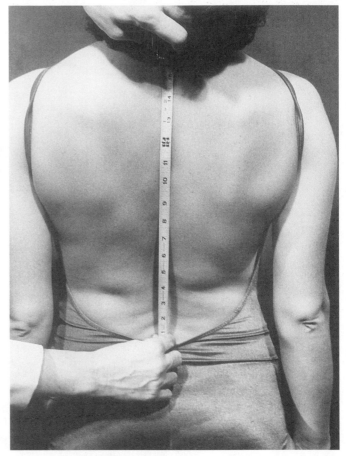

FIGURE 12–19 Tape measure alignment in the starting position for measurement of thoracic and lumbar extension range of motion. When the subject moves into extension, the tape slides into the tape measure case in the examiner's hand.

FIGURE 12–20 At the end of thoracic and lumbar extension range of motion, the distance between the two landmarks is less than it was in the starting position.

LUMBAR EXTENSION

Testing Position

Place the subject standing, with the cervical, thoracic, and lumbar spine in 0 degrees of lateral flexion and rotation.

Stabilization

Stabilize the pelvis to prevent posterior tilting.

Testing Motion

Ask the subject to extend the spine as far as possible. The end of the extension ROM occurs when the pelvis begins to tilt posteriorly.

Normal End-feel

The end feel is firm owing to stretching of the anterior longitudinal ligament, anterior fibers of the annulus fibrosus, zygapophyseal joint capsules, rectus abdominis, and external and internal oblique muscles. The end-feel may also be hard owing to contact between the spinous processes.

Measurement Method for Lumbar Extension: Modified Modified–Schober or Simplified Skin Distraction

1. Use a skin-marking pencil to place marks on the right and left posterior superior iliac spines. Use a

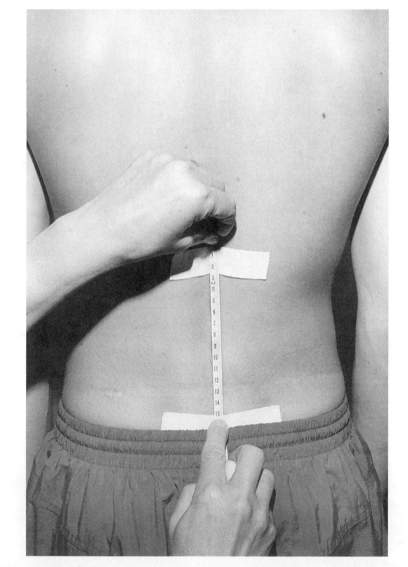

FIGURE 12–21 Tape measure alignment in the starting position for measurement of lumbar extension range of motion with use of the simplified skin distraction method (modified–modified Schober method).

ruler to locate and mark a midline point on the sacrum that is on a level with the posterior superior iliac spines. Make a mark on the lumbar spine that is 15 cm above the mark on the sacrum.

2. Align the tape measure between the superior and the inferior marks on the spine, (Fig. 12–21), and ask the subject to bend backward as far as possible.

3. At the end of the ROM, note the distance between the superior and the inferior marks (Fig. 12–22). The ROM is the difference between 15 cm and the length measured at the end of the motion.

Alternative Measurement Method for Lumbar Extension: Modified Schober Technique

Battie and coworkers[53] found a mean of 1.6 cm in 100 healthy adults.

1. Use a skin-marking pencil to place a mark at the lumbosacral junction. Place a second mark 10 cm above the first mark (measure to the nearest millimeter). Place a third mark 5 cm below the first mark (lumbosacral junction).

2. Align the tape measure between the most superior and the most inferior marks. Ask the subject to put the hands on the buttocks and to bend backward as far as possible.

3. Note the distance between the most superior and the most inferior marks at the end of the ROM and subtract the final measurement from the initial 15 cm. The ROM is the difference between 15 cm and the length measured at the end of the motion

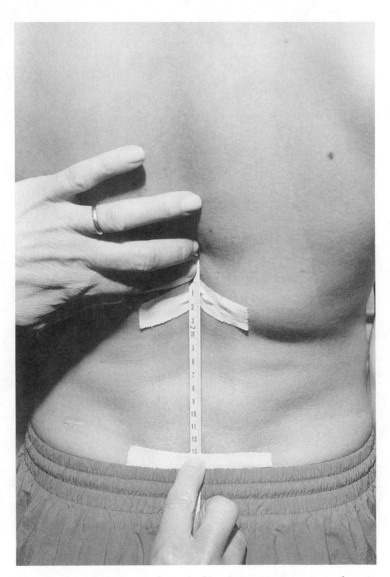

FIGURE 12–22 Tape measure alignment at the end of lumbar extension range of motion, with use of the simplified skin distraction method.

THORACIC AND LUMBAR LATERAL FLEXION

ROM ranges from 18 to 38 degrees with use of a goniometer[12] and from 5 to 7 cm with use of a tape measure.[54]

Testing Position

Place the subject standing, with the cervical, thoracic, and lumbar spine in 0 degrees of flexion, extension, and rotation.

Stabilization

Stabilize the pelvis to prevent lateral tilting.

Testing Motion

Ask the subject to bend the trunk to one side while keeping the arms in a relaxed position at the sides of the body. Keep both feet flat on the floor with the knees extended (Fig. 12–23). The end of the motion occurs when the heel begins to rise on the foot opposite to the side of the motion and the pelvis begins to tilt laterally.

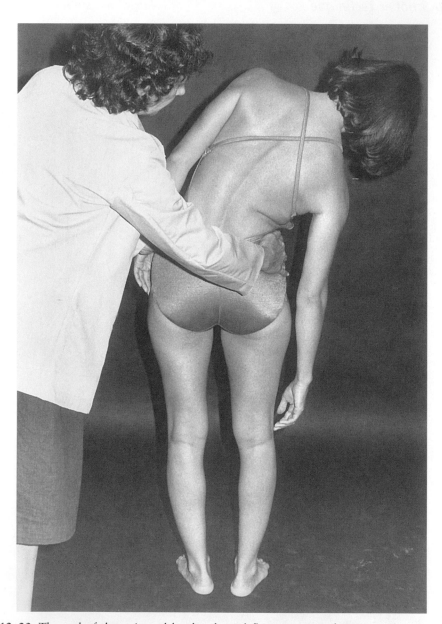

FIGURE 12–23 The end of thoracic and lumbar lateral flexion range of motion. The examiner places both hands on the subject's pelvis to prevent lateral pelvic tilting.

Normal End-feel

The end-feel is firm owing to the stretching of the contralateral fibers of the annulus fibrosus, zygapophyseal joint capsules, intertransverse ligaments, thoracolumbar fascia, and the following muscles: external and oblique abdominals, longissimus thoracis, iliocostalis lumborum and thoracis lumborum, quadratus lumborum, multifidus, spinalis thoracis, and serratus posterior inferior. The end-feel may also be hard owing to impact of the ipsilateral zygapophyseal facets (right facets when bending to the right) and the restrictions imposed by the ribs and costal joints in the upper thoracic spine.

Measurement Method for Thoracic and Lumbar Lateral Flexion: Universal Goniometer

Fitzgerald and associates[12] found that lateral flexion measured with a goniometer ranged from a mean of 37.6

degrees (in a group 20 to 29 years old) to 18.0 degrees (in a group 70 to 79 years old). See Table 12–2 for additional information.[12] According to Sahrmann,[55] more than three-quarters of thoracic and lumbar lateral flexion ROM takes place in the thoracic spine.

1. Use a skin-marking pencil to mark the spinous processes of C7 and S1.
2. Center the fulcrum of the goniometer over the posterior aspect of the spinous process of S1.
3. Align the proximal arm so that it is perpendicular to the ground.
4. Align the distal arm with the posterior aspect of the spinous process of C7 (Figs. 12–24 and 12–25).

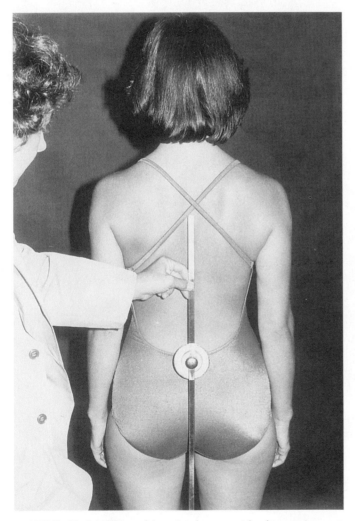

FIGURE 12–24 The subject is shown with the goniometer aligned in the starting position for measurement of thoracic and lumbar lateral flexion.

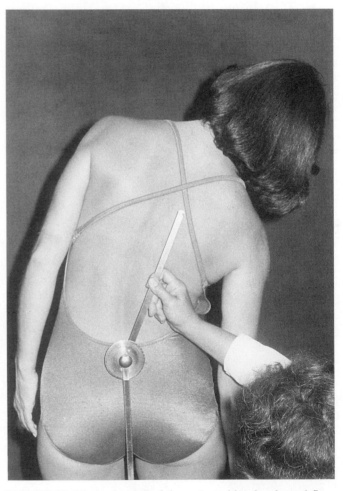

FIGURE 12–25 At the end of thoracic and lumbar lateral flexion, the examiner keeps the distal goniometer arm aligned with the subject's seventh cervical vertebra. The examiner makes no attempt to align the distal arm with the subject's vertebral column. As can be seen in the photograph, the lower thoracic and upper lumbar spine become convex to the left during right lateral flexion.

Alternative Measurement of Thoracic and Lumbar Lateral Flexion: Fingertip-to-Floor Method

1. Place the subject in the erect standing position, with the arms hanging freely at the sides of the body. Ask the subject to bend to the side as far as possible while keeping both feet flat on the ground and the knees extended.

2. At the end of the ROM, make a mark on the leg level with the tip of the middle finger. Use a tape measure to measure the distance between the mark on the leg and that on the floor (Fig. 12–26). One problem with this method is that it may be affected by the subject's body proportions. Therefore, it should be used only to compare repeated measurements for a single subject and not for comparing one subject with another subject.

In a variation of the fingertip-to-floor method, designed to account for differences in body size, Mellin[54] suggests that a mark should be made on the thigh, where the tip of the third finger rests in the starting position. A second mark should be made on the leg at the point where the tip of the third finger rests at the end of the lateral flexion ROM. The distance between the two marks is the thoracolumbar ROM. In a study involving 39 healthy subjects, Mellin[54] found that the mean ROM in lateral flexion using this technique was 22 cm (SD = 5.4 cm).

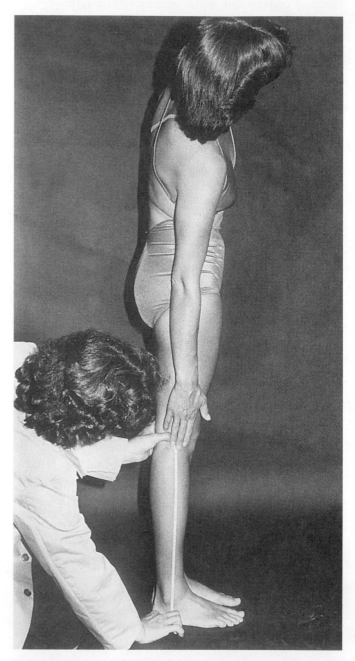

FIGURE 12–26 At the end of thoracic and lumbar lateral flexion range of motion, the examiner is using a tape measure to determine the distance from the tip of the subject's third finger to the floor. Lateral pelvic tilting should be avoided.

Alternative Measurement Method for Thoracic and Lumbar Lateral Flexion: Double Inclinometer

According to the AMA, the ROM is 25 degrees to each side of the body.[4]

1. Use a skin-marking pencil to identify locations on the spinous processes of S1 and T1.
2. Place one inclinometer over the S1 spinous process and the other over that of T1 and then zero both inclinometers (Fig. 12–27).
3. Ask the subject to bend to the side as far as possible while keeping both knees straight and both feet firmly on the ground (Fig. 12–28).
4. At the end of the ROM, note the information on the dials of both inclinometers. Calculate lateral flexion ROM by subtracting the reading on the sacral inclinometer from that on the dial of the thoracic inclinometer. Repeat the entire measurement process to measure lateral flexion on the other side.

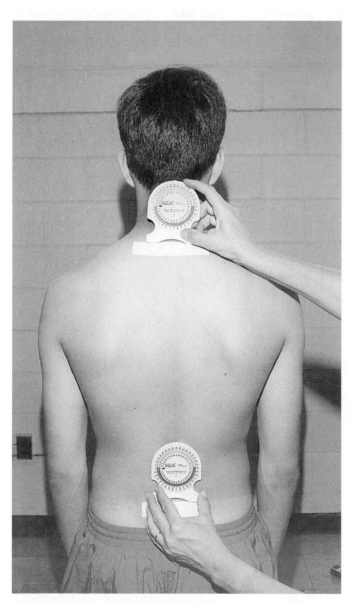

FIGURE 12–27 The subject is in the starting position for measurement of thoracic and lumbar lateral flexion with both inclinometers aligned and zeroed.

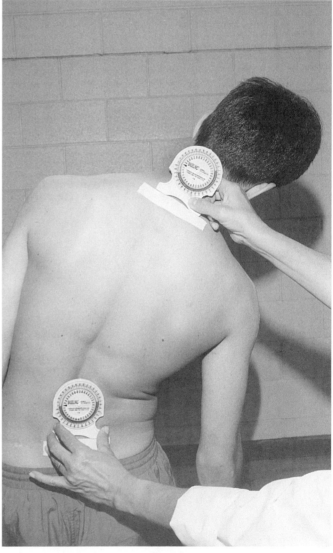

FIGURE 12–28 Inclinometer alignment at the end of thoracic and lumbar lateral flexion range of motion.

THORACIC AND LUMBAR ROTATION

Motion occurs in the transverse plane around a vertical axis.

Testing Position

Place the subject sitting, with the feet on the floor to help stabilize the pelvis. A seat without a back support is preferred so that rotation of the spine can occur freely. The cervical, thoracic, and lumbar spine are in 0 degrees of flexion, extension, and lateral flexion.

Stabilization

Stabilize the pelvis to prevent rotation. Avoid flexion, extension, and lateral flexion of the spine.

Testing Motion

Ask the subject to turn his body to one side as far as possible keeping his trunk erect and feet flat on the floor (Fig. 12–29). The end of the motion occurs when the examiner feels the pelvis start to rotate.

Normal End-feel

The end-feel is firm owing to stretching of the fibers of the contralateral annulus fibrosus and zygapophyseal joint capsules; costotransverse and costovertebral joint capsules; supraspinous, interspinous, and iliolumbar ligaments and the following muscles: rectus abdominis, external and internal obliques and multifidus, and semispinalis thoracis and rotatores. The end-feel may also be hard owing to contact between the zygapophyseal facets.

Measurement Method for Thoracic and Lumbar Rotation: Universal Goniometer

See Figures 12–30 and 12–31.

1. Center the fulcrum of the goniometer over the center of the cranial aspect of the subject's head.
2. Align the proximal arm parallel to an imaginary line between the two prominent tubercles on the iliac crests.
3. Align the distal arm with an imaginary line between the two acromial processes.

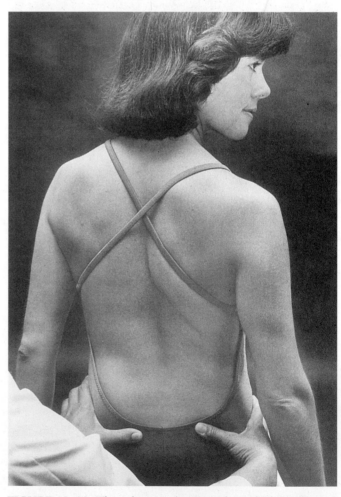

FIGURE 12–29 The subject is shown at the end of the thoracic and lumbar rotation range of motion. The subject is seated on a low stool without a back rest so that spinal movement can occur without interference. The examiner positions her hands on the subject's iliac crests to prevent pelvic rotation.

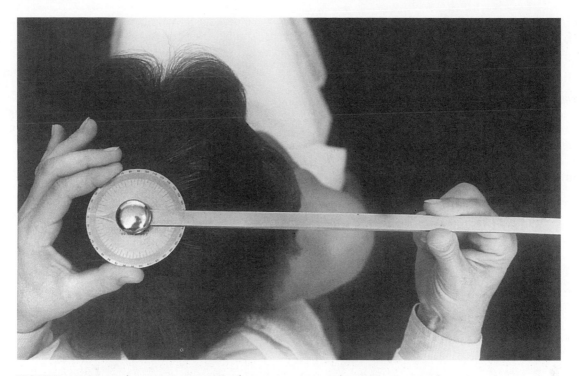

FIGURE 12–30 In the starting position for measurement of rotation range of motion, the examiner stands behind the seated subject. The examiner positions the fulcrum of the goniometer on the superior aspect of the subject's head. One of the examiner's hands is holding both arms of the goniometer aligned with the subject's acromion processes. The subject should be positioned so that the acromion processes are aligned directly over the iliac tubercles.

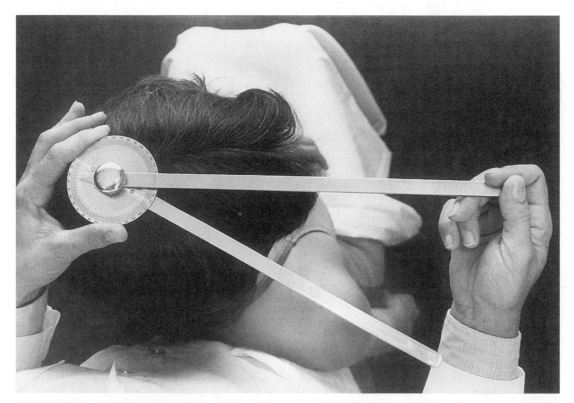

FIGURE 12–31 At the end of rotation, one of the examiner's hands keeps the proximal goniometer arm aligned with the subject's iliac tubercles while keeping the distal goniometer arm aligned with the subject's right acromion process.

Alternative Measurement Method for Thoracic and Lumbar Rotation: Double Inclinometer

According to the AMA,[4] rotation ROM measured with use of inclinometers is 30 degrees to each side.

1. Use a skin-marking pencil to place a mark over the spinous processes of S1 and the seventh cervical vertebra.
2. Place the subject in a forward-flexed standing position so that the subject's back is parallel to the ground.
3. Place one inclinometer at S1 and the other over the spinous process of the seventh cervical vertebra and zero both inclinometers (Fig. 12–32).
4. Ask the subject to rotate the trunk as far as possible without moving into extension. (Fig. 12–33).

Note the degrees shown on the inclinometers at the end of the motion. The difference between the inclinometer readings is the rotation ROM.

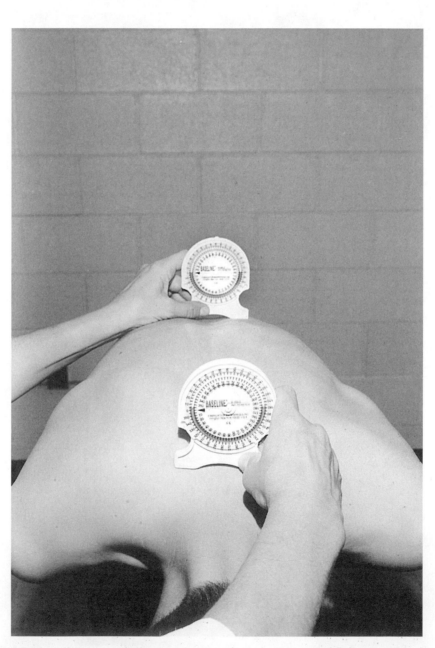

FIGURE 12–32 The subject is in the starting position for measurement of thoracic and lumbar rotation, with inclinometers aligned and zeroed.

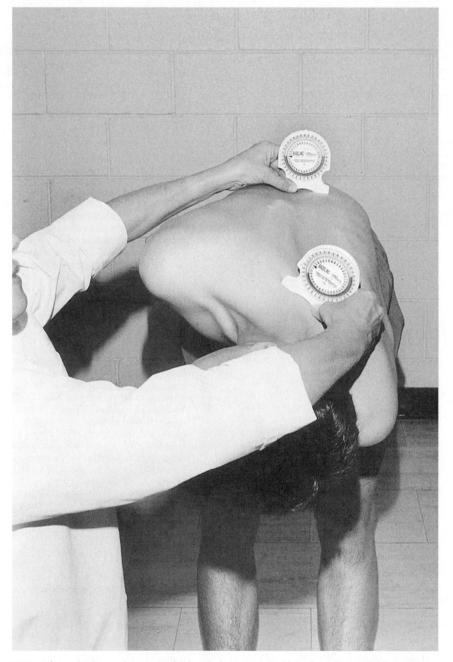

FIGURE 12–33 The subject is shown with the inclinometers aligned at the end of thoracic and lumbar rotation range of motion.

REFERENCES

1. Bogduk, N: Clinical Anatomy of the Lumbar Spine and Sacrum, ed 3. Churchill Livingstone, New York, 1997.
2. Cyriax, JH, and Cyriax, P: Illustrated Manual of Orthopaedic Medicine. Butterworths, London, 1983.
3. American Academy of Orthopaedic Surgeons: Joint Motion: Method of Measuring and Recording. AAOS, Chicago, 1965.
4. American Medical Association: Guides to the Evaluation of Permanent Impairment, ed 3. AMA, Chicago, 1988.
5. Loebl, WY: Measurement of spinal posture and range of spinal movement. Ann Phys Med 9:103, 1967.
6. Sullivan, MS, Dickinson, CE, and Troup, JDG: The influence of age and gender on lumbar spine range of motion. A study of 1126 healthy subjects. Spine 19:682, 1994.
7. Macrae, IF, and Wright, V: Measurement of back movement. Ann Rheum Dis 28:584, 1969.
8. Moll, JMH, and Wright, V: Normal range of spinal mobility: An objective clinical study. Ann Rheum Dis 30:381, 1971.
9. Anderson, JAD, and Sweetman, BJ: A combined flexi-rule hydrogoniometer for measurement of lumbar spine and its sagittal movement. Rheumatol Rehabil 14:173, 1975.
10. Gracovetsky, S, et al: A database for estimating normal spinal motion derived from non-invasive measurements. Spine 20:1036, 1995.
11. McGregor, AH, McCarthy, D and Hughes SP: Motion characteristics of the lumbar spine in the normal population. Spine 20:2421, 1995.
12. Fitzgerald, GK, et al: Objective assessment with establishment of normal values for lumbar spine range of motion. Phys Ther 63:1776, 1983.
13. Bookstein, NA, et al: Lumbar extension range of motion in elementary school children. Abstr Phys Ther 72:S35, 1992.
14. Sughara, M, et al: Epidemiological study on the change of mobility of the thoraco-lumbar spine and body height with age as indices for senility. J Hum Ergol (Tokyo) 10:49, 1981.
15. Freidrich, M, et al: Spinal posture during stooped walking under vertical space constraints. Spine 25:1118, 2000.
16. Sjolie, AN: Access to pedestrian roads, daily activities and physical performance of adolescents. Spine 25:1965, 2000.
17. Ensink, FB, et al: Lumbar range of motion. Influence of time of day and individuals factors on measurements. Spine 21:1339, 1996.
18. Sullivan, MS, Shoaf, LD, and Riddle, DL: The relationship of lumbar flexion to disability in patients with low back pain. Phys Ther 80:240, 2000.
19. Lundberg, G, and Gerdle, B: Correlations between joint and spinal mobility, spinal sagittal configuration, segmental mobility, segmental pain symptoms and disabilities in female homecare personnel. Scand J Rehab Med 32:124, 2000.
20. Kujala UM, et al: Lumbar mobility and low back pain during adolescence. A longitudinal three-year follow-up study in athletes and controls. Am J Sports Med 25:363, 1997.
21. Nattrass, CL, et al: Lumbar spine range of motion as a measure of physical and functional impairment: An investigation of validity (abstract). Clin Rehabil 13:211, 1999.
22. Shirley, FR, et al: Comparison of lumbar range of motion using three measurement devices in patients with chronic low back pain. Spine 19:779, 1994.
23. Hsieh, CY, and Pringle, RK: Range of motion of the lumbar spine required for four activities of daily living. J Manipulative Physiol Ther 17:353, 1994.
24. Patel, RS: Intratester and intertester reliability of the inclinometer in measuring lumbar flexion. Phys Ther 72:S44, 1992.
25. Williams, R, et al: Reliability of the modified–modified Schober and double inclinometer methods for measuring lumbar flexion and extension. Phys Ther 73:26, 1993.
26. Mayer, RS, et al: Variance in the measurement of sagittal lumbar range of motion among examiners, subjects, and instruments. Spine 20:1489, 1995.
27. Saur, PMM, et al: Lumbar range of motion: Reliability and validity of the inclinometer technique in the clinical measurement of trunk flexibility. Spine 21:1332, 1996.
28. Samo, DG, et al: Validity of three lumbar sagittal motion measurement methods: Surface inclinometers compared with radiographs. J Occup Environ Med 39:209, 1997.
29. Chen, SP, et al: Reliability of the lumbar sagittal motion measurement methods: Surface Inclinometers. J Occup Environ Med 39:217, 1997.
30. Mayer, TG, et al: Spinal range of motion. Accuracy and sources of error with inclinometric measurement. Spine 22:1976, 1997.
31. Nitschkje, JE, et al: Reliability of the American Medical Association Guides' Model for Measuring Spinal Range of Motion. Its implication for whole-person impairment ratings. Spine 24:262, 1999.
32. Breum, J, Wiberg, J, and Bolton, JE: Reliability and concurrent validity of the BROM II for measuring lumbar mobility. J Manipulative Physiol Ther 18:497, 1995.
33. Madson, TJ, Youdas, JW, and Suman, VJ: Reproducibility of lumbar spine range of motion measurements using the back range of motion device. J Orthop Sports Phys Ther 29:470, 1999.
34. Reynolds, PMG: Measurement of spinal mobility: A comparison of three methods. Rheumatol Rehabil 14:180, 1975.
35. Miller, MH, et al: Measurement of spinal mobility in the sagittal plane: New skin distraction technique compared with established methods. J Rheumatol 11:4, 1984.
36. Portek, I, et al: Correlation between radiographic and clinical measurement of lumbar spine movement. Br J Rheumatol 22:197, 1983.
37. Gill, K, et al: Repeatability of four clinical methods for assessment of lumbar spinal motion. Spine 13:50, 1988.
38. Van Adrichem, JAM, and van der Korst, JK: Assessment of the flexibility of the lumbar spine. A pilot study in children and adolescents. Scand J Rheumatol 2:87, 1973.
39. Greene, WB, and Heckman, JD (eds): The Clinical Measurement of Joint Motion. American Academy of Orthopaedic Surgeons. Rosemont, Ill, 1994.
40. Lindahl, O: Determination of the sagittal mobility of the lumbar spine. Acta Orthop Scand 37:241, 1966.
41. Youdas, JW, Suman, VJ and Garrett, TR: Reliability of measurements of lumbar spine sagittal mobility obtained with the flexible curve. J Orthop Sports Phys Ther 21:13, 1995.
42. Katzman, WB, Cutter, KA, and Ash, BA: Differences in reliability of the flexible ruler for the experienced and novice tester. Abstract Feb. 2000. J Orthop Sports Phys Ther 30:A9, 2000.
43. Bryan, JM, et al: Investigation of the flexible ruler as a noninvasive measure of lumbar lordosis in black and white adult female sample populations. J Orthop Sports Phys Ther 11:3, 1989.
44. Lovell, FW, Rothstein, JM, and Personius, WJ: Reliability of clinical measurements of lumbar lordosis taken with a flexible rule. Phys Ther 69:96, 1989.
45. Schenkman, M, et al: A clinical tool for measuring functional axial rotation. Phys Ther 75:151, 1995.
46. Schenkman, M, et al: Spinal movement and performance of a standing reach task in participants with and without Parkinson disease. Phys Ther 81:1400, 2001.
47. Petersen, CM, et al: Intraobserver and interobserver reliability of asymptomatic subject's thoracolumbar range of motion using the OS I CA-6000 Spine Motion Analyzer. J Orthop Sports Phys Ther 220:207, 1997.
48. Robinson, ME, et al: Intrasubject reliability of spinal range of motion and velocity determined by video motion analysis. Phys Ther 73:626, 1993.
49. Steffan, T, et al: A new technique for measuring lumbar segmental motion in vivo: method, accuracy and preliminary results. Spine 22:156, 1997.
50. Kraus, H, and Hirschland, RP: Minimum muscular fitness tests in school children. Res Q Exerc Sport 25:178, 1954.
51. Nicholas, JA: Risk factors, sports medicine and the orthopedic system: An overview. J Sports Med 3:243, 1975.
52. Brodie, DA, Bird, HA, and Wright, V: Joint laxity in selected athletic populations. Med Sci Sports Exerc 14:190, 1982.
53. Battie, MC, et al: The role of spinal flexibility in back pain complaints in industry. A prospective study. Spine 15:768, 1990.
54. Mellin, GP: Accuracy of measuring lateral flexion of the spine with a tape. Clin Biomech 1:85, 1986.
55. Sahrmann, SA: Diagnosis and Treatment of Movement Impairment Syndromes. Mosby, St Louis, 2002.

CHAPTER 13

The Temporomandibular Joint

Structure and Function

Temporomandibular Joint

Anatomy

The temporomandibular joint (TMJ) is the articulation between the mandible, the articular disc, and the temporal bone of the skull (Fig. 13–1A). The disc divides the joint into two distinct parts, which are referred to as the upper and lower joints. The larger upper joint consists of the convex articular eminence and concave mandibular fossa of the temporal bone and the superior surface of the disc. The lower joint consists of the convex surface of the mandibular condyle and the concave inferior surface of the disc.[1–3] The articular disc helps the convex mandible conform to the convex articular surface of the temporal bone (Fig. 13–1B).[2]

The TMJ capsule is described as being thin and loose above the disc but taut below the disc in the lower joint. Short capsular fibers surround the joint and extend between the mandibular condyle and the articular disc and between the disc and the temporal eminence.[3] Longer capsular fibers extend from the temporal bone to the mandible.

The primary ligaments associated with the TMJ are the temporomandibular, the stylomandibular and the sphenomandibular ligaments (Fig. 13–2). The muscles associated with the TMJ are the medial and lateral pterygoids, temporalis, masseter, digastric, stylohyoid, mylohyoid and geniohyoid.

Osteokinematics

The upper joint is an amphiarthrodial gliding joint. The lower joint is a hinge joint. The TMJ as a whole allows

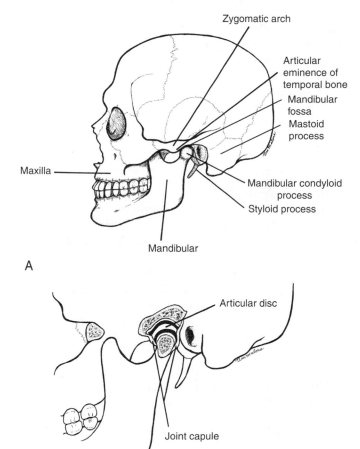

FIGURE 13–1 (A) Lateral view of the skull showing the temporomandibular joint (TMJ) and surrounding structures. (B) A lateral view of the TMJ showing the articular disc and a portion of the joint capsule.

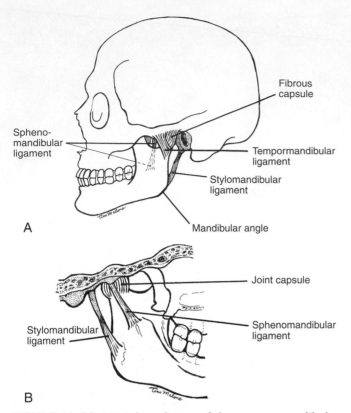

FIGURE 13–2A (A) A lateral view of the temporomandibular joint showing the oblique fibers of the temporomandibular ligament and the stylomandibular and sphenomandibular ligaments. (B) A medial view of the temporomandibular joint showing the medial portion of the joint capsule and the stylomandibular and sphenomandibular ligaments.

motions in three planes around three axes. All of the motions except mouth closing begin from the resting position of the joint in which the teeth are slightly separated (freeway space).[3,4] The amount of freeway space, which usually varies from 2 mm to 4 mm, allows free anterior, posterior, and lateral movement of the mandible. The functional motions permitted are mandibular elevation (mouth closing) and depression (mouth opening), protrusion (anterior translation) and retrusion (posterior translation), and right and left lateral deviation (excursion). Maximal contact of the teeth in mouth closing is called centric occlusion.

The oblique portion of the temporomandibular ligament limits mandibular depression, retrusion, and rotation of the condyle during mouth opening. The horizontal portion of the temporomandibular ligament limits posterior translation of the mandibular condyle in retrusion and lateral deviation of the mandible. The functions of the stylomandibular and sphenomandibular ligaments are controversial. According to Magee,[5] the ligaments keep the condyle, disc, and temporal bone in close approximation. These ligaments also may prevent

excessive protrusion, but their exact function has not been verified.

The diagastric and lateral pterygoid muscles produce mandibular depression.[1,3–5] The mylohyoid and geniohyoid muscles assist in the motion, especially against resistance.[3,5] Mandibular elevation is produced by the temporalis, masseter, and medial pterygoid muscles,[1,3–5] which are responsible for maintaining the freeway space. Mandibular protrusion is a result of bilateral action of the masseter,[1,5] medial,[1,3,5] and lateral[3–6] pterygoid muscles. The mylohyoid, stylohyoid, and digastric muscles may assist.[5] Retrusion is brought about by bilateral action of the posterior fibers of the temporalis muscles[1,3–5]; by the diagastric,[1,3–5] middle, and deep fibers of the masseter[3,5]; and by the stylohyoid , mylohyoid,[1,5] and geniohyoid[1,3,5] muscles. Mandibular deviation is produced by a unilateral contraction of the medial and lateral pterygoid muscles.[1–5] A unilateral contraction of the temporalis muscle causes deviation to the same side.

Cervical spine muscles may be activated in conjunction with TMJ muscles because a close functional relationship exists between the head and the neck.[1,4–9] Coordinated and parallel movements at the TMJ and cervical spine joints have been observed in some studies, and researchers suggest that preprogrammed neural commands may simultaneously activate both jaw and neck muscles.[7–9]

Arthrokinematics

Mandibular depression (mouth opening) occurs in the sagittal plane and is accomplished by rotation and sliding of the mandibular condyles. Condylar rotation is combined with anterior and inferior sliding of the condyles on the inferior surface of the discs, which also slide anteriorly (translate) along the temporal articular eminences. Mandibular elevation (mouth closing) is accomplished by rotation of the mandibular condyles on the discs and sliding of the discs with the condyles posteriorly and superiorly on the temporal articular eminences.

In protrusion, the bilateral condyles and discs translate together anteriorly and inferiorly along the temporal articular eminences. The movement takes place at the upper joint, and no rotation occurs during this motion. In lateral deviation, one mandibular condyle and disc slide inferiorly, anteriorly, and medially along the articular eminence. The other mandibular condyle rotates about a vertical axis and slides medially within the mandibular fossa. For example, in left lateral deviation, the left condyle spins and the right slides anteriorly.

Capsular Pattern

In the capsular pattern, mandibular depression is limited to 1 cm, with deviation toward the restricted side.[5] Protrusion is limited and accompanied by deviation

TABLE 13–1   Mouth Opening Range of Motion in Subjects 18 to 61 Years of Age: Mean Linear Distance in Millimeters

Travers et al*[13]	Lewis et al*[14]		Higbie et al[†15]		Walker et al[†11]		Gavish et al[‡16]
25–35 yrs n = 27F	25–35 yrs n = 27F	23–39 yrs n = 29M	18–54 yrs n = 20M and 20F		21–61 yrs n = 3F and 12M		15–16 yrs n = 248
			Mean	(SD)	Mean	(SD)	Mean (SD)
46.6	46.0	52.1	44.5	(5.3)	43.5	(6.1)	51.6 (6.2)

F = Females; M = males; (SD) = standard deviation.
* Measurements were obtained with an Optotrak jaw-tracking system.
† Measurements were obtained with a millimeter ruler.
‡ The instrument that was used was not reported.

toward the restricted side.[5] Lateral deviation is limited on the side opposite the restriction.[4]

Research Findings

The normal range of motion (ROM) for mouth opening is considered to be a distance sufficient for the subject to place two or three flexed proximal interphalangeal joints within the opening. That distance may range from 35 mm to 50 mm and is considered to be a measure of functional opening, although an opening of only 25 mm to 35 mm is needed for normal activities.[5] A definition of normal range of mouth opening as 40 mm to 50 mm was arrived at by consensus judgements made at a 1995 Permanent Impairment Conference by representatives of all major societies and academies whose members treat TMJ disorders.[10] Similar mean ROMs for mouth opening, from a low of 43.5 mm to a high of 52.1 mm, are presented in Table 13–1. The linear distances for protrusion and lateral deviation are presented from three sources in Table 13–2.

TABLE 13–2   Protrusion and Lateral Deviation (Deviation) Range of Motion: Mean Linear Distance in Millimeters

	Buschang et al*[12]	Walker et al[†11]	Magee[‡5]
	25–35 yrs n = 27F	21–61 yrs n = 3F and 12M	
Motion	Mean	Mean (SD)	
Protrusion	9.3	7.1 (2.3)	3–6§
L. Deviation	11.0	8.6 (2.1)	10–15
R. Deviation	11.5	9.2 (2.6)	

(SD) = Standard deviation; F = female; M = male
* Measurements were obtained with an Optotrak jaw tracking system.
† Measurements were obtained with a millimeter ruler.
‡ The instrument that was used to obtain measurements is unknown.
§ Normal values may vary depending upon the degree of overbite (greater movement) and underbite (lesser movement).

Dijkstra and coworkers[17] investigated the relationship between vertical and horizontal mandibular ROM in 91 healthy subjects (59 women and 32 men) with a mean age of 27.2 years. A mean ratio was found ranging from 6.0:1 to 6.6:1 between vertical and horizontal ROM. Individual ratios ranged from 3.6 to 15.5, and correlations between the vertical and the horizontal ROM measurements were weak. Therefore, based on the results of this study, the authors concluded that the 4:1 ratio between vertical and horizontal ROM that has been used in the past[18] should be replaced by the approximately 6:1 ratio found in this study. However, the authors found that the ratio has poor predictive value. A review of values in Tables 13–1 and 13–2 indicates that the ratio between mandibular depression (vertical ROM) and lateral deviation (horizontal ROM) is between 4:1 and 5:1. Dijkstra and coworkers'[17] measurements of incisal linear distance during mouth opening included the overbite measurement, and this addition may account for some of the differences between these authors' ratios and the ratios shown in the tables.

Effects of Age, Gender, and Other Factors

Age

Thurnwald[19] found that the ROM in all active TMJ motions except retrusion decreased with increasing age. Mouth opening decreased from a mean of 59.4 mm in the younger group to 54.3 mm in the older group. The study involved 50 males and 50 females ranging from 17 to 65 years of age. The author also found a decrease in the quality of six passive accessory movements with increasing age. Resistance to passive accessory movement and crepitus increased in the older group. A number of other studies have investigated populations of children, adolescents, and elderly individuals to determine the prevalence of TMJ disorders in these age groups.[20–24]

Gender

Studies investigating the effects of gender on temporomandibular function in a healthy population are scarce.

Thurnwald[19] determined that the subject's gender significantly affected mouth opening and lateral deviation. The 50 males in the study had a greater mean range of mouth opening (59.4 mm) than the 50 females (54.0 mm). The males also had a greater mean ROM in right lateral deviation, but the difference between genders in this instance was small. No effect of gender was apparent on passive accessory motions. Lewis, Buschang, and Throck-morton[14] found that males had significantly greater mouth opening ROM (mean = 52.1 mm) than females (mean = 46.0 mm) in the study (see Table 13–1).

In contrast to the findings of Lewis, Buschang, and Throckmorton,[14] Westling and Helkimo[25] found that the angular displacement of the mandible in relation to the cranium (angle of mouth opening) in maximal jaw opening in adolescents was slightly larger in females than in males. This finding might have been influenced by the fact that females generally reach adult ROM values by 10 years of age, whereas males do not reach an adult ROM values until 15 years of age.[26]

Mandibular Length

Dijkstra and colleagues,[27] in a study of mouth opening in 13 females and 15 males, found that the linear distance between the upper and the lower incisors during mandibular depression was significantly influenced by mandibular length. In a more recent study, Dijkstra and associates[28] investigated the relationship between incisor distances, mandibular length, and angle of mouth opening in 91 healthy subjects (59 women and 32 men) ranging from 13 to 56 years of age (mean 27.2 years). Mouth opening was influenced by both mandibular length and angle of mouth opening. Therefore, it is possible that subjects with the same mouth opening distance may differ from each other in regard to TMJ mobility. Lewis, Buschang, and Throckmorton[14] found that mandibular length accounted for some of the gender differences in mouth opening and for most of the gender differences in condylar translation in mouth opening. Westling and Helkimo[25] found that passive ROM as measured by mouth opening was strongly correlated to mandibular length.

To adjust for mandibular length, Miller and coworkers[29] conducted a study to determine whether a "mouth opening index" developed by the authors might be able to differentiate between TMJ disorders of arthrogenous origin and those of myogenous origin. Forty-seven patients and 27 healthy control subjects were included in the study. The temporomandibular opening index (TOI) was determined by employing the following formula: TOI = (PO - MVO/ PO + MVO) x 100. "PO" in the formula refers to passive opening and "MVO" refers to maximal voluntary opening. A significant difference was found between the mean TOI between the two groups of patients and between the myogenous and the control groups but not between the arthrogenous group and the

control group. The authors suggested that the TOI might be a better measure than simple linear distance measures for mouth opening. In a subsequent study, Miller and associates[30] compared the TOI in 11 patients with a disorder with the TOI in a control group of 11 individuals without TMJ disorders. Based on the results of the study, the authors concluded that the TOI appears to be independent of age, gender, and mandibular length.

Head and Neck Positions

Higbie and associates[15] investigated the effects of head position (forward, neutral, and retracted) on mouth opening in 20 healthy males and 20 healthy females between 18 and 54 years of age. Mouth opening ROM measured with a millimeter ruler was significantly different among the three positions. Mouth opening was greatest in the forward head position (mean = 44.5, SD = 5.3), less in the neutral head position (mean = 41.5, SD = 4.8), and least in the retracted head position (mean = 36.2, SD = 4.5). Day-to-day reliability was found to vary from 0.90 to 0.97, depending on head position, and the standard error of measurement (SEM) ranged from 0.77 to 1.69 mm, also depending on head position. As a result of the findings, the authors concluded that the head position should be controlled when mouth opening measurements are taken. However, the authors found that an error of 1 mm to 2 mm occurred regardless of the position in which the head was placed.

Temporomandibular Disorders

The structure of the TMJs and the fact that these joints get so much use predisposes the joints, associated ligaments, and musculature to injury, mechanical problems, and degenerative changes. For example, the articular disc may become entrapped, deformed, or torn; the capsule may become thickened; the ligaments may become shortened or lengthened; and the muscles may become inflamed, contracted, and hypertrophied. These problems may give rise to a variety of symptoms and signs that are included in the temporomandibular disorder (TMD) classification. Restricted mouth opening ROM is considered to be one of the important signs of TMD.[29] Popping or clicking noises (or both) in the joint during mouth opening and/or closing and deviation of the mandible during mouth opening and closing may be present.[16,22,24,31] Other signs and symptoms include facial pain, muscular pain,[31] and tenderness in the region of the TMJ, either unilaterally or bilaterally, headaches, and stiffness of the neck. TMDs appear to be more prevalent in females of all ages after puberty, although the actual percentages of women affected varies among investigators.[23,24,31-34] The reason for this gender preference has been attributed a number of factors including, among others, greater stress levels in women,[33] hormonal influences,[34] and habits of adolescent girls that are extremely harmful to the temporomandibular joints (e.g., intensive gum chewing, continuous arm leaning, ice crushing, nail biting, biting foreign objects, jaw play, clenching, and bruxism).[16,22]

Reliability and Validity

Most of the following studies agree that TMJ ROM measurements of the distance between the upper and the lower incisors are reliable. The validity of these ROM measurements is more controversial. Walker, Bohannon, and Cameron[11] found that measurements of incisor distances for mouth opening had construct validity. However, some authors question how differences in the length and size of the mandible affect linear distance measurements.

Walker, Bohannon, and Cameron[11] determined that six TMJ motions measured with a millimeter ruler were reliable. Measurements were taken by two testers at three sessions, each of which were separated by a week. The 30 subjects who were measured included 15 patients with a TMJ disorder (13 females and 2 males with a mean age of 35.2 years) and 15 subjects without a TMJ disorder (12 females and 3 males with a mean age of 42.9 years). The intratester reliability intraclass correlation coefficients (ICCs) for tester one ranged from 0.82 to 0.99, and the intratester reliability for tester two ranged from 0.70 to 0.90. Intertester reliability ranged from good to excellent (ICC = 0.90 to 1.0). However, only mouth opening measurements had construct validity and were useful for discriminating between subjects with and without TMJ disorders. The technical error of measurement (difference between measurements that would have to be exceeded if the measurements were to be truly different) was 2.5 mm for mouth opening measurement in subjects without a TMJ disorder. Higbie and associates[15] also found that ROM measurements of mouth opening were highly reliable with use of a millimeter ruler. Twenty males and 20 females with a mean age of 32.9 years were measured by two examiners. Intratester, intertester, and test-retest reliability ICCs ranged from 0.90 to 0.97, depending on head position. SEM values indicated that an error of 1 mm to 2 mm existed for the measurement technique used in the study. Kropmans and colleagues[35] found similar high reliability in a study of mouth opening involving 5 male and 20 female patients with painfully restricted TMJs. Intratester, intertester, and test-retest reliability varied between 0.90 and 0.96. However, in contrast to the findings of Walker, Bohannon, and Cameron[11] and those of Higbie and associates,[15] the authors found that the smallest detectable difference of maximal mouth opening in this group of subjects varied from 9 mm to 6 mm. Based on these results, a clinician would have to measure at least 9 mm of improvement in maximal mouth opening in this group of patients to say that improvement had occurred.

The following studies investigated incisor distances as a measure of mandibular condylar movements. Buschang and associates,[12] in a sample of 27 healthy females 23 to 25 years of age, found that measurements of incisor motion during protrusion and lateral deviation provided moderately reliable measures of condylar translation. The linear distances that the incisors moved during lateral deviation provided the best measure of contralateral condylar translation. Travers and coworkers,[13] in a study involving 27 females, determined that the incisor linear distance in maximal mouth opening does not provide reliable information about condylar translation, because normal individuals perform mouth opening with highly variable amounts of condylar translation. Dijkstra and colleagues,[27] in a study of 28 healthy volunteers (13 females and 15 males) between 21 and 41 years of age, found that linear distance between the central incisors in maximal mouth opening was only weakly related to condylar movement. Lewis, Buschang, and Throckmorton,[14] who studied incisor movements in mouth opening in 29 men and 27 women, concluded that incisor movements should not be used as an indicator of condylar translation.

The influence of mandibular length on incisor distance measurements in mouth opening has been well documented.[14,25,27,28] The TOI mouth opening index was developed by Miller and coworkers[29] and Miller and associates.[30] According to these authors, the index is independent of mandibular length as well as gender and age. If additional research supports the authors' claims, use of the TOI would increase the validity of incisor measurements of mouth opening. Additional information about the TOI is presented in the section on mandibular length.

Range of Motion Testing Procedures: Temporomandibular Joint

Landmarks for Ruler Alignment Measuring

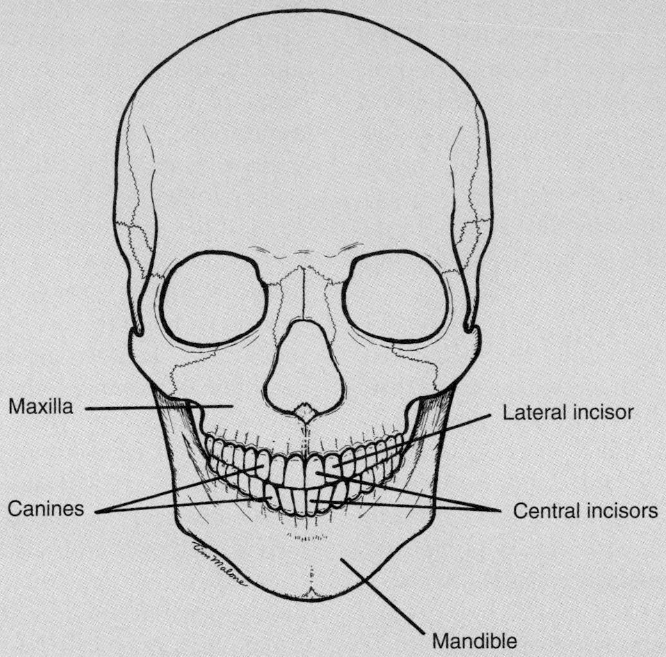

FIGURE 13–3 The adult has between 28 and 32 permanent teeth including 8 incisors, 4 canines, 8 premolars, and 8 to 12 molars. The central and lateral incisors and canines serve as landmarks for ruler placement.

DEPRESSION OF THE MANDIBLE (MOUTH OPENING)

Motion occurs in the sagittal plane around a medial-lateral axis. Functionally, the mandible is able to depress approximately 35 mm to 50 mm so that the subject's three fingers or two knuckles can be placed between the upper and the lower central incisor teeth.[5] According to the consensus judgements of the Permanent Impairment Conference, the normal ROM for mouth opening ranges between 40 mm and 50 mm.[10] The mean ROM in Table 13–1 shows ranges from 43.5 mm to 52.1 mm.

Testing Position

Place the subject sitting, with the cervical spine in 0 degrees of flexion, extension, lateral flexion, and rotation.

Stabilization

Stabilize the posterior aspect of the subject's head and neck to prevent flexion, extension, lateral flexion, and rotation of the cervical spine.

Testing Motion

Grasp the mandible so that it fits between the thumb and the index finger and pull the mandible inferiorly (Fig. 13–4). The subject may assist with the motion by opening the mouth as far as possible. The end of the motion occurs when resistance is felt and attempts to produce additional motion cause the head to nod forward (cervical flexion).

Normal End-feel

The end-feel is firm owing to stretching of the joint capsule, retrodiscal tissue, and the temporomandibular ligament, as well as the masseter, temporalis, and medial pterygoid muscles.[4,5]

Measurement Method

Measure the distance between the upper and the lower central incisor teeth with a ruler (Fig. 13–5). In normal active movement, no lateral deviation occurs during depression. If lateral deviation does occur, it may take the form of either a C-shaped or an S-shaped curve. With a C-shaped curve, the deviation is to one side and should be noted on the recording form. With an S-shaped curve, the deviation occurs first to one side and then to the opposite side.[5] A description of the deviations should be included on the recording form (Fig. 13–6).

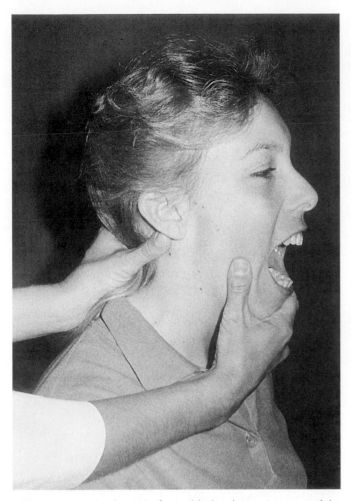

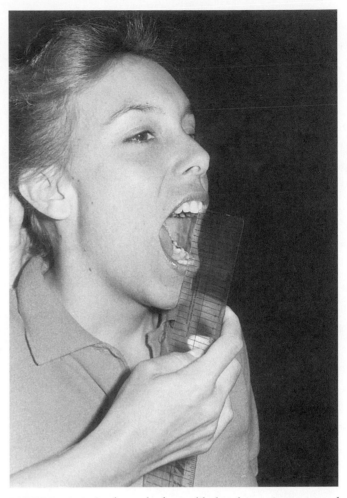

FIGURE 13–4 At the end of mandibular depression, one of the examiner's hands maintains the end of the range of motion by pulling the jaw inferiorly. The examiner's other hand holds the back of the subject's head to prevent cervical motion.

FIGURE 13–5 At the end of mandibular depression range of motion, the examiner uses the arm of a plastic goniometer to measure the distance between the subject's upper and lower central incisors.

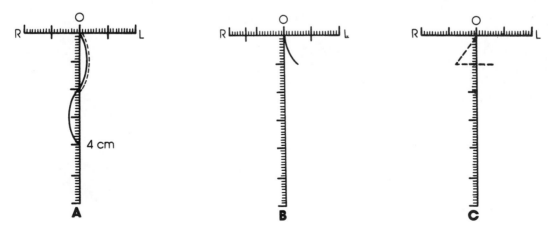

FIGURE 13–6 Examples of recording deviations in temporomandibular motions. (*A*) Deviation R and L on opening; maximum opening, 4 cm; lateral deviation equal (1 cm each direction); protrusion on functional opening (*dashed lines*). (*B*) Capsule-ligamentous pattern: opening limited to 1 cm; lateral deviation greater to R than to L; deviation to L on opening. (*C*) Protrusion is 1 cm; lateral deviation to R on protrusion (indicates weak lateral pterygoid on opposite side). (Magee, DJ: Orthopedic Physical Assessment, ed 3. WB Saunders, Philadelphia, 1997, p. 165, with permission).

PROTRUSION OF THE MANDIBLE

This translatory motion occurs in the transverse plane. Normally, the lower central incisor teeth are able to protrude 6 mm to 9 mm beyond the upper central incisor teeth. However the distance may range from 3 mm[5] to 10 mm.[4] See Table 13–2 for additional information.

Testing Position

Place the subject sitting, with the cervical spine in 0 degrees of flexion, extension, lateral flexion, and rotation. The TMJ is opened slightly.

Stabilization

Stabilize the posterior aspect of the head and neck to prevent flexion, extension, lateral flexion, and rotation of the cervical spine.

Testing Motion

Grasp the mandible between the thumb and the fingers from underneath the chin. The subject may assist with the movement by pushing the chin anteriorly as far as possible. The end of the motion occurs when resistance is felt and attempts at additional motion cause anterior motion of the head (Fig. 13–7).

Normal End-feel

The end-feel is firm owing to stretching of the joint capsule, temporomandibular, stylomandibular and sphenomandibular ligaments, as well as the temporalis, masseter, digastric, stylohyoid, mylohyoid and geniohyoid muscles.[3,5]

Measurement Method

Measure the distance between the lower central incisor and the upper central incisor teeth with a tape measure or ruler (Fig. 13–8). Alternatively, two vertical lines drawn on the upper and lower canines or lateral incisors may be used as the landmarks for measurement.[11]

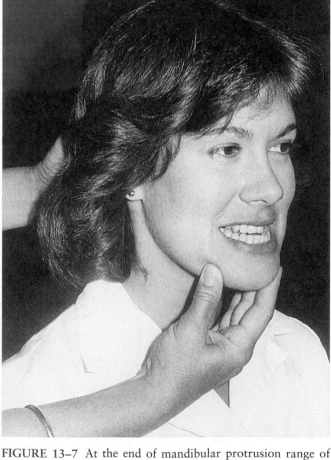

FIGURE 13–7 At the end of mandibular protrusion range of motion, the examiner uses one hand to stabilize the posterior aspect of the subject's head while her other hand moves the mandible into protrusion.

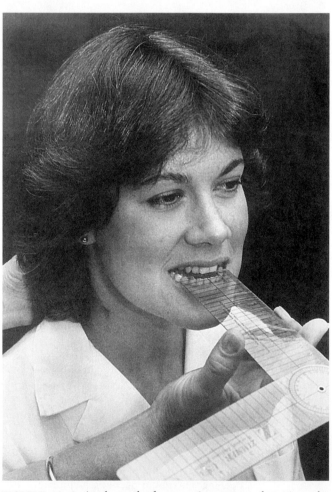

FIGURE 13–8 At the end of protrusion range of motion, the examiner uses the end of a plastic goniometer to measure the distance between the subject's upper and lower central incisors. The subject maintains the position.

LATERAL DEVIATION OF THE MANDIBLE

This translatory motion occurs in the transverse plane. The amount of lateral movement to the right and left sides should be similar, between 10 mm and 12 mm[2] but may range from 6 mm to 15 mm.[5] According to the consensus judgement of the Permanent Impairment Conference, the normal ROM is between 8 mm and 12 mm.[10] See Table 13–2 for additional information.

Testing Position

Place the subject sitting, with the cervical spine in 0 degrees of flexion, extension, lateral flexion, and rotation. The TMJ is opened slightly so that the subject's upper and lower teeth are not touching prior to the start of the motion.

Stabilization

Stabilize the posterior aspect of the head and neck to prevent flexion, extension, lateral flexion, and rotation of the cervical spine.

Testing Motion

Grasp the mandible between the fingers and the thumb and move it to the side. The end of the motion occurs when resistance is felt and attempts to produce additional motion cause lateral cervical flexion (be careful to avoid depression, elevation, and protrusion and retrusion during the movement) (Fig. 13–9).

Normal End-feel

The normal end-feel is firm owing to stretching of the joint capsule and temporomandibular ligaments, as well as the temporalis, medial, and lateral pterygoid muscles.

Measurement Method

Measure the distance between the most lateral points of the lower and the upper cuspid or the first bicuspid teeth with a tape measure or ruler (Fig. 13–10). Alternatively, two vertical lines drawn on the upper and lower central incisors may be used as landmarks for measurement.

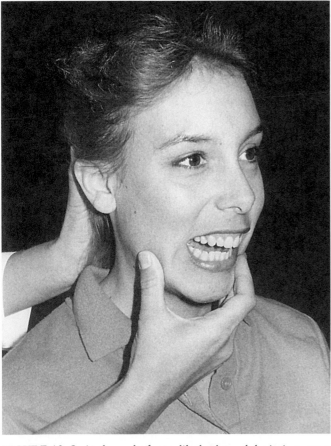

FIGURE 13–9 At the end of mandibular lateral deviation range of motion, the examiner uses one hand to prevent cervical motion and the other hand to maintain a lateral pull on the mandible.

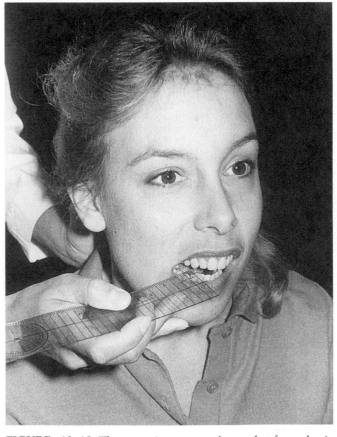

FIGURE 13–10 The examiner uses the end of a plastic goniometer to measure the distance between the upper and the lower canines.

REFERENCES

1. Perry, JF: The temporomandibular joint. In Levangie, PK, and Norkin, CC (eds): Joint Structure and Function: A Comprehensive Analysis, ed 3. FA Davis, Philadelphia, 2001.

2. Iglarsh, ZA, and Synder-Mackler, L: The temporomandibular joint and the cervical spine. In Richardson, JK, and Iglarsh, ZA (eds): Clinical Orthopaedic Physical Therapy. WB Saunders, Philadelphia, 1994.

3. Williams, PL: Gray's Anatomy, ed 38. Churchill Livingstone, New York, 1995.

4. Harrison, AL: The temporomandibular joint. In Malone, TR, McPoil, T, and Nitz, AJ (eds): Orthopedic and Sports Physical Therapy, ed 3. CV Mosby, St Louis, 1997.

5. Magee, DJ: Orthopedic Physical Assessment, ed 3. WB Saunders, Philadelphia, 1997.

6. Cailliet, R: Soft Tissue Pain and Disability, ed 3. FA Davis, Philadelphia, 1996.

7. Zafar, H, Nordh, E, and Eriksson, PO: Temporal coordination between mandibular and head-neck movements during jaw opening-closing tasks in man. Arch Oral Biol 45:675, 2000.

8. Zafar, H: Integrated jaw and neck function in man. Studies of mandibular and head-neck movements during jaw opening-closing tasks. Swed Dent J 143(Suppl):1, 2000.

9. Eriksson, PO, et al: Co-ordinated mandibular and head-neck movements during rhythmic jaw activities in man. J Dent Res 79:1378, 2000.

10. Phillips, DJ, et al: Guide to evaluation of permanent impairment of the temporomandibular joint. J Craniomandibular Pract 15:170, 1997.

11. Walker, N, Bohannon, RW, and Cameron, D: Discriminant validity of temporomandibular joint range of motion measurements obtained with a ruler. J Orthop Sports Phys Ther 30:484, 2000.

12. Buschang, PH, et al: Incisor and mandibular condylar movements of young adult females during maximum protrusion and lateratrusion of the jaw. Arch Oral Biol 46:39, 2001.

13. Travers, KH, et al: Associations between incisor and mandibular condylar movements during maximum mouth opening in humans. Arch Oral Biol 45:267, 2000.

14. Lewis, RP, Buschang, PH, and Throckmorton, GS: Sex differences in mandibular movements during opening and closing. Am J Orthod Dentofacial Orthop 120:294, 2001.

15. Higbie, EJ, et al: Effect of head position on vertical mandibular opening. J Orthop Sports Phys Ther 29:127, 1999.

16. Gavish, A, et al: Oral habits and their association with signs and symptoms of temporomandibular disorders in adolescent girls. J Oral Rehabil 27:22, 2000.

17. Dijkstra, PU, et al: Ratio between vertical and horizontal mandibular range of motion. J Oral Rehabil 25:353, 1998.

18. Hockstedler, JL, Allen, JD, and Follmar, MA: Temporomandibular joint range of motion:a ratio of intercisal opening to excursive movement in a healthy population. Cranio 14:296, 1996.

19. Thurnwald, PA: The effect of age and gender on normal temporomandibular joint motion. Physiother Theory Pract 7:209, 1991.

20. Sonmez, H, et al: Prevalence of temporomandibular dysfunction in Turkish children with mixed and permanent dentition. J Oral Rehabil 28:280, 2001

21. Alamoudi, N, et al: Temporomandibular disorders among school children. J Clin Pediatr Dent 22:323, 1998.

22. Winocur, E, et al: Oral habits among adolescent girls and their association with symptoms of temporomandibular disorders. J Oral Rehabil 28: 624, 2001.

23. Hiltunen, K, et al: Prevalence of signs of temporomandibular disorders among elderly inhabitants of Helsinki, Finland. Acta Odontol Scand 53:20, 1995.

24. Rauhala, K, et al: Facial pain and temporomandibular disorders: an epidemiological study.

25. Westling, L, and Helkimo, E: Maximum jaw opening capacity in adolescents in relation to general joint mobility. 19:485, 1992.

26. Wright, DM, and Moffat, BC, Jr: The postnatal development of the human temporomandibular joint. Am J Anat 141:235, 1974.

27. Dijkstra, PU, et al: Temporomandibular joint mobility assessment: A comparison between four methods. J Oral Rehabil 22:439, 1995.

28. Dijkstra, PU, et al: Influence of mandibular length on mouth opening. J Oral Rehabil 26: 117, 1999.

29. Miller, VJ, et al: A mouth opening index for patients with temporomandibular disorders. J Oral Rehabil 26: 534, 1999.

30. Miller, VJ, et al: The temporomandibular opening index (TOI) in patients with closed lock and a control group with no temporomandibular disorders (TMD): an initial study. J Oral Rehabil 27:815, 2000.

31. Esposito, CJ, Panucci, PJ, and Farman, AG: Associations in 425 patients having temporomandibular disorders. J Kentucky Med Assoc 98:213, 2001.

32. Le Resche, L: Epidemiology of temporomandibular disorders: implications for the investigation of etiologic factors. Crit Rev Oral Biol Med 8: 291, 1997.

33. Kutilla, M, et al: TMD treatment need in relation to age, gender, stress and diagnostic subgroup. J Orofac Pain 12:67, 1998.

34. Warren, MP, and Fried, JL: Temporomandibular disorders and hormones in women. Cells Tissues Organs 169:187, 2000.

35. Kropmans, T, et al: Smallest detectable difference of maximal mouth opening in patients with painfully restricted temporomandibular joint function. Eur J Oral Sci 108:9, 2000.

APPENDIX A

Normative Range of Motion Values

TABLE A–1	Shoulder, Elbow, Forearm, and Wrist Motion: Mean Values in Degrees						
Motion	Wanatabe et al [1] 0–2 yrs n = 45	Boone and Azen [2] 1–54 yrs n = 109 (males)	Green and Wolf [3] 18–55 yrs n = 20 (10 M, 10 F)	Walker et al [4] 68–85 yrs n = 60 (30 M, 30 F)	Downey et al [5] 61–93 yrs n = 106 (60 M, 140 F shoulders)	AAOS [6]	AMA [7]
SHOULDER COMPLEX							
Flexion	172–180	167	156	165	165	180	150
Extension	78–89	62		44		60	50
Abduction	177–181	184	168	165	158	180	180
Medial rotation	72–90	69	49	62	65	70	90
Lateral rotation	118–134	104	84	81	81	90	90
ELBOW AND FOREARM							
Flexion	148–158	143	145	143		150	140
Extension		1		−4*		0	0
Pronation	90–96	76	84	71		80	80
Supination	81–93	82	77	74		80	80
WRIST							
Flexion	88–96	76	73	64		80	60
Extension	82–89	75	65	63		70	60
Radial deviation		22	25	19		20	20
Ulnar deviation		36	39	26		30	30

AAOS = American Association of Orthopaedic Surgeons; AMA = American Medical Association; M = males; F = females.
Values obtained with a universal goniometer.
* Minus sign indicates flexed position.

TABLE A–2	Glenohumeral Motion: Mean Values in Degrees			
Motion	Ellenbecker et al [8] 11–17 yrs n = 113 (M)	Ellenbecker et al [8] 11–17 yrs n = 90 (F)	Boon & Smith [9] 12–18 yrs n = 50 (18 M, 32 F)	Lannan et al [10] 21–40 yrs n = 60 (20 M, 40 F)
GLENOHUMERAL				
Flexion				106
Extension				20
Abduction				129
Medial rotation	51	56	63	49
Lateral rotation	103	105	108	94

M = males; F = females.
Values obtained with a universal goniometer.

TABLE A–3	Finger Motions: Mean Values in Degrees				
Motion	Skarilova & Plevkova* [11] 20–25 yrs n = 200 (100 M, 100 F)	Hume et al† [12] 26–28 yrs n = 35 (M)	Mallon et al‡ [13] 18–35 yrs n = 120 (60 M, 60 F)	AAOS [6]	AMA [7]
FINGER MCP					
Flexion	91	100	95	90	90
Extension	26		20	45	20
FINGER PIP					
Flexion	108	105	105	100	100
Extension		0	7	0	0
FINGER DIP					
Flexion	85	85	68	90	70
Extension		0	8	0	0

DIP = Distal interphalangeal; MCP = metacarpophalangeal; PIP = proximal interphalangeal.
AAOS = American Association of Orthopaedic Surgeons; AMA = American Medical Association; M = Males; F = females.
* Values obtained with a metallic slide goniometer on dorsal aspect.
† Values obtained with a universal goniometer on lateral aspect.
‡ Values obtained with a digital goniometer on dorsal aspect.

TABLE A–4   Thumb Motions: Mean Values in Degrees

Motion	Skarilova and Plevkova* [11] 20–25 yrs n = 200 (100 M, 100 F) Active	Skarilova and Plevkova* [11] 20–25 yrs n = 200 (100 M, 100 F) Passive	Jenkins et al[†][14] 16–72 yrs n = 119 (50 M, 69 F) Active	DeSmet et al[‡][15] 16–83 yrs n = 101 (43 M, 58 F)	AAOS[6]	AMA[7]
THUMB CMC						
Abduction					70	
Flexion					15	
Extension					20	50
THUMB MCP						
Flexion	57	67	59	54	50	60
Extension	14	23			0	0
THUMB IP						
Flexion	79	86	67	80	80	80
Extension	23	35			20	10

CMC = carpometacarpal; F = females; IP = interphalangeal; M = males; MCP = metacarpophalangeal.
* Values obtained with a metallic slide goniometer on dorsal aspect.
† Values obtained with a computerized Greenleaf goniometer.
‡ Values obtained with a gonimeter applied to the dorsal aspect.

TABLE A–5   Hip and Knee Motions: Mean Values in Degrees

Motion	Waugh et al [16] 6–65 hrs n = 40	Drews et al [17] 12 hrs–6 days n = 54 (26 M, 28 F)	Schwarze and Denton [18] 1–3 days n = 1000 (473 M, 527 F)	Wanatabe et al [1] 8–12 mos n = 45	Phelps et al [19] 24 mos n = 18 (M and F)	Boone and Azen [2] 1–54 yrs n = 109 (109 M)	Roach and Miles [20] 25–74 yrs n = 1683 (821 M, 862 F)	AAOS[6]	AMA[7]
HIP									
Flexion						122	121	120	100
Extension	46*	28*	20*	3*	3*	10	19	20†	30
Abduction		55	78			46	42	45	40
Adduction		6	15					30	20
Medial rotation		80	58	38	52	27	32	45	50
Lateral rotation			80	79	47	47	32	45	50
KNEE									
Flexion			150	148–159		142	132	135	150
Extension	15*	20*	15*					10	

M = males; F = females.
* Values refer to extension limitations.
† A 1994 AAOS value.

TABLE A–6	Ankle and Foot Motions: Mean Values in Degrees

Motion	Waugh et al [16] 6–65 hrs n = 40 (18 M, 22 F)	Wanatabe et al [1] 4–8 mos n = 54	Boone and Azen [2] 1–54 yrs n = 109 (M)	McPoil and Cornwall [23] x = 26.1 yrs n = 27 (9 M, 18 F)	Mecagni et al [22] 64–87 yrs n = 34 (F)	AAOS [6]	AMA [7]
ANKLE							
Dorsiflexion	59	51	13	16	11	20	20
Plantar flexion	26	60	56		64	50	40
Inversion			37	19 (Subtalar)	26	35	30
Eversion			21	12 (Subtalar)	17	15	20
FIRST MTP							
Flexion						45	30
Extension				86		70	50

F = females; M = males.
All range of motion values in the table obtained with a universal goniometer.

TABLE A–7	Cervical Spine Motions: Mean Values in Centimeters and Degrees

Motion	Youdas et al* [24] 11–19 yrs n = 40 (20 M, 20 F) M	F	30–39 yrs n = 41 (20 M, 21 F) M	F	70–79 yrs n = 40 (20 M, 20 F) M	F	Lantz et al† [25] 20–39 yrs n = 63 Act	Pass	Hsieh and Young‡ [26] 14–31 yrs n = 34 (27 M, 7 F)	Balogun et al§ [27] 18–26 yrs n = 21 (15 M, 6 F)		AAOS [6]	AMA [7]
CERVICAL SPINE													
Flexion	64		47		39		60	74	01 cm	0.4 cm	32	45	50
Extension	86	84	68	78	54	55	56	53	22 cm	19 cm	64	45	60
Right lateral flexion	45	49	43	47	26	28	43	48	11 cm	13 cm	41	45	45
Right rotation	74	75	61	72	50	53	72	79	12 cm	11 cm	64	60	80

AAOS = American Association of Orthopaedic Surgeons; AMA = American Medical Association; F = female; M = male.
* Values in degrees were obtained for active range of motion using the cervical range of motion (CROM) instrument.
† Values in degrees were obtained for active (Act) and passive (Pass) range of motion with use of the OSI CA-6000 Spinal Motion Analyzer.
‡ Values in centimeters were obtained with a tape measure.
§ Values in centimeters obtained with a tape measure appear in the first column, whereas values in degrees obtained with a Myrin gravity-referenced goniometer appear in the second column.
NB: AMA values in degrees were obtained with use of a universal goniometer and AAOS values in degrees were obtained with use of an inclinometer.

TABLE A–8	Thoracic and Lumbar Spine Motions: Mean Values in Centimeters and Degrees										
	Haley et al*[29] 5–9 yrs n = 282 (140 M, 142 F)	Moll and Wright*[30] 15–75 yrs n = 237 (119 M, 118 F)	Van Adrichem and van der Korst†[31] 15–18 yrs n = 66 (34 M, 32 F)		Breum et al‡[32] 18–38 yrs n = 47 (27 M, 20 F)		McGregor et al§[33] 50–59 yrs n = 41 (21 M, 20 F)		Fitzgerald et al¶[34] 20–82 yrs n = 172 (168 M, 4 F)	AAOS[6]	AMA[7]
Motion			M	F			M	F			
Flexion	6–7 cm	5–7 cm	7 cm	6 cm	56‡	54‡	55	60		80	60
Extension					22	21	21	18	16–41	25	25
Right lateral flexion					33	31	30	30	18–38	35	25
Right rotation					8	8	26	26		45	30

AAOS = American Association of Orthopaedic Surgeons; AMA = American Medical Association; F = female; M = male

* Lumbar values obtained with use of the modified Schober method.

† Lumbar values obtained using the modified–modified Schober (simplified skin distraction) method

‡ Lumbar values in the first column were obtained with the BROM II. Lumbar values in the second column were obtained with double inclinometers.

§ Lumbar values obtained with the OSI CA-6000.

¶ Lumbar values for thoracolumbar extension and lateral flexion were obtained with a universal goniometer. Lower values are for ages 70–79 years and higher values are for ages 20–29 years.

NB: AAOS values for thoracolumbar motions were obtained with a universal goniometer. AMA values were obtained with use of the two-inclinometer method for lumbar motions of flexion, extension, and lateral flexion. The value for rotation is for the thoracolumbar spine.

TABLE A–9	Temporomandibular Motions: Mean Values in Millimeters								
	Walker, Bohannon, and Cameron*[35] 21–61 yrs n = 15 (3 M, 12 F)	Phillips et al†[36]	Higbie et al‡[37] 18–54 yrs n = 40 (20 M, 20 F)			Thurnwald§			
						17–25 yrs n = 50 (25 M, 25 F)		50–65 yrs n = 50 (25 M, 25 F)	
Motion			Head Positions Fwd Neut Retract			M	F	M	F
Opening	43	40–50	45	42	36	61	55	58	51
Left lateral Deviation	9	8–12				9	8	8	6
Right lateral Deviation	9					10	9	7	9
Protrusion	7					5	5	5	4

Fwd = Forward; Neut = neutral; Retract = retracted.

* Values were obtained for active range of motion (ROM) with an 11-cm plastic ruler marked in millimeters.

† Values represent consensus judgments of normal ROM made at the Permanent Impairment Conference.

‡ Values were obtained for active ROM with a ruler.

§ Values were obtained for active ROM with Vernier calipers as the measuring instrument.

REFERENCES

1. Wanatabe, H, et al: The range of joint motion of the extremities in healthy Japanese people: The differences according to age. (Cited in Walker, JM: Musculoskeletal development: A review. Phys Ther 71:878, 1991.)
2. Boone, DC, and Azen, SP: Normal range of motion of joints in male subjects. J Bone Joint Surg 61:756, 1979.
3. Greene, BL, and Wolf, SL: Upper extremity joint movement: Comparison of two measurement devices. Arch Phys Med Rehabil 70:288, 1989.
4. Walker, JM, et al: Active mobility of the extremities in older subjects. Phys Ther 4:919, 1984.
5. Downey, PA, Fiebert, I, and Stackpole-Brown, JB: Shoulder range of motion in persons aged sixty and older. (abstract). Phys Ther 71:S75, 1991.
6. American Academy of Orthopaedic Surgeons: Joint Motion: Method of measuring and recording. American Academy of Orthopaedic Surgeons, Chicago, 1965.
7. American Medical Association: Guides to the Evaluation of Permanent Impairment, ed 3. AMA, Chicago 1988.
8. Ellenbecker, TS, et al: Glenohumeral joint internal and external rotation range of motion in elite junior tennis players. J Orthop Sports Phys Ther 24:336, 1996.
9. Boon, AJ, and Smith, J: Manual scapular stabilization: Its effect on shoulder rotational range of motion. Arch Phys Med Rehabil 81:978, 2000.
10. Lannan, D, Lehman, T, and Toland, M: Establishment of normative data for the range of motion of the glenohumeral joint. Master of Science thesis, University of Massachusetts, Lowell, 1996.
11. Skarilova, B, and Plevkova, A: Ranges of joint motion of the adult hand. Acta Chir Plast 38:67, 1996.
12. Hume, M, et al: Functional range of motion of the joints of the hand. J Hand Surg 15A:240, 1990.
13. Mallon, WJ, Brown, HR, and Nunley JA: Digital ranges of motion: Normal values in young adults. J Hand Surg 16A:882, 1991.
14. Jenkins, M, et al: Thumb joint motion: What is normal? J Hand Surg 23B:796, 1998.
15. DeSmett, L, et al: Metacarpophalangeal and interphalangeal flexion of the thumb: Influence of sex and age, relation to ligamentous injury. Acta Orhtop Belg 59:37, 1993.
16. Waugh, KG, et al: Measurement of selected hip, knee and ankle joint motions in newborns. Phys Ther 63:1616, 1983.
17. Drews, JE, Vraciu, JK, and Pellino, G: Range of motion of the lower extremities of newborns. Phys Occup Ther Pediatr 4:49, 1884.
18. Schwarze, DJ, and Denton, JR: normal values of neonatal limbs: An evaluation of 1000 neonates. J Pediatr Orthop 13:758, 1993.
19. Phelps, E, Smith, LJ, and Hallum, A: Normal ranges of hip motion of infants between 9 and 24 months of age. Dev Med Child Neurol 27:785, 1985.
20. Roach, KE, and Miles, TP: Normal hip and knee active range of motion: The relationship of age. Phys Ther 71: 656, 1991.
21. Greene, WB, and Heckman, JD (eds): The Clinical Measurement of Joint Motion. American Academy of Orthopaedic Surgeons, Rosemont, III. 1994.
22. Mecagni, C, et al: Balance and ankle range of motion in community dwelling women aged 64–87 years: A correlational study. Phys Ther 80:1004, 2000.
23. McPoil, TG, and Cornwall, MW: The relationship between static lower extremity measurements and rearfoot motion during walking. Phys Ther 24:309, 1996.
24. Youdas, J, et al: Normal range of motion of the cervical spine: An initial goniometric study. Phys Ther 72:770, 1992.
25. Lantz, CA, Chen, J, and Buch, D: Clinical validity and stability of active and passive cervical range of motion with regard to total and uniplanar motion. Spine 24:1082, 1999.
26. Hsieh, C-Y and Yeung, BW: Active neck motion measurements with a tape measure. J Orthop Sports Phys Ther 8:88, 1986.
27. Balogun, JA, et al: Inter-and intratester reliability of measuring neck motions with tape measure and Myrin Gravity-Reference Goniometer. J Orthop Sports Phys Ther 9:248, 1989.
28. American Medical Association: Guides to the Evaluation of Permanent Impairment, ed 4. AMA, Chicago, 1993.
29. Haley, SM, Tada, WL, Carmichael, EM: Spinal mobility in young children. Phys Ther 66:1697, 1986.
30. Moll, JMH, and Wright, V: Normal range of spinal mobility: An objective clinical study. Ann Rheum Dis 30:381, 1971.
31. van Adrichem, JAM, and van der Korst, JK: Assessment of flexibility of the lumbar spine. A pilot study in children and adolescents. Scand J Rheumatol 2:87, 1973.
32. Breum, J, Wiberg, J, and Bolton, JE: Reliability and concurrent validity of the BROM II for measuring lumbar mobility. J Manipulative Physiol Ther 18:497, 1995.
33. Mcgregor, AH, MacCarthy, ID, and Hughes, SP: Motion characteristics of the lumbar spine in the normal population. Spine 20:2421, 1995.
34. Fitzgerald, GK, et al: Objective assessment with establishment of normal values for lumbar spine range of motion. Phys Ther 63:1776, 1983.
35. Walker, N, Bohannon, RW, Cameron, D: Validity of temporomandibular joint range of motion measurements obtained with a ruler. J Orthop Sports Phys Ther 30:484, 2000.
36. Phillips, DJ, et al: Guide to evaluation of permanent impairment of the temporomandibular joint. J Craniomandibular Pract 15:170, 1997.
37. Higbie, EJ, et al: Effect of head position on vertical mandibular opening. J Orthop Sports Phys Ther 29:127, 1999.
38. Thurnwald, PA: The effect of age and gender on normal temporomandibular joint movement. Physiother Theory Pract 7:209, 1991.

APPENDIX B

Joint Measurements by Body Position

	Prone	*Supine*	*Sitting*	*Standing*
Shoulder	Extension	Flexion		
		Abduction		
		Medial rotation		
		Lateral rotation		
Elbow		Flexion		
Forearm			Pronation	
			Supination	
Wrist			Flexion	
			Extension	
			Radial deviation	
			Ulnar deviation	
Hand			All motions	
Hip	Extension	Flexion	Medial rotation	
		Abduction	Lateral rotation	
		Adduction		
Knee		Flexion		
Ankle and foot	Subtalar inversion	Dorsiflexion	Dorsiflexion	
	Subtalar eversion	Plantar flexion	Plantar flexion	
		Inversion	Inversion	
		Eversion	Eversion	
		Midtarsal inversion	Midtarsal inversion	
		Midtarsal eversion	Midtarsal eversion	
Toes		All motions	All motions	
Cervical spine			Flexion	
			Extension	
			Lateral flexion	
			Rotation	
Thoracic and lumbar spine			Rotation	Flexion
				Extension
				Lateral flexion
Temporomandibular joint			Depression	
			Anterior protrusion	
			Lateral deviation	

APPENDIX C

Goniometer Price Lists

TABLE C–1	Plastic Goniometers			
Type	Size (in)	Scale (degrees)	Increments (degrees)	Cost (U.S. $)
E-Z Read JAMAR Full Circle	$12^{1}/_{2}$	0–180 and 0–360	1	19.95*
International Goniometer	$12^{1}/_{4}$	0–360	1	17.95[†]
ISOM (STFR) Goniometer Full Circle	12	0–360	1	18.49[‡]
Baseline ISOM	12	0–360		17.95[§]
				22.95[¶]
ISOM Full Circle	8	0–360	1	8.99[‡]
				10.00[§]
				9.95[¶]
Full Circle	8	0–90 and 0–180	5	5.95*
Full Circle	8	0–90 degrees and 0–180	5	8.95*
Full Circle	8	0–180	1	11.95*
International Goniometer	$7^{7}/_{8}$	0–180	5	10.95[†]
E-Z Read JAMAR Half Circle	$6^{3}/_{4}$	0–180	5	7.95*
Half Circle	$6^{3}/_{4}$	0–180	5	3.95*
E-Z Read JAMAR Full Circle	6	0–180	1	9.95*
ISOM Full Circle	6	0–360	1	7.49[‡]
				7.95[¶]
				8.00[§]
Pocket Goniometer		0–180		4.49[†]
Devore Pocket Finger Goniometer	$4 \times 2^{1}/_{8}$	0–180	1	17.50[†]
Roylan Finger Goniometer		30 of hyperextension to 129 of flexion		10.29**
Roylan Finger/Toe Goniometer		30 of hyperextension to 120 of flexion		20.49**
Digit Goniometer		Measures 110 of flexion and 40 of hyperextension	5	25.99[‡]

All prices are from 2002 catalogs except those for Sammons-Preston and Best Priced Products, which are from 2001 catalogs.
* Sammons Preston 1–800–323–5547.
[†] North Coast Medical 1–800–821–9391.
[‡] Best Priced Products 1–800–824–2939.
[§] Pro-Med Products 1–800–542–9297.
[¶] American 3-B Scientific 1–888–326–6335.
** Smith-Nephew 1–800–558–8633.

TABLE C–2	Metal Goniometers			
Type	*Size (in)*	*Scale (degrees)*	*Increments (degrees)*	*Cost (U.S. $)*
Full Circle Stainless Steel Goniometer	14	0–360, 0–180, and 180–0	1 (thumb knob varies tension in arms)	31.99*
Half Circle Stainless Steel Goniometer	14	0–180, and 180–0	1 (nonlocking friction arm)	35.95[†] 27.99* 34.95[‡]
Full Circle Stainless Steel Goniometer	14	0–360, 0–180, 180–0	1 (knob varies tension in arms and locks)	39.95[†]
Black Aluminum X-Ray Goniometer	14	0–180 and 180–0	$2^1/_2$ (white radiopaque markings)	35.99*
Half Circle Stainless Steel Goniometer	8	0–180 and 180–0	1 (thumb knob varies tension in arms)	15.99*
Stainless Steel Metal Goniometer	8	0–180	1 (thumb knob varies tension in arms and locks)	20.95[†] 22.50*
Black Aluminum X-Ray Goniometer	8	0–180 and 180–0	$2^1/_2$ (white radiopaque markings)	27.99*
Robinson Pocket Goniometer	7	0–180	5	15.95[†]
	7.25	0–180	5	13.95[‡]
	6	0–180	5	17.95[§] 11.99*
Standard Stainless Steel Finger Goniometer	6	0–180 and 180–0	5	23.99* 27.95[†]
Deluxe Stainless Steel Finger Goniometer	6	0–180 and 180–0	5	31.99*
Deluxe Small Joint Stainless Steel Goniometer	$5^1/_2$	0–150	5	32.95[†]
Stainless Steel Finger Goniometer	$5^1/_2$		5	25.95[§] 34.50[‡] 45.99[¶]
Stainless Steel Finger Goniometer	4	0–150	5	29.95[†]
Small Stainless Steel Finger Goniometer	$3^1/_2$		5	23.99*

* Sammons Preston 1–800–323–5547.
[†] Flag House 1–800–793–7900.
[‡] North Coast Medical 1–800–821–9319.
[§] Best Priced Products 1–800–824–2939.
[¶] Smith-Nephew 1–800–558–8633.

TABLE C–3	Inclinometers	
Type	**Features**	**Cost (U.S. $)**
Universal Inclinometer (fluid based)	Available with clip or headband	59.99*
Universal Inclinometer (fluid based)	Available with two interchangeable bases	69.99[†]
Baseline Bubble Inclinometer	Size 4″ × 3″ with 360-degree rotating dial	59.99* 79.00[‡] 99.00[§]
MIE Inclinometer (Bubble Inclinometer)	Size 4″ × 3″ with 360-degree rotating dial	95.00[¶] 105.00** 129.95[††]
PROsupinator Gravity Based Fluid Inclinometer	Measures supination and pronation and ulnar and radial deviation on a 5-degree, 360 scale	64.95** 49.95[§]
Unilevel Dual Scale Inclinometer	1-degree increments on one side and 2-degree increments on the other side	115.00[¶]
Baseline Digital Inclinometer		239.00[‡]
Saunders Digital Inclinometer (methods, guides and protocol)	Arch attachment for measuring irregular surfaces and ruler for radiographs and sacral base angles. On/off, alternate 0, and hold buttons	299.99[†] 319.95[††]
CROM (Cervical Range of Motion Instrument) includes storage case and a manual with normal values	Measures flexion/extension, rotation, lateral tilt, and protraction/retraction	379.95[††] 349.99[†]
BROM (lumbar range of motion instrument)	Measures lumbar range of motion	475.95[††]

* Best Priced Products 1–800–824–2939
[†] The Saunders Group 1–800–966–3138
[‡] American 3B Scientific 1–888–326–6335
[¶] ProMed products 1–800–542–9297
[§] North Coast Medical 1–800–821–9319
** FlagHouse 1–800–793–7900
[††] Sammons Preston 1–800–323–5547

Numerical Recording Forms

			Range of Motion—TMJ and Spine			
Patient's Name				Date of Birth		
	Left				Right	
			Date			
			Examiner's Initials			
			Temporomandibular Joint			
			Depression			
			Anterior Protrusion			
			Lateral Deviation—Right			
			Lateral Deviation—Left			
			Comments:			
			Cervical Spine			
			Flexion			
			Extension			
			Lateral Flexion—Right			
			Lateral Flexion—Left			
			Rotation—Right			
			Rotation—Left			
			Comments:			
			Thoracolumbar Spine			
			Flexion			
			Extension			
			Lateral Flexion—Right			
			Lateral Flexion—Left			
			Rotation—Right			
			Rotation—Left			
			Comments:			
			Lumbar Spine			
			Flexion			
			Extension			
			Comments:			

			Range of Motion—Upper Extremity			
	Left		Patient's Name _____ Date of Birth _____ Right			
			Date			
			Examiner's Initials			
			Shoulder Complex			
			Flexion			
			Extension			
			Abduction			
			Medial Rotation			
			Lateral Rotation			
			Comments:			
			Glenohumeral			
			Flexion			
			Extension			
			Abduction			
			Medial Rotation			
			Lateral Rotation			
			Comments:			
			Elbow and Forearm			
			Flexion			
			Supination			
			Pronation			
			Comments:			
			Wrist			
			Flexion			
			Extension			
			Ulnar Deviation			
			Radial Deviation			
			Comments:			

Range of Motion—Hand

Patient's Name _____ Date of Birth _____

Left				Right		
			Date			
			Examiner's Initials			
			Thumb			
			CMC Flexion			
			CMC Extension			
			CMC Abduction			
			CMC Opposition			
			MCP Flexion			
			IP Flexion			
			IP Extension			
			Index Finger			
			MCP Flexion			
			MCP Extension			
			MCP Abduction			
			PIP Flexion			
			DIP Flexion			
			Middle Finger			
			MCP Flexion			
			MCP Extension			
			MCP Radial Abduction			
			MCP Ulnar Abduction			
			PIP Flexion			
			DIP Flexion			
			Ring Finger			
			MCP Flexion			
			MCP Extension			
			MCP Abduction			
			PIP Flexion			
			DIP Flexion			
			Little Finger			
			MCP Flexion			
			MCP Extension			
			MCP Abduction			
			PIP Flexion			
			DIP Flexion			
			Comments:			

			Range of Motion—Lower Extremity			
Patient's Name _____ Date of Birth _____						
Left						Right
			Date			
			Examiner's Initials			
			Hip			
			Flexion			
			Extension			
			Abduction			
			Adduction			
			Medial Rotation			
			Lateral Rotation			
			Knee			
			Flexion			
			Ankle			
			Dorsiflexion			
			Plantarflexion			
			Inversion—Tarsal			
			Eversion—Tarsal			
			Inversion—Subtalar			
			Eversion—Subtalar			
			Inversion—Midtarsal			
			Eversion—Midtarsal			
			Great Toe			
			MTP Flexion			
			MTP Extension			
			MTP Abduction			
			IP Flexion			
			Toe _____			
			MTP Flexion			
			MTP Extension			
			MTP Abduction			
			PIP Flexion			
			DIP Flexion			
			DIP Extension			
			Comments:			

Muscle Length

Patient's Name _____ Date of Birth _____

	Left				Right	
			Date			
			Examiner's Initials			
			Upper Extremity			
			Biceps Brachii			
			Triceps Brachii			
			Flexor Digitorum Profundus & Superficialis			
			Extensor Digitorum			
			Lumbricals			
			Comments:			
			Lower Extremity			
			Hip Flexors—Thomas Test			
			Rectus Femoris—Ely Test			
			Hamstrings—SLR			
			Hamstrings—Distal Hamstring Length Test			
			Tensor Fascia Lata—Ober Test			
			Gastrocnemius			
			Comments:			

Index

A "b" following a page number indicates a box; an "f" indicates a figure, and a "t" indicates a table.

A

Abduction. *See* specific joints
Achilles tendon
  anatomy of, 288, 288f
Acromioclavicular joint
  anatomy of, 59, 59f
  arthrokinematics of, 60
  osteokinematics of, 59–60
Active range of motion. *See also* Range of
  motion
  defined, 6–7
  testing of, 7
Activities of daily living
  functional range of motion in
    ankle and foot, 250–252, 251f–252f, 251t
    cervical spine, 302f–303f, 302–303
    elbow, 96t, 96–97, 97f–98f
    hand, 143f, 143–144, 144t
    hip, 189f–190f, 189t, 189–192
    knee, 225, 226f–227f, 226t
    shoulder, 63, 64f–65f, 64t
    thoracic/lumbar spine, 337f–338f,
      337–338
    wrist, 115t–116t, 115–117, 116f–117f
Adduction. *See* specific joints
Adductor longus and brevis muscles
  anatomy of, 207
  in Thomas test, 206f–211f, 206–211
Adolescents
  low-back pain in, 337
  range of motion in
    ankle and foot, 247t
    cervical spine, 298t–299t
    elbow, 94, 94t
    hip, 184t, 186t
    knee, 224, 224t
    shoulder, 61, 61t
    thoracic and lumbar spine, 334,
      335t–336t, 336
    wrist, 113t, 113–114
  temporomandibular joint disorders in,
    368–369
  urban *versus* rural, 336
Adults
  range of motion in, 11
    ankle and foot, 247t–248t, 247–248

    cervical spine, 298t–299t, 298–299
    elbow, 94–95, 95t
    hand, 142
    hip, 184t, 184–187, 186t
    knee, 223t–224t, 224–225
    shoulder, 61t, 61–62
    temporomandibular joint, 367, 367t
    thoracic and lumbar spine, 334,
      335t–336t
    wrist, 113t, 113–114
Age
  range of motion and, 11–12
    ankle and foot, 247, 247t–249t
    cervical spine, 297–299, 298t–299t
    elbow, 94t–95t, 94–95
    hand, 141
    hip, 184–187, 185t–186t
    knee, 223t–224t, 223–225
    shoulder, 61t, 61–62
    temporomandibular joint, 367, 367t
    thoracic and lumbar spine, 333–334,
      335t–336t
    wrist, 112f, 112–113
Alignment
  in ankle and foot testing
    for toe abduction, 285, 285f
    anatomical landmarks for, 255f, 263f,
      269f, 279f
    for dorsiflexion, 257f–259f, 257–258
    for eversion, 267, 267f–268f, 273, 273f,
      277f–278f, 277–278
    for toe extension, 282, 283f
    for toe flexion, 280, 281f, 286–287
    for inversion, 265, 265f, 271, 271f, 274,
      275f
    for muscle length, 290, 290f
    for plantarflexion, 261, 262f
  in cervical spine testing
    anatomical landmarks for, 307f–309f
    for extension, 314f–317f, 315–317
    for flexion, 310f–313f, 311–313,
    for lateral flexion, 318, 319f–323f,
      321–323
    for rotation, 324, 325f–328f, 326, 328
  in elbow testing
    anatomical landmarks for, 99, 99f

    for extension, 102
    for flexion, 100, 101f
    of muscle length, 107, 107f, 109, 109f
    for pronation, 103, 103f
    for supination, 105, 105f
  general procedures for, 27f–29f, 27–30
    exercise for, 30
  in hand testing
    for abduction, 150, 151f, 164, 165f
    for adduction, 152, 153f
    anatomical landmarks for, 145f
    for extension, 148, 149f, 154, 158, 162,
      163f, 172, 175
    for flexion, 146, 147f, 156, 156f–157f,
      160, 161f, 170, 171f, 173, 174f
    for muscle length, 178, 179f
    for opposition, 168, 168f–169f
  in hip testing
    for abduction, 198, 199f
    for adduction, 201, 201f
    anatomical landmarks for, 192f–193f
    for extension, 196, 197f
    for flexion, 194, 195f
    for lateral rotation, 205, 205f
    for medial rotation, 203, 203f
    for muscle length, 210, 211f, 214, 215f,
      218, 219f
  in knee testing
    anatomical landmarks for, 229f
    for extension, 232
    for flexion, 230, 231f
    for muscle length, 232, 235, 235f, 239,
      239f
  in shoulder testing, 68, 68f–69f
    for abduction, 80, 80f–81f
    anatomical landmarks for, 68f–69f
    for extension, 76, 76f–77f
    for flexion, 72, 72f–73f
    for lateral rotation, 88, 88f–89f
    for medial rotation, 84, 84f–85f
  in temporomandibular joint testing
    anatomical landmarks for, 370f
    for depression, 370, 371f
    for lateral deviation, 373, 373f
    for protrusion, 372, 372f
  in thoracic and lumbar spine testing

Alignment (Continued)
    anatomical landmarks for, 343f
        for extension, 357f–359f, 357–359
        for flexion, 346, 346f–347f, 350f–351f,
            350–351
        for rotation, 360, 361f–363f, 362
    in wrist testing
        anatomical landmarks for, 119f
        for extension, 122, 123f
        for flexion, 120, 121f
        of muscle length, 131, 131f, 135,
            135f
        for radial deviation, 124, 125f
        for ulnar deviation, 126, 127f
American Academy of Orthopaedic
    Surgeons
    range of motion findings of
        ankle, 246, 246t, 378t
        elbow, 94, 94t, 375t
        foot, 246, 246t, 378t
        hand, 140t, 140–141, 376t–377t
        hip, 184, 184t, 377t
        knee, 224, 377t
        shoulder, 60, 60t, 375t
        spine, 333, 334t, 378t–379t
        wrist, 112t, 112–113, 375t
American Medical Association
    range of motion findings of
        ankle, 246, 246t, 378t
        elbow, 94, 94t, 375t
        foot, 246, 246t, 378t
        hand, 140t, 140–141, 376t–377t
        hip, 184, 184t, 377t
        knee, 223t, 223–224, 377t
        shoulder, 60, 60t, 375t
        spine, 298t, 333, 334t, 378t–379t
        wrist, 112t, 112–113, 375t
    recording guide of, 34
Anatomical landmarks
    goniometer alignment using, 27, 27f
        ankle, 255f, 263f, 269f
        cervical spine, 307f–309f
        elbow, 99, 99f
        foot, 255f, 263f, 269f, 279f
        hand, 145f, 159f
        hip, 192f–193f
        knee, 229f
        shoulder, 68f–69f
        temporomandibular joint, 370f
        thoracic and lumbar spine, 343f
        wrist, 119f
Anatomy
    ankle and foot, 241, 242f–246f, 243–245
    cervical spine, 295f–297f, 295–296
    elbow, 91f–93f, 91–93
    hand, 137f–139f, 137–139
    hip, 183f–184f, 183–184
    knee, 221f–222f, 221–222
    shoulder, 57–60, 58f–59f
    temporomandibular joint, 365, 365f–366f
    thoracic and lumbar spine, 331–333,
        332f–333f
    wrist, 111f–112f, 111–112
Ankle. See also Foot
    anatomical landmarks of, 255f, 263f, 269f
    anatomy of, 241–244, 242f–244f
    arthrokinematics of, 241, 243–245

capsular pattern in, 241
dorsiflexion of
    end-feel determinations and, 20
    functional range of motion in, 250–252,
        251f–252f, 251t
    reliability of testing of, 253, 253t
    research findings in, 248t–249t, 248–249
    talocrural testing of, 256f–259f, 256–259
eversion of
    reliability of testing of, 253, 254t
    subtalar testing of, 272f–273f, 272–273
    tarsal testing of, 266f–268f, 266–268
inversion of
    reliability of testing of, 253, 254t
    subtalar testing of, 270f–271f, 270–271
    tarsal testing of, 264f–265f, 264–265
osteokinematics of, 241, 243–244
plantarflexion of
    functional range of motion in, 250–252,
        251f, 251t
    reliability of testing of, 253, 253t
    talocrural testing of, 260f–262f, 260–262
range of motion of
    age and, 247, 247f
    disease and, 250
    functional, 250–252, 251f–252f, 251t
    gender and, 248t, 248–249
    injury and, 250
    normative values for, 378t
    numerical recording form for, 390f
    reliability and validity in testing of,
        252–254, 253t–254t
    research findings in, 246t–248t, 246–247
subtalar eversion of
    testing of, 272f–273f, 272–273
subtalar inversion of
    testing of, 270f–271f, 270–271
talocrural dorsiflexion of
    testing of, 256f–259f, 256–259
talocrural plantarflexion of
    testing of, 260f–262f, 260–262
tarsal eversion of
    testing of, 266f–268f, 266–268
tarsal inversion of
    testing of, 264f–265f, 264–265
Ankylosis
    sagittal-frontal-transverse-rotation
        method of recording, 34
Anterior-posterior axis
    defined, 4, 5f
Arm. See also specific joints; Upper-
    extremity testing
    muscle length testing in, 106f–109f,
        106–107
    range of motion of, 99f–105f, 99–105
    structure and function of, 91f–93f, 91–93,
        106f, 108f
Arthrokinematics
    of acromioclavicular joint, 60
    of atlanto-occipital and atlantoaxial joints,
        296
    of carpometacarpal joint, 138–139
    defined, 4
    of glenohumeral joint, 57–58
    of humeroulnar and humeroradial joints,
        92
    of iliofemoral joint, 184

of interphalangeal joints
    toes, 246
    fingers, 138
    thumb, 140
of intervertebral and zygapophyseal
    joints, 297
of lumbar spine, 333
of metacarpophalangeal joints, 138–139
of metatarsophalangeal joints, 245
of midtarsal joint, 245
of radioulnar joints, 93
of scapulothoracic joint, 60
of sternoclavicular joint, 59
of subtalar joint, 243–244
of talocrural joint, 241
of tarsometatarsal joints, 245
of temporomandibular joint, 366
of thoracic spine, 332
of tibiofemoral and patellofemoral joints,
    222
of tibiofibular joints, 241
of wrist, 112
Ascending stairs
    range of motion necessary for
        ankle and foot, 251, 251f, 251t
        hip, 189, 189f, 189t
        knee, 225, 226f, 226t
Athletes
    ankle sprains in, 250
    low-back pain in, 337
Atlantoaxial joint. See also Cervical spine
    anatomy of, 295, 295f
    arthrokinematics of, 296
    osteokinematics of, 295–296
Atlanto-occipital joint. See also Cervical
    spine
    anatomy of, 295, 295f
    arthrokinematics of, 296
    capsular pattern in, 296
    osteokinematics of, 295–296
Axes
    in osteokinematics, 4, 5f

B

Back Range of Motion Device
    price of, 385t
    reliability of, 339t, 340
Ballet
    range of motion of hip and, 188
Baseball players
    shoulder rotation in, 62–63
Basic concepts, 3–14
Beighton hypermobility score, 10, 11t
Benign joint hypermobility syndrome
    defined, 10
Biceps brachii muscle
    muscle length testing of, 106f–107f,
        106–107
Biceps femoris muscle
    anatomy of, 212, 212f, 236, 236f
    in distal hamstring length test, 236f–239f,
        236–239
    in straight leg test, 212f–215f, 212–215
Biological variation
    standard deviation indicating, 44, 44t
Body position

joint measurements and, 381t
Body size
    range of motion and
        ankle and foot, 250
        cervical spine, 302
Body-mass index
    range of motion and
        elbow, 95
        hip, 187
        knee, 225
        shoulder, 62
Bubble goniometers, 24–25, 25f

C

CA-6000 Spine Motion Analyzer
    in cervical spine testing
        reliability of, 305
        testing position and, 301–302
    in thoracic and lumbar spine testing
        of functional activities, 337
        reliability of, 339t, 341–342
Calcaneus
    anatomy of, 288, 288f
Capsular fibrosis
    capsular pattern in, 10
Capsular pattern of restricted motion
    of atlanto-occipital and atlantoaxial joints,
        296
    of carpometacarpal joint, 139
    defined, 9
    example of, 9b
    of glenohumeral joint, 58
    of humeroulnar and humeroradial joints,
        92
    of iliofemoral joint, 184
    of interphalangeal joints
        fingers, 138
        thumb, 140
    of intervertebral and zygapophyseal
        joints, 297
    of lumbar spine, 333
    of metacarpophalangeal joints, 138–139
    of metatarsophalangeal joints, 245–246
    of midtarsal joint, 245
    of radioulnar joints, 93
    in range of motion testing, 9t, 9–10
    of subtalar joint, 244
    of talocrural joint, 241
    of temporomandibular joint, 366–367
    of thoracic spine, 332
    of tibiofemoral and patellofemoral joints,
        222
    of tibiofibular joints, 241
    of wrist, 112
Carpal tunnel syndrome
    wrist position and, 117
Carpometacarpal joints. *See also* Hand
    anatomy of, 137f, 138
    arthrokinematics of, 138–139
    capsular pattern of, 139
    osteokinematics of, 138
    range of motion of, 140–141, 141t
        normative values for, 377t
Carrying angle
    elbow, 91–92
Cervical Range of Motion Device

in cervical spine testing
    of extension, 316–317, 317f
    of flexion, 312–313, 313f
    of lateral flexion, 322–323, 323f
    reliability of, 304t, 304–306
    research findings in, 298, 299t
    of rotation, 328, 328f
    price of, 385t
Cervical spine, 295–328
    anatomical landmarks of, 307f–309f
    anatomy of, 295f–297f, 295–297
    arthrokinematics of, 296–297
    capsular pattern in, 296–297
    extension of
        age and, 299–301, 300t–301t
        testing of, 314f–317f, 314–317
    flexion of
        age and, 299t–301t, 299–300
        testing of, 310f–313f, 310–313
    lateral flexion of
        testing of, 318f–323f, 318–323
    osteokinematics of, 295–297
    range of motion of
        age and, 297–299, 299t–301t
        body size and, 302
        functional, 302f–303f, 302–303
        gender and, 299t–301t, 299–301
        normative values for, 378t
        numerical recording form for, 387f
        reliability and validity of testing of,
            303–306, 304t
        research findings in, 297, 298t
        testing position and, 301–302, 381t
    rotation of
        age and, 300, 300t–301t
        testing of, 324f–328f, 324–328
Children
    range of motion in, 11
        ankle and foot, 247t, 247–248
        cervical spine, 299t
        elbow, 94, 94t
        hip, 184t–186t, 184–186
        knee, 223t–224t, 223–224
        shoulder, 61, 61t
        wrist, 113, 113t
Clavicle
    as shoulder anatomical landmark, 68f
Coefficients
    correlation, 45–47, 46t
        intraclass, 46–47
    of variation
        in reliability evaluation, 45
        of replication, 45
Collateral ligaments
    elbow, 91, 92f
Concurrent validity
    criterion-related validity and, 39
Construct validity
    applications of, 40–41
    defined, 40
Content validity
    defined, 39
Correlation coefficients
    intraclass, 46–47
        Pearson product moment, 46, 46t
        in reliability evaluation, 45–47, 46t
Criterion-related validity, 39–40

of extremity joint studies, 40
    of spinal studies, 40
Cup holding
    range of motion necessary for
        hand, 143, 143f
Cybex inclinometer
    in thoracic and lumbar spine testing,
        340

D

Degrees of freedom of motion
    defined, 6
Depression
    testing of mandibular, 370, 371f
Descending stairs
    range of motion necessary for
        ankle and foot, 251, 251f, 251t
        hip, 189, 189f, 189t
        knee, 225, 226f, 226t
Deviation. *See* specific joints
Devore goniometer
    price of, 383t
    reliability of, 144
Dexter Hand Evaluation and Treatment
    System
    reliability of, 145
Diabetes mellitus
    ankle and foot range of motion in, 250
Disability
    range of motion and
        hip, 188–189
        thoracic and lumbar spine, 337
Disorders. *See also* specific conditions
    ankle and foot, 250
    temporomandibular joint, 368–369
Distal goniometer arm
    defined, 28–29, 29f
Distal hamstring length test, 236f–239f,
    236–239
Distal interphalangeal joints. *See*
    Interphalangeal joints
Distal tibiofibular joint. *See* Tibiofibular
    joints
Doorknob turning
    range of motion necessary for
        wrist, 115, 115t, 116f
Dorsal interossei muscles
    muscle length testing in, 176f–179f,
        176–179
Dorsiflexion. *See* Ankle; Foot
Double inclinometers
    in cervical spine testing
        of extension, 316, 316f
        of flexion, 312, 312f
        of lateral flexion, 322, 322f
        of rotation, 326, 327f
    in thoracic and lumbar spine testing
        age and, 334
        disability and, 334
        of flexion, 346, 346f–347f, 351, 351f
        of lateral flexion, 359, 359f
        reliability of, 339t, 339–340
        of rotation, 362, 362f–363f
Down syndrome
    hypermobility in, 10
Drinking

range of motion necessary for
  cervical spine, 302
  elbow, 96t, 96–97, 97f
  hand, 144
  shoulder, 63, 64t, 65f
  wrist, 115t, 116–117
Driving
  range of motion necessary for
    cervical spine, 303, 303f
Duchenne's muscular dystrophy
  testing reliability in, 65
Dynamometers
  potentiometers and, 25

E

Eating
  range of motion necessary for
    cervical spine, 302
    elbow, 96t, 96–97
    hand, 144
    shoulder, 63, 64t, 65f
    wrist, 115t, 116–117
Elbow. *See also* specific joints
  anatomical landmarks of, 99, 99f
  anatomy of, 91f–93f, 91–93
  arthrokinematics of, 92–93
  capsular pattern in, 92–93
  carrying angle of, 91–92
  extension of
    end-feel determinations and, 21
    recording of, 31–32, 32f
    testing of, 102
  flexion of
    end-feel determinations and, 20
    exercise for, 30
    goniometer alignment for, 27f–28f,
      30
    recording of, 31, 31f, 34b
    reliability studies of, 41
    testing of, 36, 100, 100f
  hyperextension of
    recording of, 31–32, 32f
  ligaments of, 91, 92f
  muscle length testing in, 106f–109f,
    106–109
  osteokinematics of, 92–93
  pronation of
    testing of, 102f–103f, 102–103
  range of motion
    testing position and, 381t
  range of motion of, 99f–105f, 99–105
    age and, 94t–95t, 94–95
    body-mass index and, 95
    example of, 12b, 13f, 14b, 14f
    functional, 96t, 96–97, 97f–98f
    gender and, 95
    normative values for, 375t
    numerical recording form for, 388f
    reliability and validity in testing of,
      97–98
    research findings in, 94t–95t, 94–96
    right *versus* left side and, 95
    sports and, 95–96
  supination of
    testing of, 104f–105f, 104–105
Elderly adults

range of motion in, 11
  ankle and foot, 247t–248t, 247–248
  cervical spine, 289–299, 299t
  elbow, 95, 95t
  hip, 184t, 186t, 186–187
  knee, 223t–224t, 224–225
  shoulder, 61
  thoracic and lumbar spine, 334,
    335t–336t
  wrist, 113
Electrogoniometers
  in elbow testing, 98
  overview of, 25–26
Ely test
  of rectus femoris muscle length, 232–235,
    233f–235f
End-feels
  abnormal, 8t
  in ankle and foot
    abduction of, 284
    dorsiflexion of, 20, 257
    eversion of, 267, 273, 277
    extension of, 282
    flexion of, 280, 286–287
    inversion of, 265, 271, 274
    muscle length testing in, 289
    plantarflexion of, 261
  in cervical spine
    extension of, 314–315
    flexion of, 310
    lateral flexion of, 318
    rotation of, 324
  defined, 8
  in elbow
    extension of, 21, 102
    flexion of, 20, 100
    muscle length testing in, 107, 109
    pronation of, 102
    supination of, 105
  in hand
    abduction of, 150, 164
    adduction of, 152
    extension of, 148, 154, 158, 162, 172, 175
    flexion of, 146, 156, 160, 170, 173
    muscle length testing in, 176, 178
    opposition of, 168
  in hip
    abduction of, 198
    adduction of, 201
    extension of, 196
    flexion of, 194
    muscle length testing in, 210, 213–214,
      218
    rotation of, 203, 205
  in knee
    extension of, 232
    flexion of, 230
    muscle length testing in, 238
  normal, 8t
    in ankle and foot testing, 257, 261,
      265, 267, 271, 273–274, 277, 280, 282,
      284
    in cervical spine testing, 310–311,
      314–315, 318, 324
    in elbow testing, 100, 102, 105, 107,
      109
    in hand testing, 146, 148, 150, 152, 154,

      156, 160, 162, 164, 168, 170, 172–173
    in hip testing, 194, 196, 198, 201, 203,
      205, 210, 213, 218
    in knee testing, 230, 232, 238
    in shoulder testing, 72, 76, 80, 84, 88
    in temporomandibular joint testing,
      370, 371–373
    in thoracic and lumbar spine testing,
      344, 348, 352, 354, 357, 360
    in wrist testing, 120, 122, 126
  in range of motion testing, 8, 8t
    general procedures for, 20–21
  in shoulder
    abduction of, 80
    extension of, 76
    flexion of, 72
    lateral rotation of, 88
    medial rotation of, 84
  in temporomandibular joint
    depression of, 370
    lateral deviation of, 373
    protrusion of, 372
  in thoracic and lumbar spine
    extension of, 352, 354
    flexion of, 344
    lateral flexion of, 348, 357
    rotation of, 360
  in wrist
    extension of, 122
    flexion of, 120
    muscle length testing in, 130, 133
    radial deviation of, 124
    ulnar deviation of, 126
Errors
  measurement, 29, 41, 43
Eversion. *See* Ankle; Foot
Exos Handmaster
  reliability of, 144
Explanation procedures, 34–35
  example of, 34–35
  exercise for, 36
Extension. *See* specific joints
Extensor digiti minimi muscle
  muscle length testing of, 132f–135,
    132–135
Extensor digitorum muscle
  muscle length testing of, 132f–135,
    132–135
Extensor indicis muscle
  muscle length testing of, 132f–135,
    132–135
Extremity joint studies
  criterion-related validity of, 40

F

Face validity
  types of, 39
FASTRAK system
  in thoracic and lumbar spine testing,
    341–342
Finger. *See also* Hand
  anatomy of, 137f–139f, 137–139
  arthrokinematics of, 138
  capsular pattern in, 138
  osteokinematics of, 137–138
  range of motion of, 140, 140t–141t

functional, 143–144, 144t
    normative values for, 376t
    numerical recording form for, 389f
Fingertip-to-floor method
    in thoracic and lumbar spine testing
        of flexion, 345
        of lateral flexion, 358, 358f
        reliability of, 340–341
Fishermen
    lumbar and thoracic spine testing in,
        335–336
Flexible rulers
    in cervical spine testing
        reliability of, 306
    in thoracic and lumbar spine testing
        age and, 334
        reliability of, 341
Flexion. See specific joints
Flexor digitorum muscles
    muscle length testing in, 128f–131f,
        128–131
Flexor muscles of hip
    anatomy of, 206f, 206–207
    muscle length testing in, 206f–211f,
        206–211
Fluid goniometers, 24–25, 25f
    reliability of
        in elbow testing, 98
        in knee testing, 228
Foot. See also Ankle
    anatomical landmarks of, 255f, 263f, 269f,
        279f
    anatomy of, 241–245, 242f–245f
    arthrokinematics of, 245
    dorsiflexion of
        functional range of motion in, 250–252,
            251f
        reliability of testing of, 253, 253t
    eversion of
        reliability of testing of, 253, 254t
        transverse tarsal testing of, 276f–278f,
            276–278
    interphalangeal extension of
        testing of, 287
    interphalangeal flexion of
        testing of, 287
    inversion of
        reliability of testing of, 253, 254t
        transverse tarsal testing of, 274f–275f,
            274–275
    metatarsophalangeal abduction of
        testing of, 284f–285f, 284–285
    metatarsophalangeal adduction of
        testing of, 286
    metatarsophalangeal extension of
        testing of, 282f–283f, 282–283
    metatarsophalangeal flexion of
        testing of, 280f–281f, 280–281
    osteokinematics of, 245–246
    plantarflexion of
        functional range of motion in, 250,
            251f
        reliability of testing of, 253, 253t
    range of motion of
        age and, 247, 247f
        disease and, 250
        functional, 250–252, 251f

gender and, 248t, 248–249
    injury and, 250
    normative values for, 378t
    numerical recording form for, 390f
    reliability and validity in testing of,
        252–254, 253t–254t
    research findings in, 246t, 246–247
    testing position and, 249t, 249–250,
        381t
    transverse tarsal eversion of
        testing of, 276f–278f, 276–278
    transverse tarsal inversion of
        testing of, 274f–275f, 274–275
Forearm, 91–109. See also Elbow
    anatomical landmarks of, 99, 99f
    range of motion
        testing position and, 381t
    range of motion of, 99f–105f, 99–105
        normative values for, 375t
        numerical recording form for, 388f
    structure and function of, 91f–93f, 91–92
Forefoot. See also Foot
    in transverse tarsal eversion testing,
        276f–278f, 276–278
    in transverse tarsal inversion testing,
        274f–275f, 274–275
Freedom of motion degrees
    defined, 6
Frontal plane
    defined, 4, 5f
Fulcrum
    in goniometer alignment, 29
Functional axial rotation device
    in thoracic and lumbar spine testing,
        341
Functional range of motion
    ankle and foot, 250–252, 251f–252f, 251t
    cervical spine, 302f–303f, 302–303
    elbow, 96t, 96–97, 97f–98f
    hand, 143f, 143–144, 144t
    hip, 189f–190f, 189t, 189–192
    knee, 225, 226f–227f, 226t
    shoulder, 63, 64f–65f, 64t
    thoracic and lumbar spine, 337f–338f,
        337–338
    wrist, 115t–116t, 115–117, 116f–117f

G

Gastrocnemius muscle
    anatomy of, 288, 288f
    muscle length testing in, 288f–291f,
        288–291
Gender
    range of motion and, 12
        ankle and foot, 248t, 248–249
        cervical spine, 299t–300t, 299–301
        elbow, 95
        hand, 141, 141t
        hip, 186t, 187
        knee, 225
        shoulder, 60t, 61–62
        temporomandibular joint, 367–368
        thoracic and lumbar spine, 334–335,
            335t–336t
        wrist, 114
Glenohumeral joint

anatomy of, 57, 57f–58f
    arthrokinematics of, 57–58
    capsular pattern of, 58
    osteokinematics of, 57
    range of motion of
        abduction in, 78, 79f, 80
        extension in, 74, 75f, 76
        flexion in, 70, 71f, 72
        lateral rotation in, 86, 87f, 88
        medial rotation in, 82, 83f, 84
        normative values for, 376t
        numerical recording form for, 388f
        research findings in, 60t, 60–61
Goniometers, 21–27, 22f–25f. See also
    specific types of instruments
    alignment of, 27f–29f, 27–29. See also
        Alignment
    electrogoniometers as, 25–26
    fluid (bubble), 24–25, 25f
    gravity-dependent, 24–25, 25f
    measurement errors with, 29
    metal, 22
    pendulum, 24, 25f
    plastic, 22
    price lists for, 383t–385t
    proximal and distal arms of, 28–29, 29f
    recording of measurements with, 29–34,
        31f–33f
    reliability of, 41–43, 43t
        in ankle and foot testing, 252–254,
            253t–254t
        in cervical spine testing, 303–306, 304t
        in elbow testing, 98
        in hand testing, 144–145
        in hip testing, 190–192, 191t
        in knee testing, 227t, 227–228
        in shoulder testing, 66–67
        in temporomandibular joint testing,
            369
        in thoracic and lumbar spine testing,
            338–342, 339t
        in wrist testing, 117–119
    universal, 21–24, 22f–24f. See also
        Universal goniometer
    visual estimation versus, 26–27
Goniometry
    basic concepts in, 3f, 3–14, 5f–7f, 8t–9t,
        11t, 13f–14f
    basic objectives in, 1
    defined, 3
    example of, 3b, 3f
    explanation procedure for, 34–36
    indications for, 4
    testing procedures in, 35–36
Gravity-dependent goniometers
    overview of, 24–25, 25f
    reliability of
        in cervical spine testing, 303, 306
        in thoracic and lumbar spine testing,
            340–341
Gripping
    range of motion necessary for
        hand, 143f, 143–144
Grooming. See Personal care activities
Guides to the Evaluation of Permanent
    Impairment, 34

H

Hamstrings
  muscle length testing in, 212f–215f,
    212–215
    distal, 236f–239f, 236–239
Hand, 137–179
  anatomical landmarks of, 145f, 159f
  anatomy of, 137f–139f, 137–139
  arthrokinematics of, 138–140
  capsular pattern in, 138–140
  carpometacarpal abduction of
    testing of, 164, 164f–165f
  carpometacarpal adduction of
    testing of, 166
  carpometacarpal extension of
    testing of, 162, 162f–163f
  carpometacarpal flexion of
    testing of, 160, 160f–161f
  carpometacarpal opposition of, 166,
    167f–169f, 168
  interphalangeal extension of
    testing of, 154, 158, 175
  interphalangeal flexion of
    testing of, 152, 152f–153f, 155,
      155f–157f, 173, 173f–174f
  metacarpophalangeal abduction of
    testing of, 150, 150f–151f
  metacarpophalangeal adduction of
    testing of, 152
  metacarpophalangeal extension of
    testing of, 148, 148f–149f, 172
  metacarpophalangeal flexion of
    testing of, 146, 146f–147f, 170,
      170f–171f
  muscle length testing in, 176f–179f,
    176–179
  osteokinematics of, 137–140
  range of motion of, 140–175
    age and, 140–142
    functional, 143f, 143–144, 144t
    gender and, 140–142, 141t
    normative values for, 376t–377t
    numerical recording form for, 389f
    reliability and validity in testing of,
      144–145
    research findings in, 140t–141t,
      140–144, 143f, 144t
    right *versus* left sides and, 142
    testing position and, 142–143,
      381t
Head. *See also* Cervical spine;
  Temporomandibular joint
  temporomandibular joint and position of,
    368
Hereditary disorders
  hypermobility in, 10
Hip
  abduction of
    testing of, 198, 198f–199f
  adduction of
    testing of, 200, 200f–201f
  anatomical landmarks of, 192f–193f
  anatomy of, 183f–184f, 183–184
  arthrokinematics of, 184
  capsular pattern in, 184
  extension of
    testing of, 195, 196f–197f

flexion of
  recordings of, 33f
  testing of, 194, 194f–195f
  lateral rotation of
    testing of, 204, 204f–205f
  medial rotation of
    testing of, 202, 202f–203f
  muscle length testing in
    of flexors, 206f–211f, 206–211
    of hamstrings, 212f–215f, 212–215
    Ober test in, 216f–219f, 216–219
    straight leg test in, 212f–215f,
      212–215
    of tensor fasciae latae, 216f–219f,
      216–219
    Thomas test in, 206f–211f, 206–211
  osteokinematics of, 183–184
  positioning of
    example of, 18b, 19f
  range of motion of
    age and, 184t–186t, 184–187
    ballet and, 188
    body-mass index and, 187
    disability and, 188–189
    example of, 12b, 13f
    functional, 189f–190f, 189t, 189–190
    gender and, 187
    normative values for, 377t
    numerical recording form for, 390f
    reliability and validity in testing of,
      190–192, 191t
    research findings in, 184t–186t, 184–189
    sagittal-frontal-transverse-rotation
      method of recording, 33b–34b
    sports and, 188
    testing position and, 187–188, 188t, 381t
House painting
  range of motion necessary for
    cervical spine, 303
Humeroradial joint. *See also* Elbow
  anatomy of, 91f–92f, 91–92
  arthrokinematics of, 92
  osteokinematics of, 92
Humeroulnar joint. *See also* Elbow
  anatomy of, 91f–92f, 91–92
  arthrokinematics of, 92
  osteokinematics of, 92
Humerus
  as shoulder anatomical landmark, 68f–69f
Hydrogoniometers
  in shoulder testing, 67
  in thoracic and lumbar spine testing
    age and, 334
Hypermobility
  causes of, 10
  defined, 10
  in range of motion testing, 10, 11t
Hypermobility syndrome
  defined, 10
Hypomobility
  causes of, 9
  defined, 8–9
  in range of motion testing, 8–10, 9t
  sagittal-frontal-transverse-rotation
    method of recording, 34

I

Iliacus muscle
  anatomy of, 206, 206f
  in Thomas test, 206f–211f, 206–211
Iliofemoral joint
  anatomy of, 183f–184f, 183–184
  arthrokinematics of, 184
  capsular pattern in, 184
  osteokinematics of, 183–184
Iliotibial band
  anatomy of, 216, 216f
  Ober test, 216f–219f, 216–219
Inclinometers
  in cervical spine testing
    of extension, 316, 316f
    of flexion, 312, 312f
    of lateral flexion, 322, 322f
    of rotation, 326, 327f
  overview of, 24–25, 25f
  price list for, 385t
  reliability of, 42
    in ankle and foot testing, 252
    in hip testing, 192
    in shoulder testing, 67
    in thoracic and lumbar spine testing,
      338–340, 339t
  in thoracic and lumbar spine testing
    age and, 334
    disability and, 334
    of flexion, 346, 346f–347f, 351, 351f
    of lateral flexion, 359, 359f
    of rotation, 362, 362f–363f
Index finger. *See also* Hand
  range of motion of, 141t
    numerical recording form for, 389f
Infants. *See also* Children
  range of motion in, 11
Injury
  ankle and foot, 250
  repetitive wrist, 117
Instruments, 21–27, 22f–25f. *See also* specific
    instruments
  electrogoniometers as, 25–26
  gravity-dependent goniometers as, 24–25,
    25f
  universal goniometer as, 21–24, 22f–24f,
    26
  visual estimation *versus*, 26–27
Interossei muscles
  muscle length testing in, 176f–179f,
    176–179
Interphalangeal joints
  foot. *See also* Foot
    anatomy of, 246, 246f
    arthrokinematics of, 246
    extension of, 287
    flexion of, 287
    osteokinematics of, 246
  hand. *See also* Hand
    anatomy of, 137f–139f, 138–139
    arthrokinematics of, 138, 140
    capsular pattern of, 138, 140
    extension of, 154, 158, 175
    flexion of, 152, 152f–153f, 155,
      155f–157f, 173, 173f–174f
    osteokinematics of, 138, 140
    range of motion of, 140, 140t–141t,

142
range of motion of
normative values for, 376t–377t
Intertester reliability
evaluation of, 42
in ankle and foot testing, 252–254,
253t–254t
in cervical spine testing, 303–306, 304t
in elbow testing, 98
exercise for, 50–51
in hand testing, 144
in hip testing, 191t, 191–192
in knee testing, 227t, 227–228
in shoulder testing, 63, 65
in temporomandibular joint testing, 369
in thoracic and lumbar spine testing,
338–342, 339t
in wrist testing, 118–119
Intervertebral joints. See also Cervical spine
anatomy of, 296, 296f
arthrokinematics of, 297
capsular pattern in, 297
osteokinematics of, 296–297
Intraclass correlation coefficient
in reliability evaluation, 46–47
Intratester reliability
evaluation of, 42
in ankle and foot testing, 252–254,
253t–254t
in cervical spine testing, 303–306, 304t
in elbow testing, 98
exercise for, 48–49
in hip testing, 190–191, 191t
in knee testing, 227t, 227–228
in shoulder testing, 63, 65
in temporomandibular joint testing, 369
in thoracic and lumbar spine testing,
338–342, 339t
in wrist testing, 118–119
Inversion. See Ankle; Foot

J

Jaw. See Temporomandibular joint
Joint effusions
capsular pattern in, 10
Joint measurements
body position and, 381t
Joint motion testing
basic concepts in, 4–6, 5f
body position and, 18t
criterion-related validity of, 40
reliability studies of, 41–43

K

Knee
anatomical landmarks of, 229f
anatomy of, 221f, 221–222
arthrokinematics of, 222
capsular pattern in, 222
extension of
testing of, 232
flexion of
testing of, 230, 230f–231f
goniometer for
example of, 24b, 24f

muscle length testing in
distal hamstring length test in,
236f–239f, 236–239
Ely test in, 232–235, 233f–235f
osteokinematics of, 222
range of motion of
age and, 223t–224t, 223–225
body-mass index and, 225
functional, 225, 226f, 226t–227f
gender and, 225
normative values for, 377t
numerical recording form for, 390f
reliability and validity in testing of,
227t, 227–228
research findings in, 223t–224t, 223–225
testing position for, 18b, 381t
Kyphometers
in thoracic and lumbar spine testing, 339
Kyphosis
occupational, 336–337

L

Landmarks
anatomical. See Anatomical landmarks
Lifestyle
in temporomandibular joint disorders,
368–369
thoracic and lumbar spine range of
motion and, 335–337
Ligaments
elbow, 91, 92f
wrist, 111f–112f, 111–112
Little finger. See also Hand
range of motion of, 141t
numerical recording form for, 389f
Looking upward
range of motion necessary for
cervical spine, 302, 302f
Lordosis
occupational, 336–337
Low-back pain
range of motion and, 337
Lower-extremity testing, 181–291. See also
specific structures
ankle and foot in, 241–291
hip in, 183–219
knee in, 221–239
numerical recording forms for, 390f–391f
objectives in, 181
reliability studies of, 41–42
Lumbar spine
anatomical landmarks of, 343f
anatomy of, 332–333, 333f
arthrokinematics of, 333
capsular pattern in, 333
extension of
testing of, 352f–355f, 352–355
flexion of
testing of, 344f–351f, 344–351
lateral flexion of
testing of, 356f–359f, 356–359
osteokinematics of, 333
range of motion
testing position and, 381t
range of motion of
age and, 333–334, 335t–336t

disability and, 337
functional, 337f–338f, 337–338
gender and, 334–335, 335t–336t
lifestyle and, 335–337
normative values for, 379t
numerical recording form for, 387f
occupation and, 335–337
reliability and validity of testing of,
338–342, 339t
research findings in, 333–337, 334t–336t
rotation of
testing of, 360f–363f, 360–363
Lumbrical muscles
muscle length testing in, 176f–179f,
176–179

M

Mandibular length. See also
Temporomandibular joint
range of motion and, 368–369
Mean
defined, 43
standard error of, 47
Measurement
standard error of, 47–48
Measurement errors
defined, 43
goniometer-related, 29
reliability and, 41
standard deviation indicating, 44–45,
45t
Measurement instruments, 21–27, 22f–25f.
See also Goniometers; Instruments; other
instruments
Medial-lateral axis
defined, 4, 5f
Men. See Adults; Gender
Metacarpophalangeal joints. See also Hand
anatomy of, 137, 137f–139f, 139
arthrokinematics of, 138–139
capsular pattern of, 138–139
osteokinematics of, 137–139
range of motion of, 140, 140t–141t
age and, 11, 12, 142
gender and, 142
normative values for, 376t–377t
testing position and, 142–143
Metal goniometers
price list for, 384t
Metatarsals
in transverse tarsal eversion testing,
276f–278f, 276–278
in transverse tarsal inversion testing,
274f–275f, 274–275
Metatarsophalangeal joints. See also Foot
abduction of
testing of, 284f–285f, 284–285
adduction of
testing of, 286
anatomical landmarks of, 279f
anatomy of, 245, 246f
arthrokinematics of, 245
capsular pattern in, 245–246
extension of
normative values for, 378t
testing of, 282f–283f, 282–283

flexion of
normative values for, 378t
testing of, 280f–281f, 280–281
osteokinematics of, 245
Midcarpal joint. *See also* Wrist
anatomy of, 111f–112f, 111–112
arthrokinematics of, 112
osteokinematics of, 112
Middle finger. *See also* Hand
range of motion of, 141t
numerical recording form for, 389f
Midtarsal joint. *See also* Ankle
anatomy of, 244, 244f
arthrokinematics of, 245
capsular pattern in, 245
osteokinematics of, 244
Modified Schober test
in thoracic and lumbar spine testing
of extension, 355
of flexion, 350, 350f
reliability of, 340–341
Modified-modified Schober test
in thoracic and lumbar spine testing
of extension, 354f, 354–355
of flexion, 348f–349f, 348–349
procedure for, 343
Motion
range of. *See* Range of motion; specific
joints
testing. *See* Testing motion
Mouth opening
in temporomandibular joint
disorders of, 368–369
head and neck positions and, 368
mandibular length and, 368–369
testing of, 370, 371f
Muscle length
defined, 12
testing of, 12–14, 13f–14f
of biceps brachii, 106f–107f,
106–107
examples of, 12b, 13f, 14, 14f
of extensor digitorum, indicis, and
digiti minimi, 132f–135f, 132–135
of flexor digitorum muscles, 128f–131f,
128–131
of gastrocnemius, 288f–291f, 288–291
of hamstrings, 212f–215f, 212–215,
236f–239f, 236–239
of lumbricals and interossei, 176f–179f,
176–179
numerical recording form for,
391f
of rectus femoris, 232–235, 233f–235f
of tensor fasciae latae, 216f–219f,
216–219
of triceps brachii, 108f–109f, 108–109
Myrin OB Goniometer, 25

N

Neck. *See also* Cervical spine;
Temporomandibular joint
temporomandibular joint and position of,
368
Neutral zero method
in range of motion testing, 6, 6f–7f
NK Hand Assessment System
reliability of, 145
Noncapsular pattern of restricted motion
defined, 10
example of, 10b
in range of motion testing, 10
Normative values
range of motion
ankle and foot, 378t
cervical spine, 378t
elbow and forearm, 375t
finger, 376t
glenohumeral joint, 376t
hip, 377t
knee, 377t
shoulder, 375t
temporomandibular joint, 379t
thoracic and lumbar spine, 379t
thumb, 377t
wrist, 375t
Numerical recording forms
instructions for completing, 32, 32f
for muscle length, 391f
for range of motion, 387f–391f
of ankle and foot, 390f
of elbow and forearm, 388f
of hand, 389f
of hip, 390f
of knee, 390f
of shoulder, 388f
of spine, 387f
of temporomandibular joint, 387f
of wrist, 388f

O

OB Myrin gravity goniometer
in thoracic and lumbar spine testing
reliability of, 340–341
Ober test
of tensor fasciae latae muscle length,
216f–219f, 216–219
Occupation
range of motion and
cervical spine, 303
thoracic and lumbar spine, 335–337
Opposition
thumb, 166, 167f–169f, 168
Optotrak motion analysis system
in knee testing, 228
Orthoranger goniometer
reliability of
in ankle and foot testing, 252
in elbow testing, 98
in hip testing, 190–191
in shoulder testing, 66
in wrist testing, 118
Osteokinematics
of acromioclavicular joint, 59–60
of atlanto-occipital and atlantoaxial joints,
295–295
of carpometacarpal joint, 138
defined, 4
of glenohumeral joint, 57
of humeroulnar and humeroradial joints,
92
of iliofemoral joint, 183–184
of interphalangeal joints
foot, 246
hand, 138
thumb, 140
of intervertebral and zygapophyseal
joints, 296–197
of lumbar spine, 333
of metacarpophalangeal joints, 137–139
of metatarsophalangeal joints, 245
of midtarsal joint, 244
planes and axes in, 4–6, 5f
of radioulnar joints, 93
of scapulothoracic joint, 60
of sternoclavicular joint, 58
of subtalar joint, 243
of talocrural joint, 241
of tarsometatarsal joints, 245
of temporomandibular joint, 365–366
of thoracic spine, 331–332
of tibiofemoral and patellofemoral joints,
222
of tibiofibular joints, 241
of wrist, 112

P

Pain
causes in passive range of motion of,
7–8
low-back, 337
Palmar interossei muscles
muscle length testing in, 176f–179f,
176–179
Passive insufficiency
defined, 12
Passive range of motion. *See also* Range of
motion
defined, 7
testing of, 7–8
example of, 7b
Pearson product moment correlation
coefficient
in reliability evaluation, 46, 46t
Pectineus muscle
anatomy of, 207
in Thomas test, 206f–211f, 206–211
Pendulum goniometers, 24, 25f
reliability of
in cervical spine testing, 305–306
in elbow testing, 98
Peripheral neuropathy
ankle and foot range of motion in, 250
Personal care activities
range of motion necessary for
cervical spine, 302
shoulder, 63, 64f, 64t
wrist, 116t, 116–117, 117f
Picking up coin
range of motion necessary for
hand, 143, 143f
Picking up object from the floor
range of motion necessary for
lumbar, 338, 338f
Pictorial charts

in goniometry recordings, 32, 33f
Planes
    in osteokinematics, 4–6, 5f
Plantarflexion. *See* Ankle; Foot
Plastic goniometers
    price list for, 383t
Pleurimeter inclinometer
    reliability of
        in hip testing, 192
        in thoracic and lumbar spine testing, 339
Plumb line and skin markings
    in thoracic and lumbar spine testing
        age and, 334
        reliability of, 340
Positioning. *See also* Testing positions
    general procedures for, 17–18, 18t
        example of, 17
    importance of, 17
    joint measurements and, 381t
    in range of motion testing, 18t
    reliability and, 43t
Positions
    testing. *See* Positioning; Testing positions
Posture
    spinal
        disability and, 337
        effects of stooped, 336–337
Potentiometers, 25–26
Pouring from pitcher
    range of motion necessary for
        wrist, 115t, 116
Power lifters
    elbow range of motion in, 96
    shoulder rotation in, 63
Price lists
    goniometer, 383t–385t
Procedures, 17–36
    for alignment, 27f–29f, 27–30
    for end-feel testing, 20–21
    explanation of, 34–36
    instruments in, 21–27, 22f–25f. *See also*
        Goniometers; Instruments; other
        instruments
    for positioning, 17–18, 18t
    for range of motion testing, 20–21. *See also*
        specific joints and structures
    for recording, 29–34, 31f–33f
    reliability and, 42
    for stabilization, 18–19, 19f
    testing, 35–36
Pronation. *See* Elbow
Protrusion
    testing of mandibular, 372, 372f
Proximal goniometer arm
    defined, 28, 29f
Proximal interphalangeal joints. *See*
    Interphalangeal joints
Proximal tibiofibular joint. *See* Tibiofibular
    joints
Psoas major muscle
    anatomy of, 206, 206f
    in Thomas test, 206f–211f, 206–211
Putting on socks
    range of motion necessary for
        hip, 190, 190f

knee, 227f
lumbar, 338, 338f

R

Radiocarpal joint. *See also* Wrist
    anatomy of, 111f–112f, 111–112
    arthrokinematics of, 112
    osteokinematics of, 112
Radiography
    in knee testing, 228
Radioulnar joint. *See also* Elbow
    anatomy of, 92f–93f, 92–93
    arthrokinematics of, 93
    osteokinematics of, 93
Range of motion. *See also* specific joints
    active, 6–7
    basic concepts in, 6–12
    defined, 6
    end-feels in, 8, 8t
    factors affecting, 10–12
    functional. *See* Functional range of
        motion
    hypermobility in, 10, 11t
    hypomobility in, 8–10, 9t
    neutral zero method of testing, 6,
        6f–7f
        example of, 6b
    normative values for, 375t–379t
    notation systems for, 6
    numerical recording forms for,
        387f–391f
    passive, 7–8
    recording of, 29–34, 31f–33f
    reliability studies of, 41–43
        exercises for, 48–52
        statistical methods in, 43–48
    testing procedures for, 20–21
    validity studies of, 40
Reaching
    range of motion necessary for
        elbow, 96, 96t
        shoulder, 63, 64f–65f, 64t
        wrist, 116t, 116–117, 117f
Reading a newspaper
    range of motion necessary for
        elbow, 96, 96t, 98f
Rearfoot. *See* Subtalar joint
Recordings
    numerical forms for, 387f–391f
        instructions for, 32, 32f
    procedures for, 29–34, 31f–33f
        AMA guides in, 34
        numerical forms in, 32, 32f
        pictorial charts in, 32, 33f
        sagittal-frontal-transverse-rotation
            method in, 33–34
Rectus femoris muscle
    anatomy of, 206, 206f, 232, 233f
    in Ely test, 232–235, 233f–235f
    in Thomas test, 206f–211f, 206–211
Reliability, 41–51
    of ankle and foot testing, 252–254,
        253t–254t
    of cervical spine testing, 303–306, 304t
    defined, 41

of elbow testing, 97–98
    evaluation of, 43–51
        coefficient of variation in, 45
        correlation coefficients in, 45–47, 46t
        exercises for, 48–51
        intertester, 50–51
        intratester, 48–49
        standard deviation in, 43–45, 44t–45t
        standard error of measurement in,
            47–48
    goniometric study summary of, 31–43
    of hand testing, 144–145
    of hip testing, 190–192, 191t
    of knee testing, 227t, 227–228
    recommendations for improving, 42–43,
        43t
    of shoulder testing, 63, 65–67
    of temporomandibular joint testing,
        369
    of thoracic and lumbar spine testing,
        338–342, 339t
    of wrist testing, 117–119
Repetitive injury
    wrist, 117
Replication
    coefficient of variation of, 45
Right *versus* left side
    range of motion and
        elbow, 95
        hand, 141
        shoulder, 62–63
        wrist, 114
Ring finger. *See also* Hand
    range of motion of, 141t
        numerical recording form for, 389f
Rising from chair
    range of motion necessary for
        ankle and foot, 251, 252f
        elbow, 96, 96t, 97f
        knee, 226f, 226t
        wrist, 115t, 116
Rotation. *See also* specific joints
    sagittal-frontal-transverse-rotation
        method of recording, 33
Rulers
    flexible. *See* Flexible rulers
    in temporomandibular joint testing
        of lateral deviation, 373, 373f
        of mouth opening, 370, 371f
        of protrusion, 372, 372f
        reliability of, 369
Running
    range of motion necessary for
        ankle and foot, 251

S

Sagittal plane
    defined, 4, 5f
Sagittal-frontal-transverse-rotation method
    in goniometry recordings, 33–34
Sartorius muscle
    anatomy of, 206, 206f
    in Thomas test, 206f–211f, 206–211
Scapula
    as shoulder anatomical landmark, 68f

Scapulothoracic joint
  anatomy of, 60
  arthrokinematics of, 60
  osteokinematics of, 60
Schober test
  modified-modified, 343, 348f–349f,
    348–349, 354f, 354–355
  of thoracic and lumbar spine
    modified, 340–341, 350, 350f, 355
    modified-modified, 343, 348–349, 349f,
      354f, 354–355
    reliability of, 339t, 340
School bus use
  low-back mobility and, 336
Semimembranosus muscle
  anatomy of, 212, 212f, 236, 236f
  in distal hamstring length test, 236f–239f,
    236–239
  in straight leg test, 212f–215f, 212–215
Semitendinosus muscle
  anatomy of, 212, 212f, 236, 236f
  in distal hamstring length test, 236f–239f,
    236–239
  in straight leg test, 212f–215f, 212–215
Sewer workers
  stooped posture in, 336–337
Shoulder, 57–89. *See also* specific joints
  abduction of
    testing of, 78–80, 79f–81f
  adduction of
    testing of, 82
  anatomical landmarks of, 68f–69f
  anatomy and function of, 57–60
    of acromioclavicular joint, 59f, 59–60
    of glenohumeral joint, 57f–58f, 57–58
    of scapulothoracic joint, 60
    of sternoclavicular joint, 58f, 58–59
  extension of
    testing of, 6, 7f, 74–76, 75f–77f
  flexion of
    testing of, 6, 7f, 70–73, 71f–73f
  range of motion of
    age and, 11, 12, 61t, 61–62
    alignment for testing of, 68, 68f–69f
    body-mass index and, 62
    functional, 63, 64f–65f, 64t
    gender and, 60t, 61–62
    normative values for, 375t
    numerical recording form for, 388f
    reliability and validity in testing of, 63,
      65–67
    research findings in, 60t–61t, 60–63
    sagittal-frontal-transverse-rotation
      method of recording, 33b
    sports and, 62–63
    testing position and, 62, 381t
  rotation of
    lateral (external), 86–88, 87f–89f
    medial (internal), 82–84, 83f–85f
    reliability studies of, 41
    sports and, 62–63
Simplified skin distraction method
  in thoracic and lumbar spine testing
    of extension, 354f, 354–355
    of flexion, 348f, 348–349
    procedure for, 343

reliability of, 341
Sit to stand
  range of motion necessary for
    lumbar, 337–338, 338f
Sitting
  range of motion necessary for
    hip, 190, 190f
    knee, 225, 226t
Skin markings and plumb line
  in thoracic and lumbar spine testing
    age and, 334
    reliability of, 340
Spinal posture
  disability and, 337
  effects of stooped, 336–337
Spine
  cervical, 295–328. *See also* Cervical spine
  range of motion of
    age and, 11, 12
    numerical recording form for, 387f
    reliability studies of, 42
  studies of
    criterion-related validity of, 40
    reliability, 42
  testing objectives in, 293
  thoracic and lumbar, 331–363. *See also*
    Lumbar spine; Thoracic spine
SPINETRAK system
  in thoracic and lumbar spine testing
    disability and, 337
    reliability of, 341–342
Spinometer
  in thoracic and lumbar spine testing
    age and occupation and, 335–336
Spondylometers
  in thoracic and lumbar spine testing,
    340
Sports
  range of motion and
    cervical spine, 302–303
    elbow, 95–96
    hip, 189
    shoulder, 62–63
  wrist injuries in, 117
Stabilization
  procedures for, 18–19, 19f
    ankle and foot, 256, 260, 264, 266, 270,
      272, 274, 276, 280, 282, 284
    cervical spine, 310, 314, 318, 324
    elbow, 100, 102, 104, 107–108
    example of, 18b, 19f
    hand, 146, 148, 150, 152, 154–155, 158,
      160, 162, 164, 166, 170, 172
    hip, 194, 196, 198, 200, 202, 204, 208,
      213, 216
    knee, 230, 232, 237
    shoulder, 70, 74, 78, 82, 86
    temporomandibular joint, 370, 371–373
    thoracic and lumbar spine, 344, 348,
      352, 354, 356, 360
    wrist, 120, 122, 124, 126
Stair ascent and descent
  range of motion necessary for
    ankle and foot, 251, 251f, 251t
    hip, 189, 189f, 189t
    knee, 225, 226f, 226t

Standard deviation
  defined, 43
  formulas for, 43
  in reliability evaluation, 43–45, 44t–45t
    biological variation and, 44, 44t
    determination of mean and, 44, 44t
    measurement error and, 44–45, 45t
Standard error of mean
  standard error of measurement *versus*,
    47
Standard error of measurement
  in reliability evaluation, 47–48
  in shoulder testing, 66–67
Standing on tiptoe
  range of motion necessary for
    ankle and foot, 250–251, 251f
Steering wheel turning
  range of motion necessary for
    wrist, 115t, 116
Sternoclavicular joint
  anatomy of, 58, 58f
  arthrokinematics of, 59
  osteokinematics of, 58
Sternum
  as shoulder anatomical landmark, 68f
Stooped posture
  spinal effects of, 336–337
Straight leg test
  of hamstring muscle length, 212f–215f,
    212–215
Subtalar joint. *See also* Ankle
  anatomical landmarks of, 269f
  anatomy of, 243, 243f
  arthrokinematics of, 243–244
  capsular pattern in, 243
  eversion of
    testing of, 272f–273f, 272–273
  inversion of
    testing of, 270f–271f, 270–271
  neutral position of
    reliability of testing and, 253–254
  osteokinematics of, 243
Supination. *See* Elbow
Swimming
  range of motion and
    cervical spine, 303
Synovial inflammation
  capsular pattern in, 10

T

Talocrural joint. *See also* Ankle
  anatomical landmarks of, 255f
  anatomy of, 241, 242f–243f
  arthrokinematics of, 241
  capsular pattern in, 241
  dorsiflexion of
    testing of, 256f–259f, 256–259
  osteokinematics of, 241
  plantarflexion of
    testing of, 260f–262f, 260–262
Tape measure
  in cervical spine testing
    of extension, 315, 315f
    of flexion, 311, 311f
    of lateral flexion, 321, 321f

reliability of, 306
research findings in, 298t
of rotation, 326, 326f
in thoracic and lumbar spine testing
age and gender and, 335
of extension, 353f–355f, 353–355
of flexion, 345, 345f, 348f–349f, 348–350
of lateral flexion, 358, 358f
reliability of, 339t, 340–341
Tarsal joints. *See also* Ankle; Foot
anatomical landmarks of, 263f
eversion of
testing of, 266f–268f, 266–268
inversion of
testing of, 264f–265f, 264–265
Tarsometatarsal joints. *See also* Foot
anatomy of, 245, 245f
arthrokinematics of, 245
capsular pattern in, 245
osteokinematics of, 245
Telephone use
range of motion necessary for
cervical spine, 302
elbow, 96, 96t
hand, 144
wrist, 115, 115t, 116f
Temporal variation
defined, 43
Temporomandibular joint, 365–373
anatomical landmarks of, 370f
anatomy of, 365, 365f–366f
arthrokinematics of, 366
capsular pattern in, 366–367
disorders of, 368–369
lateral deviation of
testing of, 373, 373f
mandibular depression of
testing of, 370, 371f
mandibular protrusion of
testing of, 372, 372f
objectives in testing of, 293
osteokinematics of, 365–366
range of motion
testing position and, 381t
range of motion of
age and, 367, 367t
disorders and, 368–369
gender and, 367–368
head and neck positions and, 368
mandibular length and, 268
normative values for, 379t
numerical recording form for, 387f
recording of, 370, 371f
reliability and validity of testing of, 369
research findings in, 367t, 367–369
Tendinitis
wrist, 117
Tendo-Achilles lengthening procedure
range of motion and, 250
Tennis players
elbow range of motion in, 95–96
shoulder rotation in, 63
Tensor fasciae latae muscle
anatomy of, 206f, 207, 216, 216f
in Ober test, 216f–219f, 216–219

in Thomas test, 206f–211f, 206–211
Testing motion
ankle and foot
abduction of, 284, 284f
dorsiflexion of, 256f, 256–257
eversion of, 267, 267f, 272f, 272–273, 276, 276f
extension of, 282, 282f
flexion of, 280, 280f, 286–287
inversion of, 264, 264f, 270, 270f, 274, 274f
muscle length in, 289f, 289–290, 291f
plantarflexion of, 260, 260f
cervical spine
extension of, 314, 314f, 316f–317f, 316–317
flexion of, 310, 310f, 313, 313f, 318, 318f, 322f–323f, 322–323
rotation of, 324, 324f, 326, 328
elbow
extension of, 102
flexion of, 100, 100f
muscle length in, 107, 107f, 109, 109f
pronation of, 102, 102f
supination of, 104, 104f
hand
abduction of, 150, 150f, 164, 164f
adduction of
extension of, 148, 148f, 154, 158, 162, 162f, 172, 175
flexion of, 146, 146f, 152, 152f, 155, 155f, 160, 160f, 170, 170f, 173, 173f
muscle length in, 178, 178f–179f
opposition of, 166, 167f
hip
abduction of, 198, 198f
adduction of, 200, 200f
extension of, 196, 196f
flexion of, 194, 194f
muscle length in, 208, 209f, 213, 214f–215f, 216, 217f–219f
rotation of, 202, 202f, 204, 204f
knee
flexion of, 230, 230f
muscle length in, 234f–235f, 235, 238, 238f
shoulder
abduction of, 78, 79f
adduction of, 82
extension of, 74, 75f
flexion of, 70, 71f
lateral rotation of, 86, 87f
medial rotation of, 82, 83f
temporomandibular joint
depression of, 370, 371f
lateral deviation of, 373, 373f
protrusion of, 372, 372f
thoracic and lumbar spine
extension of, 352, 352f, 354
flexion of, 344, 344f, 348, 350–351, 356, 356f
rotation of, 360, 360f
wrist
extension of, 122, 122f
flexion of, 120, 120f
muscle length in, 130, 130f, 133, 134f

radial deviation of, 124, 124f
ulnar deviation of, 126, 126f
Testing positions
cervical spine, 301–302
defined, 17–18
hand, 142–143
hip, 187–188, 188t
knee, 249–250
shoulder, 62
wrist, 114–115
Testing procedures. *See* Procedures; specific procedures and structures
Thomas test
of hip flexor muscle length, 206f–212f, 206–212
Thoracic spine
anatomical landmarks of, 343f
anatomy of, 331, 332f
arthrokinematics of, 332
capsular pattern in, 332
extension of
testing of, 352f–353f, 352–353
flexion of
testing of, 344, 344f–347f, 347
lateral flexion of
testing of, 356f–359f, 356–359
osteokinematics of, 331–332
range of motion of
age and, 333–334, 335t–336t
disability and, 337
functional, 337f–338f, 337–338
gender and, 334–335, 335t–336t
lifestyle and, 335–337
normative values for, 379t
numerical recording form for, 387f
occupation and, 335–337
reliability and validity of testing of, 338–342, 339t
research findings 333–337, 334t–336tn
testing position and, 381t
rotation of
testing of, 360f–363f, 360–363
Three-dimensional (3-D) Space System
in cervical spine testing, 305
Thumb. *See also* Hand
anatomical landmarks of, 159f
anatomy of, 139, 139f
arthrokinematics of, 139
capsular pattern in, 139
carpometacarpal joint testing, 160, 160f–161f, 162, 162f–163f, 164, 164f–165f, 166, 167f–169f, 168
interphalangeal joint testing, 173, 173f–174f, 175
metacarpophalangeal joint testing, 170, 170f–171f, 172
osteokinematics of, 139
range of motion of, 140, 141t
age and, 142
functional, 143–144, 144t
gender and, 142
normative values for, 377t
numerical recording form for, 389f
Tibiofibular joints. *See also* Ankle
anatomy of, 241, 242f
arthrokinematics of, 241

capsular pattern in, 241
osteokinematics of, 241
Toe. *See also* Foot
  anatomy of, 246, 246f
  arthrokinematics of, 246
  osteokinematics of, 246
  range of motion of
    interphalangeal joint testing in, 287
    numerical recording form for, 390f
    research findings in, 246, 246t
    testing position and, 250, 381t
Transverse plane
  defined, 4–5, 5f
Transverse tarsal eversion
  testing of, 276f–278f, 276–278
Transverse tarsal inversion
  testing of, 274f–275f, 274–275
Transverse tarsal joint. *See also* Ankle
  anatomy of, 244, 244f
  arthrokinematics of, 245
  capsular pattern in, 245
  osteokinematics of, 244
Triceps brachii
  muscle length testing of, 108f–109f,
    108–109
True biological variation
  defined, 43

U

Universal goniometer, 21–24, 22f–24f
  components of, 22f–23f, 22–23
  example of, 24b, 24f
  exercise for, 26
  metal, 22, 22f
  plastic, 22, 22f
  reliability of, 41–43
    in ankle and foot testing, 252–254
    in cervical spine testing, 303–304
    in elbow testing, 98
    in hip testing, 192
    in knee testing, 227–228
    in shoulder testing, 66–67
    in thoracic and lumbar spine testing,
      357, 357f, 360, 361f
    in wrist testing, 118
  uses of, 21
Upper-extremity testing, 55–179. *See also*
  specific structures
  elbow and forearm in, 91–109
  hand in, 137–179
  numerical recording forms for, 388f–389f,
    391f
  objectives in, 55

reliability studies of, 41
shoulder in, 57–89
wrist in, 111–135

V

Validity, 39–41
  of ankle and foot testing, 252–254
  of cervical spine testing, 303
  concurrent, 39
  construct, 40–41
  content, 39
  criterion-related, 39–40
  defined, 39
  of elbow testing, 97–98
  face, 39
  of hand testing, 144–145
  of hip testing, 190–192
  of knee testing, 227–228
  of shoulder testing, 63, 65–67
  of temporomandibular testing, 369
  of thoracic and lumbar spine testing,
    338–342
  of wrist testing, 117–119
Variation
  coefficient of, 45
Vertebrae. *See also* Cervical spine; Lumbar
  spine; Thoracic spine
  anatomy of, 295, 295f–296f, 331–333,
    332f–333f
Vertical axis
  defined, 4, 5f
Visual estimation
  goniometer use *versus*, 26–27
  reliability of
    in cervical spine testing, 304–306
    in knee testing, 228

W

Walking
  low-back mobility and, 336
  range of motion necessary for
    ankle and foot, 250–252, 251t
    hip, 189, 189f, 189t
    knee, 226, 226t, 227t
Wallpapering
  range of motion necessary for
    cervical spine, 303
Women. *See* Adults; Gender
Wrist, 111–135. *See also* specific joints
  anatomical landmarks of, 119f
  anatomy of, 111f–112f, 111–112
  arthrokinematics of, 112

capsular pattern in, 112
extension of
  testing of, 122, 122f–123f
flexion of
  reliability studies of, 41
  testing of, 120, 120f–121f
muscle length testing in, 128f–135f,
  128–135
osteokinematics of, 112
radial deviation of
  testing of, 124, 124f–125f
range of motion of
  age and, 113f, 113–114
  functional, 115t–116t, 115–117, 116f–117f
  gender and, 114
  normative values for, 375t
  numerical recording form for, 388f
  reliability and validity in testing of,
    117–119
  research findings in, 112t–113t,
    112–115
  right *versus* left sides and, 114
  testing position and, 114–115, 381t
ulnar deviation of
  testing of, 126, 126f–127f
Writing
  range of motion necessary for
    hand, 143, 143f

Z

Zygapophyseal joints. *See also* Cervical
  spine
  anatomy of, 296, 297f
  arthrokinematics of, 297
  capsular pattern in, 297
  osteokinematics of, 296–297